Computational Tools and Techniques for Biomedical Signal Processing

Butta Singh
Guru Nanak Dev University, India

A volume in the Advances in Bioinformatics and Biomedical Engineering (ABBE) Book Series

IGI Global
DISSEMINATOR OF KNOWLEDGE

www.igi-global.com

Published in the United States of America by
IGI Global
Medical Information Science Reference (an imprint of IGI Global)
701 E. Chocolate Avenue
Hershey PA, USA 17033
Tel: 717-533-8845
Fax: 717-533-8661
E-mail: cust@igi-global.com
Web site: http://www.igi-global.com

Library of Congress Cataloging-in-Publication Data

Names: Singh, Butta, 1981- editor.
Title: Computational tools and techniques for biomedical signal processing / Butta Singh, editor.
Description: Hershey, PA : Medical Information Science Reference, [2017] | Series: Advances in bioinformatics and biomedical engineering | Includes bibliographical references and index.
Identifiers: LCCN 2016024900| ISBN 9781522506607 (hardcover) | ISBN 9781522506614 (ebook)
Subjects: LCSH: Signal processing. | Biomedical engineering.
Classification: LCC R857.S47 C66 2017 | DDC 610.28--dc23 LC record available at https://lccn.loc.gov/2016024900

This book is published in the IGI Global book series Advances in Bioinformatics and Biomedical Engineering (ABBE) (ISSN: 2327-7033; eISSN: 2327-7041)

British Cataloguing in Publication Data
A Cataloguing in Publication record for this book is available from the British Library.

For electronic access to this publication, please contact: eresources@igi-global.com.

Advances in Bioinformatics and Biomedical Engineering (ABBE) Book Series

Ahmad Taher Azar
Benha University, Egypt

ISSN: 2327-7033
EISSN: 2327-7041

Mission

The fields of biology and medicine are constantly changing as research evolves and novel engineering applications and methods of data analysis are developed. Continued research in the areas of bioinformatics and biomedical engineering is essential to continuing to advance the available knowledge and tools available to medical and healthcare professionals.

The **Advances in Bioinformatics and Biomedical Engineering (ABBE) Book Series** publishes research on all areas of bioinformatics and bioengineering including the development and testing of new computational methods, the management and analysis of biological data, and the implementation of novel engineering applications in all areas of medicine and biology. Through showcasing the latest in bioinformatics and biomedical engineering research, ABBE aims to be an essential resource for healthcare and medical professionals.

Coverage

- DNA Structure
- Data Analysis
- Tissue Engineering
- Nucleic Acids
- Orthopedic Bioengineering
- Robotics and Medicine
- Data Mining
- Algorithms
- DNA Sequencing
- Molecular Simulations

IGI Global is currently accepting manuscripts for publication within this series. To submit a proposal for a volume in this series, please contact our Acquisition Editors at Acquisitions@igi-global.com or visit: http://www.igi-global.com/publish/.

The Advances in Bioinformatics and Biomedical Engineering (ABBE) Book Series (ISSN 2327-7033) is published by IGI Global, 701 E. Chocolate Avenue, Hershey, PA 17033-1240, USA, www.igi-global.com. This series is composed of titles available for purchase individually; each title is edited to be contextually exclusive from any other title within the series. For pricing and ordering information please visit http://www.igi-global.com/book-series/advances-bioinformatics-biomedical-engineering-abbe/73671. Postmaster: Send all address changes to above address.

Titles in this Series

For a list of additional titles in this series, please visit: www.igi-global.com

Handbook of Research on Computational Intelligence Applications in Bioinformatics
Sujata Dash (North Orissa University, India) and Bidyadhar Subudhi (National Institute of Technology, India)
Medical Information Science Reference • copyright 2016 • 514pp • H/C (ISBN: 9781522504276) • US $230.00 (our price)

Applying Business Intelligence to Clinical and Healthcare Organizations
José Machado (University of Minho, Portugal) and António Abelha (University of Minho, Portugal)
Medical Information Science Reference • copyright 2016 • 347pp • H/C (ISBN: 9781466698826) • US $165.00 (our price)

Biomedical Image Analysis and Mining Techniques for Improved Health Outcomes
Wahiba Ben Abdessalem Karâa (Taif University, Saudi Arabia & RIADI-GDL Laboratory, ENSI, Tunisia) and Nilanjan Dey (Department of Information Technology, Techno India College of Technology, Kolkata, India)
Medical Information Science Reference • copyright 2016 • 414pp • H/C (ISBN: 9781466688117) • US $225.00 (our price)

Big Data Analytics in Bioinformatics and Healthcare
Baoying Wang (Waynesburg University, USA) Ruowang Li (Pennsylvania State University, USA) and William Perrizo (North Dakota State University, USA)
Medical Information Science Reference • copyright 2015 • 528pp • H/C (ISBN: 9781466666115) • US $255.00 (our price)

Emerging Theory and Practice in Neuroprosthetics
Ganesh R. Naik (University of Technology Sydney (UTS), Australia) and Yina Guo (Taiyuan University of Science and Technology, China)
Medical Information Science Reference • copyright 2014 • 377pp • H/C (ISBN: 9781466660946) • US $265.00 (our price)

Technological Advancements in Biomedicine for Healthcare Applications
Jinglong Wu (Okayama University, Japan)
Medical Information Science Reference • copyright 2013 • 382pp • H/C (ISBN: 9781466621961) • US $245.00 (our price)

Biomedical Engineering and Cognitive Neuroscience for Healthcare Interdisciplinary Applications
Jinglong Wu (Okayama University, Japan)
Medical Information Science Reference • copyright 2013 • 472pp • H/C (ISBN: 9781466621138) • US $245.00 (our price)

IGI GLOBAL
DISSEMINATOR OF KNOWLEDGE
www.igi-global.com

701 E. Chocolate Ave., Hershey, PA 17033
Order online at www.igi-global.com or call 717-533-8845 x100
To place a standing order for titles released in this series, contact: cust@igi-global.com
Mon-Fri 8:00 am - 5:00 pm (est) or fax 24 hours a day 717-533-8661

To my family for their abundant support and love.
To my teacher Prof (Dr.) Dilbag Singh for his dedication to education and for serving as an inspirational role model.

Table of Contents

Detailed Table of Contents

Cardiovascular Disease (CVD) is globally acknowledged research problem. The continuous Electrocardiogram (ECG) monitoring can assist in tackling the problem of CVD. The redundancy in the monitoring of ECG signal is reduced by various signal processing techniques either in 1D or 2D domain. This chapter is having the sole objective of reviewing the existing 2D ECG data compression techniques and comparing it with the 1D compression techniques. Furthermore, proposing a novel nonlinear complexity sorting approach for 2D ECG data compression. The broad basic steps involved in the procedure are preprocessing, transformation and encoding. The preprocessing steps includes QRS detection, 2D ECG image formulation, Dc quantization and complexity sorting. The second stage of transformation includes the various decomposition techniques. At encoding stage, standard image codec (JPEG2000) can be employed. The performance evaluation of the proposed complexity sorting algorithm is performed on records of Massachusetts Institute of Technology – Beth Israel Hospital arrhythmia database.

Blood pressure monitoring is essential in hospital and home monitoring scenarios, with applications requiring on-line beat-to-beat blood pressure estimation, such as tele-monitoring of neurally mediated syncope. This chapter presents a comprehensive review of investigated approaches and reported performance, using different noninvasive correlates of the circulatory and cardiovascular system. Papers of interest were located in Scopus, IEEE Xplore and PubMed databases. The resulting pool of papers was then methodologically reviewed using 5 thematic taxonomies developed: 1) pulse arrival time and pulse transit time, 2) vascular transit time, 3) RS2 time, 4) heart sound characteristics, 5) PPG characteristics. The status of evidence in the literature demonstrates that cardiovascular signals such as the electrocardiogram, photoplethysmogram, and phonocardiogram contain important information for the estimation of blood pressure. Still, there are open issues regarding the validity, reliability and stability of these methods.

The current study deals with the investigation of the effect of long-term endurance training on the autonomic nervous system of healthy adults. ECG was recorded for 5 min under resting condition in a sitting position using an ECG acquisition device for 25 swimmers and 25 age-matched sedentary controls. Heart Rate Variability (HRV) parameters of the volunteers were used for statistical analysis and classification using binary classification trees and artificial neural networks. The LF/HF ratio for swimmers and sedentary controls was found to be 0.89 ± 0.32 and 0.94 ± 0.46, respectively. This may be attributed to the vagal dominance due to endurance training in the swimmers. Statistical ECG signal processing and db06 wavelet based processing were performed to understand the effect of swimming on the cardiac health. The signal classification results indicated that both the HRV and the processed ECG signal features may be used for the classification of the swimmers and the sedentary controls using CART, Boosted tree, Random Forest and neural network algorithms.

Parameter estimation is a central issue in mathematical modelling of biomedical systems and for the development of patient specific models. The technique of estimating parameters helps in obtaining diagnostic information from computational models of biological systems. However, in most of the biomedical systems, the estimation of model parameters is a challenging task due to the nonlinearity of mathematical models. In this chapter, the method of estimation of nonlinear model parameters from measurements of state variables, using the extended Kalman filter, is extensively explained using an example of the three-dimensional model of the HIV/AIDS system.

Here, we present a multi-scale two-directional two-dimensional principal component analysis (MS2D2PCA) method for the efficient and effective extraction of essential feature information from signals. Time-invariant multi-scale matrices are constructed in the first step. The two-directional two-dimensional principal component analysis then operates on the multi-scale matrices to reduce the dimension, rather than vectors in conventional PCA. Results are presented from an experiment to classify twenty hand motions using 89-channel EMG signals recorded in stroke survivors, which illustrates the efficiency and effectiveness of the proposed method for biomedical signal analysis. With this multi-scale two-directional two-dimensional principal component analysis for high-dimensional signal classification, spatial-time-frequency discriminant information from high-dimensional EMG electrode array can be effectively extracted and reduced using the proposed method. Compared with the time domain feature extraction in conjunction with PCA, MS2D2PCA performed better with higher classification accuracy and less PCs in EMG classification. The efficiency and effectiveness of the method can be further validated by using high-dimensional EEG, MEG, fMRI signals. Although the present study focuses on high-dimensional signal pattern classification, based on the PCs obtained at multiple scales, it is relatively straightforward to expand MS2D2PCA for high-dimensional signal compression, denoising, component extraction, and other related tasks.

Medical image enhancement improves the quality and facilitates diagnosis. This chapter investigates three methods of medical image enhancement by exploiting useful edge information. Since edges have higher perceptual importance, the edge information based enhancement process is always of interest. But determination of edge information is not an easy job. The edge information is obtained from various approaches such as differential hyperbolic function, Haar filters and morphological functions. The effectively determined edge information is used for enhancement process. The retinal image enhancement method given in this chapter improves the visual quality of the vessels in the optic region. X-ray image enhancement method presented here is to increase the visibility of the bones. These algorithms are used to enhance the computer tomography, chest x-ray, retinal, and mammogram images. These images are obtained from standard datasets and experimented. The performance of these enhancement methods are quantitatively evaluated.

During the last decades, the call for Information and Communication Technologies (ICTs) in healthcare has been augmented to endow with healthcare services at a global scale and to trim down medical errors that cost human lives. Enriched with explosive computing and high communicating power, ICTs like

Internet, mobile telephony, and other enabled gadgets plays a prominent role in our day-to-day activities. With the potential to provide access to service for patients in difficult-to reach areas and facilitating medical record keeping and information sharing are the main considerations of leveraging ICTs in realm of clinical care. The insurgence of these innovating technologies into healthcare sectors is not only blurring the boundaries for the emergence of other new technologies but also causing a paradigm shift in providing acute and preventative care in public health. The main goal of this chapter is to offer readers an insight into how the emergence of ICTs have transformed healthcare sector by delivering cost-efficient and quality of care to patients.

These days most of the Blood Pressure (BP) measuring devices are having inflatable cuff that is needed to be occluded on the patient's arm for measuring blood pressure. This technique is not suitable in cases where continuous measurement of BP is required. Therefore, this work is aimed at designing of non-invasive and continuously monitors the blood pressure by using Pulse Transit Time (PTT) technique. For taking out PTT both of the signals are extracted from the body of the patient with the help of bio sensors i.e. Electrocardiogram (ECG) sensor and Photoplethysmogram (PPG) sensor. PTT was measured by taking the peak to peak time difference of ECG signal and PPG signal and this PTT is indirectly correlated with blood pressure, based on which Systolic Blood Pressure (SBP) and Diastolic Blood Pressure (DBP) is calculated.

Signal processing in biomedical engineering is essentially required for classification while serving mainly two aims. The first is noise removal and the second is signal representation. Signal representation deals with transforming the signal in such a way that the signal is most informative in that particular domain for the application at hand. This chapter will describe signal processing methods like spectrogram with specific applications to locomotion and transition classification using Electromyography (EMG) data. A wavelet analysis application on foot acceleration signals for automatic identification of toe off in locomotion and the ramp transition is also shown. Finally, the performance of EMG and accelerometer performance across different time windows of a gait cycle in locomotion and transition classification is presented with an emphasis on fusing the data from both sensors for better classification.

The nanoelectronic circuits based on single electronics would revolutionise the new generation electronic bio-medical gadgets. The high speed nanoelectronic devices would make these gadgets faster and more accurate. The nanoelectronic integrated circuits would be a boon for power saving along with advanced portability. As the scaling down of silicon based integrated circuits is limited in nanometer regime alternative materials like organic molecules, polymers, carbon nanotubes and graphene are focal point of research. These materials exhibit various electrical, electronic and mechanical properties, flexibility being one of very significant ones. Flexible nanelectronic integrated circuits would make biomedical applications very patient friendly. The in-vivo examination and diagnosis would be less injurious to the body. Also the flexible nature will increase the maneuverability of the device by the operator. It will improve the targeted diagnosis and targeted drug delivery procedures. This would further facilitate system-on- chip (soc) that will integrate multiple biomedical signal acquisition (ECG, EEG, EP, and respiration-related signals) with on-chip digital signal processing.

Every woman experiences an extensive fluctuation in HRV during her menstrual cycle and even after menopause. A woman who lives long enough will experience menopause as a normal physiologic event. The study of the influence of premenopausal and postmenopausal symptoms on HRV has not been adequate. During this period, health management is an important factor to be considered as it affects the entire quality of women life. Many women having diverse physical, behavioural as well as psychological symptoms at the time of menopause and even after the menopause. Thus, HRV analysis is an appropriate tool to examine the physiological effects of the menstrual cycle in young healthy women and the postmenopause in old women. This chapter intends to study the influence of the menstrual cycle, and postmenopause on autonomic modulation of heart with a perspective of signal processing approach.

Diabetic retinopathy is proved to be one of the most important eye disorders in recent decades that late diagnosis of it may cause low vision or even blindness. Specialist are able to detect retinopathy in retinal images using machine learning as a decision support system which helps accelerate and facilitate the diagnosis. The automated diabetic retinopathy is a difficult computer vision problem –with the goal of detecting features of retinopathy. The present chapter is written with the purpose of analyzing and comparing different feature extraction methods to evaluate the best algorithm for detection retinopathy with least error. Extracted features using these methods are used to classify images into normal and altered groups.

Preface

The knowledge pool of various disciplines have been enhanced by the advent of high-performance computing techniques in achieving practical solutions to their problems and the area of biomedical signal processing is no exception to this. Electronics, computers and subsequently computational tools, have become integral components of biomedical engineering in particular biomedical signal analysis, performing a variety of tasks from data acquisition and preprocessing for removal of artifacts to feature extraction and interpretation.

This edited book should be of interest to a broad spectrum of medical practitioners and engineers associated with biomedical domain. Many of the chapters cover topics that can be adequately covered only in a book dedicated solely to these areas. In this sense, every chapter represents a serious compromise with respect to comprehensive coverage of the associated topics. Practicing biomedical engineers, computer scientists, information technologists, medical physicists, and data-processing specialists working in diverse areas of biomedical signal applications, and hospital information systems may find this edited book valuable in their quest to learn advanced techniques for biomedical signal processing.

In Chapter 1, authors proposed a lossy ECG data compression technique based on converting the ECG signal into 2D ECG image. A period sorting preprocessing technique was introduced, which consists of a length-based ordering of all periods. The authors exploited inter- and intra-beat dependencies to compress irregular ECG signals. A preprocessing technique consists of QRS detector, period length normalization, Dc equalization, approximate entropy based complexity sorting and image transform was proposed. The technique focused on the preprocessing stage by reducing the vertical high frequency content of the 2D image. The performance evaluation of ECG data compression technique was investigated through six parameters 1) Compression ratio (CR), 2) Percent root mean square difference (PRD), 3) Percent root mean square difference normalized (PRDN), 4) Root mean square (RMS) error, 5) Signal to noise ratio (SNR) and 6) Quality score (QS) on MIT-BIH database.

Chapter 2 presents a review of approaches for the noninvasive blood pressure estimation based on noninvasive surrogate metrics of the cardiovascular state. Recent developments in the noninvasive estimation of cardiovascular function are presented, with especial focus on the estimation of blood pressure. The methods to estimate the several important features of the cardiovascular system have been demonstrated through the relations between the signals measured on the body surface (e. g. blood pressure and cardiac output), translating electrical and mechanical cardiovascular activity with promising results.

Incorporation of physical exercise in the lifestyle of a person has been given an emphasis across the globe in recent years. This is due to the health benefits accrued by doing physical exercises. Hence, various researchers are studying the effect of different modalities of exercise and the health benefits associated with it. Swimming has evolved as one of the most popular physical exercises not only in the developed countries but also in the developing countries. Chapter 3 focused to understand the effect of long-term swimming on the autonomic nervous system and the cardiac health of healthy volunteers. ECG was recorded for 5 min under resting condition in a sitting position using an ECG acquisition device for 25 swimmers and 25 age-matched sedentary controls. Heart rate variability (HRV) parameters of the volunteers are used for statistical analysis and classification using binary classification trees and artificial neural networks.

Chapter 4 demonstrated the Extended Kalman Filter and its applicability in parameter estimation using the three dimensional HIV model. Parameter estimation is an important issue for development of patient specific models of physiological and biological processes. However, the online estimation of model parameters in biomedical systems is a challenging task due to the nonlinear and chaotic nature of such systems. Further, the measurements obtained from biomedical systems such as biosignals are often corrupted by random noises and artifacts. A Kalman filter is an optimal estimator which estimates certain parameters of interest from indirect, inaccurate and uncertain observations. It is a recursive algorithm and hence new measurements are processed as they arrive. The adopted model consists of three state variables namely the CD4 cell population, CD8 cell population and the HIV-1 viral load. The model accurately maps the interaction between the human immunodeficiency virus and the human immune system. Also, this model has been proved to be an efficient tool for viral load estimation and therapy planning in HIV/AIDS patients.

In conventional array-based Principal Component Analysis (PCA), a 2D time-frequency feature matrix is usually transformed into a 1D vector and modelled as a point in a high-dimensional vector space. However, this approach leads to several issues, such as the "curse of dimensionality" dilemma and the small sample size problem, leading to numerical instability, as well as high computational complexity and storage requirements in classification. Chapter 5 aimed at the problem of high volume feature space and a novel multi-scale two-directional two-dimensional principal component analysis has been proposed. For investigation, this approach employed to extract and classify specific STF patterns in 89-channel EMG signals from the stroke subjects for identification of 20 hand movements, which illustrates the efficiency and effectiveness of the proposed method for biomedical signal analysis.

Image enhancement technique is an appealing and powerful tool in medical image processing and the main purpose is to bring out hidden detail in an image and help diagnosing. Enhancing contrast, edges etc. are some common image pre-processing algorithms used by physicians to visualize the medical images for diagnosis. Chapter 6 described the hyperbolic filter based CT, retinal and mammogram enhancement algorithm. It also analyzed a hyperbolic filter based unsharp filter for retinal image enhancement, edge enhancement of chest x-ray image by Haar filters and the enhancement of vasculature in optic disc region based on edge information along with morphological operators. Enhancement Measure (EME), Structural Similarity Measure (SSIM), Mean Squared Error (MSE), and figure of merit (F) are used as performance evaluation parameters.

Chapter 7 focused diverse technologies such as cloud-computing, big data analytics, mobile computing, IoT and sensor technologies that support ICTs emergence in healthcare realm and their potential to deliver timely, cost-effective, remote access and quality of healthcare services to patients has been explored. In addition, some of the opportunities and controversies regarding ICTs development along with the future research directions were laid out. The insurgence of these innovating technologies into healthcare sectors is not only blurring the boundaries for the emergence of other new technologies but also causing a paradigm shift in providing acute and preventative care in public health.

Chapter 8 presents a method to develop Pulse Transit Time (PTT) technique based non-invasive continuous blood pressure monitoring device. This chapter includes Electrocardiogram (ECG) and Photoplethysmogram (PPG) sensors and their interfacing with the PIC microcontroller. The ECG sensor used here is producing an analog output so this analog signal must be converted into digital signals. From analog to digital conversion, ECG sensor is interfaced with the analog channel of PIC18F452. PIC18 microcontroller is used because it consists of a 10 bit analog to digital converter, which can be easily used for further processing. PPG sensor is connected with interrupt input of a microcontroller

In Chapter 9, the signal processing methods like spectrogram and wavelet have been presented with application to locomotion and transition classification. Frequency domain representation, spectrogram, proved to be successful in classifying the locomotion and the transition. A wavelet analysis application on foot acceleration signals for automatic identification of toe off in locomotion and the ramp transition is also shown. Finally, the performance of EMG and accelerometer performance across different time windows of a gait cycle in locomotion and transition classification is presented with an emphasis on fusing the data from both sensors for better classification.

Chapter 10 focused on the significance of nanoelectronics in biomedical applications. The various avenues of biomedical applications are directly or indirectly dependent upon electronic circuitry. The better the electronics more is the reliability of the electronic applications. Reducing device sizes and higher component densities are making electronic circuits and computational systems more efficient. Flexible nanelectronic integrated circuits would make biomedical applications very patient friendly. The in-vivo examination and diagnosis would be less injurious to the body. Also the flexible nature will increase the maneuverability of the device by the operator. It will improve the targeted diagnosis and targeted drug delivery procedures. This would further facilitate system-on- chip (soc) that will integrate multiple biomedical signal acquisition (ECG, EEG, EP, and respiration-related signals) with on-chip digital signal processing.

Chapter 11 is dedicated to application of linear HRV analysis methods for detecting the HRV variations during the menstrual cycle phases in the lying postures. In time domain methods such as (nn50) number of pairs of adjacent NN intervals differing by more than 50ms), and (TINN) Triangular Interpolation of NN intervals are analyzed and implemented on preprocessed menstrual cycle HRV dataset of 74 young women in the menstrual, follicular and luteal phases. nn50 and TINN are used to examine the effects of the menstrual, follicular and luteal phases of the menstrual cycle. In the second phase of this chapter, the linear time domain methods are applied on HRV dataset comprising 20 postmenopausal women in the lying postures. Further, a comparative study was made between 74 premenopausal women in the follicular phase of the menstrual cycle and 20 postmenopausal women.

Chapter 12 presented some predictive techniques for diabetic retinopathy detection. For this purpose, different texture based feature extraction techniques such as statistical features of histogram, grey level co-occurrence matrix, grey level run length matrix, wavelet transform features, gabor filter and local binary pattern has been considered. The results of classification of diabetic retinopathy images are compared. Specialist are able to detect retinopathy in retinal images using machine learning as a decision support system which helps accelerate and facilitate the diagnosis. The automated diabetic retinopathy is a difficult computer vision problem –with the goal of detecting features of retinopathy.

For continuous monitoring of patient's health status, the ECG signal is recorded for long time durations typically for several hours or few days. The storage of such huge volume of data requires large memory space, for example, a three-channel ECG signal sampled at a frequency of 1 kHz with 11 bits of resolution in three lead system of a particular patient, recorded for 24 h requires 928 MB of memory size per channel without any overhead. Such huge volume of data is also expected to have inter and intra beat correlation or inherent sparsity. The ECG data compression methods can also be broadly divided into three categories namely direct method, transformed method and parameter extraction method. In Chapter 13, a brief analysis of algorithms, mathematical background and its simulation implementation using MATLAB, for ECG data compression is discussed. The selected techniques from direct ECG compression methods are TP, AZTEC, Fan, and Cortes. Moreover selected techniques from transformed ECG compression methods are Walsh Transform, DCT, and Wavelet transform.

Chapter 14 proposed an effective ECG signal optimization and propagation framework using particle swarm optimization, Genetic Algorithm, ZigBee wireless environment, discrete wavelet transform, noise removal filters and signal drift removal filter techniques. All of the technologies have been combined on one platform to increase the performance of the ECG signal recording using body wearable wireless sensors for ECG monitoring and low energy propagation of the ECG signal by compressing the signal using optimization techniques. Compressed and Optimized ECG data has been transferred over Zigbee IEEE 802.15.4 saving energy implicating it on a hardware chip.

Chapter 15 discussed different partitional, fuzzy clustering and Maximum Entropy methods and optimization using PSO, QPSO and WQPSO. A nature inspired meta heuristics swarm intelligence methods particularly PSO and its variants improve the performance of conventional clustering methods in terms of quality of clusters and convergence speed. The experiments on these methods were conducted on Medical images, liver disorder and breast cancer datasets and the analysis reveals that the optimized clustering produces better clustering results than standard clustering in terms of validity measures. The proposed clustering methods are well suited to detect the patterns of interest from diverse data types of biomedical datasets particularly to deal with medical disorders.

Butta Singh
Guru Nanak Dev University Regional Campus, India

Acknowledgment

I am extremely happy to express my thanks to the Worthy Vice Chancellor, Guru Nanak Dev University, India for providing the academic environment to carry out the editing of this book. I would like to thank my teacher Dr Dilbag Singh, Head of Department Instrumentation and Control Engineering, National Institute of Technology Jalandhar India for his continuous moral support and constant encouragement. He has, by setting examples, instilled a great appreciation of good work ethic, curiosity, creativity and honesty towards work that are so essential for success and enjoyment for a career in academics.

My warmest thanks are due to all chapter authors, reviewers and publisher for their support and contribution to this book. Special thanks to Mr Anukul Pandey, Research Scholar, for extending help in various ways throughout this work.

Last but not least I would like to thank those who directly or indirectly involved in bringing up this book successfully. I wish to express my warmest thanks to my parents for their unselfish efforts to help their son in all fields of life. Finally, many thanks to my life companion Savita and my dear brother Er Varinder Singh, Renu and my sweet children Mehak, Love and Noor for their support, care and sacrifices.

Chapter 1
Nonlinear Complexity Sorting Approach for 2D ECG Data Compression

Anukul Pandey
Dr. B. R. Ambedkar National Institute of Technology, India

Barjinder Singh Saini
Dr. B. R. Ambedkar National Institute of Technology, India

Butta Singh
Guru Nanak Dev University Regional Campus, India

Neetu Sood
Dr. B. R. Ambedkar National Institute of Technology, India

ABSTRACT

Cardiovascular Disease (CVD) is globally acknowledged research problem. The continuous Electrocardiogram (ECG) monitoring can assist in tackling the problem of CVD. The redundancy in the monitoring of ECG signal is reduced by various signal processing techniques either in 1D or 2D domain. This chapter is having the sole objective of reviewing the existing 2D ECG data compression techniques and comparing it with the 1D compression techniques. Furthermore, proposing a novel nonlinear complexity sorting approach for 2D ECG data compression. The broad basic steps involved in the procedure are preprocessing, transformation and encoding. The preprocessing steps includes QRS detection, 2D ECG image formulation, Dc quantization and complexity sorting. The second stage of transformation includes the various decomposition techniques. At encoding stage, standard image codec (JPEG2000) can be employed. The performance evaluation of the proposed complexity sorting algorithm is performed on records of Massachusetts Institute of Technology – Beth Israel Hospital arrhythmia database.

INTRODUCTION

In the modern era, Cardiovascular Diseases (CVD) had emerged as one of the vital causes of mortality in both urban and rural areas (S. Gupta, Gudapati, Gaurav, & Bhise, 2013; Nichols, Townsend, Scarborough, & Rayner, 2014). The electrocardiogram (ECG) monitoring facilitates in providing clinical health

DOI: 10.4018/978-1-5225-0660-7.ch001

status of the concerned patient to the healthcare center in case of the hostile cardiac behavior (Alesanco & Garcia, 2010). It is broadly adopted in the 24-h Holter monitoring, the clinical ECG workstation handling and telemedicine applications. Cardiac monitoring using ECG signal is the best representative of heart electrical functionality and had proven to be useful in the diagnosis of most of the heart disease.

The ECG signal which monitors the electrical activity of heart is usually characterized by its various set points (P, QRS, T) and intervals (PR interval, QT interval and RR interval) that reflects the rhythmic electrical depolarisation and repolarisation of atria and ventricles. ECG is having the possibility of reduction of redundant information through inter- and intra-beat correlation, which is the basic cause of its compression. In general, ECG signal compression techniques widely fall under three categories of the direct method, transformed method, and parameter extraction method. The direct data compression method (V. Kumar, Saxena, & Giri, 2006) openly analyzes and reduces data points in the time domain, and the example includes turning point (TP), amplitude zone time epoch coding (AZTEC), Improved Modified AZTEC technique, coordinate reduction time encoding system (CORTES), the delta algorithm, the Fan algorithm (Jalaleddine, Hutchens, Strattan, & Coberly, 1990; Sabarimalai Sur & Dandapat, 2014), and the ASCII character encoding (S K Mukhopadhyay, Mitra, & Mitra, 2012). The transformed method analyzes energy distribution by converting the time domain to some other domain and example includes Fourier transform, Fourier descriptor (Reddy & Murthy, 1986), Karhunen–Loeve transform (KLT), the Walsh transform, the discrete cosine transform (DCT) (Batista, Melcher, & Carvalho, 2001; Benzid, Messaoudi, & Boussaad, 2008), DCT with modified stages and wavelet transform, and the compressed sensing. The parameter extraction method is based upon dominant feature extraction from the raw signal; examples include neural based or syntactic methods, peak picking, and linear prediction method. For such data reduction, compression techniques are designed, which are classified as lossless or lossy techniques. To combat a huge growth rate of memory requirement and data sparsity, many ECG compression and decompression algorithms had already developed to represent the raw ECG in the processed format.

The storage of such huge volume of data requires large memory space, for example, a three-channel ECG signal sampled at a frequency of 1 kHz with 11 bits of resolution in three lead system of a particular patient, recorded for 24 h requires 928 MB of memory size per channel without any overhead. Such huge volume of data is expected to have inter and intra beat correlation or inherent sparsity.

The lossless data compression guarantees the integrity of reconstructed data at a compromised CR, typically CR level of 2 to 1 with exact replication of original ECG while the lossy data compression achieves a high compression ratio with varying level of reconstruction error (Koski, 1997). Many researchers have proposed ECG compression techniques by treating ECG signal as a two-dimensional (2D) image (H. Lee & Buckley, 1999; Wang & Meng, 2008) and exploiting the inter- and intra-beat correlations by the encoder (Sabarimalai Sur & Dandapat, 2014). The "cut and align beats approach and 2D DCT" and "period normalization and truncated SVD algorithm" (Wei, Chang, Chou, & Jan, 2001) are available preprocessing techniques to get good compression results in ECG. This kind of preprocessing steps is also often associated with the use of state-of-the-art image encoders, like JPEG2000 (Taubman, Marcellin, & Rabbani, 2002). The preprocessing technique proposed in this chapter is a modification of techniques presented in (Chou, Chen, Shiau, & Kuo, 2006; Filho, Rodrigues, da Silva, Faria, & Carvalho, 2008). In this chapter, authors proposed a lossy ECG data compression technique based on converting the ECG signal into 2D ECG image. A period sorting preprocessing technique was introduced, which consists of a length-based ordering of all periods. The authors exploited inter- and intra-beat dependencies to compress irregular ECG signals.

Another preprocessing technique consists of QRS detector, period length normalization, Dc equalization, complexity sorting and image transform was proposed. The technique focused on the preprocessing stage by reducing the vertical high frequency content of the 2D image.

Although the vertical high-frequency content of the resulting image has been reduced by Dc equalization and variance based linear complexity sorting techniques, but adjacent lines may still be very dissimilar after this preprocessing stage, does not guarantee the maximum resemblance across adjacent rows.

A 2D ECG image compression falls in the category of lossy compression technique that is formulated through the 1D ECG signal. The conversion procedure comprises of QRS detection, period length normalization, Dc equalization, complexity sorting, transformation and image codec represented in Figure 1.

In this chapter a detailed discussion and each and every step of conversion procedure from 1D ECG to 2D ECG image were illustrated. Out of five distinct stage of conversion process, the horizontal and vertical uniformity in 2D ECG were achieved from period normalization, Dc equalization and complexity sorting. To form the equal universal period length of all periods and to better exploit the interbeat dependencies, period normalization was applied. Depending upon compression efficiency universal period length can be its maximum or average length of formulated 2D ECG. The linear and nonlinear complexity sorting can be applied to achieve the high vertical smoothness that future assists the image encoder in achieving optimum compression efficiency. The linear complexity sorting includes variance based vertical sorting whereas nonlinear complexity includes entropy based sorting.

The major advantage in 2D ECG compression compared to 1D ECG were higher compression efficiency at the trade-off of its formulation and processing time delay. Processing delay can be further reduced by means high processing speed and also by selection of an optimized number of ECG beats.

The performance evaluation of any ECG data compression techniques can be broadly assessed through following six parameters namely:

1. Compression ratio (CR),
2. Percent root mean square difference (PRD),
3. Percent root mean square difference normalized (PRDN),
4. Root mean square (RMS) error,
5. Signal to noise ratio (SNR),
6. Quality score (QS).

Figure 1. Generalized 2D ECG data compression flowchart

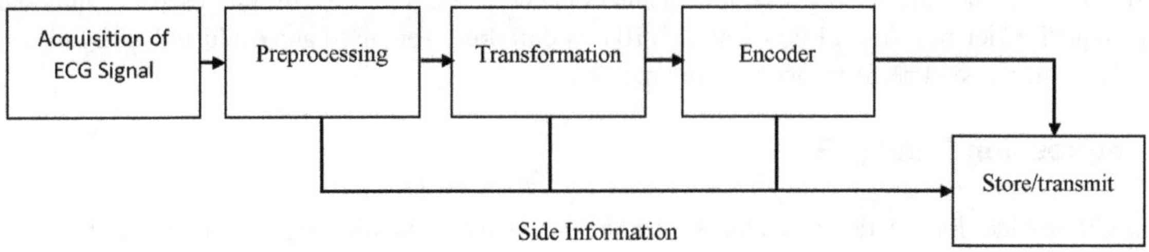

These six qualitative performance evaluation parameters mentioned above are extensively used in literature for accessing the efficiency of any of the compression techniques. The degree of distortion measure in reconstructed ECG signal is primarily computed with respect to the original data, based on the visual as well the qualitative evaluation. The six qualitative performance evaluation parameters mentioned above are extensively used in literature for the comparison purpose.

The comparison of existing ECG compression methods using the above-mentioned performance measures can be carried out, by performing experimentations over most cited Massachusetts Institute of Technology - Beth Israel Hospital (MIT-BIH) database (Goldberger et al., 2000).

Ultimately after compression via either 2D or 1D the main purpose lies in monitoring the critical cardiac patients, ambulatory patients, and the person under cardiac surveillance. The ECG is recorded continuously, and the recorded data becomes so voluminous that it becomes practically impossible to handle them without compression. The central goal of any data compression technique is to achieve maximum data volume reduction while preserving the significant signal morphology on reconstruction. Conceptually, data compression is a process of detecting and eliminating redundancies in a given set of information. Since the size of the data reduces considerably, compression of the data results in resourceful deployment of memory space for permanent storage of digitized ECG in the computer.

The rest of the chapter is organized as follows by discussing the database and performance measure used in literature. Followed by Need of 2D ECG data compression is presented. In due course proposed non-linear complexity sorting approach for 2D ECG data compression is illustrated. Afterward the results for comparative study of 2D ECG compression is presented with respect to 1D ECG compression. Discussion section has been provided to illustrate advantage and disadvantage of 2D ECG compression schemes. Finally, the conclusion is made based on the results.

DATABASE AND PERFORMANCE MEASURE

In the emerging field of medical engineering, research subjects like cardiac arrhythmia detection, heart rate variability, cardiovascular and pulmonary dynamics, artificial intelligence based medical decision support and ECG compression, etc. are of major interest (Pincus, 1991). The Massachusetts Institute of Technology (MIT) supplies some invaluable resources for such research projects. These resources include databases containing recorded physiological signals and software for analyzing, viewing and creating such recordings. In the present study, ECG samples from Arrhythmia Database (Goldberger et al., 2000) (http://ecg.mit.edu) have been taken for investigation of the efficiency of the various methods. The Database contains 48 half-hour excerpts of two-channel ambulatory ECG recordings, obtained from 47 subjects studied by the BIH Arrhythmia Laboratory. The 11-bit resolutions over 10 mV range with a sampling frequency of 360 Hz per sample channel were recorded. To access the proposed pre-processing technique's efficiency, first 21,600 samples (10 min duration) were used and evaluated with following six data compression performance measure metric.

Compression Ratio (CR)

The CR provides information about the degree by which the compression algorithm removes the redundant data. Higher the *CR* less number of bits required to store or transmits the data that can be defined as

$$CR = \frac{B_0}{B_c} \tag{1}$$

where, B_0 is the total number of bits required to represent original data and B_c total number of bits required to represent compressed data along with the side information needed for retrieval of original data. In our database setting

$$CR = \frac{11 \times f_s \times N}{B_{c2d} + B_s} \tag{2}$$

where f_s is the sampling frequency, N is the total number of samples in 1D ECG signal, B_{c2d} is the total number of bits in compressed 2D ECG and B_s are the bits required to store the side information

Percentage Root Mean Square Difference (PRD)

It is a measure of acceptable fidelity and degree of distortion introduced during compression and decompression algorithm. Usually, the clinical acceptability of reconstructed signal after decompression is determined through visual inspection. The numerical evaluation of level the level of distortion in reconstructed signal in comparison to original signal can be carried out via PRD measure, defined as

$$PRD(\%) = 100 \times \sqrt{\frac{\sum_{n=1}^{N} (X_s(n) - X_r(n))^2}{\sum_{n=1}^{N} (X_s(n))^2}} \tag{3}$$

Percentage Root Mean Square Difference, Normalized (PRDN)

It is a normalized version of PRD, is PRDN, which does not depend on the mean signal value $\bar{X}$. For any signal, the information lies in its variance. The mean value of the data does not actively contribute to the reconstructed signal fidelity issue. PRDN provides better error estimation in reconstructed signal than PRD.

$$PRDN(\%) = 100 \times \sqrt{\frac{\sum_{n=1}^{N} (X_s(n) - X_r(n))^2}{\sum_{n=1}^{N} (X_s(n) - \bar{X})^2}} \tag{4}$$

Percentage Root Mean Square Difference, Normalized with Respect to Database (PRD_1024)

As for storage purpose, MIT-BIH database adds a 1024 in the original signal, to evaluate the fidelity of reconstructed signal 1024 must be subtracted from the original signal.

$$\mathrm{PRD\_1024}(\%) = 100 \times \sqrt{\frac{\sum_{n=1}^{N} (X_s(n) - X_r(n))^2}{\sum_{n=1}^{N} (X_s(n) - 1024)^2}} \tag{5}$$

Root Mean Square Error (RMS)

It provides a measure of error in are constructed signal with respect to original signal with respect to signal length.

$$RMS = \sqrt{\frac{\sum_{n=1}^{N} (X_s(n) - X_r(n))^2}{(N-1)}} \tag{6}$$

Signal to Noise Ratio (SNR)

SNR, measure of degree of noise energy introduced by compression in decibel (dB) scale

$$SNR = 10 \times \log\left(\frac{\sum_{n=1}^{N} (X_s(n) - \bar{X})^2}{\sum_{n=1}^{N} (X_s(n) - X_r(n))^2}\right) \tag{7}$$

All the six measures are simultaneously used in literature for accessing the efficacy of any ECG compression algorithm.

NEED OF 2D ECG DATA COMPRESSION

Conceptually, data compression is a process of detecting and eliminating redundancies in a given set of information. The key goal of any data compression technique is to achieve maximum data volume reduction while preserving the significant signal morphology on reconstruction. In other words, improvement in CR over existing methods for comparable PRD. The reason for switching from 1D ECG data compression to 2D ECG data compression is to exploit the correlation among inter and intra-beat.

However, most existing ECG compression techniques (Batista et al., 2001; Borsali & Na, 2004; H. Lee & Buckley, 1999) did not utilize such correlation between intra beats. To decorrelate the inherent intra and inter-beat similarity in ECG signal 2D ECG compression is needed.

BASICS OF 2D ECG DATA COMPRESSION

Several 2D compression techniques (Huang, Wang, & Chen, 2009; H. Lee & Buckley, 1999; Wang & Meng, 2008) of ECG signals have been proposed, which utilize both intra and interbeat correlations and achieve superior performance. The broad basic steps involved in the 2D ECG data compression procedure are preprocessing, 2D transformation and encoding. The preprocessing steps involves QRS detection, Dc equalization and complexity sorting. Whereas in 2D transformation includes stacking (ECG image formulation), cosine, wavelet, and singular decomposition, etc. At encoding stage, any standard image codec (JPEG2000) or video codec (H.264/AVC) can be employed. The each of the steps is described below

Preprocessing for 2D ECG Compression

The preprocessing step for 2D ECG compression methods is essential for significant improvements in exploitation of inter- and intra-beat correlation the broad steps involved are

1. QRS detection and 2D ECG Formulation,
2. Period Normalization,
3. Dc equalization,
4. Complexity sorting.

QRS Detection and 2D ECG Formulation

The mapping of signal to image (1D ECG to 2D ECG) achieved through QRS detection step. The location of R-wave peak is identified via any appropriate and the efficient QRS detection algorithm present in the literature (Pan & Tompkins, 1985; Ramakrishnan, Prathosh, & Ananthapadmanabha, 2014; Sandryhaila, Saba, & Kovacevic, 2012; Zidelmal, Amirou, Moukadem, & Dieterlen, 2014). After detection of R wave in ECG, the researchers have segmented the ECG Signal in various ways to for formulate 2D ECG.

In (Filho et al., 2008) authors have segmented the ECG signal via locating the maxima of QRS complex that is the location of R-wave. This location is treated as the segmentation boundary, leaving half peak at each end of row vector in 2D ECG image. The assembly of a cut and aligned ECG data is illustrated by authors of (Wang & Meng, 2008). Detected QRS complex is cut and aligned according to each identified R-wave to formulate 2D ECG. This algorithm demands proper alignment of QRS complex for maximum use of the beat to beat correlation.

Furthermore, a cut and aligned method was also employed by authors of (Huang et al., 2009). The ECG signals are cut at every 80^{th}sample prior to each R-wave, which avoids cutting at QRS peak and causing in a large border.

In (Chou et al., 2006) authors used to cut the 1D ECG signals 130^{th}sample prior to each R wave with the same reasoning mentioned above to avoid large boundary values. The advantage of prior cutting is by avoiding the larger row boundary ends makes 2D ECG smoother row vectors. This results makes the 2D array easy to compress.

Figure 2. The four existing methods for 2D ECG array formulation from 1D ECG data

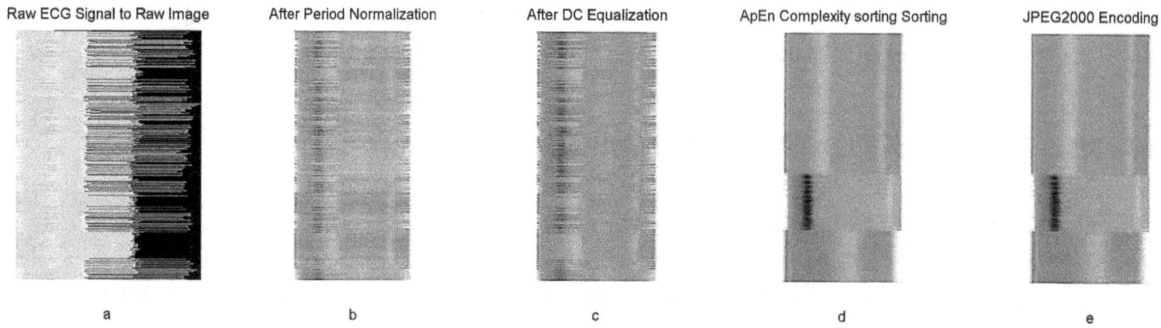

All the four methods for 2D ECG formulation discussed above is depicted in Figure 2.

The methods for 2D ECG array formulation heavily dependent upon the accuracy of QRS detection algorithm. The error in QRS algorithm affects the compression efficiency. In other words, higher the R-peak detection accuracy better the compression efficiency. The first and foremost demand for better compression efficiency in 2D ECG compression is accurate, fast, computationally efficient and reliable QRS detection algorithm.

Period Normalization

To match the length of the detected R-wave in 2D ECG array (Wei et al., 2001) proposed the period normalization also adopted by (Bilgin, Marcellin, & Altbach, 2003; Filho et al., 2008). Interpolation or decimation achieve the clamping to the common value of the columns in 2D ECG array to its normalized period. Cubic spline interpolation is employed for period normalization to normalized period (N_p). The selection of period length is open research issue. Mostly the maximum or mean value of period over entire row vector is considered as the N_p.

$$I_k = cubic\ spline\left(V_i, N_p\right) \tag{8}$$

where V_i represents the particular row vector, i=1, 2, R. R is the number of row vector in 2D ECG array. I_k is the period normalized row vectors $k \in 1{:}R$.

Similar to period normalization, an additional period sorting is also introduced in (Chou et al., 2006) which employed sorted (ascending/ descending) the row vector of 2D ECG array based on the column length. This type of period sorting finds application in irregular ECG data compression. The period sorting may compromise with the vertical correlation factor in the case of dynamic RR intervals. That may affect 2D coder efficiency.

Dc Equalization

Filho *et al.* proposes the Dc equalization (Filho et al., 2008). Which neutralizes the different dc levels present in the row vectors. The high-frequency present in the period normalized this step minimizes 2d ECG array. The mathematical representation of Dc equalization is as follows

$$Dc_k = \lfloor Average(I_k) \rfloor \tag{9}$$

where I_k are signal samples of kth normalized row and Dc_k is the average of all the signal samples averaged over the normalized length. The $\lfloor \ \rfloor$ operation represents the least integer function that make the 2D ECG array integer. Based on Dc_k, minimum Dc level and an offset, all the segments are clamped to the minimum Dc level

Complexity Sorting

Though Dc equalization reduces the vertical high frequency but still there is the scope of maximization of correlation among the rows in the 2D ECG array. Which can be achieved by the complexity sorting approach. The variance based complexity sorting was implemented by Filho (Filho et al., 2008). in which low variance based ascending order sorting was arranged by assuming the ECG as a stationary signal.

In each and every preprocessing step (QRS detection, period normalization, Dc equalization or complexity sorting) the previous location is necessary for an inverse process that is considered as side information. Which are very minimal with respect to overall data.

PROPOSED NON-LINEAR COMPLEXITY SORTING APPROACH FOR 2D ECG DATA COMPRESSION

As in 2D ECG array each and every row contain one beat of ECG data. After the period normalization and Dc equalization nonlinear complexity, sorting provides better inter-beat correlation because entropy can capture randomness in data better than the variance. In other words, the correlation in adjacent row can be quantified better by use of approximate entropy (*ApEn*) (Pincus, Goldberger, Steven, & Goldberger, 1994; Pincus, 1991) based than variance because of in apart from visual high degree of randomness variance fails to distinguish the suitable degree of correlation. Therefore, in this chapter, application of *ApEn* based nonlinear complexity sorting for 2D ECG data compression is proposed for minimization of vertical high-frequency content. Given a signal $u(1), u(2), \ldots u(N)$, where, *N*is the total number of data points. Fix *m*, a positive integer and *r*, a positive real number. For our study we have chosen r equal to 20% of standard deviation and *m*=2. *ApEn* algorithm can be summarized (Singh, Singh, Jaryal, & Deepak, 2012) as

Step 1: Form *m* vectors *X* defined as with length *N*-*m*+1:

$$X(i) = \left[u_i u_{i+1} \ldots u_{i+m-1} \right] 1 \le i \le N - m + 1$$

Step 2: Calculation of distance between two vector d_m:

$$d_m[X(i), X(j)] = \max\left|u_{i+k-1} - u_{j+k-1}\right| k = 0,1,...m$$

Step 3: Define for each *i*, for *i* =1, 2, ..., *N*-*m*+1:

$$C_i^m(r) = \frac{v^m(i)}{N - m + 1}$$

where $v^m(i) =$ number of $d_m[X(i), X(j)] \leq r$

Step 4: Taking natural logarithm of each $C_i^m(r)$ along with mean value over *i*:

$$\phi^m(r) = \frac{1}{N - m + 1}\sum_{i=1}^{N-m+1} \ln C_i^m(r)$$

Step 5: Increase the dimension to *m*+1 and repeat 1 to 4.
Step 6: Calculate *ApEn* value for a finite data length of *N:*

$$ApEn(m, r, N) = \phi^m(r) - \phi^{m+1}(r)$$

The degree of the regularity of given data can be quantified as m similar points are likely to be similar to m+1 similar points in subspace. Whereas irregular data points do not follow these characteristics. Thus, high regularity quantities low values of *ApEn*. *ApEn* is a regularity, not a magnitude statistic (Richman & Moorman, 2000). The ascending order row-wise *ApEn* complexity sorting is carried out for vertical high frequency removal.

Transformation and Encoding

The 2D transformation (DCT, DWT, SVD, etc.) been utilized for improvement in compression efficiency. In the proposed work JPEG2000 by MATLAB 2012a software tool has been successfully employed as a image compression standard due to its ability to simultaneously address the need for progressive transmission by quality and spatial locality (Taubman et al., 2002), (Bilgin et al., 2003). The quantization step was fixed to a value of 1.5259×10^{-05}. Default parameters of JPEG 2000 were employed with the targeted compression ratio 180.

The incorporated transformation and its coefficient coding used in the state of art literature (Sabarimalai Sur & Dandapat, 2014) is represented in Table 1.

Table 1. Different transform and coefficient coding used in 2D ECG data compression

Reference/Author and Year	Transform	Coefficient Coding
(H. Lee & Buckley, 1999)	CAB and 2-D DCT	Uniform quantization (UQ) and run-length coding
(Wei et al., 2001)	SVD	Uniform quantization
(Bilgin et al., 2003)	DWT	JPEG2000 and differential coding
(Wang & Meng, 2008)	DWT	CAB and modified SPIHT
Approach 1 (Chou et al., 2006)	DWT	JPEG2000
Approach 2 (Chou et al., 2006)	DWT	JPEG2000
(Wang & Meng, 2008)	DWT	VQ with DCCR and DPCM
(Huang et al., 2009)	DWT	CAB, USDZQ, ROI mask adaptive arithmetic encoder
(Filho et al., 2008)	-	JPEG2000 and H.264/AVC intraframe encoder

DCT: Discrete cosine transform
DWT: Discrete wavelet transform
SVD: Singular value decomposition
USDZQ: uniform scalar deadzone quantizer
ROI: region of interest
Most of 2D ECG array compressor uses DWT for transformation and JPEG2000 coefficient encoding.

RESULTS

To evaluate the efficiency of the 2D ECG compression algorithm experiments are completed on all the 48 records of MIT-BIH Arrhythmia ECG database have been tested. It is subtly assumed that the ECG reconstructed signals have been subjectively validated through visual inspection by the physician. The dataset from the data base divided according to the literature (Bilgin, Marcellin, & Altbach, 2004; Huang et al., 2009) into three categories.

1. All records.
2. The first dataset consists of record numbers 100; 101; 102; 103; 107; 109; 111; 115; 117; 118; and 119.
3. Second datasetis formulated via collection of record numbers 104; 107; 111; 112; 115; 116; 117; 118; 119; 201; 207; 208; 209; 212; 213; 214; 228; 231 and 232.

The original signal and its reconstructed signal along with error is shown in Figure 3. For record 119.

Table 2 shows the performance measure in terms of CR, PRD_1024, PRD, PRDN, RMS, SNR and QS for all records of MIT-BIH arrhythmia database. The mean values of CR, PRD, PRDN, RMS, SNR and QS of 48 subjects were 43.51, 12.59, 1.19, 16.37, 11.46, 16.37 and 47.133 respectively.

The graphical comparison between *PRD* versus *CR* for the various state of art ECG compressor with proposed method is depicted in Figure 4. Lower the slope of *PRD* –*CR* curves better the compression efficiency results in a higher value of *QS*.

Table 3 shows the performance comparison of proposed 2D ECG compression technique for average values for a database with respect to the state of art 1D ECG compression methods.

Table 4 shows the experimental results over performance measure for various existing 2D ECG compression technique. Based on different approaches applied in the algorithm the performance of compressor

Figure 3. (a) Original ECG from MIT-BIH database of record 119, (b) reconstructed ECG signal and (c) reconstruction error signal with CR=33.18 and PRD=0.70

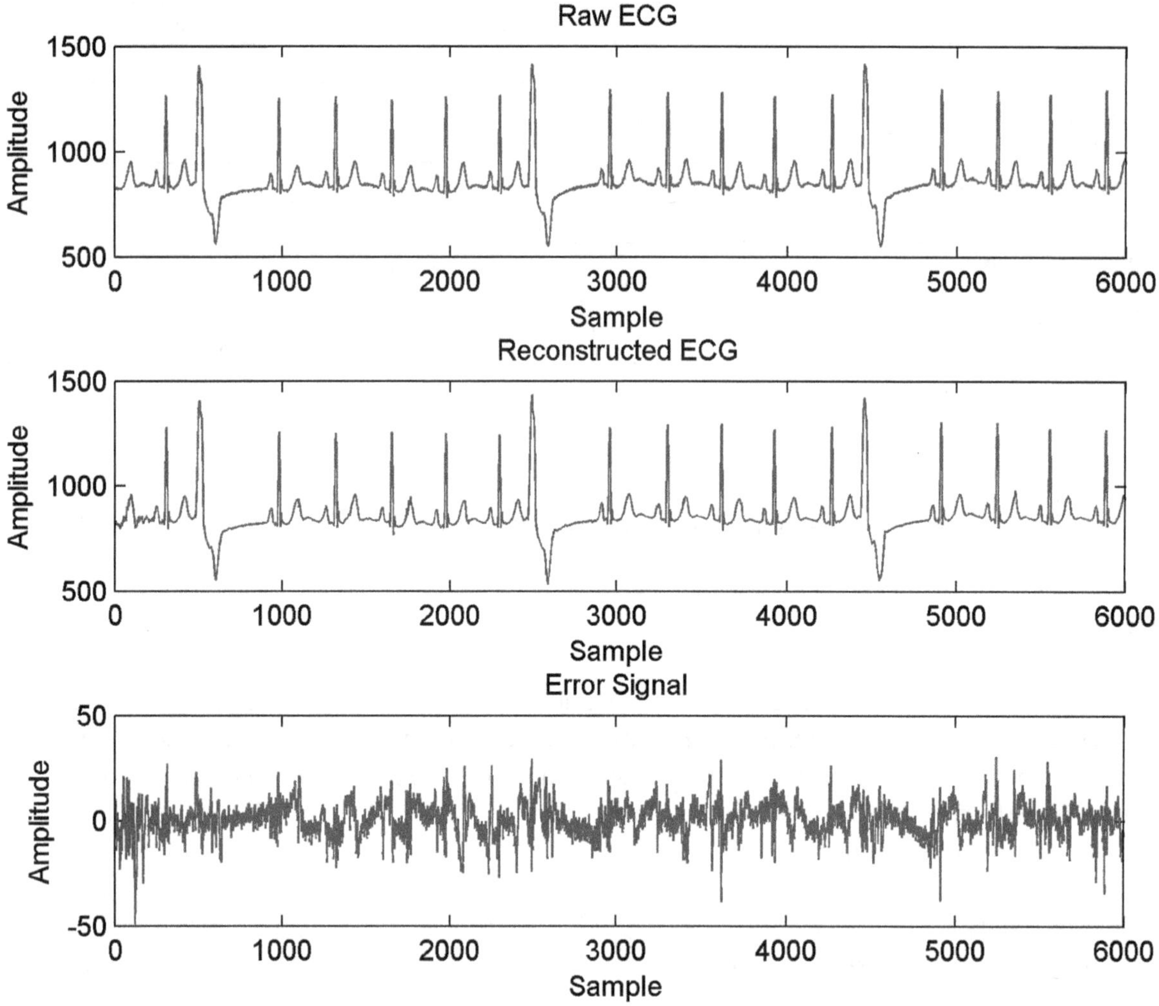

is achieved according. The inherent irregularity in ECG may affect the compressor efficiency because of the requirement of interpolation in period normalization step.

Table 5 shows the experimental results of the performance measure for various existing 1D ECG compression techniques.

DISCUSSION

In this chapter, we presented 2D ECG compression technique based on nonlinear complexity sorting which carefully designed to apply before JPEG200. Our results show that this nonlinear complexity sorting was successfully adapted for ECG signals. Results obtained by successively the compressor over the ten minutes of lead II of the 48 records of the MIT-BIH Arrhythmia Database.

Table 2. Performance measures of proposed technique for 48 ECG records from MIT-BIH arrhythmia database

Records	CR	PRD_1024	PRD	PRDN	RMS	SNR	QS
100	43.05	6.30	0.48	12.77	4.57	17.87	90.48
101	45.41	9.46	0.81	13.01	7.82	17.72	56.31
102	43.92	12.66	0.83	21.03	8.07	13.54	52.99
103	44.32	6.41	0.52	7.93	5.06	22.01	85.79
104	43.45	24.52	1.83	31.35	17.9	10.07	23.78
105	41.69	7.93	0.62	9.67	6.10	20.29	67.10
106	45.55	21.44	1.68	24.02	16.62	12.39	27.18
107	44.70	13.40	2.33	13.92	23.10	17.13	19.18
108	48.23	15.12	0.96	22.33	9.40	13.02	50.25
109	41.54	7.39	0.74	8.38	7.26	21.53	56.16
111	44.70	14.36	0.86	16.77	8.57	15.51	51.85
112	41.57	2.97	0.60	11.12	5.14	19.08	69.40
113	46.59	12.97	1.22	13.80	12.16	17.20	38.15
114	47.19	14.63	0.65	21.28	6.44	13.44	72.79
115	45.46	6.37	0.83	10.99	7.71	19.18	54.70
116	42.42	5.82	1.58	10.49	13.33	19.58	26.83
117	48.63	3.19	0.65	11.71	5.60	18.63	74.43
118	43.64	6.54	1.47	14.36	12.62	16.86	29.62
119	45.09	3.82	0.89	7.22	7.69	22.83	50.41
121	46.39	3.41	0.68	10.82	5.88	19.31	68.04
122	41.70	3.46	0.74	8.70	6.38	21.21	56.02
123	48.44	3.93	0.78	11.37	6.73	18.89	62.27
124	48.09	5.92	1.34	10.54	11.60	19.55	36.01
200	41.09	30.16	2.35	31.62	23.60	10.00	17.47
201	43.13	13.40	0.68	18.26	6.75	14.77	63.33
202	47.79	8.95	0.54	11.02	5.30	19.16	89.30
203	39.25	28.23	3.20	29.61	31.88	10.57	12.26
205	40.76	6.66	0.52	13.13	5.02	17.64	77.99
207	43.92	25.13	2.30	26.96	22.86	11.39	19.11
208	39.41	23.28	2.30	24.60	22.90	12.18	17.15
209	38.86	16.56	1.02	19.63	10.17	14.14	37.92
210	41.21	13.41	0.81	15.86	8.06	16.00	50.81
212	40.20	19.03	1.40	20.99	13.89	13.56	28.81
213	37.52	13.79	1.99	14.92	19.46	16.53	18.87
214	43.79	14.96	1.45	15.76	14.44	16.05	30.27
215	37.20	18.68	1.18	21.02	11.78	13.55	31.46
217	43.97	13.14	1.64	13.61	16.40	17.32	26.79

continued on following page

Table 2 Continued

Records	CR	PRD_1024	PRD	PRDN	RMS	SNR	QS
219	43.22	9.24	1.58	14.9	14.33	16.53	27.37
220	44.33	5.38	0.75	10.95	6.90	19.21	58.79
221	42.31	15.43	1.08	17.38	10.73	15.20	39.20
222	43.57	16.20	0.71	23.57	7.08	12.55	61.13
223	42.14	6.26	0.86	10.78	7.90	19.35	49.27
228	45.91	22.3	1.79	23.89	17.88	12.44	25.63
230	44.25	15.66	1.21	17.43	12.04	15.18	36.49
231	49.22	10.69	0.70	12.81	6.91	17.85	70.53
232	44.81	16.64	0.72	22.37	7.13	13.01	62.59
233	38.72	22.44	2.57	23.33	25.64	12.64	15.09
234	40.29	7.030	0.54	7.72	5.36	22.25	74.83

Figure 4. Graphical comparative analysis of proposed method and existing ECG compressor

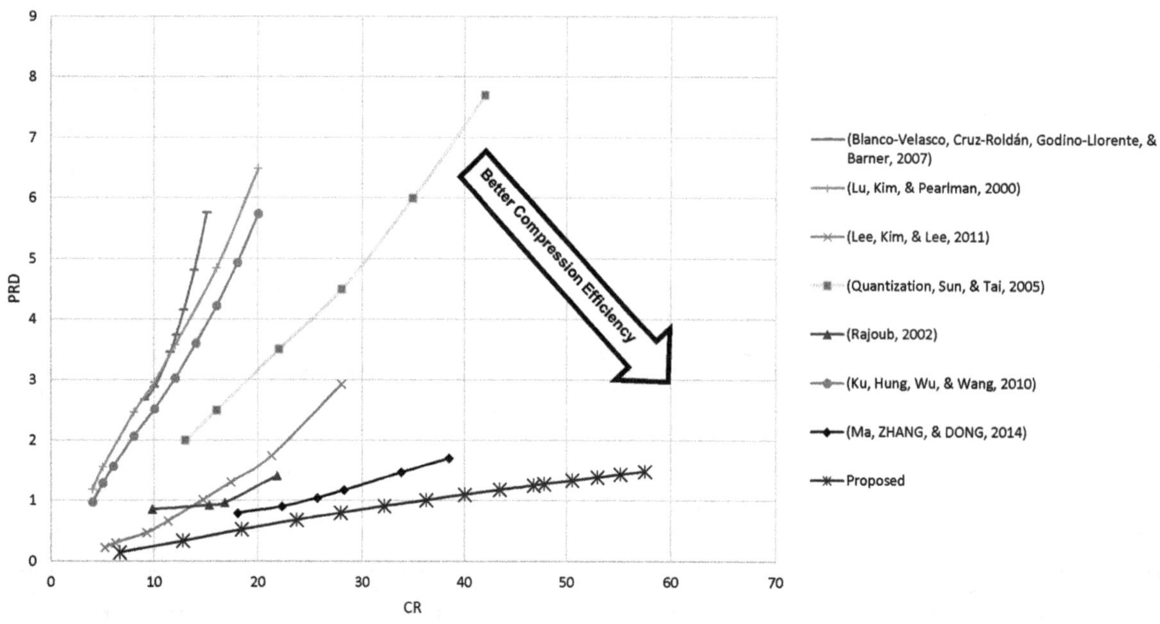

Table 3. Performance comparison of proposed 2D ECG compression technique for average values for database with respect to state of art 1D ECG compression methods

Algorithm	PRD	CR	QS
m-AZTEC (Vinod Kumar, Saxena, Giri, & Singh, 2005)	25.5	5.6	0.22
Perceptual Masks (Duarte, Matos, & Batista, 2007)	1.24	3.5	2.82
SPIHT (Lu, Kim, & Pearlman, 2000)	1.18	8	6.78
Al-Shrouf (Al-Shrouf, Abo-Zahhad, & Ahmed, 2003)	5.3	11.6	2.19
Mukhopadhy(S.K. Mukhopadhyay, Mitra, & Mitra, 2011)	0.023	7.18	312.17
Mukhopadhy(S K Mukhopadhyay et al., 2012)	7.89	15.72	20.60
Bilgin(Bilgin et al., 2003)	3.26	20	6.13
Hilton (Hilton, 1997)	2.6	8	3.08
Johan (A. Djohan, T.Q. Nguyen, Djohan, Nguyen, & Tompkins, 1995)	3.9	8	2.05
Fira and Goras (Fira& Goras, 2008)	0.61	12.74	20.89
USZZQ and Huffman coding of DSM (Manikandan & Dandapat, 2006)	2.73	11.06	4.05
Proposed	**1.18**	**43.51**	**36.87**

Table 4. Experimental results over performance measure for existing 2D ECG compression methods

Reference/Author and Year	CR	PRD	PRD_1024	Record
(H. Lee & Buckley, 1999)	24	8.1	-	100
(Wei et al., 2001)	10	1.18	-	117
(Bilgin et al., 2003)	20	3.26	-	First Datasets
	20	4.8	-	Second Datasets
(Wang & Meng, 2008)	24	3.85	-	100
Approach 1 (Chou et al., 2006)	10	-	1.15	119
Approach 2 (Chou et al., 2006)	10	-	1.03	
(Wang & Meng, 2008)	36	5.8±2.60	-	First Datasets
(Huang et al., 2009) Approach 1	24	3.58	-	First Datasets
Approach 2	24	3.51	-	First Datasets
Approach 3	24	3.43	-	First Datasets
(Filho et al., 2008) Type 1-JPEG2000	24	-	4.10	100
Type 2-JPEG2000	24	-	5.16	100
Type 2-JPEG2000	24	-	3.95	100
Proposed	32	0.40	5.30	100
	33.08	0.70	2.99	119
	35.40	0.53	2.59	117
	32.86	0.74	6.48	First Datasets

Table 5. CR and PRD for various prevailing1D ECG data compression methods

ECG Compressor/Author	From Literature			Test Condition (MIT-BIH Arrhythmia Database)
	CR	PRD	QS	
(Hilton, 1997)	8	2.6	3.08	Data instance of record 117
(S. Lee, Kim, & Lee, 2011)	 27.98 21.30 9.28	 2.93 1.75 0.48	 10.24 12.17 19.33	30-min of one lead data instance of 48 records. 15% Window Size 20% Window Size 50% Window Size
(Batista et al., 2001)	 6.20 7.90 9.30 10.9	 1.5 2.0 2.5 3.0	 4.13 3.95 3.72 3.63	Averaged CR and PRD for composed of 96 signals (both leads from MIT-BIH database), with 43,200 samples each, (2 min duration)
(R. Gupta & Mitra, 2014)	 10.02 5.65 31.27 6.74 15.81 18.87 19.82 8.967 26.35 13.91 18.46	 6.745 6.071 6.497 2.795 4.001 6.446 3.023 2.5 6.019 5.239 2.444	 1.49 0.93 4.81 2.41 3.95 2.93 6.56 3.59 4.38 2.66 7.55	Data instance of 11 ECG records with lead namely: 100-v5 105-v1 109-v1 113-v1 115-v1 119-v1 121-v1 122-v1 124-v4 201-v1 205-v1
(Ku, Hung, Wu, & Wang, 2010)	4 8 14 20	0.98 2.07 3.60 5.74	4.08 3.86 3.89 3.48	Average CR and PRD over 11 ECG records from MIT-BIH database namely 100, 101, 102, 103, 107, 109, 111, 115, 117, 118, and 119 of duration 10-min
(Aggarwal & Patterh, 2012)	24.01 13.19	2.01 1.05	11.94 12.56	3.0341-min of each channel of 16 ECG records from MIT-BIH database
(S. Lee et al., 2011)	17.34	1.31	13.23	All 48 records

Advantages

- Maximum utilization of inter and intra but correlation results better compressor efficiency.
- Wide applicability in monitoring purpose.
- By reducing buffering time duration possibility of real time deployment of technology.
- Simple and elegant algorithm designed algorithm procedure.

Disadvantages

- Requirement of accurate QRS detection which may affected by various artefacts and by varying morphologies.
- Buffer delay in 2D image formulation.

Sur and Dandapat *et al.* (Sabarimalai Sur & Dandapat, 2014) presented a prospective review of various ECG data compression methods like Fourier transform, Fourier descriptor, Karhunen–Loeve Transform (KLT), the Walsh transform, the Discrete Cosine Transform (DCT) and the wavelet transform. In order to efficiently explore inter and intra beat correlations at the encoder, processing techniques for 2D ECG image were also discussed by the authors. In two-dimensional ECG compression methods, transformation are applied on 2D representation of 1D ECG signals to improve the compression efficiency.

For 1D ECG compressor the following literature presents the state of art algorithm.

Reddy *et al.* (Reddy & Murthy, 1986) devised fourier descriptor based ECG data compression. The advantage of the proposed method was its capability to handle noisy records without any requirement of the post processing, which was duly justified by the value of on an average CR =7 and PRD=7, making it suitable for the morphological study.

Batista *et al.* (Batista et al., 2001) developed an effective compression technique which was based on optimized quantization of DCT coefficients. The efficiency of the technique was verified on all 48 records of MIT-BIH arrhythmia database. The results of CR and PRD using the proposed technique for 100th record were 10.2 and 3 respectively.

Lee *et al.* (S. Lee et al., 2011) formulated a new real time ECG compression method. This method comprised of reduction of the ECG signal to half its original sampling rate followed by the application of sample differencing and R peak detection. The accumulated errors were computed when DCT was applied on two consecutive ECG periods followed by the use of Huffman coding as an entropy coding mechanism. The proposed approach showed that the CR was 27.9 and the PRD was 2.93 on an average for 48 data records with a 15% window size.

The Jalaleddine *et al.* (Jalaleddine et al., 1990) had surveyed various direct data ECG compression schemes which includes Turning Point (TP), Amplitude Zone Time Epoch Coding (AZTEC), improved modified AZTEC technique, Co-ordinate Reduction Time Encoding System (CORTES), the delta algorithm and the Fan algorithm.

Cox *et al.* (Cox, Nolle, Fozzard, & Oliver, 1968) proposed AZTECH algorithm rhythm analysis the advantage of this method lies in its ability of high data reduction ratio but suffers from loss of data fidelity due to the presence of discontinuity that occurs in the reconstructed ECG waveform. Kumar *et al.* (Vinod Kumar et al., 2005) developed improved modified AZTECH technique in which the statistical parameters of the signal to be compressed are computed and they adjust themselves to the nature of the signal by recalculating the threshold value. The authors have concluded that using least square polynomial smoothing filter a significant reduction in PRD was obtained for a typical value of CR=2.76, threshold value of 0.010, PRD value with and without smoothing filter were 4.54 and 6.56 respectively.

Kumar *et al.* (V. Kumar et al., 2006) had surved AZTECH, modified AZTECH, Fan and Scan Along Polygonal Approximation (SAPA) techniques. The authors had also suggested some modifications in them, thereby making suitable for telemedicine purposes. In the modified version the CR value is high and PRD value had gone considerably low for the same value of threshold.

Recently, Mukhopadhyay*et al.* (S K Mukhopadhyay et al., 2012; S.K. Mukhopadhyay et al., 2011; S.K. Mukhopadhyay, Mitra, & Mitra, 2013) proposed ASCII based encoding methods are also employed for compression due to its simplicity, which enables them to be used in portable and mobile data ECG data monitoring systems.

Transmission of ECG data through appropriate channel (internet, wired or wireless), or stored in semiconductor/magnetic memory are prone to some kind of error. The effect of random noise in ECG over isoelectric line is tolerable whereas the loss of information in the typical P, QRS and T wave amplitude or its interval is quite significant.

CONCLUSION

In this chapter, a brief review for existing 2D ECG data compression is presented. The 2D ECG compression can successfully access the correlation among inter and intra-beat. For maximum utilization of inter-beat correlation nonlinear *ApEn* based complexity sorting and JPEG2000 encoding is presented. The performance measure computed over several records in the MIT-BIH arrhythmia database. Through comparative analysis with 1D ECG data compression, it can be concluded that 2D ECG compressor provides a better result with the only disadvantage of higher computational demand with accurate QRS detection. The most recent developments in the estimation of cardiovascular representative i.e. ECG noninvasively with especial focus on the assessment of maximum compression efficiency.

REFERENCES

Aggarwal, V., & Patterh, M. S. (2012). Quality controlled ECG compression using essentially non-oscillatory point-value decomposition (ENOPV) technique. *Digital Signal Processing*, *22*(1), 878–884. doi:10.1016/j.dsp.2012.06.010

Al-Shrouf, A., Abo-Zahhad, M., & Ahmed, S. M. (2003). A novel compression algorithm for electrocardiogram signals based on the linear prediction of the wavelet coefficients. *Digital Signal Processing*, *13*(4), 604–622. doi:10.1016/S1051-2004(02)00031-3

Alesanco, A., & Garcia, J. (2010). Clinical assessment of wireless ECG transmission in real-time cardiac telemonitoring. *IEEE Transactions on Information Technology in Biomedicine*, *14*(5), 1144–1152. doi:10.1109/TITB.2010.2047650 PMID:20378476

Batista, L. V., Melcher, E. U. K., & Carvalho, L. C. (2001). Compression of ECG signals by optimized quantization of discrete cosine transform coefficients. *Medical Engineering & Physics*, *23*(2), 127–134. doi:10.1016/S1350-4533(01)00030-3 PMID:11413065

Benzid, R., Messaoudi, A., & Boussaad, A. (2008). Constrained ECG compression algorithm using the block-based discrete cosine transform. *Digital Signal Processing*, *18*(1), 56–64. doi:10.1016/j.dsp.2007.08.003

Bilgin, A., Marcellin, M. W., & Altbach, M. I. (2003). Compression of electrocardiogram signals using JPEG2000. *IEEE Transactions on Consumer Electronics*, *49*(4), 833–840. doi:10.1109/TCE.2003.1261162

Bilgin, A., Marcellin, M. W., & Altbach, M. I. (2004). Wavelet compression of ECG signals by JPEG2000. *Data Compression Conference, 2004. Proceedings*. http://doi.org/ doi:10.1109/DCC.2004.1281503

Borsali, R., & Na, A. (2004). *ECG Compression Using an Ensemble Polynomial Modeling: Comparison With the DCT Based Technique*. Academic Press.

Chou, H.-H., Chen, Y.-J., Shiau, Y.-C., & Kuo, T.-S. (2006). An effective and efficient compression algorithm for ECG signals with irregular periods. *IEEE Transactions on Bio-Medical Engineering*, *53*(6), 1198–1205. doi:10.1109/TBME.2005.863961 PMID:16761849

Cox, J. R., Nolle, F. M., Fozzard, H. A., & Oliver, G. C. (1968). AZTEC, a preprocessing program for real-time ECG rhythm analysis. *IEEE Transactions on Bio-Medical Engineering*, *15*(April), 128–129. doi:10.1109/TBME.1968.4502549 PMID:5648088

Djohan, A., Nguyen, T. Q. W. J. T., Djohan, A., Nguyen, T. Q., & Tompkins, W. J. (1995). ECG compression using discrete symmetric wavelet transform. In IEEE -EMBC and CMBEC (pp. 167–168). Montreal, Canada: IEEE.

Duarte, R. C. M., Matos, F. M., & Batista, L. V. (2007). Near-lossless compression of ECG signals using perceptual masks in the DCT domain. In *IV Latin American Congress on Biomedical Engineering IFMBE Proceedings 18* (pp. 229–231). IFMBE. doi:10.1007/978-3-540-74471-9_53

Filho, E. B. L., Rodrigues, N. M. M., & da Silva, E. A. B. (1923–1926). da, Faria, S´. M. M. de, & Carvalho, M. B. de. (2008). ECG signal compression based on Dc equalization and complexity sorting. *IEEE Transactions on Bio-Medical Engineering*, *55*(7).

Fira, C. M., & Goras, L. (2008). An ECG signals compression method and its validation using NNs. *IEEE Transactions on Bio-Medical Engineering*, *55*(4), 1319–1326. doi:10.1109/TBME.2008.918465 PMID:18390322

Goldberger, A. L., Amaral, L. A., Glass, L., Hausdorff, J. M., Ivanov, P. C., Mark, R. G., & Stanley, H. E. et al. (2000). PhysioBank, PhysioToolkit, and PhysioNet: Components of a new research resource for complex physiologic signals. *Circulation*, *101*(23), e215–e220. doi:10.1161/01.CIR.101.23.e215 PMID:10851218

Gupta, R., & Mitra, M. (2014). Wireless electrocardiogram transmission in ISM Band: An approach towards telecardiology. *Journal of Medical Systems*, *38*(10), 90. doi:10.1007/s10916-014-0090-5 PMID:25085695

Gupta, S., Gudapati, R., Gaurav, K., & Bhise, M. (2013). Emerging risk factors for cardiovascular diseases: Indian context. *Indian Journal of Endocrinology and Metabolism*, *17*(5), 806–814. doi:10.4103/2230-8210.117212 PMID:24083161

Hilton, M. L. (1997). Wavelet and wavelet packet compression of electrocardiograms. *IEEE Transactions on Bio-Medical Engineering*, *44*(5), 394–402. doi:10.1109/10.568915 PMID:9125824

Huang, B., Wang, Y., & Chen, J. (2009). 2-D compression of ECG signals using ROI mask and conditional entropy coding. *IEEE Transactions on Bio-Medical Engineering*, *56*(4), 1261–1263. doi:10.1109/TBME.2008.2009643 PMID:19272868

Jalaleddine, S. M., Hutchens, C. G., Strattan, R. D., & Coberly, W. A. (1990). ECG data compression techniques-a unified approach. *IEEE Transactions on Bio-Medical Engineering*, *37*(4), 329–343. doi:10.1109/10.52340 PMID:2186997

Koski, A. (1997). Lossless ECG encoding. *Computer Methods and Programs in Biomedicine*, *52*(1), 23–33. doi:10.1016/S0169-2607(96)01779-8 PMID:9034667

Ku, C., Hung, K., Wu, T., & Wang, H. (2010). Wavelet-based ECG data compression system with linear quality control scheme. *IEEE Transactions on Bio-Medical Engineering*, *57*(6), 1399–1409. doi:10.1109/TBME.2009.2037605 PMID:20142155

Kumar, V., Saxena, S. C., & Giri, V. K. (2006). Direct data compression of ECG signal for telemedicine. *International Journal of Systems Science*, *37*(1), 45–63. doi:10.1080/00319100500412337

Kumar, V., Saxena, S. C., Giri, V. K., & Singh, D. (2005). Improved modified AZTEC technique for ECG data compression: Effect of length of parabolic filter on reconstructed signal. *Computers & Electrical Engineering*, *31*(4-5), 334–344. doi:10.1016/j.compeleceng.2005.02.002

Lee, H., & Buckley, K. M. (1999). ECG data compression using cut and align beats approach and 2-D transforms. *IEEE Transactions on Bio-Medical Engineering*, *46*(5), 556–564. doi:10.1109/10.759056 PMID:10230134

Lee, S., Kim, J., & Lee, M. (2011). A real-time ECG data compression and transmission algorithm for an e-health device. *IEEE Transactions on Bio-Medical Engineering*, *58*(9), 2448–2455. doi:10.1109/TBME.2011.2156794 PMID:21606020

Lu, Z., Kim, D. Y., & Pearlman, W. A. P. (2000). Wavelet compression of ECG signals by set partitioning in hierarchical trees algorithm. *IEEE Transactions on Bio-Medical Engineering*, *47*(7), 849–856. doi:10.1109/10.846678 PMID:10916255

Manikandan, M. S., & Dandapat, S. (2006). Wavelet threshold based ECG compression using USZZQ and Huffman coding of DSM. *Biomedical Signal Processing and Control*, *1*(4), 261–270. doi:10.1016/j.bspc.2006.11.003

Mukhopadhyay, S. K., Mitra, S., & Mitra, M. (2011). A lossless ECG data compression technique using ASCII character encoding. *Computers & Electrical Engineering*, *37*(4), 486–497. doi:10.1016/j.compeleceng.2011.05.004

Mukhopadhyay, S. K., Mitra, S., & Mitra, M. (2012). An ECG signal compression technique using ASCII character encoding. *Measurement*, *45*(6), 1651–1660. doi:10.1016/j.measurement.2012.01.017

Mukhopadhyay, S. K., Mitra, S., & Mitra, M. (2013). ECG signal compression using ASCII character encoding and transmission via SMS. *Biomedical Signal Processing and Control*, *8*(4), 354–363. doi:10.1016/j.bspc.2013.02.007

Nichols, M., Townsend, N., Scarborough, P., & Rayner, M. (2014). Cardiovascular disease in Europe: Epidemiological update. *European Heart Journal*, *35*(42), 3028–3034. doi:10.1093/eurheartj/ehu299 PMID:24014390

Pan, J., & Tompkins, W. J. (1985). A real-time QRS detection algorithm. *IEEE Transactions on Bio-Medical Engineering*, *32*(3), 230–236. doi:10.1109/TBME.1985.325532 PMID:3997178

Pincus, S. M. (1991). Approximate entropy as a measure of system complexity. *Proc. Natl Acad.*, *88*(March), 2297–2301. doi:10.1073/pnas.88.6.2297 PMID:11607165

Pincus, S. M., Goldberger, A. L. R. Y. L., Steven, M., & Goldberger, A. L. R. Y. L. (1994). Physiological time-series analysis: What does regularity quantify? *The American Journal of Physiology*, *266*(4 Pt 2), H1643–H1656. Retrieved from http://www.pubmedcentral.nih.gov/articlerender.fcgi?artid=1332574&tool=pmcentrez&rendertype=abstract PMID:8184944

Ramakrishnan, A. G., Prathosh, A. P., & Ananthapadmanabha, T. V. (2014). Threshold-independent QRS detection using the dynamic plosion index. *IEEE Signal Processing Letters*, *21*(5), 554–558. doi:10.1109/LSP.2014.2308591

Reddy, B. R. S., & Murthy, I. S. N. (1986). ECG data compression using Fourier descriptors. *IEEE Transactions on Bio-Medical Engineering*, *33*(4), 428–434. doi:10.1109/TBME.1986.325799 PMID:3957398

Richman, J. S., & Moorman, J. R. (2000). Physiological time-series analysis using approximate entropy and sample entropy. *American Journal of Physiology. Heart and Circulatory Physiology*, *278*(6), 2039–2049. PMID:10843903

Sabarimalai Sur, M., & Dandapat, S. (2014). Wavelet-based electrocardiogram signal compression methods and their performances: A prospective review. *Biomedical Signal Processing and Control*, *14*(1), 73–107. Retrieved from http://linkinghub.elsevier.com/retrieve/pii/S1746809414000998

Sandryhaila, A., Saba, S., & Kovacevic, J. (2012). Efficient Compression of QRS Complexes Using Hermite Expansion. *IEEE Transactions on Signal Processing*, *60*(2), 947–955. doi:10.1109/TSP.2011.2173336

Singh, B., Singh, D., Jaryal, A. K., & Deepak, K. K. (2012). Ectopic beats in approximate entropy and sample entropy-based HRV assessment. *International Journal of Systems Science*, *43*(5), 884–893. doi:10.1080/00207721.2010.543478

Taubman, D. S., Marcellin, M. W., & Rabbani, M. (2002). JPEG2000: Image compression fundamentals, standards and practice. *Journal of Electronic Imaging*, *11*(2), 286. doi:10.1117/1.1469618

Wang, X., & Meng, J. (2008). A 2-D ECG compression algorithm based on wavelet transform and vector quantization. *Digital Signal Processing*, *18*(2), 179–188. doi:10.1016/j.dsp.2007.03.003

Wei, J. J., Chang, C. J., Chou, N. K., & Jan, G. J. (2001). ECG data compression using truncated singular value decomposition. *IEEE Transactions on Information Technology in Biomedicine*, *5*(4), 290–299. doi:10.1109/4233.966104 PMID:11759835

Chapter 2
A Review on Noninvasive Beat-to-Beat Systemic and Pulmonary Blood Pressure Estimation through Surrogate Cardiovascular Signals

Ana Castro
Universidade do Porto, Portugal

Jens Muehlsteff
Philips Research Europe, The Netherlands

Paulo de Carvalho
University of Coimbra, Portugal

Sandra S. Mattos
Unidade de Cardiologia e Medicina Fetal, Brazil

Miguel Coimbra
Universidade do Porto, Portugal

ABSTRACT

Blood pressure monitoring is essential in hospital and home monitoring scenarios, with applications requiring on-line beat-to-beat blood pressure estimation, such as tele-monitoring of neurally mediated syncope. This chapter presents a comprehensive review of investigated approaches and reported performance, using different noninvasive correlates of the circulatory and cardiovascular system. Papers of interest were located in Scopus, IEEE Xplore and PubMed databases. The resulting pool of papers was then methodologically reviewed using 5 thematic taxonomies developed: 1) pulse arrival time and pulse transit time, 2) vascular transit time, 3) RS2 time, 4) heart sound characteristics, 5) PPG characteristics. The status of evidence in the literature demonstrates that cardiovascular signals such as the electrocardiogram, photoplethysmogram, and phonocardiogram contain important information for the estimation of blood pressure. Still, there are open issues regarding the validity, reliability and stability of these methods.

DOI: 10.4018/978-1-5225-0660-7.ch002

INTRODUCTION

Cardiovascular system monitoring includes a myriad of tools and methodological approaches for the adequate diagnosis, treatment of patients, and preventive medicine (Webster, 2006; Akay, 2006). The cardiovascular system is a complex network centered on the heart, a self-paced organ that pumps blood through the pulmonary and systemic circulations. Heart activity may be analyzed via various physiological signals that are related such as the electrocardiogram (ECG), impedance cardiogram (ICG), the phonocardiogram (PCG), or blood pressure (BP). These different signals represent different information, related to electrical and hemodynamic processes (Guyton and Hall,2006).

Reliable, noninvasive and continuous assessment of the cardiovascular state is extremely important in clinical practice since the cardiovascular state may shift rapidly e.g. in anesthesia care or neurally mediated syncope onset (Meyer et al., 2011). The advantages of noninvasive physiological signal analysis have long been known (Lewis et al., 1977), but recent studies have focused in the noninvasive signal analysis of the cardiovascular state to estimate hemodynamic variables such as BP and Cardiac Output (Smith and Ventura, 2013; Couceiro et al., 2011). Noninvasive monitoring of the cardiovascular state of a patient is gaining a lot of interest for a safer, continuous, and comfortable patient assessment, in clinical and home-based scenarios (Zheng et al., 2014; Ha et al., 2014).

Two reviews on noninvasive methods to estimate BP were recently published: (Peter et al., 2014) focused on the noninvasive estimations using the auscultatory, oscillometric and tonometry techniques, as well as on pulse wave velocity and pulse transit/arrival time as BP surrogates; in (Buxi et al., 2015), the authors focused on pulse transit/arrival time methodologies, discussing calibration, acquisition and processing of the non-invasive signals, and the design of measurement systems. This chapter focuses on the review of the noninvasive surrogate cardiovascular signals only, addressing not only the pulse transit/arrival time methodologies, but also the combined and individual use of heart sound (PCG) and photoplethysmography (PPG), discussing their limitations.

The use of surrogate measures for BP inference is gaining commercial traction and products for clinical use are already available (Nihon Kohden, 2015; Sotera Wireless, 2015). Pulse wave transit time calculated from the ECG and the PPG is analyzed to detect changes in the BP in order to trigger a cuff-based BP measure (PWTT, Nihon Kohden) (Nihon Kohden, 2015). Recently, a first system was approved by the FDA for BP monitoring in general ward based on pulse arrival time (ViSi Mobile, Sotera Wireless), which requires intermittent recalibration by standard cuff-based BP measurements (Sotera Wireless, 2015). Due to this market interest, the need in the standardized characterization of these new BP measurement approaches has been addressed by a first IEEE-standard for wearable cuffless blood pressure measurement devices dealing with the calibration issue and performance evaluation (IEEE-SA, 2014).

This chapter presents a review of approaches for the noninvasive BP estimation based on noninvasive surrogate metrics of the cardiovascular state. It is organized in the following sections: Blood Pressure Monitoring, where current methods in clinical use will be briefly described; Physiology of the Cardiovascular System, where basic principles and their relations to different noninvasive signals are presented, as well as BP regulation mechanisms are discussed; Methodological Review, where the main approaches for the noninvasive BP estimation will be described with a review on the most relevant studies; and finally, a critical Discussion is presented.

BLOOD PRESSURE MONITORING

BP assessment is a standard procedure in all clinical care settings. Established and widely used BP measurement methods are based on few main techniques: the analysis of Korotkoff sounds, oscillometry, pressure measurement via invasive arterial lines, tonometry, and the volume clamp method.

Intermittent Measures

Cuff-based methods are most often used in daily clinical practice, which analyze the blood pulse in a peripheral artery (arm or leg), and use a cuff to hamper the blood passage with an increase in cuff pressure sufficient to stop blood flow completely. A sphygmomanometer provides the pressure during cuff deflation and as soon as blood flow starts again characteristics sounds due to turbulent blood flow can be heard - so called Korotkoff sounds - and the associated pressure is interpreted as systolic blood pressure. The pressure at which audible sounds disappear corresponds to the moment when blood flow returns to laminar and is associated with the diastolic pressure. A different method, but employing the oscillometry technique, may be used to detect points of oscillation in the artery, and capture the corresponding pressures. Cuff-based methods are the gold standard for noninvasive BP measurement, however they do not provide continuous monitoring, and may be uncomfortable for long-term monitoring. Therefore, research to address these issues continues, aiming for desirable noninvasive, continuous BP measurement methods.

Continuous Measures

Established approaches for continuous noninvasive BP assessment are the volume clamp method (Penaz et al.,1973) and tonometry (Kemmotsu et al., 1991). These methods allow continuous BP monitoring, either using finger cuffs to measure pressure that is necessary to maintain a constant vascular volume (clamp method), or and facilitate the applanation of the radial artery at the wrist to measure the pressure transmitted to the skin (tonometry) (Webster, 2006). A comprehensive review on the history of blood pressure measurement, and the methods in clinical use is provided in (Chung et al., 2013).

In intensive care setting, where cardiovascular function of the patient may alter quickly, or during anesthesia and noxious stimulation, an invasive arterial catheter is often used to acquire the BP wave, and monitor beat-to-beat BP. In these scenarios the insertion of an arterial catheter outpaces associated risks such as infection or thrombosis. Still, this method is restricted for high acuity settings only. An extensive review of studies analyzing radial artery cannulation, anatomical considerations, and complications is provided in (Brzezinski et al., 2009), and recommendations for BP measurement in different patient populations is presented in (Pickering et al., 2005).

Commercially available noninvasive continuous BP measurements for clinical application still have limitations in clinical practice, e.g. in combination with vasopressors, or in cold environments, highly sensitive to motion artifacts as well as they are bulky, which limits their use for ambulatory patients (Webster, 2006).

Besides systemic BP, Pulmonary Arterial Pressure (PAP) is also an important parameter of the cardiovascular function that needs to be monitored, especially in Pulmonary Arterial Hypertension (PAH) patients. PAP can be estimated noninvasively by an echocardiogram, however this estimation is not reliable, and in many cases is difficult to obtain (Smith and Ventura, 2013; Testani et al., 2010). For precise measurements of PAP, patients are usually submitted to a right heart catheterization, an invasive procedure associated with high risks and high costs. Noninvasive and regular assessment of PAP trough noninvasive methods has been addressed by (Xu et al., 2002; Smith and Ventura,2013), with encouraging results.

A recent review on continuous noninvasive BP monitoring describes some of these methods in detail, providing indication of solutions commercially available, as well as a critical discussion on the new approaches using pulse transit time (Peter et al., 2014). The errors reported in comparison to the invasive measurements, described in the following section, were of 3±1.16/1.4±1.36 mmHg for the auscultatory method, -2.6±9/6.1±7 mmHg for the oscillometric method, -1.1±4.1/-0.5±2.1 mmHg for the tonometry, and 6.5±2.6/5.4±2.9 mmHg for the volume clamp (SBP/DBP).

The next section provides a brief overview of the physiology of the cardiovascular system and BP regulation mechanisms. For a more detailed review of the mechanisms, please refer to (Guyton and Hall, 2006).

PHYSIOLOGY OF THE CARDIOVASCULAR SYSTEM

The heart is a self-paced pump (Figure 1), in which the right ventricle directs deoxygenated blood to the lungs for gas exchange (pulmonary circulation), and the left ventricle pumps oxygenated blood from the lungs to all body parts for nutrient and oxygen intake (systemic circulation).

The cardiovascular system is regulated by the humoral and autonomic nervous system (sympathetic/parasympathetic balance), with slow and fast action of the regulating systems (Guyton and Hall, 2006).

Figure 1. Heart chambers: right atria (RA), left atria (LA), right ventricle (RV), left ventricle (LV), and aortic (AV), pulmonary (PV), tricuspid(TV) and mitral (MV) valves

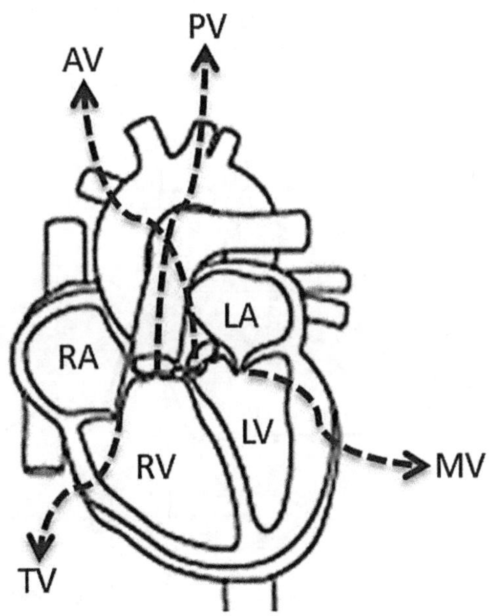

Cardiovascular Signals

The Electrocardiogram (ECG) depicts the electrical activity of the heart, containing information on the timing of sinoatrial and atrioventricular nodes' activation, conduction properties, and tissue viability. Electrical activity of the heart is initiated by the sinoatrial node, resulting in the atria contraction, which results in a blood flow to the ventricles; a short pause follows in electrical conductance, and consecutive the atrioventricular node triggers discharge of the ventricle contraction. Figure 2 shows the P, Q, R, S and T waves of the ECG: the P wave is the depolarization spread through the atria, followed by the atria contraction; about 0.16 s after the onset of the P wave, the QRS waves appear, corresponding to the depolarization of the ventricles, and their contraction (ventricular systole); finally, the Twave, corresponding to the repolarization of the ventricles, is observed (Guyton and Hall, 2006). Simultaneously, this electrical activation results in mechanical processes, which are audible and can be registered using a stethoscope this signal is called phonocardiogram (PCG). It contains information on the mechanical response of the heart contraction as well as blood flow through the heart chambers and great arteries. Typical PCG of healthy subjects is characterized by two main sounds, composed of four components (see Figure 2): the first heart sound, corresponding mainly to the closure of the atrioventricular valves, is low in pitch and relatively long-lasting. When the aortic and pulmonary valves close at the end of the systole, a rapid snap may be heard since these valves close rapidly (Figures 1 and 2), and the surroundings vibrate for a short period (Figure 1) (Guyton and Hall, 2006). In pathological cases heart sound might exhibit further components (see e.g. (Bickley, 2009; Tavel, 2006; Smith and Ventura, 2013)).

Figure 2. Cardiovascular signals and time intervals

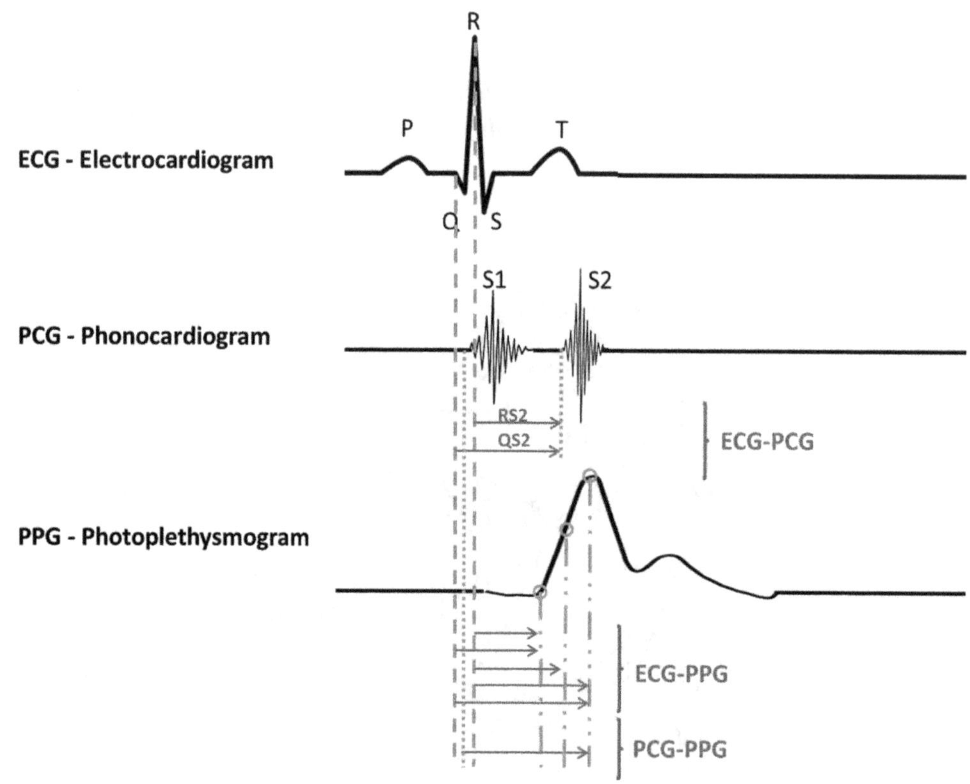

The Photoplethysmography (PPG) is sensitive to blood volume changes detected by infrared light absorption through the tissue (Akay, 2006). It is an indirect way of noninvasively measuring the pulse in the periphery and provides insight on the blood flow and arterial wall stiffness. This information has been used for example the estimation of vasoconstriction in response to noxious stimulation (Paloheimo et al., 2010). The PPG is used as a marker of the arrival of a pressure pulse in the periphery and its timing in relation to the electrical or mechanical onsets of the heart has been linked to the BP. A review of the applications of PPG in clinical monitoring is given in (Allen, 2007).

The transthoracic Impedance Cardiogram (ICG) is a technique to detect blood flow and blood volume changes in the thorax, by impedance measurements (Sherwood, Chair). The impedance of the thorax Z can be recorded by passing a high frequency low amplitude current between two electrodes and recording the resulting voltage. The impedance cardiogram is a recording of the first time derivative of Z (dZ/dt) and varies according to the beating heart; several points in this wave are used to characterize the pumping of the heart such as the pre-ejection period (PEP, defined as time interval from the beginning of electrical stimulation of the ventricles to the opening of the aortic valve, Q-peak in ECG to point B), as shown in Figure 3, or the left ventricular ejection time (LVET, point of aortic valve opening to closure). It is observed that as soon as the left ventricle pressure (LVP) is high enough, the aortic valve opens letting the blood flow to all body parts, and the first derivative point B (see Figure 3) may be used to estimate the PEP noninvasively (Johnston et al., 1998).

Blood Pressure and Regulation Mechanisms

The BP wave shape is the result of the coupling of the ventricular activity and the vascular bed, meaning the result of CO (stroke volume and heart rate) and total peripheral resistance (compliance, vasoconstriction/dilation) (Guyton and Hall, 2006). BP waveform changes continuously in response to external interferences, and internal autonomic and humoral regulation (Akay, 2006). BP variations are related to the respiratory cycle (high frequency band), and low frequency oscillations (central oscillators modulating sympathetic efferences). BP is therefore influenced by changes in Heart Rate (HR), ventricle contractility, venous return, arterial stiffness and peripheral resistance. All these factors are regulated by three distinct mechanisms: local autoregulation, neural control regulation, and humoral regulation. A well-established marker for arterial stiffness is the carotid-femoral pulse wave velocity, as described in (Millasseau et al., 2005).

Blood flow to tissues is strongly controlled by local regulation to meet the metabolic needs by vasoconstriction/dilation, and depends on the local conditions such as PO_2, PCO_2, and temperature. Regulation from the nervous system is achieved by integrating descending input from higher neural areas and afferent information arriving from mechanical and chemical sensitive receptors, located throughout the body, and responding to changes in BP (baroreflex) and blood constitution (chemoreflex), in order to control the pH value and maintain an adequate flow of oxygenated blood. Several studies have analyzed the relation between the ECG and the BP wave variability to assess the baroreflex function, using time and frequency domain techniques (Akay, 2006; La Rovere et al., 2008; Logier et al., 2011). Finally, there is the humoral regulation that through the secretion of hormones such as angiotensin II and antidiuretic hormone, regulates the BP levels (usually slower responses than the remaining regulating mechanisms). All these mechanisms result in homeostasis especially in challenging tasks such as posture change and exercise.

Figure 3. Pulse arrival time (PAT), pulse transit time (PTT), and pre-ejection period (PEP) schematic representation

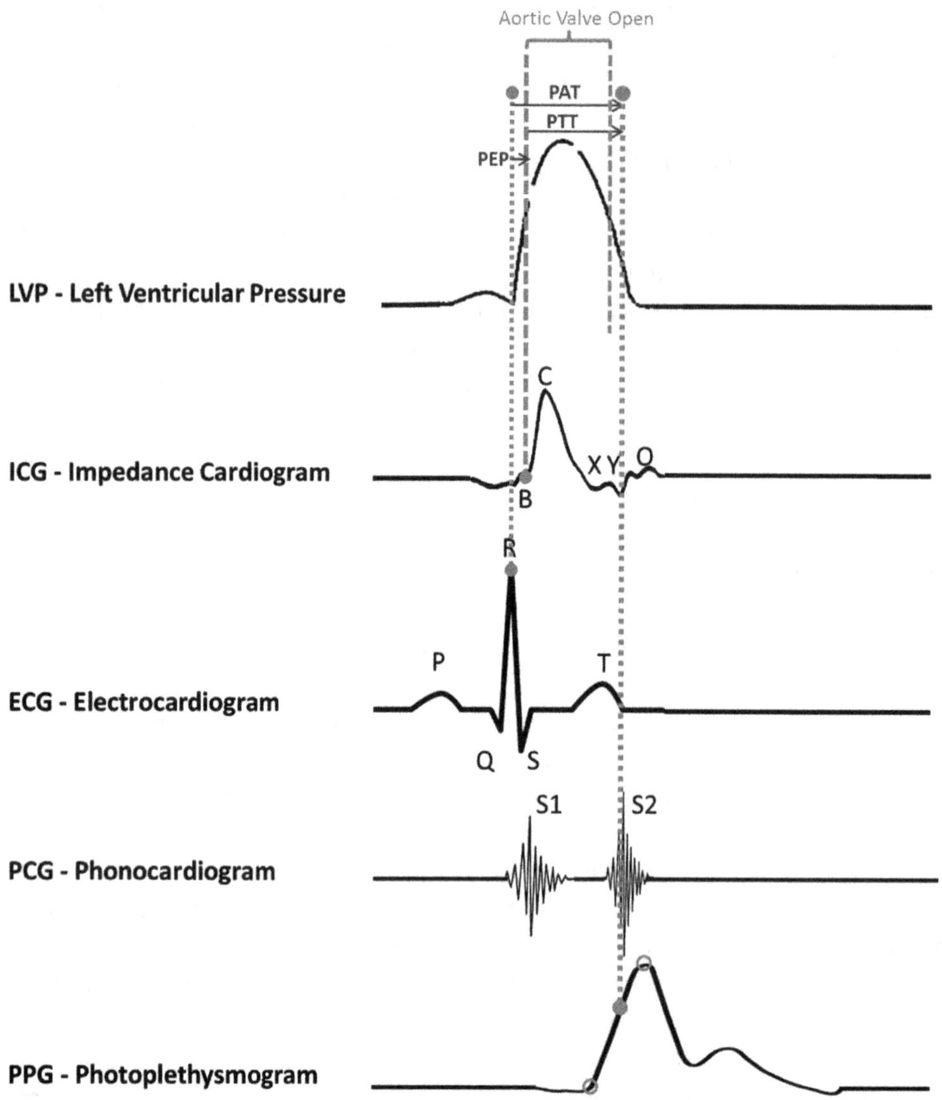

Besides the clinical value of its absolute BP measurements, BP pulse contour analysis has been explored for assessing heart and vascular functions, e.g. for the estimation of the CO as alternative to the standard more risky pulmonary arterial catheter technique (Drummond and Murphy, 2011).

Multivariate Cardiovascular Assessment

The center of the cardiovascular system is the heart, with the electrical activation and blood ejection through the systemic and pulmonary circulations. Figures 2 and 3 show relations of cardiovascular signals, which can be easily acquired noninvasively and synchronously and encode the complex interactions conditioned by sympathetic/parasympathetic and humoral activities. Sympathetic/parasympathetic balance is difficult to comprehensively assess based on a single cardiovascular signal only, such as the baroreflex gain estimation, therefore several studies have addressed this issue with multivariate approaches (La Rovere et al., 2008; Logier et al., 2011). Since focus is on BP assessment, it is described how these signals may be used to produce better noninvasive estimates of the BP.

Cardiac Output (CO) is defined as the blood volume pumped by the heart each minute; it is a function of Stroke Volume (SV) and Heart Rate (HR) (Equation 1) (Guyton and Hall, 2006).

$$CO\ (l/min) = SV \times HR \tag{1}$$

SV is determined by the preload (end-diastolic pressure) and afterload (end-systolic pressure), which is significantly associated with the Systemic Vascular Resistance (SVR, Equation 2).

$$SVR \propto \frac{\Delta P}{CO}. \tag{2}$$

Changes in afterload with resulting changes in isovolumetric pressure directly alter the PEP, also greatly correlated with mean arterial pressure (P), which is affected by SV, HR, SVR and central venous pressure (CVP) - Equation 3.

$$P = \left(CO \cdot SVR\right) + CVP. \tag{3}$$

Left Ventricular Ejection Time (LVET, time interval from the opening to the closing of the aortic valve) is correlated to the obstruction to left ventricular outflow, and therefore directly affects SV. Age is another variable that highly influences CO. CO output gradually decreases with age with diminished SV.

Pulse Wave Velocity (PWV) may be modeled by the Moens-Korteweg equation (Bramwell and Hill, 1922):

$$PWV = \sqrt{\frac{E_{Inc} \cdot h}{2r\rho}}. \tag{4}$$

where E_{Inc} is the incremental elastic modulus of the vessel wall, given a constant ratio of wall thickness (h), with a radius r, and blood density ρ, assuming an isotropic arterial wall with isovolumetric change with pulse pressure.

BP and PWV are interconnected since according to Equation 5:

$$E = E_0 e^{\alpha P}. \tag{5}$$

where $\alpha \approx 0.017\ mmHg^{-1}$(Hughes et al., 1979; Proença et al., 2010).

Pulse Transit Time (PTT) is given by the quotient of the distance traveled by the pressure wave and PWV. By combining the Hughes equation and the Moens-Korteweg equation, a calibration function can be derived, which leads to a logarithmic dependency of the form:

$$P = A \ln\left(PTT\right) + B . \quad (6)$$

and a quadratic relationship by linearizing the exponential as $E \approx E_0\left(1+\alpha P\right)$. $E \approx E_0\left(1+\alpha P\right)$:

$$P = \frac{A}{PTT^2} + B . \quad (7)$$

This framework does not provide a clear solution as to how the systolic and diastolic phases should be handled.

Calibration parameters A and B are subject dependent and can change over time when the patient status changes. More detailed information on the joint model simplifications may be found in (Proença et al., 2010; Peter et al., 2014).

METHODOLOGICAL REVIEW

Papers of interest were located in Scopus, IEEE Xplore and PubMed databases using the keywords blood pressure, noninvasive, monitoring, and beat-to-beat. No constraints were applied to the publication year. The resulting pool of papers was then methodologically reviewed using 5 thematic taxonomies developed in this section:

1. Pulse arrival time and pulse transit time,
2. Vascular transit time,
3. RS2 time,
4. Heart sound characteristics,
5. PPG characteristics.

Table 1 presents a summary of studies discussing noninvasive methods for BP beat-to-beat estimation, and their classification according to the scheme above.

Pulse Arrival Time and Pulse Transit Time

The PAT and PTT analysis is the most explored in the literature, so for readability, this section will be divided into clusters according to the studies' main focus.

PAT vs. PTT

The most popular measurement setup comprises a one-lead ECG and a PPG clip at a finger, toe or ear, because the ECG is more easily accessible. The ECG R peak of the QRS complex provides the time of each heartbeat, and the foot of the PPG volume pulse gives the arrival time. The definition of electrical activation and pulse onset varies between studies, but usually the R peak is used since it can be obtained more accurately than the Q wave onset, and the point of arrival in the PPG is usually an intermediate

Table 1. Comparison of noninvasive blood pressure estimation approaches in the literature

Article	Estimated Arterial Pressure		Features Extracted						Physiological Signals			
	Systemic	Pulmonary	PAT	PTT	VTT	RS2	PCG Feat.	PPG Feat.	PCG	ECG	ICG	PPG
Lane (1983)	●	○	●	●	○	○	○	○	○	●	○	○
Forouzanfar (2013)*	●	○	●	○	○	○	○	○	○	●	○	○
Ahmad (2012)*	●	○	●	○	○	○	○	○	○	●	○	○
Muehlsteff (2006)	●	○	●	●	○	○	○	○	○	●	●	●
Muehlsteff (2008)	●	○	●	●	○	○	○	○	○	●	●	●
Proenca (2010)	●	○	●	●	○	○	○	○	○	●	●	●
Sharwood-Smith (2006)	●	○	●	○	○	○	○	○	○	●	○	●
Pitson (1998)	●	○	●	○	○	○	○	○	○	●	○	●
Chen (2000)	●	○	●	○	○	○	○	○	○	●	○	●
Poon (2005)#	●	○	●	○	○	○	○	○	○	●	○	●
Pandian (2008)	●	○	●	○	○	○	○	○	○	●	○	●
Meigas (2007)	●	○	●	○	○	○	○	○	○	●	○	●
Lass (2004)	●	○	●	○	○	○	○	○	○	●	○	●
Wong (2005)	●	○	●	○	○	○	○	○	○	●	○	●
Gesche (2012)	●	○	●	○	○	○	○	○	○	●	○	●
Wong (2009)	●	○	●	○	○	○	○	○	○	●	○	●
Fung (2004)	●	○	●	○	○	○	○	○	○	●	○	●
Gu (2008)	●	○	●	○	○	○	○	●	○	●	○	●
Yoon (2009)	●	○	●	○	○	○	○	●	○	●	○	●
Mase (2011)	●	○	●	○	○	○	○	○	○	●	○	●
Kim (2008)	●	○	●	○	○	○	○	●	○	●	○	●
Baek (2010)	●	○	●	○	○	○	○	●	○	●	○	●
Spulak (2011)	●	○	●	○	○	○	○	●	○	●	○	●
Ahlstrom (2005)	●	○	●	○	●	○	○	○	●	●	○	●
Sola (2011)	●	○	●	●	○	○	○	○	●	●	●	●
Sola (2013)	●	○	●	●	○	○	○	○	○	●	●	●
Chandrasekaran (2013)#	●	○	○	○	●	○	○	○	●	○	○	●
Liu (2014)	●	○	●	○	○	○	○	○	○	●	○	●
Zheng (2014b)	●	○	●	○	○	○	○	○	○	●	○	●
Foo (2006)	●	○	○	○	●	○	○	○	●	○	○	●
Wong (2006)	●	○	●	○	○	●	●	○	●	○	○	●
Zhang (2006)+	●	○	○	○	○	●	○	○	●	●	○	○
Zhang (2008)	○	●	○	○	○	●	○	○	●	●	○	○
Chen (1996)	○	●	○	○	○	○	●	○	●	●	○	○

continued on following page

Table 1. Continued

Article	Estimated Arterial Pressure		Features Extracted						Physiological Signals			
	Systemic	Pulmonary	PAT	PTT	VTT	RS2	PCG Feat.	PPG Feat.	PCG	ECG	ICG	PPG
Smith (2013)	○	●	○	○	○	○	●	○	●	●	○	○
Xu (2002)	○	●	○	○	○	○	●	○	●	○	○	○
Peretto (2011)	○	●	○	○	○	○	●	○	●	●	○	○
Tranulis (2002)	○	●	○	○	○	○	●	○	●	●	○	○
Dennis (2010)	○	●	○	○	○	○	●	○	●	●	○	○
Longhini (1991)	○	●	○	○	○	○	●	○	●	○	○	○
Bartels (1992)	●	○	○	○	○	○	●	○	●	○	○	○
Lim (2013)++	●	○	○	○	○	○	●	○	●	○	○	○
Chua (2010)	●	○	●	○	○	○	○	●	○	●	○	●
Teng (2003)	●	○	○	○	○	○	○	●	○	○	○	●
Suzuki (2008)	●	○	○	○	○	○	○	●	○	○	○	●
Suzuki (2009)	●	○	○	○	○	○	○	●	○	○	○	●
Monte-Moreno (2011)	●	○	○	○	○	○	○	●	○	○	○	●
Lee (2013)	●	○	○	○	○	○	○	●	○	○	○	●
Kurylyak (2013)	●	○	○	○	○	○	○	●	○	○	○	●
Fukushima (2013)	●	○	○	○	○	○	○	●	○	○	○	●
Visvanathan (2013) #	●	○	○	○	○	○	○	●	○	○	○	●

* Pulse Oscillometry, # SmartPhones, + SimulationStudy, ++ Esophageal Stethoscope.

point between the onset and the peak since it is more stable and accurate (Figure 3) (Proença et al., 2010). However, this leads to the estimation of a Pulse Arrival Time (PAT) made up of two parts (see Figure 4):

$$PAT = PEP + PTT \tag{8}$$

In contrast to the PTT measure introduced before, as the time span between the blood ejection through the aorticvalve and its arrival at a peripheral site, PAT behaves differently vs PTT due to the PEP. PEP contributions are discussed e.g. (Zhang et al., 2011; Payne et al., 2005). In this section the PAT/PTT terminology will be used according to this definition.

To remove the influence of the PEP from the PAT there are several strategies proposed: using two PPG-setup (e.g. one at the ear, another at the finger) or using an additional signal to estimate the PEP such as from HS (identification of the onset of the opening phase of the aortic valve), from the HS and PPG (estimation of the LVET from PPG and subtracting it to the QS2 interval) or from ICG (ECG R peak to B-point). A typical issue of these approaches is the achieved accuracy and error propagation (Carvalho et al., 2010).

There is non-consistent terminology in the definition and interpretation of PAT in the literature, but it may be broadly defined as the time between a specific event in the ECG, such as the QRS complex, to a specific point of the blood pulse in a different body location, for example rise of the blood pulse. Figure 2 presents different PAT definitions explored in the literature.

Figure 4. Pulse arrival time (PAT), pulse transit time (PTT), and pre-ejection period (PEP) schematic representation: time intervals between electrical onset, aortic valve opening and pulse wave in the periphery

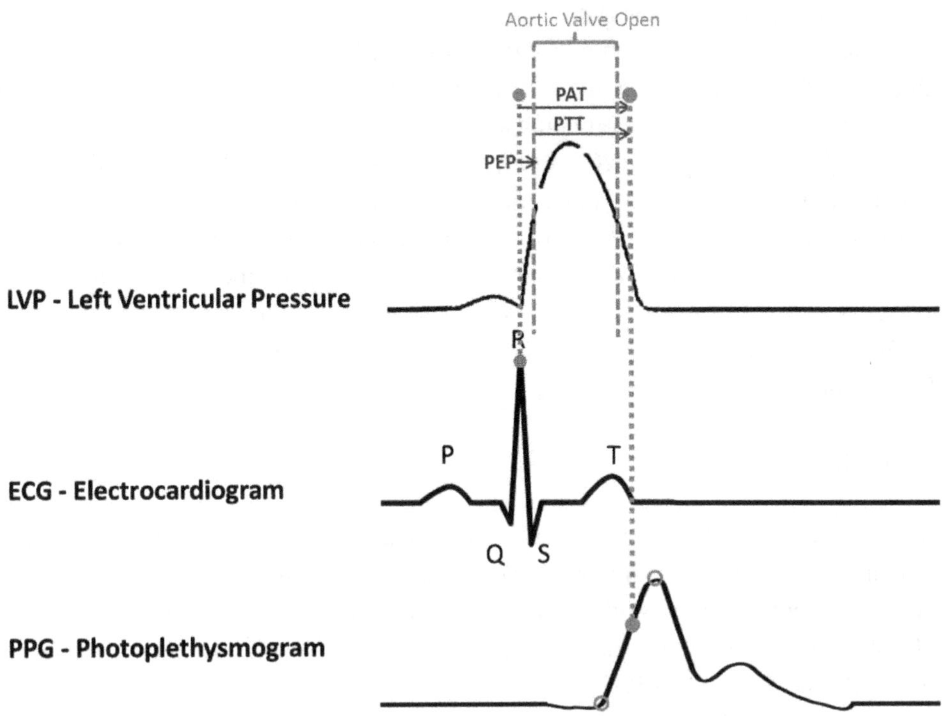

In (Newlin, 1981; Payne et al., 2005) the authors analyzed the relation between PAT and PEP on blood pressure, and concluded that this may not be a good feature to measure BP due to the inconsistent medication responses of PEP. In (Payne et al., 2005) vasoactive drugs were used to induce hemodynamic changes. Although it was considered a good metric to assess BP variability, it may not serve as a reliable BP estimate due to the influence of PEP, with a wide error band if no calibration is used. Using the PAT minus the PEP estimated using the cardiac bioimpedance presented better results (Equation 8).

In (Pollak and Obrist, 1983) the authors estimated the time between ECG Q wave and the beginning of the blood pulse (QPI), from the Q-wave to S2 (QS2), from the beginning of the pulse to the incisura of BP wave (left-ventricular ejection time, LVET), from S2 to the incisura of the BP, and PEP was estimated as the difference between the QS2 and the LVET. It was observed that separating PEP, and determining the different interactions of different sets of physiological mechanisms may be very useful. The author argues that PTT may provide important information about behavior-related changes in arterial stiffness, and PEP may provide important information about normal and abnormal behaviorally-related changes in left ventricular function.

Static Conditions

In (Lane et al., 1983), a study with 4 human subjects, relationships between PTT and intra-arterial BP were analyzed. PTT was obtained from the ECG R wave and two peripheral pulses (brachial and radial), and the difference between them obtained. Also, the pulse location was defined at three different locations (peak, foot and slope). A correlation analysis demonstrated that PTT was moderately correlated with SBP, but not DBP, and that a large portion of the variance could not be explained by PTT alone, with wide inter and intra-individual variability.

In (Ahmad et al., 2012) the authors propose to measure PAT to improve the cuff-based measurement of the BP, although still using the cuff to measure the BP, obtaining errors below the recommended range of 5 mmHg in more than 70% of the estimations.

Researchers in (Forouzanfar et al., 2013) propose a theoretical model of the cardiovascular system describing the relations between signals and allowing the estimation of the BP; a 3-D finite-element upper arm model encompassing the effect of arm soft tissue, muscle, brachial artery, and humerus mechanical properties on oscillometric measurements was used; the model was later validated in an experimental study with 10 volunteers. Results were encouraging, with errors of 5.31 and 4.51 mmHg for SBP and DBP respectively, although this method was still cuff-dependent to detect the pulse in the periphery (oscillometry).

Dynamic Conditions

T-wave amplitudes of the ECG, HR and PAT were used to assess responses to psychological and physiological challenges (arithmetic task and cycling) (Furedy et al., 1996). The authors observed that PAT decreased with the exercise effort. With increasing levels of exercise, oxygen consumption increases, leading to elevated CO, SV (Guyton and Hall, 2006), and BP (Sullivan et al., 1989), which accounts for the elevation in HR and decrease in PAT.

The impact of exercise on PAT was also studied (Wong and Zhang, 2005). The participants performed a treadmill test while ECG, PPG and BP were monitored. PATs were calculated using the R wave as marker and two different points in the PPG (curve onset and peak). The authors observed that the two PATs decreased with increasing physical effort, with a corresponding increase in the systolic and diastolic BPs. This was also observed during cardiopulmonary exercise tests on a bicycle (Wibmer et al., 2014; Gesche et al., 2012; Muehlsteff et al., 2006). In (Muehlsteff et al.,2006) it was observed that in short-term physical stress tests, PEP dominates PTT variations raising.

In (Lass et al., 2004) the authors studied the PAT as a surrogate of BP in resting and exercise conditions. They observe that PAT may be used as a beat-to-beat SBP surrogate as measured by the Finapress (12.2±5.5 mmHg error and 9.6±5.4 mmHg through the auscultatory method), although individual calibration is necessary: for example, PAT is higher with increasing age. This was also reported in (Meigas et al., 2007). In their paper the authors used a previously validated method to detect R peaks from ECG and starting front of the PPG pulse, calculating the PWTT between ECG R-peak and50% rising front of PPG pulse.

PAT analysis is in several studies limited to static conditions, but in (Fung et al., 2004) the authors investigated the impact of hemodynamic changes during surgery in the PTT based estimation of the systolic BP, using a model of the kinetic energy of the wave and the gravitational potential energy (Equations 9 and 10) with an error of -0.08±11.32 mmHg.

$$BP = \frac{A}{PTT^2} + B. \tag{9}$$

where

$$A = \left(0.6 \times height\right)^3 \times \frac{\rho}{1.4}. \quad (10)$$

where ρ is the average blood density.

In this study the authors also employed recalibration for the model offset B, using the cuff-based measures. Limitations of PTT such as the PEP which may have greater impact in lower HRs, movement artifacts, and synchronization between the different monitors are also discussed. In a different study, PAT and PPG wave characteristics were also explored to calibrate and estimate BP; the authors observed that rest and exercise conditions change the PPG waveform, and this information may be used to improve the estimation of the BP, with individually calibration through the relative amplitude of the secondary peak of the PPG (Gu et al., 2008).

Another important feature is the cardiovascular feedback control, that can be assessed by small variations of BP and HR (baroreflex). In (Ma and Zhang, 2005) the authors performed a correlation analysis between the PAT and the systemic systolic BP variability. PAT was determined as the difference between the R peak, and the PPG wave onset (foot) and peak, concluding that BP variability may be assessed using the PAT measured on the PPG wave onset (foot).

The PAT was also closely linked to the systemic BP in patients submitted to obstetric spinal anesthesia, with more than 50% of the variation explained by the BP. Remaining variation may be explained by other factors, such as patient size, variation in accuracy of estimates of both arterial pressure and PAT, and individual variations in vessel wall characteristics, but argue that this may not be a problem for measurements within the same individual, allowing to assess moment-to-moment changes (Sharwood-Smith et al., 2006).

In (Liu et al., 2014) the authors used the PAT for the estimation of SBP under exercise conditions, and analyzed the estimations' hysteresis. They observed that for the same systolic SBP, PAT measured during exercise was significantly larger than PAT measured during recovery for all subject groups, which may be a result of changes in the tone of the vascular smooth muscle, which is altered during exercise and may not be disregarded for this application.

Home Monitoring

Most interesting is to get rid of the cuff in home monitoring scenarios in particular during sleep which is assessed in (Budinger, 2003; Pitson and Stradling, 1998). (Pitson and Stradling, 1998) report good results to estimate disease severity using PAT and the setup was easier to use. Consistent relation of BP vs. PAT were observed: a BP decrease due to inspiratory effort or arousal was accompanied by a PAT increase. A review of the applications of the PAT/PTT in sleep disorder patients is given in (Smith et al., 1999). The authors also emphasize on issues using PAT such as the interpatient variability, measuring technique, clinical validation and calibration stability. Calibration of noninvasive cuffless BP monitoring is a recurring issue. Individual and intermittent recalibration has been discussed (Bartels and Harder, 1992; Yoon et al., 2009; Sola et al., 2013) since baseline conditions may alter even due to simple daily life activities such as a posture change (Muehlsteff et al., 2008).

The search for small, noninvasive and unobtrusive monitors is of great importance to monitor daily activities, especially for wearable systems. In (Pandian et al., 2008) the authors propose a wearable vest for multi-parameter physiological monitoring with ECG, PPG, BP, body temperature, and galvanic skin response. This system was used to estimate PAT and to assess if it may be used to estimate the BP in static and walking conditions, also with estimations of HR and QT intervals. More recently Zheng et al. (2014b) explored the feasibility of a 24-hour BP monitoring cuffless device using PAT, with promising results in the estimation of the overnight averaged SBP over long periods.

Calibration and Repeatability Analysis

Intrapatient variability of the PAT-BP relation has been addressed by individual calibration and periodical recalibration in time (Chen et al., 2000). BP measurements were obtained by a cuff-based method during a surgical procedure. A correlation of 0.97 and an error within 10% range in 97.8% of the monitoring time was obtained. A different approach without the use of cuff-based calibration in different experimental conditions was evaluated in (Poon and Zhang, 2005) producing biased estimations of the BP (SBP and DBP errors of 0.6±9.8 mmHg and0.9±5.6 mmHg), with a proposed implementation on a PDA and a smartphone. The method proposed in (Chen et al.,2000) was also used in the estimation of BP in dialysis patients (Ahlstrom et al., 2005); the Vascular Transit Time (VTT) was also obtained in this study using PCG monitoring and defined as the time between the S1 and the PPG onset, estimating PEP and its influence in the BP estimates (more detailed information on VTT in the following section). PAT and PEP had better correlation to the BP than VTT, and the authors observed that the PAT allowed to detect hypotension episodes due to hypervolemia better than hypertension episodes.

Individual calibration for BP using PAT as a surrogate seems to be necessary to improve estimation results, although good correlation is observed between the estimated BP and the ground truth, errors are inferior with individual models, rather than with a general population model (Yoon et al., 2009). This was also observed in (Masè et al., 2011), where the authors suggest that this may be a feasible approach to monitor patients during stress tests, allowing the beat-to-beat monitoring of BP with ECG and PPG.

In (Mico and Carmen, 2009) the authors evaluated their technique with PAT to estimate BP (Wong and Zhang,2005) in normotensive subjects with repeatability analysis; the authors conclude that the regression obtained in the first test was not valid in the repeat test (1.4±10.2 and 2.1±7.3 mmHg), although good results could be obtained if the regression coefficients were readjusted (0.0±5.3 and 0.0±2.9 mmHg).

In (Sola et al., 2011) the blood wave velocity was estimated using PCG, ECG and ICG. PCG first heart sound was used to guide detection of the B point in the ICG; Periods of ICG and PCG were ensemble averaged (2 minutes) using the R-wave of the simultaneously recorded ECG as synchronization trigger. B-point identification wasper formed by selecting the local maximum of the ensemble averaged third derivate of the ICG signal occurring the closest to the global maximum of the ensemble-averaged PCG envelope (see Figure 3). The estimation of blood velocity was used to assess arterial wall stiffness. PTT and PEP estimations were used to estimate the pulse wave velocity with high correlation to the measured on the carotid to femoral arteries (ρ=0.88). This work was expanded in (Sola et al.,2013) where the authors propose a noninvasive estimation of the mean BP through a chest sensor (central site), incorporating information from all the sources described and with individual calibration. Six different strategies of individual calibration were investigated, and the best calibration strategy was a subject-dependent calibration based on the data of the first day with an offset correction (mean error 0.7±5.1 mmHg). It should be highlighted that the calibration was made on the first experiment, and on the repetition two weeks later, the estimator still presented still a good performance.

Confounding Factors

Foo et al studied the use of PAT in children (Foo et al., 2005b,a) and adult (Foo et al., 2005c) populations to noninvasively assess arterial compliance and blood pressure, and how age and limb position may affect these values. PAT may be used to assess BP, but also different related variables. For example, Foo reviewed the use of PAT as an indicator of respiratory distress in children for sleep disorders studies (Foo, 2007). In his review the author determined that the PAT was used in several studies with success on detecting inspiratory effort in children through a noninvasive method, but also for calibration/personalization. The major limitation of PAT monitoring was seen in motion artifacts and calibration/personalization. This was confirmed in Naschitz et al, where the feasibility of PAT to monitor sleep studies is stated (Naschitz et al., 2004). An approach to overcome the problem of artifacts is proposed in (Sola et al., 2009) with parametric modeling of the PPG wave. PTT was also used by Foo et al in a children population to assess the ankle brachial index through a PAT ratio between upper and lower limbs, demonstrating that, besides information on the arterial stiffness and blood pressure, PTT may be used as a surrogate of the ankle brachial index (Foo et al., 2007). The relation between VTT and BP was also explored in a study that will be described in the next subsection (Foo et al., 2006).

The concern on PAT changes in different daily activities and postural changes is especially important in ambulatory monitoring. The impact of postural changes in PEP, PAT, and systolic BP was studied in (Muehlsteff et al., 2008), that demonstrated that it is difficult to infer BP using simple calibration strategies of PAT only. In this paper, the PAT was defined as the time delay between the R-peak of the ECG, detected by a modified Pan-Tompkins algorithm, and the pulse-foot of the PPG-signal. It was observed that posture changes have a significant subject-specific effect in healthy subjects, and that from sitting to lying conditions the PEP changes up to 40 ms (Equation 8). This makes simple calibration functions, such as those derived from the Moens- Korteweg model (Equation 4), to fail when inferring BP during postural changes, making this another challenge for individual calibration under different constraints.

In (Baek et al., 2010) the authors assessed the impact of confounding factors HR and arterial stiffness index (time interval from maximum derivative point to the maximum of the dicrotic notch in the PPG), in patients submitted to general anesthesia and volunteers. The maximum first derivative point was selected from the PPG signal, with range determined from consecutive R-peak indexes of the ECG signal. The SBP and DBP values were calculated from the maximum and minimum points of the BP signal, with range determined by R-peak index points. The authors observed that models taking into account HR and the arterial stiffness index provided better estimations of the BP rather than the PAT alone, as described in previous studies (Kim et al., 2008). Other confounding factors, such as biometric data (e.g. weight and height) of the patient, have also been suggested to improve BP estimations (Kim et al., 2005).

The different definitions in the literature of the PAT/PTT seem to suggest that the information contained in the PPG curve might be of value to the determination of the BP; this was explored in (Spulak et al., 2011), where different PATs and PPG wave amplitudes were used in an exploratory study to assess which variable better correlated to MBP. Inconsistent results were observed, although correlation values were fairly low in this exploratory study, it was high in some volunteers, depending on the input parameters. Also the results were improved if the extracted metrics were an average of several cardiac cycles.

Most authors defend that the PAT, because of the influence of the PEP, is not a good estimator of BP. In (Wagner et al., 2010) the authors studied the impact of cardiovascular disease in the PAT performance in BP estimation. PAT was found to be altered in patients with heart failure.

Vascular Transit Time

The long recognized influence of PEP on the estimations of BP has led researchers to the search of more robust metrics for the noninvasive estimation of BP. The definition of vascular transit time (VTT) is slightly different from the PAT since instead of beginning temporal interval at the onset of the heart electrical activity, the S1 is used instead (closure of the AV valves). S1 may be seen as an approximation of the moment of aortic valve opening although it is not accurate (Figure 5). The reason to differentiate these two is the fact that the PAT includes the PEP that may be altered by many factors such as BP, and ventricular stroke volume, in some coexisting cardiac diseases (Lewis et al., 1977; Pollak and Obrist, 1983). Knowing this, a few authors suggest to use VTT instead, as a surrogate of BP (Foo et al., 2006; Chandrasekaran et al., 2013).

In a clinical study with 31 healthy volunteers, the authors propose the use of a synchronized analysis of PCG and PPG in the determination of the VTT and its relation to the BP. BP was collected using a sphygmomanometer, and the VTT related to it, for three postural exercises. It was demonstrated that the VTT changes in accordance to BP. An increase in SBP and DBP was accompanied by a decrease in VTT.

Figure 5. Schematic representation of RS2 and VTT in detail

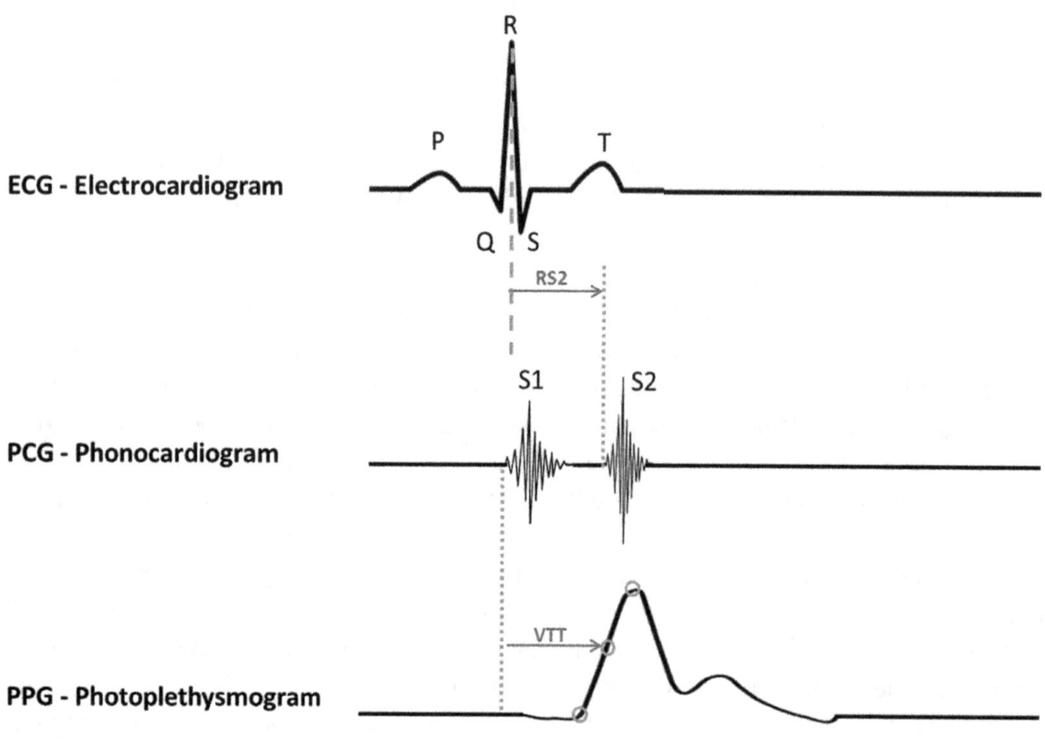

VTT detects abrupt changes of BP, and the authors suggest that this may be useful in monitoring geriatric and pediatric populations (Foo et al., 2006). The estimation of BP is in this study given by Equation 11.

$$\Delta SBP = -0.425 \times \Delta VTT \,. \tag{11}$$

This model resulted in a correlation of 0.82. However, the individuals were at rest and only two posture changes were observed (limited relative SBP change). Using the same argument, (Chandrasekaran et al., 2013) used the VTT to estimate the aortic pressure, and assess its applicability in smart phones. Two approaches were studied, using two smart phones linked (one for PCG and the other for PPG), and a smart phone connected to a diaphragm and microphone in the subject's chest. VTT was determined in the two experimental setups, and SBP estimated using Equation 11 (Foo et al., 2006). To estimate SBP and DBP, the authors employed the stroke volume (SV) and pulse pressure (PP) formulation as described in (Cohn et al., 1995); the authors analyzed the estimated BP using the traditional methods in a Bland-Altman analysis (Bland and Altman, 1986), and reporting good results according to the available guidelines (O'Brien et al., 2002, 2010).

RS2 Time: Electrical to Mechanical

The RS2 timing (Figure 5), and its relation to BP was addressed in few studies. RS2 reflects the time from ventricles contraction and closure of the aortic valve. In (Zhang and Zhang, 2006) the authors studied the theoretical basis of the connections between heart sound and BP, in a simulation study. A model for the left heart circulation was proposed, considering the ventricular pressure as a function of time and ventricular volume (Palladino et al., 1996), and the effect of ejection and heart rate (Danielsen and Ottesen, 2001; Ottesen and Danielsen, 2003; Li et al., 1990); (Zhang and Zhang, 2006) proposed a modified model, coupling a nonlinear model of the arterial system including characteristic impedance of the proximal aorta, total peripheral resistance, and a pressure dependent compliance. The authors did a simulation study of the modified model, reporting the effect of changing the model parameters (peripheral resistance, arterial compliance, heart rate, contractility, and end-diastolic volume). It was demonstrated that RS2 changed inversely with BP for different peripheral resistance, heart rate and contractility.

Experimental results with RS2 estimation using ECG and PCG in 66 normal and 19 abnormal patients confirmed the theoretical assumptions, and were compared with results by (Poon and Zhang, 2005) using PTT (ECG, PPG), with similar outcome. No predictive analysis was performed (Wong et al., 2006). These results were expanded in (Zhang et al., 2008), with the implementation of the left ventricular-arterial interaction model for the aortic blood pressure, with a simulation and an experimental validation study of the model. RS2 was shown to correlate with BP measurements in all subjects during resting and exercise conditions.

Heart Sound Characteristics

Heart sounds are related to the mechanical processes of blood flow and turbulence, and the second heart sound is a combination of these mechanical phenomena, including the closure of the aortic and pulmonary valves. Heart sound spectral characteristics have been studied and connected to the blood pressure (Arnott et al., 1984).

The spectral characteristics of S2 were demonstrated to vary with BP, and it was demonstrated that SBP may be determined on normal subjects using these features, since the short-term spectral power spectrum of S2 shifts towards higher frequency bands with increasing BP. In (Bartels and Harder, 1992) the normalized spectrum of S2 was used to estimate SBP, and demonstrated a good correlation between the intra-arterial BP measurements and the estimated pressure via the acoustic method proposed (MRE of 6%). These results were obtained following a learning phase, in which some measurements in the patient were used for calibration.

The S1 and S2 amplitudes and the S1/S2 ratio have also been studied in relation to the blood pressure in normal subjects, demonstrating that S1/S2 was correlated to intravascular BP measurements (Lim et al., 2013).

As referred earlier, besides systemic hypertension, pulmonary hypertension is a problem that requires a follow-up and invasive measurement of the pulmonary circulation status. Pulmonary hypertension is usually detected through auscultation, and hyperphonesis of the P2 in S2. A very interesting study shows the use of auscultation to estimate PAP using the method described in (Leier, 2001), with a significant correlation (r=0.64, p=0,01) between the PAP estimated by the echocardiogram and the systolic PAP estimated using the auscultatory method (mean difference7.6±7.6 mmHg) (McNab et al., 2010). The method is based on the distance on the patient's chest from the pulmonary auscultation site, and the relative loudness of the A2 and P2 components of S2: the distance at which the A2 and P2 loudness are equal allows the estimation of the systolic PAP. These results were obtained through clinical assessment, without the use of PCG signal processing, therefore, automatic methods to separate and analyze S2 components have been under the scientific community scope, and noninvasive PAP estimation through the heart sound analysis has been explored in several studies (Longhini et al., 1991; Chen et al., 1996; Peretto et al., 2011; Xu et al., 2001; Dennis et al.,2010; Smith and Ventura, 2013).

Separation of A2 and P2 components was explored in (Xu et al., 2001), in which a methodology for spectral characterization and separation of A2 and P2 was proposed using a Wigner-Ville distribution. The method presented good results when A2 and P2 were well separated (increased split, characteristic of pulmonary hypertension), although it required manual intervention to model and extract the characteristics of the chirp models. The method was further developed and applied in a combined study with animal and human subjects, where the dechirping method described in (Xu et al., 2001) was applied to estimate the split interval between A2 and P2 (SI) (Xu et al., 2002). Since the SI is affected by HR, a normalization was applied to each SI (NS I) as given by Equation 12. In this study ECG was used as a marker for S2 detection, limiting the PCG segmentation problem.

$$NSI = \frac{SI \times HR}{600}. \tag{12}$$

The results presented a good correlation with the invasive PAP measures, SEE 5.3 mmHg in pigs and 7.8 mmHg in patients. The authors also refer that hypertension has low impact on the NS I, and therefore on the estimation of the pulmonary pressure. This is important since spectral characteristics of S2 may be altered in hypertensive patients.

In (Longhini et al., 1991) the authors studied the relation between S2 spectrum characteristics and the measured PAP in patients with indication for a heart catheterization. They concluded that the changes in PAP were reflected in the features of the pulmonary component spectrum of S2 (peak frequency and quality of resonance), and may be used in its noninvasive estimation, with better results for the estimation of the systolic PAP (Equation 13).

$$PAP = A + B \cdot F_n + C \cdot Q . \tag{13}$$

where A, B, and C are constants.

The spectral features of S2 were also used in (Chen et al., 1996) to estimate PAP and compared them to the standard noninvasive echocardiography assessment in patients with bioprosthetic heart valves (aortic and mitral). ECG was used as marker, and S2 with maximum split (inspiration) for each subject were manually selected, and through a correlation analysis, a template for each patient selected. This was then used to extract the features from A2 and P2 components of S2 for each patient, consisting of dominant frequencies of S2, A2 and P2, quality of resonance (Q) of A2 and P2, and the ratio between dominant frequencies and quality of resonance of A2 and P2. Direct application of Equation 13 presented poor results. Since the systems were different, the authors reproduced the regression with the same features obtaining better results (r=0.65, SEE 7 mmHg), and a multivariate regression with the features described previously presented even better results, with the best performance including F p, Q p, F p/Fa, and F s (r=0.84, SEE 5.6 mmHg).

The authors in (Peretto et al., 2011) presented a comparison of two indirect estimations of PAP using echocardiography and PCG, and compared the results of the two methods. Although echocardiography may be used to estimate PAP, this technique may not always be available, it requires specialized training, and also in some patients' measurements may not be obtained because of physiological constraints (Xu et al., 2002). The authors studied 40 subjects during echocardiography assessment; ECG and PCG were analyzed in conjunction. S2 was identified using ECG as a marker, and directly split into A2 as P2 as described in (Longhini et al., 1991). Frequency of the maximum amplitude of P2 spectrum (Fn) and quality of resonance (Q) were extracted, to estimate PAP as given by Equation 13 (Longhini et al., 1991). A, B, and C in Equation 13 were 2.0, 0.5 and 18.9, respectively. The PCG based method presented a systematic bias of 4 mmHg (parameters not adjusted to this population), that was corrected prior comparisons; PCG based and echocardiography based estimations were concordant between subjects, and the authors conclude this method may be useful in a first-stage diagnosis.

A few studies addressed the issue of noninvasive PAP estimation, using additional features from the heart sound (Tranulis et al., 2002; Dennis et al., 2010; Smith and Ventura, 2013). In (Tranulis et al., 2002) PAP was estimated using S2 characteristics, employing ECG as a marker for PCG segmentation. Since S2 is a non-stationary signal, the authors suggest to use joint time-frequency representations instead of classical Fourier analysis. In this study Wigner-Ville distribution was used to manually extract three features (start frequency of A2 and P2 components), and splitting time (SI), and wavelet analysis resulting in 21 features corresponding to a 7 scales decomposition (18th Coiflet), squared for each scale, the maximum value was registered as well as the sum of the decomposition coefficients. These features were then used to train a neural network to estimate PAP, and compared to the catheter measurements through a correlation analysis and SEE (r=0.86, 8.4 mmHg for systolic PAP, and r=0.89, 6.0 mmHg for mean PAP). This study was conducted on only 9 pigs, and therefore has limited applicability, and also there was no separation between individual data from training and test sets, resulting in a overly optimistic estimation of accuracy (Dennis et al., 2010). In (Dennis et al., 2010) the authors analyze a set of heart sound features, and ECG based timing of events to diagnose PAP (normal vs pulmonary hypertension), including systole durations, dominant frequencies of S1, S2 and A2, P2, among others. These features were extracted with a commercially available tool (Audicor, Inovise Medical, Inc.), that records ECG and PCG simultaneously (proprietary features). Data was collected from 51 patients (20 for training and 31 for testing). The authors present an approach similar to (Tranulis et al., 2002), surpassing the limitation of using same patient data to train and test the neural network. The results were compared to invasive measurements of PAP, features were ranked according to their importance in PAP estimation, and the best location to collect heart sound for the diagnosis tool was analyzed. The authors concluded that the system provided a good performance in disease detection (77% accuracy), and although the objective was not to obtain good results in PAP estimation, a SEE of 11.7 mmHg was observed. Regarding the range of pulmonary blood pressure, this is a high estimation error, even higher than the recommended for systemic blood pressure (O'Brien et al., 2002, 2010). Whole heart sound features were little predictive of pulmonary hypertension, percentage of heartbeat ventricular systole was helpful, and the more predictive feature was the ration between A2 and P2 powers, as would be clinically expected. This work was further developed in (Smith and Ventura, 2013), where PAP was estimated using the same approach and different algorithms, (38 features and 109 patients, non-overlapping training and test sets), with a SEE of 8.3 mmHg for the MLP algorithm.

Photoplethysmography Wave Characteristics

Besides the use of PPG to mark the pulse arrival in the periphery, as described in the previous sections and illustrated in Figure 3, more recently several authors suggest that the PPG curve characteristics may also be used to improve PTT estimation earlier referred (Mico and Carmen, 2009; Gu et al., 2008; Baek et al., 2010; Yoon et al.,2009; Spulak et al., 2011), or per se as will be described in this section, since the PPG wave reflects the characteristics of the vascular bed and blood flow in the periphery (Allen, 2007). Figure 6 presents some of the different features that may be extracted from the PPG to estimate BP.

In (Teng and Zhang, 2003) the authors propose to estimate the systolic and diastolic BP using the PPG wave properties in a linear regression (upstroke and diastolic time, and 2/3 and 1/2 amplitude wave

Figure 6. Some of the features extracted from the photoplethysmogram: dPPGM corresponding to the point of maximum derivative of the PPG ascending curve; PPG amplitudes (PPGA, PPGa); time to 1/2 and 2/3 of the relative amplitude (T1/2 and T2/3) and dicrotic notch (TN); PPG onset (PPG0); PPG maximum amplitude (PPGM)

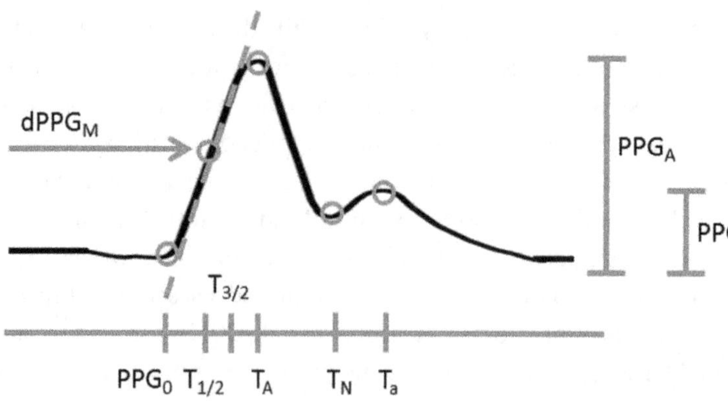

duration). Although diastolic time presented the best results (0.21±7.32 and 0.02±4.39 mmHg error for SBP and DBP respectively), the PPG wave is prone to interference such as movement, interindividual variability, or respiration cycle (Lázaro et al.,2013).

Several classification approaches are used, as well as different PPG features are proposed in the estimation of the BP. (Kurylyak et al., 2013) use an extensive list of amplitudes and time intervals based on the relative amplitude of the PPG, and neural networks to estimate the BP, although the results present a high variability, the database is composed of individuals with different ages, not taken into account. The impact of age on the PPG characteristics was analyzed in (Suzuki and Oguri, 2008), demonstrating that dividing patients in age group improved the estimation results. In (Suzuki and Oguri, 2009) the AdaBoost method was adopted with an error of -1.2±11.7 mmHg in the test set (1.3±5.1 mmHg in the training set).

An exploratory study is presented in (Monte-Moreno, 2011), where the author proposes to use a submodule that computes the feature vector, a decision function based on a linear classifier; and a finite state automaton; the author estimates SBP, DBP and blood glucose level from the PPG characteristics, exploring several machine learning techniques such as neural networks and support vector machines, and feature selection; the best results were obtained with the random forest technique, and errors below the recommended target range for these monitors (absolute error below 15 mmHg in more than 90% of the measurements) (O'Brien et al., 2010).

A comparison of the PPG features versus PAT to estimate BP during sleep studies is presented in (Chua et al., 2010); the results in this study show that the PPG amplitude presented better results than the PAT to estimate SBP, with a higher coherence, and significantly lower estimation errors.

The information in the PPG was also used in (Fukushima et al., 2013) to assess the CO and SVR in the estimation of BP. The authors propose to use the accelerated PPG (double differentiation) to extract information form the new wave, including the HR variability metrics (ratio between low and high frequency bands of the beat-to-beat interval). Only correlation values between BP estimation and measured by conventional methods were presented ($\rho = 0.71$). In (Lee et al., 2013) the PPG was also used to estimate CO and SVR in intensive care patients (errors of -0.01±2.70 L/min for CO and -0.87±412 dyn.s.cm5 for SVR) using PPG features only (see Equation 3).

The authors in (Visvanathan et al., 2013) propose to integrate this method for BP estimation in a smartphone, using the camera to capture the blood pulse in the finger. A model is adjusted to a training set, and then it is used to estimate the BP using the PPG collected by the smartphone camera. Several features including systolic peak amplitude, dicrotic notch amplitude, area under the curve of the different components among others, are extracted from the PPG curve and used in linear regression and SVM to estimate the BP, with good results. Estimation results were improved when using anthropometric data from the subject (age, weight, and height).

DISCUSSION

Research in the field of noninvasive blood pressure estimation promises a great impact on the remote monitoring of the population, including home care patients, elderly, or athletes. Also, beat-to-beat noninvasive cuffless pressure estimations would improve patient care in hospitals, allowing for a more continuous monitoring of the cardiovascular function of the patients with improved safety and comfort.

Even with the limitations presented, PAT is the most explored feature in the noninvasive BP estimation, since it is an easy to obtain measure based on easy to acquire ECG and PPG signals. PTT in many studies was obtained through the estimation of the PAT which encompasses a variable error in the PEP, a factor that may not be disregarded. Also the Moens-Korteweg model, used in several studies, has been derived from a simplified mechanical model assuming that there are insignificant variations of vessel radius and section, which may not be the case in real scenarios such as during exercise (Proença et al., 2010).

Changes in blood volemia, posture, vasoconstriction/dilation due to environmental changes such as temperature or emotional responses, may also affect the assumptions of many of the proposed methods. Although a lot of important clinical situations are on static conditions, applications such as ambulatory monitoring may not disregard the importance of posture changes, the baroreceptor feedback control and induced vasoconstriction/dilation that require access to context information (Muehlsteff et al., 2008). All these issues may serve as a motivation for introducing individual calibration or recalibration in the estimation, which is actually the method used in the first FDA approved monitor available in the market for the noninvasive BP estimation with surrogate cardiovascular signals (ViSi Mobile, Sotera Wireless) (Sotera Wireless, 2015). The recent IEEE standard defines that such a monitor should describe the recalibration period, and ensure good estimations within this interval, not only in steady-state but also for BP changes (IEEE-SA, 2014).

The interest in the mechanical events in relation to the BP has been gaining more interest, especially in the estimation of the pulmonary circulation BP. The use of PCG and PPG combined, or the analysis of the PCG characteristics presents a fairly unexplored avenue. High resolution time-frequency techniques may aid in the separation of the S2 components and assess its relation to the systemic and pulmonary blood pressure.

CONCLUSION AND FUTURE SCOPE

In this review, the most recent developments in the estimation of cardiovascular function noninvasively are presented, with especial focus on the estimation of blood pressure. The methods presented in the literature demonstrate that several important features of the cardiovascular system may be estimated through the relations between the signals measured on the body surface (e. g. blood pressure and cardiac output), translating electrical and mechanical cardiovascular activity with promising results considering the minimum errors defined in the standards (IEEE-SA, 2014; O'Brien et al., 2002, 2010; Bland and Altman, 1986).

As limitations in this field, although there are different strategies for the noninvasive BP assessment, few studies compared the different methods, few used biometric data to improve models, and there is a lack of repeatability analysis. Also, the majority of the presented methods are focused on the estimation of the systolic BP, although the diastolic BP is also of important clinical value and this should be subject of further studies. Finally, the calibration/recalibration methodology is an important issue, not only for individualization since results demonstrate that general models do not provide good individual results, but also taking into account hemodynamic changes that may alter the individual calibration functions throughout long monitoring periods, and should be the addressed in future studies.

ACKNOWLEDGMENT

This work was partially funded by the Fundação para a Ciência e Tecnologia (FCT, Portuguese Foundation for Science and Technology) under the reference Heart Safe PTDC/EEI-PRO/2857/2012; Project NanoSTIMA, NORTE-01-0145-FEDER-000016; Project I-CITY - ICT for Future Health/Faculdade de Engenharia da Universidade do Porto, NORTE-07-0124-FEDER-000068, funded by the Fundo Europeu de Desenvolvimento Regional (FEDER) through the Programa Operacional do Norte (ON2) and by national funds through FCT/MEC (PIDDAC).

REFERENCES

Ahlstrom, C., Johansson, A., Uhlin, F., Lnne, T., & Ask, P. (2005). Noninvasive investigation of blood pressure changes using the pulse wave transit time: A novel approach in the monitoring of hemodialysis patients. *Journal of Artificial Organs*, *8*(3), 192–197. PMID:16235036

Ahmad, S., Chen, S., Soueidan, K., Batkin, I., Bolic, M., Dajani, H., & Groza, V. (2012). Electrocardiogram-assisted blood pressure estimation. Biomedical Engineering. *IEEE Transactions on*, *59*(3), 608–618.

Akay, M. (Ed.). (2006). *Wiley Encyclopedia of Biomedical Engineering*. Wiley-Interscience.

Allen, J. (2007). Photoplethysmography and its application in clinical physiological measurement. *Physiological Measurement*, *28*(3), R1. PMID:17322588

Arnott, P., Pfeiffer, G., & Tavel, M. (1984). Spectral analysis of heart sounds: Relationships between some physical characteristics and frequency spectra of first and second heart sounds in normals and hypertensives. *Journal of Biomedical Engineering*, *6*(2), 121–128. PMID:6708485

Baek, H. J., Kim, K. K., Kim, J. S., Lee, B., & Park, K. S. (2010). Enhancing the estimation of blood pressure using pulse arrival time and two confounding factors. *Physiological Measurement*, *31*(2), 145. PMID:20009186

Bartels, A., & Harder, D. (1992). Non-invasive determination of systolic blood pressure by heart sound pattern analysis. *Clinical Physics and Physiological Measurement*, *13*(3), 249–256. PMID:1424474

Bickley, L. S. (Ed.). (2009). *Bates' Guide to Physical Examination and History Taking* (11th ed.). Lippincott Williams & Wilkins.

Bland, J. M., & Altman, D. G. (1986). Statistical methods for assessing agreement between two methods of clinical measurement. *Lancet*, *1*, 307–310. PMID:2868172

Bramwell, J. C., & Hill, A. V. (1922). The velocity of the pulse wave in man. *Proceedings of the Royal Society of London. Series B, Containing Papers of a Biological Character*.

Brzezinski, M., Luisetti, T., & London, M. J. (2009). Radial artery cannulation: A comprehensive review of recent anatomic and physiologic investigations. *Anesthesia and Analgesia*, *109*(6), 1763–1781. PMID:19923502

Budinger, T. F. (2003). Biomonitoring with wireless communications. *Annual Review of Biomedical Engineering*, *5*(1), 383–412. PMID:14527317

Buxi, D., Redout, J.-M., & Yuce, M. R. (2015). A survey on signals and systems in ambulatory blood pressure monitoring using pulse transit time. *Physiological Measurement*, *36*(3), R1. PMID:25694235

Carvalho, P., Paiva, R., Couceiro, R., Henriques, J., Antunes, M., Quintal, I., Muehlsteff, J., & Aubert, X. (2010). Comparison of systolic time interval measurement modalities for portable devices. In *Engineering in Medicine and Biology Society (EMBC), 2010 Annual International Conference of the IEEE.*

Chandrasekaran, V., Dantu, R., Jonnada, S., Thiyagaraja, S., & Subbu, K. (2013). Cuffless differential blood pressure estimation using smart phones. Biomedical Engineering. *IEEE Transactions on*, *60*(4), 1080–1089.

Chen, D., Pibarot, P., Honos, G., & Durand, L.-G. (1996). Estimation of pulmonary artery pressure by spectral analysis of the second heart sound. *The American Journal of Cardiology*, *78*(7), 785–789. PMID:8857483

Chen, W., Kobayashi, T., Ichikawa, S., Takeuchi, Y., & Togawa, T. (2000). Continuous estimation of systolic blood pressure using the pulse arrival time and intermittent calibration. *Medical & Biological Engineering & Computing*, *38*(5), 569–574. PMID:11094816

Chua, E.-P., Redmond, S., McDarby, G., & Heneghan, C. (2010). Towards using photoplethysmogram amplitude to measure blood pressure during sleep. *Annals of Biomedical Engineering*, *38*(3), 945–954. PMID:20049639

Chung, E., Chen, G., Alexander, B., & Cannesson, M. (2013). Non-invasive continuous blood pressure monitoring: A review of current applications. *Frontiers of Medicine*, *7*(1), 91–101. PMID:23345112

Cohn, J. N., Finkelstein, S., McVeigh, G., Morga, D., LeMay, L., Robinson, J., & Mock, J. (1995). Noninvasive pulse wave analysis for the early detection of vascular disease. *Hypertension*, *26*(3), 503–508. PMID:7649589

Couceiro, R., Carvalho, P., Paiva, R., Henriques, J., Antunes, M., & Quintal, I. andMuehlsteff, J. (2011). Beat-to-beat cardiac output inference using heart sounds. In *Engineering in Medicine and Biology Society,EMBC, 2011 Annual International Conference of the IEEE.*

Danielsen, M., & Ottesen, J. (2001). Describing the pumping heart as a pressure source. *Journal of Theoretical Biology*, *212*(1), 71–81. PMID:11527446

Dennis, A., Michaels, A. D., Arand, P., & Ventura, D. (2010). Noninvasive diagnosis of pulmonary hypertension using heart sound analysis. *Computers in Biology and Medicine*, *40*(9), 758–764. PMID:20691967

Drummond, K. E., & Murphy, E. (2011). *Minimally invasive cardiac output monitors*. Continuing Education in Anaesthesia, Critical Care &Pain.

Foo, J. Y. A. (2007). Pulse transit time in paediatric respiratory sleep studies. *Medical Engineering & Physics*, *29*(1), 17–25. PMID:16495120

Foo, J. Y. A., Lim, C. S., & Wang, P. (2006). Evaluation of blood pressure changes using vascular transit time. *Physiological Measurement*, *27*(8), 685. PMID:16772667

Foo, J. Y. A., Lim, C. S., Wilson, S. J., Williams, G. R., Harris, M.-A., & Cooper, D. M. (2007). Pulse transit time ratio as a potential marker for paediatriccrural and brachial blood pressure index. *Physiological Measurement*, *21*, 415–417. PMID:17287846

Foo, J. Y. A., Wilson, S. J., Williams, G. R., Coates, A., Harris, M.-A., & Cooper, D. M. (2005a). Predictive regression equations and clinical uses of peripheral pulse timing characteristics in children. *Physiological Measurement*, *26*(3), 317. PMID:15798305

Foo, J. Y. A., Wilson, S. J., Williams, G. R., Harris, M.-A., & Cooper, D. M. (2005b). Pulse transit time as a derived noninvasive mean to monitor arterial distensibility changes in children. *Journal of Human Hypertension*, *19*, 723–729. PMID:15920454

Foo, J. Y. A., Wilson, S. J., Williams, G. R., Harris, M.-A., & Cooper, D. M. (2005c). Pulse transit time changes observed with different limb positions. *Physiological Measurement*, *26*(6), 1093. PMID:16311456

Forouzanfar, M., Ahmad, S., Batkin, I., Dajani, H., Groza, V., & Bolic, M. (2013). Coefficient-free blood pressure estimation based on pulse transit time; cuff pressure dependence. Biomedical Engineering. *IEEE Transactions on*, *60*(7), 1814–1824.

Fukushima, H., Kawanaka, H., Bhuiyan, M., & Oguri, K. (2013). Cuffless blood pressure estimation using only photoplethysmography based on cardiovascular parameters. In *Engineering in Medicine and Biology Society (EMBC), 2013 35th Annual International Conference of the IEEE.*

Fung, P., Dumont, G., Ries, C., Mott, C., & Ansermino, M. (2004). Continuous noninvasive blood pressure measurement by pulse transit time. In *Engineering in Medicine and Biology Society, 2004. IEMBS '04. 26th Annual International Conference of the IEEE.*

Furedy, J. J., Szabo, A., & Pronnet, F. (1996). Effects of psychological and physiological challenges on heart rate, t-wave amplitude, and pulse-transit time. *International Journal of Psychophysiology*, *22*(3), 173–183. PMID:8835625

Gesche, H., Grosskurth, D., Kchler, G., & Patzak, A. (2012). Continuous blood pressure measurement by using the pulse transit time: Comparison to a cuff-based method. *European Journal of Applied Physiology*, *112*(1), 309–315. PMID:21556814

Gu, W., Poon, C., & Zhang, Y. (2008). A novel parameter from ppgdicrotic notch for estimation of systolic blood pressure using pulse transit time. In *Medical Devices and Biosensors, 2008. ISSS-MDBS 2008. 5th International Summer School and Symposium on.*

Guyton, A., & Hall, J. E. (Eds.). (2006). *Textbook of Medical Physiology* (11th ed.). Elsevier Saunders.

Ha, S., Kim, C., Chi, Y., Akinin, A., Maier, C., Ueno, A., & Cauwenberghs, G. (2014). Integrated circuits and electrode interfaces for noninvasive physiological monitoring. Biomedical Engineering. *IEEE Transactions on*, *61*(5), 1522–1537.

Hughes, D., Babbs, C., & Geddes, L., & Bo. (n.d.). Measurements of young's modulus of elasticity of the canine aorta with ultrasound. *Ultrasonic Imaging*, *1*(4):356 – 367. PMID:575833

IEEE-SA. (2014). *IEEE standard for wearable cuffless blood pressure measuring devices*. IEEE P1708/D04.

Johnston, P., Imam, Z., Dempsey, G., Anderson, J., & Adgey, A. (1998). The transthoracic impedance cardiogram is a potential haemodynamic sensor for an automated external defibrillator. *European Heart Journal, 19*(12), 1879–1888. PMID:9886732

Kemmotsu, O., Ueda, M., Otsuka, H., Yamamura, T., Winter, D., & Eckerle, J. (1991). Arterial tonometry for noninvasive, continuous blood pressure monitoring during anesthesia. *Anesthesiology, 75*(2), 333–340. PMID:1859020

Kim, J. Y., Cho, B. H., Im, S. M., Jeon, M. J., Kim, I. Y., & Kim, S. I. (2005). Comparative study on artificial neural network with multiple regressions for continuous estimation of blood pressure. In *Engineering in Medicine and Biology Society, 2005. IEEE-EMBS 2005. 27th Annual International Conference of the.*

Kim, J. S., Kim, K. K., Baek, H. J., & Park, K. S. (2008). *Comparable parameter related to arterial stiffness in blood pressure estimation method.* Academic Press.

Kurylyak, Y., Lamonaca, F., & Grimaldi, D. (2013). A neural network-based method for continuous blood pressure estimation from a ppg signal. In *Instrumentation and Measurement Technology Conference (I2MTC), 2013 IEEE International.*

La Rovere, M. T., Pinna, G. D., & Raczak, G. (2008). Baroreflex sensitivity: Measurement and clinical implications. *Annals of Noninvasive Electrocardiology, 13*(2), 191–207. PMID:18426445

Lane, J. D., Greenstadt, L., Shapiro, D., & Rubinstein, E. (1983). Pulse transit time and blood pressure: An intensive analysis. *Psychophysiology, 20*(1), 45–49. PMID:6828611

Lass, J., Meigas, K., Karai, D., Kattai, R., Kaik, J., & Rossmann, M. (2004). Continuous blood pressure monitoring during exercise using pulse wave transit time measurement. In *Engineering in Medicine and Biology Society, 2004. IEMBS '04. 26th Annual International Conference of the IEEE.*

Lázaro, J., Gil, E., Bailn, R., Minchol, A., & Laguna, P. (2013). Deriving respiration from photoplethysmographic pulse width. *Medical & Biological Engineering & Computing, 51*(1-2), 233–242. PMID:22996834

Lee, Q. Y., Redmond, S. J., Chan, G. S., Middleton, P. M., Steel, E., Malouf, P., & …, Lovell, N. H. (2013). Estimation of cardiac output and systemic vascular resistance using a multivariate regression model with features selected from the finger photoplethysmogram and routine cardiovascular measurements. *Biomedical Engineering Online, 12*(19), 16. PMID:23452705

Leier, C. V. (2001). Nuggets, pearls, and vignettes of master heart failure clinicians. *Congestive Heart Failure (Greenwich, Conn.), 7*(6), 297–308. PMID:11828174

Lewis, R. P., Rittogers, S. E., Froester, W. F., & Boudoulas, H. (1977). A critical review of the systolic time intervals. *Circulation, 56*(2), 146–158. PMID:872305

Li, J. K.-J., Cui, T., & Drzewiecki, G. (1990). A nonlinear model of the arterial system incorporating a pressure-dependent compliance. Biomedical Engineering. *IEEE Transactions on, 37*(7), 673–678.

Lim, K. H., Shin, Y. D., Park, S. H., Bae, J. H., Lee, H. J., Kim, S. J., & Choi, Y. J. et al. (2013). Correlation of blood pressure and the ratio of s1 to s2 as measured by esophageal stethoscope and wireless bluetooth transmission. *Pakistan Journal of Medical Sciences*, *4*(29), 1023–1027. PMID:24353680

Liu, Q., Yan, B., Yu, C.-M., Zhang, Y.-T., & Poon, C. (2014). Attenuation of systolic blood pressure and pulse transit time hysteresis during exercise and recovery in cardiovascular patients. Biomedical Engineering. *IEEE Transactions on*, *61*(2), 346–352.

Logier, R., De Jonckheere, J., Delecroix, M., Keribedj, A., Jeanne, M., Jounwaz, R., & Tavernier, B. (2011). Heart rate variability analysis for arterial hypertension etiological diagnosis during surgical procedures under tourniquet. In *Engineering in Medicine and Biology Society,EMBC, 2011 Annual International Conference of the IEEE.*

Longhini, C., Baracca, E., Brunazzi, C., Vaccari, M., Longhini, L., & Barbaresi, F. (1991). A new noninvasive method for estimation of pulmonary arterial pressure in mitral stenosis. *The American Journal of Cardiology*, *68*(4), 398–401. PMID:1858684

Ma, T., & Zhang, Y. (2005). A correlation study on the variabilities in pulse transit time, blood pressure, and heart rate recorded simultaneously from healthy subjects. In *Engineering in Medicine and Biology Society, 2005. IEEE-EMBS 2005. 27th Annual International Conference of the.*

Masè, M., Mattei, W., Cucino, R., Faes, L., & Nollo, G. (2011). Feasibility of cuff-free measurement of systolic and diastolic arterial blood pressure. *Journal of Electrocardiology*, *44*(2), 201–207. PMID:21353067

McNab, P., Castro, P., Verdejo, H., & Martinez, G. (2010). Estimacionauscultatoria de la presionsistolica dearteria pulmonar: Esfactible? correlacioncondeterminacionecocardiografica. *Revista Medica de Chile*, *138*, 1351–1356. PMID:21279246

Meigas, K., Lass, J., Karai, D., Kattai, R., & Kaik, J. (2007). Pulse wave velocity in continuous blood pressure measurements. In *World Congress on Medical Physics and Biomedical Engineering 2006*. Springer Berlin Heidelberg.

Meyer, C., Morren, G., Muehlsteff, J., Heiss, C., Lauer, T., Schauerte, P., & Kelm, M. et al. (2011). Predicting neurally mediated syncope based on pulse arrival time: Algorithm development and preliminary results. *Journal of Cardiovascular Electrophysiology*, *22*(9), 1042–1048. PMID:21410580

Mico, W., & Carmen, P. (2009). An evaluation of the cuffless blood pressure estimation based on pulse transit time technique: A half year study on normotensive subjects. *Cardiovascular Engineering: An International Journal*, *9*(1), 32–38. PMID:19381806

Millasseau, S. C., Stewart, A. D., Patel, S. J., Redwood, S. R., & Chowienczyk, P. J. (2005). Evaluation of carotid-femoral pulse wave velocity influence of timing algorithm and heart rate. *Hypertension*, *45*(2), 222–226. PMID:15642772

Monte-Moreno, E. (2011). Non-invasive estimate of blood glucose and blood pressure from a photoplethysmograph by means of machine learning techniques. *Artificial Intelligence in Medicine*, *53*(2), 127–138. PMID:21696930

Muehlsteff, J., Aubert, X., & Morren, G. (2008). Continuous cuff-less blood pressure monitoring based on the pulse arrival time approach: The impact of posture. In *Engineering in Medicine and Biology Society, 2008. EMBS 2008. 30th Annual International Conference of the IEEE.*

Muehlsteff, J., Aubert, X., & Schuett, M. (2006). Cuffless estimation of systolic blood pressure for short effort bicycle tests: The prominent role of the pre-ejection period. In *Engineering in Medicine and Biology Society, 2006. EMBS '06. 28th Annual International Conference of the IEEE.*

Naschitz, J., Bezobchuk, S., Mussafia-Priselac, R., Sundick, S., Dreyfuss, D., Khorshidi, I., & Gaitini, L. et al. (2004). Pulse transit time by r-wave-gated infrared photoplethysmography: Review of the literature and personal experience. *Journal of Clinical Monitoring and Computing*, *18*(5-6), 333–342. PMID:15957624

Newlin, D. B. (1981). Relationships of pulse transmission times to pre-ejection period and blood pressure. *Psychophysiology, 18*, 316-321.

O'Brien, E., Atkins, N., Stergiou, G., Karpettas, N., Parati, G., Asmar, R., & Shennan, A. et al. (2010). on behalf of the working group on blood pressure monitoring of the european society of hypertension, european society of hypertension international protocol revision 2010 for the validation of blood pressure measuring devices in adults. *Blood Pressure Monitoring*, *15*(1), 23–38. PMID:20110786

O'Brien, E., Pickering, T., Asmar, R., Myers, M., Parati, G., Staessen, J., & Palatini, P. et al. (2002). on behalf of the working group on blood pressure monitoring of the european society of hypertension, working group on blood pressure monitoring of the european society of hypertension international protocol for validation of blood pressure measuring devices in adults. *Blood Pressure Monitoring*, *7*(1), 3–17. PMID:12040236

Ottesen, J., & Danielsen, M. (2003). Modeling ventricular contraction with heart rate changes. *Journal of Theoretical Biology*, *222*(3), 337–346. PMID:12732480

Palladino, J., Mulier, J., & Noordergraaf, A. (1996). An alternative to time-varying elastance descriptions of the heart. In *Engineering in Medicine and Biology Society, 1996. Bridging Disciplines for Biomedicine.Proceedings of the 18th Annual International Conference of the IEEE.*

Paloheimo, M. P. J., Sahanne, S., & Uutela, K. H. (2010). Autonomic nervous system state: The effect of general anaesthesia and bilateral tonsillectomy after unilateral infiltration of lidocaine. *British Journal of Anaesthesia*, *104*(5), 587–895. PMID:20354006

Pandian, P., Mohanavelu, K., Safeer, K., Kotresh, T., Shakunthala, D., Gopal, P., & Padaki, V. (2008). Smart vest: Wearable multi-parameter remote physiological monitoring system. *Medical Engineering & Physics*, *30*(4), 466–477. PMID:17869159

Payne, R. A., Symeonides, C. N., Webb, D. J., & Maxwell, S. R. J. (2005). Pulse transit time measured from the ecg: An unreliable marker of beat-to-beat blood pressure. *Journal of Applied Physiology*, *100*(1), 136–141. PMID:16141378

Penaz, J., ... (1973). Photoelectric measurement of blood pressure, volume and flow in the finger. In *Digest of the 10th international conference on medical and biological engineering*. International Federation for Medical and Biological Engineering.

Peretto, L., Poletti, G., Longhini, L., Vitolo, A., & Santini, C. (2011). A comparison study of two indirect methods for measuring the systolic pulmonary arterial pressure. In *Medical Measurements and Applications Proceedings (MeMeA), 2011 IEEE International Workshop on.*

Peter, L., Noury, N., & Cerny, M. (2014). A review of methods for non-invasive and continuous blood pressure monitoring: Pulse transit time method is promising?. *IRBM*, *35*(5), 271–282.

Pickering, T. G., Hall, J. E., Appel, L. J., Falkner, B. E., Graves, J., Hill, M. N., & Roccella, E. J. et al. (2005). Recommendations for blood pressure measurement in humans and experimental animals: Part 1: Blood pressure measurement in humans: A statement for professionals from the subcommittee of professional and public education of the American heart association council on high blood pressure research. *Hypertension*, *45*(1), 142–161. PMID:15611362

Pitson, D., & Stradling. (1998). Value of beat-to-beat blood pressure changes, detected by pulse transit time, in the management of the obstructive sleep apnoea/hypopnoea syndrome. *The European Respiratory Journal*, *12*(3), 685–692. PMID:9762800

Pollak, M. H., & Obrist, P. A. (1983). Aortic-radial pulse transit time and ecg q-wave to radial pulse wave interval as indices of beat-by-beat blood pressure change. *Psychophysiology*, *20*, 21–28. PMID:6828608

Poon, C. C. Y., & Zhang, Y. (2005). Cuff-less and noninvasive measurements of arterial blood pressure by pulse transit time. In *Engineering in Medicine and Biology Society, 2005. IEEE-EMBS 2005. 27th Annual International Conference of the.*

Proença, J., Muehlsteff, J., Aubert, X., & Carvalho, P. (2010). Is pulse transit time a good indicator of blood pressure changes during short physical exercise in a young population? In *Engineering in Medicine and Biology Society (EMBC), 2010 Annual International Conference of the IEEE.*

Sharwood-Smith, G., Bruce, J., & Drummond, G. (2006). Assessment of pulse transit time to indicate cardiovascular changes during obstetric spinal anaesthesia. *British Journal of Anaesthesia*, *96*(1), 100–105. PMID:16257996

Sherwood, A., Allen, M. T., Fahrenberg, J., Kelsey, R. M., Lovallo, W. R., & van Doornen, L. J. (1990). Methodological guidelines for impedance cardiography. *Psychophysiology*, *27*(1), 1–23. PMID:2187214

Smith, R., & Ventura, D. (2013). A general model for continuous noninvasive pulmonary artery pressure estimation. *Computers in Biology and Medicine*, *43*(7), 904–913. PMID:23746733

Smith, R. P., Argod, J., Ppin, J.-L., & Lvy, P. A. (1999). Pulse transit time: An appraisal of potential clinical applications. *Thorax*, *54*(5), 452–457. PMID:10212114

Sola, J., Chetelat, O., Sartori, C., Allemann, Y., & Rimoldi, S. (2011). Chest pulse-wave velocity: A novel approach to assess arterial stiffness. Biomedical Engineering. *IEEE Transactions on*, *58*(1), 215–223.

Sola, J., Proenc¸a, M., Ferrario, D., Porchet, J.-A., Falhi, A., Grossenbacher, O., & Sartori, C. et al. (2013). Noninvasive and nonocclusive blood pressure estimation via a chest sensor. Biomedical Engineering. *IEEE Transactions on*, *60*(12), 3505–3513.

Sola, J., Vetter, R., Renevey, P., Chatelat, O., Sartori, C., & Rimoldi, S. F. (2009). Parametric estimation of pulse arrival time: A robust approach to pulse wave velocity. *Physiological Measurement*, *30*(7), 603. PMID:19491457

SoteraWireless (2015). *Visi mobile*. Author.

Spulak, D., Cmejla, R., & Fabian, V. (2011). Parameters for mean blood pressure estimation based on electrocardiography and photoplethysmography. In *Applied Electronics (AE), 2011 International Conference on*.

Sullivan, M. J., & Knight, J. D., & Cobb, F. R. (1989). Relation between central and peripheral hemodynamics during exercise in patients with chronic heart failure. muscle blood flow is reduced with maintenance of arterial perfusion pressure. *Circulation*, *80*, 769–781. PMID:2791242

Suzuki, S., & Oguri, K. (2008). Cuffless and non-invasive systolic blood pressure estimation for aged class by using a photoplethysmograph. In *Engineering in Medicine and Biology Society, 2008. EMBS 2008. 30th Annual International Conference of the IEEE*.

Suzuki, S., & Oguri, K. (2009). Cuffless blood pressure estimation by error-correcting output coding method based on an aggregation of adaboost with a photoplethysmograph sensor. In *Engineering in Medicine and Biology Society, 2009. EMBC 2009. Annual International Conference of the IEEE*.

Tavel, M. E. (2006). Cardiac auscultation: A glorious pastand it does have a future! *Circulation*, *113*(9), 1255–1259. PMID:16520426

Teng, X. F., & Zhang, Y. T. (2003). Continuous and noninvasive estimation of arterial blood pressure using a photoplethysmographic approach. In *Engineering in Medicine and Biology Society, 2003.Proceedings of the 25th Annual International Conference of the IEEE*.

Testani, J. M., Sutton, M. G. S. J., Wiegers, S. E., Khera, A. V., Shannon, R. P., & Kirkpatrick, J. N. (2010). Accuracy of noninvasively determined pulmonary artery systolic pressure. *The American Journal of Cardiology*, *105*(8), 1192–1197. PMID:20381676

Tranulis, C., Durand, L., Senhadji, L., & Pibarot, P. (2002). Estimation of pulmonary arterial pressure by a neural network analysis using features based on time-frequency representations of the second heart sound. *Medical & Biological Engineering & Computing*, *40*(2), 205–212. PMID:12043802

Visvanathan, A., Sinha, A., & Pal, A. (2013). Estimation of blood pressure levels from reflective photoplethysmograph using smart phones. In *Bioinformatics and Bioengineering (BIBE), 2013 IEEE 13th International Conference on*.

Wagner, D., Roesch, N., Harpes, P., Krtke, H., Plumer, P., Saberin, A., & Bhm, M. et al. (2010). Relationship between pulse transit time and blood pressure is impaired in patients with chronic heart failure. *Clinical Research in Cardiology; Official Journal of the German Cardiac Society*, *99*(10), 657–664. PMID:20473677

Webster, J. G. (Ed.). (2006). *Encyclopedia of Medical Devices and Instrumentation* (2nd ed.). Wiley-Interscience.

Wibmer, T., Doering, K., Kropf-Sanchen, C., Rdiger, S., Blanta, I., Stoiber, K., & Schumann, C. et al. (2014). Pulse transit time and blood pressure during cardiopulmonary exercise tests. *Physiological Research, 63*(3), 287–296. PMID:24564606

Wong, M., Zhang, X., & Zhang, Y. (2006). The cuffless arterial blood pressure estimation based on the timing- characteristics of second heart sound. In *Engineering in Medicine and Biology Society, 2006. EMBS '06. 28th Annual International Conference of the IEEE.*

Wong, Y., & Zhang, Y. (2005). The effects of exercises on the relationship between pulse transit time and arterial blood pressure. In *Engineering in Medicine and Biology Society, 2005. IEEE-EMBS 2005. 27th Annual International Conference of the.*

Xu, J., Durand, L.-G., & Pibarot, P. (2001). Extraction of the aortic and pulmonary components of the second heart sound using a nonlinear transient chirp signal model. Biomedical Engineering. *IEEE Transactions on*, *48*(3), 277–283.

Xu, J., Durand, L.-G., & Pibarot, P. (2002). A new, simple, and accurate method for non-invasive estimation of pulmonary arterial pressure. *Heart (British Cardiac Society)*, *88*, 76–80. PMID:12067952

Yoon, Y., Cho, J., & Yoon, G. (2009). Non-constrained blood pressure monitoring using ecg and ppg for personal healthcare. *Journal of Medical Systems*, *33*(4), 261–266. PMID:19697692

Zhang, G., Gao, M., Xu, D., Olivier, N. B., & Mukkamala, R. (2011). Pulse arrival time is not an adequate surrogate for pulse transit time as a marker of blood pressure. *Journal of Applied Physiology*, *111*(6), 1681–1686. PMID:21960657

Zhang, X.-Y., MacPherson, E., & Zhang, Y.-T. (2008). Relations between the timing of the second heart sound and aortic blood pressure. Biomedical Engineering. *IEEE Transactions on*, *55*(4), 1291–1297.

Zhang, X.-Y., & Zhang, Y.-T. (2006). A model-based study of relationship between timing of second heart sound and systolic blood pressure. In *Engineering in Medicine and Biology Society, 2006. EMBS '06. 28th Annual International Conference of the IEEE.*

Zheng, Y.-L., Ding, X.-R., Poon, C., Lo, B., Zhang, H., Zhou, X.-L., & Zhang, Y.-T. et al. (2014). Unobtrusive sensing and wearable devices for health informatics. Biomedical Engineering. *IEEE Transactions on*, *61*(5), 1538–1554.

Zheng, Y.-L., Yan, B., Zhang, Y.-T., & Poon, C. (2014b). An armband wearable device for overnight and cuffless blood pressure measurement. Biomedical Engineering. *IEEE Transactions on*, *61*(7), 2179–2186.

ADDITIONAL READING

Castro, A., Mattos, S. S., & Coimbra, M. T. (2014, August). Noninvasive blood pressure and the second heart sound analysis. In Engineering in Medicine and Biology Society (EMBC), 2014 36th Annual International Conference of the IEEE (pp. 5494-5497). IEEE.

MacMahon, S., Peto, R., Collins, R., Godwin, J., Cutler, J., Sorlie, P., & Stamler, J. et al. (1990). Blood pressure, stroke, and coronary heart disease: part 1, prolonged differences in blood pressure: prospective observational studies corrected for the regression dilution bias. *Lancet*, *335*(8692), 765–774. PMID:1969518

Nkomo, V. T., Gardin, J. M., Skelton, T. N., Gottdiener, J. S., Scott, C. G., & Enriquez-Sarano, M. (2006). Burden of valvular heart diseases: A population-based study. *Lancet*, *368*(9540), 1005–1011. PMID:16980116

Parati, G., Stergiou, G. S., Asmar, R., Bilo, G., de Leeuw, P., & Imai, Y. et al. & ESH Working Group on Blood Pressure Monitoring. (2008). European Society of Hypertension guidelines for blood pressure monitoring at home: A summary report of the Second International Consensus Conference on Home Blood Pressure Monitoring. *Journal of Hypertension*, *26*(8), 1505–1526. PMID:18622223

Pedrosa, J., Castro, A., & Vinhoza, T. T. (2014, August). Automatic heart sound segmentation and murmur detection in pediatric phonocardiograms. In Engineering in Medicine and Biology Society (EMBC), 2014 36th Annual International Conference of the IEEE (pp. 2294-2297). IEEE.

Sörnmo, L., & Laguna, P. (2005). *Bioelectrical signal processing in cardiac and neurological applications*. Academic Press.

World Health Organization; International Society of Hypertension Writing Group. (2003). 2003 World Health Organization (WHO)/International Society of Hypertension (ISH) statement on management of hypertension. *Journal of Hypertension*, *21*(11), 1983–1992. PMID:14597836

KEY TERMS AND DEFINITIONS

Blood Pressure: Representation of the blood pressure wave within the circulation system. Usually two circulations are considered: right ventricle directs deoxygenated blood to the lungs for gas exchange (pulmonary circulation), and the left ventricle pumps oxygenated blood from the lungs to all body parts for nutrient and oxygen intake (systemic circulation).

Electrocardiogram: The register of the heart electrical activity measured on the body surface. It depicts the electrical activity of the heart, containing information on the timing of sinoatrial and atrioventricular nodes' activation, conduction properties, and tissue viability.

Phonocardiogram: The heart electrical activation results in mechanical processes, which are audible and can be registered using a stethoscope. The register of the heart sound is called a phonocardiogram. The first heart sound results of the closure of the mitral and tricuspid valves closure, and the second heart sound results from the closure of the aortic and pulmonary valves.

Photoplethysmogram: The register of the blood pulse wave; it may be observed as the blood volume changes detected by infrared light absorption through the tissue, for example.

Pre-Ejection Period: Time interval between the beginning of the ventricles' electrical stimulation, to the opening of the aortic valve and blood ejection.

Pulse Arrival Time: The time between electrical activation and pulse onset on the periphery. The definition varies between studies, and it encompasses the pre-ejection period and the pulse transit time.

Pulse Transit Time: The time span between the blood ejection through the aortic valve and its arrival at a peripheral site.

Vascular Transit Time: The definition of vascular transit time is slightly different from the pulse arrival time since instead of beginning temporal interval at the onset of the heart electrical activity, the first heart sound is used instead (closure of the AV valves). The first heart sound may be seen as an approximation of the moment of aortic valve opening although it is not accurate.

Chapter 3
Non-Linear Analysis of Heart Rate Variability and ECG Signal Features of Swimmers from NIT-Rourkela: A Case Study

Anupama Ray
Indian Institute of Technology Delhi, India

Biswajeet Champaty
National Institute of Technology Rourkela, India

Suraj Kumar Nayak
National Institute of Technology Rourkela, India

D. N. Tibarewala
Jadavpur University, India

Kunal Pal
National Institute of Technology Rourkela, India

ABSTRACT

The current study deals with the investigation of the effect of long-term endurance training on the autonomic nervous system of healthy adults. ECG was recorded for 5 min under resting condition in a sitting position using an ECG acquisition device for 25 swimmers and 25 age-matched sedentary controls. Heart Rate Variability (HRV) parameters of the volunteers were used for statistical analysis and classification using binary classification trees and artificial neural networks. The LF/HF ratio for swimmers and sedentary controls was found to be 0.89 ± 0.32 and 0.94 ± 0.46, respectively. This may be attributed to the vagal dominance due to endurance training in the swimmers. Statistical ECG signal processing and db06 wavelet based processing were performed to understand the effect of swimming on the cardiac health. The signal classification results indicated that both the HRV and the processed ECG signal features may be used for the classification of the swimmers and the sedentary controls using CART, Boosted tree, Random Forest and neural network algorithms.

DOI: 10.4018/978-1-5225-0660-7.ch003

INTRODUCTION

Recent advances in the biosignal processing techniques allow relating the activity of the autonomic nervous system (ANS) with the cardiovascular mortality, diabetic neuropathy, myocardial infarction and congestive heart failure (Maestri, et al., 2007). Though the efficiency of the ANS may be predicted by performing various biochemical (Richards, et al., 1999), cardiovascular reflex and scintigraphic tests, analysis of ANS activity from the electrocardiogram (ECG)-based non-invasive tests, viz. heart rate variability (HRV), baro-reflex sensitivity, QT interval and heart rate turbulence, are being studied extensively (Katona, McLean, Dighton, & Guz, 1982). Amongst the ECG-based non-invasive tests, the analysis of the HRV is the simplest method to study the sympathovagal balance (Sztajzel, 2004). Continuous HRV monitoring and analysis of the patients may allow the early detection of the above-mentioned diseases, which in turn, help in preventing significant pathophysiological alterations in the patients (Aliberti, et al., 2013).

Athletes have been found to have sinus bradycardia, which may be attributed to the increase in the efficiency of their heart to pump more blood (Ho, Brotherton, Lewis, & Uzunyan, 2014). This helps the sports-persons (e.g. athletes and swimmers) to adapt their body to lack of oxygen during physical strains (Brosnan, et al., 2014). This adaptability of the body have been related to the vagal predominance of the ANS and better synchronization amongst the functioning of the circulatory and the respiratory organs (Aubert, et al., 1996; Baselli, et al.). In the present study, an attempt was made to study the suitability of the parameters obtained from HRV analysis for classifying swimmers from that of sedentary persons. Few studies have been conducted on the effect of the intensive swimming training in prepubertal swimmers (Vinet, Beck, Nottin, & Obert, 2005), training performance enhancement (Atlaoui, et al., 2007) and variation in performance at different altitudes (Schmitt, et al., 2006). The conclusions derived from these studies could not be generalized because the number of subjects in these studies was less. The present study, therefore, aims to compare the effect of swimming on the HRV and its relationship with ANS in long-term trained swimmers with age-matched sedentary controls.

The calculated HRV features were preliminarily screened using t-test, which analyses the variation in the means of different groups. It is considered as a linear classifier. The significantly different features were identified. Subsequently, Classification and Regression Tree (CART), Boosted Tree (BT) and Random Forest (RF) were used to figure out the importance of each feature during classification. Most of the features used in this study were not normally distributed. In other words, the features had high degrees of variances and were dependent on each other. Such data cannot be classified using traditional statistical classifiers but can be handled by CART (Lewis, 2000). The efficiency of the BT classifier is higher as compared to CART classifier. This may be attributed to the fact that BT classifier prevents the over-fitting of data, thereby, increasing the accuracy of the classifier (Lewicki & Hill, 2006). RF classifier has shown better performance as compared to CART and BT classifiers. It uses a series of decision trees which helps improving the classification efficiency (Rodriguez-Galiano, Ghimire, Rogan, Chica-Olmo, & Rigol-Sanchez, 2012). The important features obtained from the above classifiers were used for further classifications using Artificial Neural Networks (ANN). ANN has been extensively used in medical industry for pattern recognition problems (Cortes & Vapnik, 1995). In addition to this, attempts were also made to analyze the ECG signal using statistical parameters in the time and wavelet domains (Adochiei & David, 2012). Wavelet-based signal decomposition and reconstruction of the signals help in effective removal of the noise without any distortion of the original signal (Singh & Tiwari, 2006). Daubechies 6 (db06) has been selected as the analysis wavelet because of its similarity in terms of shape with the QRS complex of ECG (Mahmoodabadi, Ahmadian, Abolhasani, Eslami, & Bidgoli, 2006). The energy spectrum of db06 lies around the low frequencies and its scaling function is similar to that of the QRS complex (Paul, 2002). Multiresolution wavelet analysis was used in this study because it builds a set of linear phase band-pass filters that help in noise suppression and has been used extensively in ECG signal processing (Meste, Rix, Jané, & Caminal, 1991). The time domain and wavelet domain statistical features obtained from the non-stationary ECG signals were subsequently studied for probable classification using CART, BT, RF and ANN (Ghosh, Midya, Koley, & Purkait, 2005; Moavenian & Khorrami, 2010).

BACKGROUND

Incorporation of physical exercise in the lifestyle of a person has been given an emphasis across the globe in recent years. This is due to the health benefits accrued by doing physical exercises. Hence, various researchers are studying the effect of different modalities of exercise and the health benefits associated with it (Sawane & Gupta, 2015; Shimamoto, Adachi, Takahashi, & Tanaka, 1998). Swimming has evolved as one of the most popular physical exercises not only in the developed countries but also in the developing countries (Vaz de Almeida, et al., 1999). It differs from other modalities of exercise in many ways. Some of them include the posture of the human being and involvement of both upper and lower parts of the body. Since swimming involves immersion of the body under water, it helps regulating the body temperature. Chase *et al.* (2008) revealed many health benefits of swimming (Chase, Sui, & Blair, 2008). Swimming has been reported not only in preventing but also in treating various diseases (e.g. cardiovascular diseases and respiratory diseases like asthma) (Nualnim, et al., 2012; Rosimini, 2003). Valentine *et al.* (2001) reported that swimming has been associated with improved mental health (better than singing) (Valentine & Evans, 2001). These advantages have motivated the researchers to investigate the effect swimming on various physiological activities (e.g. metabolic, cardiovascular and endocrinological) of the body. In earlier days, the research on exercise physiology was mainly focused on the mechanisms of muscle fatigue. However, the current-day research pays attention on the analysis of the nervous system as it is reported that the nervous system has a great influence on the exercise physiology (Okano, et al., 2013).

MAIN FOCUS OF THE CHAPTER

The main focus of this study is to understand the effect of long-term swimming on the ANS and the cardiac health of healthy volunteers. In order to achieve this goal, ECG was recorded from swimmers and age-matched sedentary volunteers. HRV analysis, time domain signal processing and wavelet-based signal processing of the ECG signals were carried out. The features obtained from the above analyses were used for probable non-linear classification using ANN.

VOLUNTEERS AND METHODS

Volunteers

Student volunteers studying at National Institute of Technology, Rourkela, India were invited for the study. The volunteers were asked to fill up a questionnaire. Out of a pool of 74 volunteers, 50 volunteers (25 swimmers and 25 age-matched sedentary controls), having a mean age of 21.3 ± 3 years, were chosen for the study. Smokers and alcoholics were excluded from the study. Since there were not sufficient number of girl volunteers, who were regular in swimming, girls were excluded from the control group.

Data Acquisition

ECG data acquisition device (working in the Lead-I configuration) was used for recording the ECG of the volunteers in sitting position for a period of 5 min (Ambrosio, Guevara, Silva, Heredia, & Moreno, 2014). The ECG signals were stored as LabVIEW measurement (LVM) file for further analysis. The ECG was recorded at same hour of the day. The recordings were done before swimming to avoid any physiological variations.

HRV Analysis

Biomedical start-up kit (v 3.0) developed by National Instruments, USA was used to calculate the RR intervals (Pan & Tompkins, 1985). The HRV parameters, viz. mean heart rate (HR), mean RR, mean NN, standard deviation of RR intervals (SDNN), root mean square of successive difference (RMSSD), number of NN intervals that differ more than 50 ms (NN50), percentage of number of successive NN intervals differing more than 50 ms (pNN50), triangular interpolation of NN intervals (TINN) and the standard deviation of the points perpendicular to the line of identity (SD1) and the standard deviation of the points along the line of identity (SD2) of Poincare plot, were calculated using the software (Zhang, de Peuter, Kamphuisen, & Karemaker, 2013). The HRV features were statistically analyzed using trial version of STATISTICA software (Statsoft Inc., Hamburg, Germany) to understand whether there is a definite pattern of HRV features which can segregate the swimmers from the sedentary group. The features were initially analyzed using t-test. The non-linear statistical analysis was done using CART, BT and RF algorithms, which gave an indication about the important HRV features. The important features, obtained by the linear and non-linear statistical analysis, were fed into ANN algorithms for probable classification. 80% of the data has been used for training while the rest 20% was used for testing (Azuaje, et al., 1997; Güler & Koçer, 2005; Vu & Park, 2010; Yang, 2004). A flowchart showing working methodology of HRV analysis is shown in Figure 1.

ECG Analysis

ECG signal analysis was done using 5 sec ECG recording extracted from the raw data. The various statistical features, viz. mean, mode, summation, standard deviation (SD), kurtosis and log energy entropy (LEE), of the time domain ECG signals were calculated. Also, the ECG signal was decomposed into 8 levels using db06 wavelet of Multi-resolution analysis. The signal was reconstructed using the combination of d7 and d8 coefficients and was then used for the extraction of the features. The extracted features,

Figure 1. Flowchart of HRV feature classification

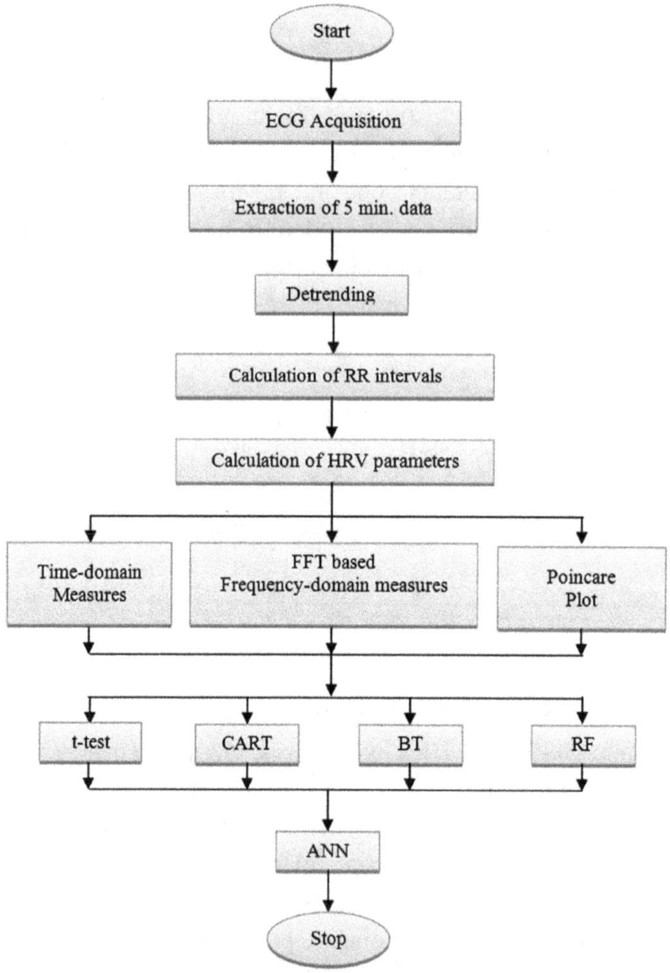

both from the time domain ECG signal and the wavelet reconstructed ECG signal, were used for the linear (t-test) and the non-linear (CART, BT and RF) classifications. The important features obtained from these classifiers were then used for pattern matching using ANN. A detailed flowchart showing the various steps towards ECG analysis is shown in Figure 2.

RESULTS

HRV Analysis

The heart rates of the control and the swimmer groups were found to be statistically insignificant. The RRTI, pNN50 and TINN features were found to be significantly different (Table 1). These features were lower in swimmers. RRTI is regarded as triangular index, whereas TINN is regarded as the triangular interpolation of the NN interval histogram. These features are obtained from the histogram plotted amongst

Figure 2. Flowchart of ECG signal feature classification

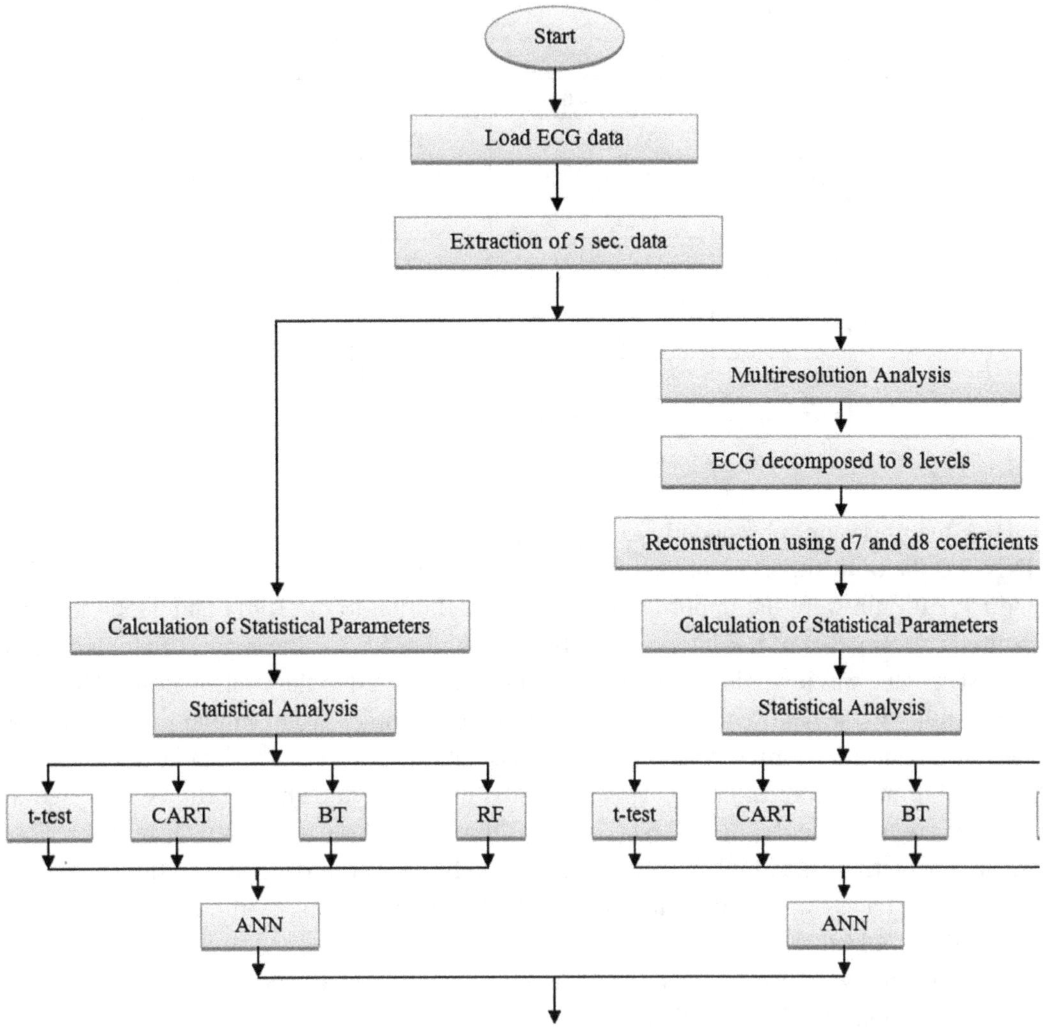

the length of the RR interval (X-axis) and the frequency of occurrence of the RR interval (Y-axis). RRTI is calculated by dividing the number of RR intervals used for the determination of the histogram by the RR interval value which has predominantly appeared during the HRV analysis (de Carvalho, et al., 2011). The TINN feature is calculated from the base of the above mentioned histogram. These features (RRTI and TINN) provide information about the overall RR-interval variability (de Abreu, et al., 2014). From the results, it was observed that RRTI and TINN were much lower in swimmer group as compared to the control (sedentary group). This can be explained by the fact that the adaptability under low oxygen condition (during physical activities) is better in swimmers due to the vagal dominance. Like RRTI and TINN features, pNN50 was also found to be lower in swimmers. Previous reports suggest that pNN50 (number of the RR-interval differences of successive RR-intervals greater than 50 msec divided by the total number of RR intervals) is inversely related to the parasympathetic dominance (Finkelstein, 2014). In the swimmers, it is interesting to note that all the statistically significant features (TINN, RRTI and pNN50) are time domain features. No frequency domain features were found to be statistically different.

Table 1. Important predictors from HRV features

Classifiers	HRV Features	Mean ± SD		p-Value	Predictor Importance
		Group-C	Group-S		
t-test	RRTI	12.39±4.03	8.61±3.60	0.001039	--
	pNN50	35.88±21.59	17.55±14.45	0.000939	--
	TINN	192.29±67.21	128.23±57.99	0.000734	--
CART	TINN	192.29±67.21	128.23±57.99	--	1.00
BT	RRTI	12.39±4.03	8.61±3.60	--	0.97
	TINN	192.29±67.21	128.23±57.99	--	0.99
	SD2	90.50±43.18	67.70±52.62	--	1.00
	LF/HF ratio	0.94±0.46	0.88±0.31	--	0.97
RF	LF Power	1206.36±954.56	1762.62±4210.68	--	1.00

The HRV features were subsequently analyzed using CART, BT and RF. The CART analysis showed that TINN was the only important predictor. BT classifier suggested that SD2 (obtained from Poincare plot) and LF/HF ratio were the important predictors in addition to the RRTI and TINN features. The SD2 feature is also marker of RR interval variability. A higher SD2 value suggests a higher variability. The mean SD2 value was lower in the swimmer group as compared to the control group. This suggested that the variability in the heart rate was much lower in the swimmer group similar results also observed form the significant time domain features. The LF/HF ratio (a marker of sympathovagal activity) was found to be high in the control group. This suggested that the sympathetic activity was predominant in the control group (since the LF/HF ratio was less than 1.3) (Arai, et al., 2011). In other words, the parasympathetic activity was higher in swimmers. The LF power was greater in the swimmer group indicating that the parasympathetic dominance was higher in this group (swimmers) (Rahman, Pechnik, Gross, Sewell, & Goldstein, 2011).

The above features were used in various combinations as categorical inputs to ANN. The t-test showed that RRTI, TINN and pNN50 were significantly different from each other. A classification efficiency of 96% was obtained when all the three features were used as the categorical inputs for MLP network. The properties of the MLP network have been given in Table 2 and the confusion matrix for the classification has been shown in Table 3.

On the contrary, when the same features were used as the categorical inputs for the RBF network, a classification efficiency of 100% was achieved. The properties of the RBF algorithm have been tabulated in Table 4 and the corresponding confusion matrix has been shown in Table 5.

The non-linear classifiers suggested that the important features were TINN, RRTI, SD2, LF/HF ratio and LF power. These features were used in various combinations as input for ANN networks. It was

Table 2. Properties of the MLP 3-21-2 network

Features	Network	Classification Efficiency	Training Algorithm	Error Function	Hidden Activation	Output Activation
RRTI, pNN50, TINN	MLP 3-21-2	96.00	BFGS 67	Entropy	Exponential	Softmax

Table 3. Confusion matrix of the MLP 3-21-2 network

	Group-C	Group-S	Overall
Total	25.00	25.00	50.00
Correct	24.00	24.00	48.00
Incorrect	1.00	1.00	2.00
Correct (%)	96.00	96.00	96.00
Incorrect (%)	4.00	4.00	4.00

Table 4. Properties of the RBF 3-22-2 network

Features	Network	Classification Efficiency	Training Algorithm	Error Function	Hidden Activation	Output Activation
RRTI, pNN50, TINN	RBF 3-22-2	100.00	RBFT	Entropy	Gaussian	Softmax

Table 5. Confusion matrix of the RBF 3-22-2 network

	Group-C	Group-S	Overall
Total	25.00	25.00	50.00
Correct	25.00	25.0000	50.00
Incorrect	0.00	0.00	0.00
Correct (%)	100.00	100.00	100.00
Incorrect (%)	0.00	0.00	0.00

Table 6. Properties of the MLP 3-30-2 network

Features	Network	Classification Efficiency	Training Algorithm	Error Function	Hidden Activation	Output Activation
SD2, L/H ratio, LF Power	MLP 3-30-2	86.00	BFGS 32	Entropy	Logistic	Softmax

found that the best classification efficiency was obtained when SD2, LF/HF power and LF power were used. Classification efficiencies of 86% and 94% were achieved using MLP and RBF algorithms. The properties and the confusion matrix for the MLP network have been tabulated in Tables 6 and 7. The properties and the confusion matrix for the RBF network have been tabulated in Tables 8 and 9.

Time-Domain Analysis of ECG Signal

Statistical features (e.g. AM, RMS, SD, variance, kurtosis, mode, median, summation and skewness) for the ECG signal of the volunteers were calculated using LabVIEW-2010 software and were tabulated in the worksheet of the STATISTICA software. None of the features were found to be significantly differ-

Table 7. Confusion matrix of the MLP 3-30-2 network

	Group-C	Group-S	Overall
Total	25.00	25.00	50.00
Correct	21.00	22.00	43.00
Incorrect	4.00	3.00	7.00
Correct (%)	84.00	88.00	86.00
Incorrect (%)	16.00	12.00	14.00

Table 8. Properties of the RBF 3-20-2 network

Features	Network	Classification Efficiency	Training Algorithm	Error Function	Hidden Activation	Output Activation
SD2, L/H ratio, LF Power	RBF 3-20-2	94.00	RBFT	Entropy	Gaussian	Softmax

Table 9. Confusion matrix of the RBF 3-20-2 network

	Group-C	Group-S	Overall
Total	25.00	25.00	50.00
Correct	24.00	23.00	47.00
Incorrect	1.00	2.00	3.00
Correct (%)	96.00	92.00	94.00
Incorrect (%)	4.00	8.00	6.00

Table 10. Important predictors from time domain features

Classifiers	Time Domain Features	Mean±SD		Predictor Importance
		Group-C	Group-S	
CART	kurtosis	6.97±4.25	9.148±4.69	1.00
BT	RMS	0.0059±0.0019	0.0061±0.0017	1.00
	SD	0.0056±0.0015	0.0059±0.0015	1.00
	Variance	0.00003±0.00002	0.00004±0.000018	1.00
RF	Median	-0.00164±0.00242	-0.0015±0.0017	1.00

ent. Subsequently, the features were classified and the important features were predicted using CART, BT and RF (Table 10).

CART analysis suggested that kurtosis was the only important predictor. The mean value of kurtosis was higher in the swimmer group. This indicated that there was a distinct peak near the mean, which repeats itself proving regularity of the HRV and, in turn, may allow the detection of the sharp R- peaks (Ghaffari, Homaeinezhad, Khazraee, & Daevaeiha, 2010). The BT classifier suggested that RMS, SD and variance were the important features. All the features were higher in swimmers. The analysis of the features using RF suggested that the median feature was the important predictor. It was also found to be higher in swimmers.

The use of all the above mentioned parameters (kurtosis, RMS, SD, variance, median) for the classification using ANN network showed that classification efficiencies of 88% and 100% were achieved when MLP and RBF algorithms were used, respectively. The properties and the confusion matrix for the MLP network have been tabulated in Tables 11 and 12. The properties and the confusion matrix for the RBF network have been tabulated in Tables 13 and 14.

Subsequently, the classification was tried using RMS, SD and variance as the categorical inputs. Similar to the previous trials, higher classification efficiency was achieved when RBF algorithm (94%)

Table 11. Properties of the MLP 5-35-2 network

Features	Network	Classification Efficiency	Training Algorithm	Error Function	Hidden Activation	Output Activation
Kurtosis, RMS, SD, variance, Median	MLP 5-35-2	88.00	BFGS 27	SOS	Tanh	Logistic

Table 12. Confusion matrix of the MLP 5-35-2 network

	Group-C	Group-S	Overall
Total	25.00	25.00	50.00
Correct	19.00	25.00	44.00
Incorrect	6.00	0.00	6.00
Correct (%)	76.00	100.00	88.00
Incorrect (%)	24.00	0.00	12.00

Table 13. Properties of the RBF 5-33-2 network

Features	Network	Classification Efficiency	Training Algorithm	Error Function	Hidden Activation	Output Activation
Kurtosis, RMS, SD, variance, Median	RBF 5-33-2	100.00	RBFT	Entropy	Gaussian	Softmax

Table 14. Confusion matrix of the RBF 5-33-2 network

	Group-C	Group-S	Overall
Total	25.00	25.00	50.00
Correct	25.000	25.00	50.00
Incorrect	0.00	0.00	0.00
Correct (%)	100.00	100.00	100.00
Incorrect (%)	0.00	0.00	0.00

Table 15. Properties of the MLP 3-35-2 network

Features	Network	Classification Efficiency	Training Algorithm	Error Function	Hidden Activation	Output Activation
RMS, SD, Variance	MLP 3-35-2	74.00	BFGS 71	SOS	Logistic	Logistic

Table 16. Confusion matrix of the MLP 3-35-2 network

	Group-C	Group-S	Overall
Total	25.00	25.00	50.00
Correct	16.00	21.00	37.00
Incorrect	9.00	4.00	13.00
Correct (%)	64.00	84.00	74.00
Incorrect (%)	36.00	16.00	26.00

Table 17. Properties of the RBF 5-33-2 network

Features	Network	Classification Efficiency	Training Algorithm	Error Function	Hidden Activation	Output Activation
Kurtosis, RMS, SD, variance, Median	RBF 5-33-2	94.00	RBFT	Entropy	Gaussian	Softmax

Table 18. Confusion matrix of the RBF 5-33-2 network

	Group-C	Group-S	Overall
Total	25.00	25.00	50.00
Correct	23.00	24.00	47.00
Incorrect	2.00	1.00	3.00
Correct (%)	92.00	96.00	94.00
Incorrect (%)	8.00	4.00	6.00

was used as compared to the MLP algorithm (74%). The properties and the confusion matrix for the MLP network have been tabulated in Tables 15 and 16. The properties and the confusion matrix for the RBF network have been tabulated in Tables 17 and 18.

Wavelet-Based Analysis of ECG Signals

The ECG signals of the volunteers were decomposed using Daubechies orthogonal wavelet db06 at d1 to d8 levels. The signal was reconstructed using a combination of d7 and d8 coefficients and was used for feature extraction (Figure 3). This is due to the fact that the reconstructed signal obtained by the combination of d7 and d8 coefficients matched best with normal patterns of ECG signal (Gavrovska, Jevtic, & Reljin, 2009; Rodriguez, Jane, & Brooks, 2000).

The various features (e.g. mean, mode, variance, standard deviation, summation, kurtosis and log energy entropy) of the reconstructed signal were calculated and analyzed using CART, BT, RF and ANN. Similar to the time-domain ECG signal analysis, no statistically significant features were found using t-test. Analysis of the features using CART, BT and RF suggested that median and RMS were the important predictors (Table 19). Both the features were used for classification using ANN. A classification efficiency of 76% was observed using MLP algorithm. Properties and confusion matrix of the MLP algorithm have been tabulated in Tables 20 and 21.

On the contrary, a classification efficiency of 98% was observed using RBF algorithm. The properties and the confusion matrix for the RBF network have been tabulated in Tables 22 and 23.

Figure 3. Wavelet decomposition and reconstruction of the ECG signal

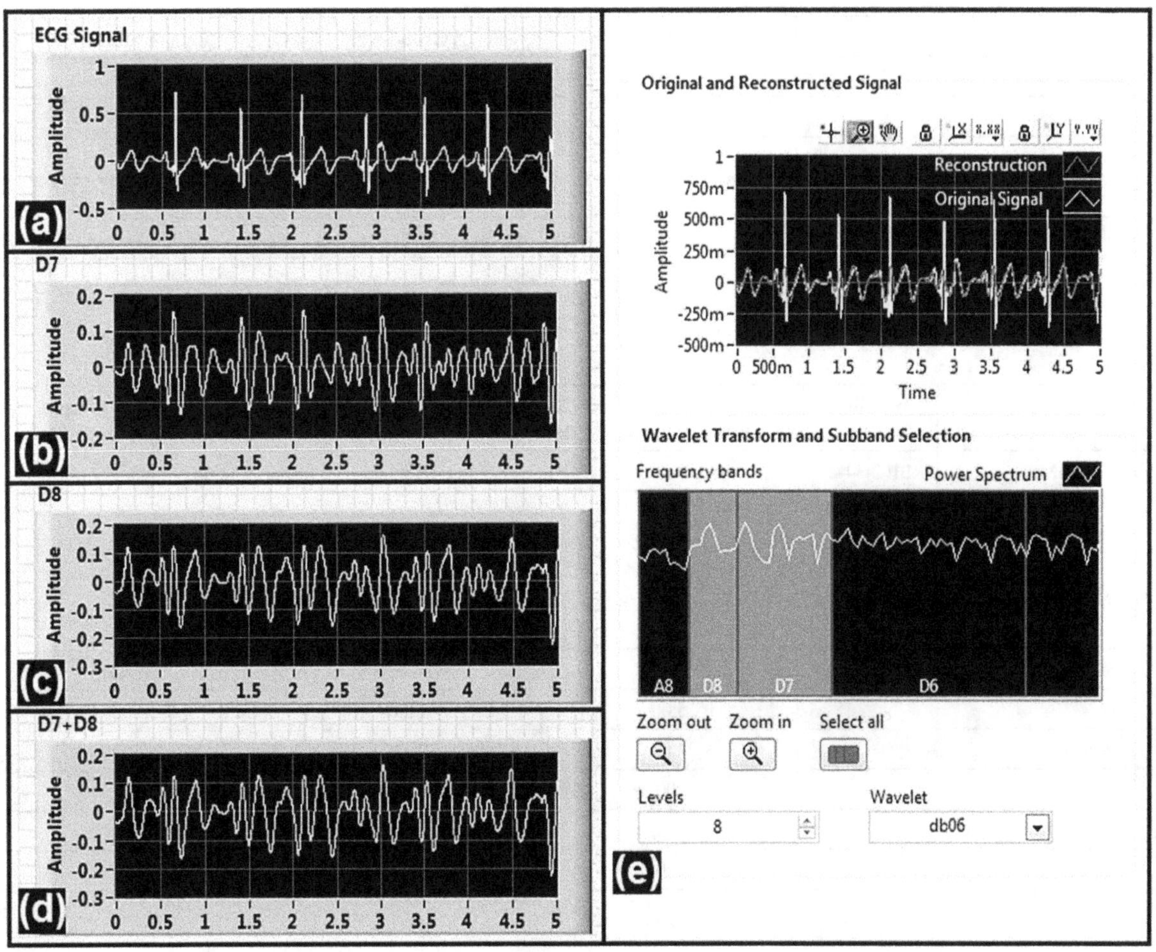

Table 19. Important predictors from time domain wavelet features

Classifiers	Wavelet Features	Mean±SD		Predictor Importance
		Group-C	Group-S	
CART	Median	-0.00004±0.000179	-0.00013±0.000219	1.00
BT	Median	-0.00004±0.000179	-0.00013±0.000219	1.00
RF	RMS	0.00299±0.000985	0.00332±0.000951	1.00

Table 20. Properties of the MLP 2-35-2 network

Features	Network	Classification Efficiency	Training Algorithm	Error Function	Hidden Activation	Output Activation
Median, RMS	MLP 2-35-2	76.00	BFGS 64	Entropy	Exponential	Softmax

Table 21. Confusion matrix of the MLP 2-35-2 network

	Group-C	Group-S	Overall
Total	25.00	25.00	50.00
Correct	22.00	16.00	38.00
Incorrect	3.00	9.00	12.00
Correct (%)	88.00	64.00	76.00
Incorrect (%)	12.00	36.00	24.00

Table 22. Properties of the RBF 2-34-2 network

Features	Network	Classification Efficiency	Training Algorithm	Error Function	Hidden Activation	Output Activation
Median, RMS	RBF 2-34-2	98.00	RBFT	Entropy	Gaussian	Softmax

Table 23. Confusion matrix of the RBF 2-34-2 network

	Group-C	Group-S	Overall
Total	25.00	25.00	50.00
Correct	24.00	25.00	49.00
Incorrect	1.00	0.00	1.00
Correct (%)	96.00	100.00	98.00
Incorrect (%)	4.00	0.00	2.00

DISCUSSION

The HRV features have often been related to the sympathetic and parasympathetic balance of the ANS. In this study, pNN50, RRTI and TINN were found to be the statistically significant predictors using t-test. RRTI and TINN have been found to provide information about the overall RR interval variability. pNN50 gives an indication of the variation in the short-term components in the HRV analysis. pNN50 provides information about the beat to beat variations, estimating the parasympathetic regulation of the heart (DeGiorgio, Miller, Meymandi, Chin, & Epps, 2010). The frequency domain HRV parameter, LF power, obtained from the FFT analysis was found to be an important feature for the prediction between the swimmer and the sedentary groups. In the study, we found that the pNN50 and the LF power of the swimmer group were higher as compared to the control group. This is in accordance to the general observation in the physically active and sedentary group individuals (Blásquez, Font, & Ortís, 2009). The higher mean value of HF power in comparison to LF power in swimmers (Table 1) and significant pNN50 prove a parasympathetic dominance over the sympathetic nervous system in the swimmer group (Aubert, Beckers, & Ramaekers, 2001; Shin, Minamitani, Onishi, Yamazaki, & Lee, 1993). The high frequency components of the HRV are associated with the parasympathetic control, whereas the low frequency components are associated with both sympathetic and parasympathetic nervous system (Winchell & Hoyt, 1996). The SD1 and SD2 features of the Poincare plot analysis indicate the short-term (due to respiratory sinus arrhythmia) and long-term variability of the heart rate, respectively (Guzik, et al., 2005; Niskanen, Tarvainen, Ranta-Aho, & Karjalainen, 2004). SD2 was significantly different in the sedentary control and the active groups. The results indicated that the short-term variability in the swimmer volunteers were lower as compared to the sedentary control volunteers. This may be accounted to the long-term endurance training of the swimmers.

The shape, size and the statistical features of the ECG and the HR give an indication about the cardiac health of an individual (Ceylan & Özbay, 2007). Amongst the statistical parameters obtained from time-domain analysis of the ECG, the most important features, as suggested by CART and BT algorithms for classification, were kurtosis, RMS, SD, variance and median. ANN classification of the features indicated that the best classification was achieved when all the features were used for pattern recognition. Wavelet-based ECG feature extraction was done using db06 wavelet. Daubechies family of wavelet was selected due to its symmetrical nature and less computational complexities (Gavrovska, et al., 2009). In the current study, a combination of d7 and d8 levels was used to reconstruct the ECG because the reconstructed signal was in close proximity of the conventional ECG. The use of Multi-resolution wavelet analysis enabled signal representation in both large scale (low frequency) and small scale (high frequency) components, which help in the study of the dynamic changes of the signal (Thakor, Gramatikov, & Mita, 1993).

CART, BT and RF algorithms have been used to find the important features for classification. In CART, the groups are split into binary trees where each node splits to form next binary tree until the groups are completely separated (Breiman, 1984). But it suffers from misclassification error, the only drawback of binary trees. Boosting is a numerical optimization technique which is known to reduce misclassification costs by adding a new tree at every step thereby reducing misclassification (Mease, Wyner, & Buja, 2007). Though binary tree classifiers are simple and easy to implement, ANN is preferred for classification over them. In the HRV study, the ANN classifier showed an accuracy of 100% when RBF algorithm was used. In the time-domain ECG signal analysis, the ANN classifier also showed an accuracy of 100% when RBF algorithm was used. On the other hand, in the wavelet-based ECG analysis the RBF-based ANN showed a predictability of 98%. ANN determines the optimal performance depending upon the trial and the error based training (Kim, et al., 2011). Thus, by repeated trials and recursive training, supervised learning ANN becomes a highly reliable classifier. ANN is a non-linear classifier in which the data distribution requires no particular requirements (Chen, Hsu, Chiu, & Rau, 2011). Apart from the above, ANN is fault tolerable provided the data set for learning is larger. The results of ANN prove that this technique of classification was highly accurate and may be used for classification of disease condition from the HRV or from ECG signal features. Amongst MLP and RBF models, higher accuracy has been consistently shown by RBF networks. MLP networks usually have more than one hidden layers and outputs of one unit are the inputs of the next layer. Each layer calculates the weighted sum of the inputs, adds the threshold weights and passes through the activation function of the particular layer and weights are calculated using back propagation algorithm (Ozyilmaz & Yildirim, 2003). RBF network consists of only one hidden layer and the neuron output is calculated using the basis function on the distance between the input vector and the neuron centre. The parameters of the RBF network are the position and inverse of width of basis function and weights of the output neurons. RBF networks need less computational speed during learning because of their localized neural connections (Park, Harley, & Venayagamoorthy, 2002). MLP converges very slowly thereby increasing the computational time without achieving high accuracy during learning as compared to the RBF networks (Er, Wu, Lu, & Toh, 2002). RBF networks have generally been used for pattern recognition where the size of the data set is small (Er, et al., 2002; Moody & Darken, 1989). This explains the higher accuracy of the RBF networks in comparison to MLP networks.

FUTURE RESEARCH DIRECTION

The current study was focused in analyzing the effect of long-term swimming on the activity of the ANS and cardiac conduction pathway of healthy individuals. Future research can be performed to investigate the effect of swimming on other physiological parameters like blood pressure, breathing, muscle toning, body weight, sleep and mental state. Studies can be performed to find out techniques of improving swimming performance for maximizing the performance in competitions. Comparative study of swimming with other modalities of exercise such as running and cycling can also be done to analyze the physiological activities in swimmers and persons doing other types of exercise.

CONCLUSION

HRV parameters were statistically analyzed to extract the features which may help classifying the state of the ANS of swimmer and sedentary groups. Classification trees and boosted classification trees were used for classification. The RF and BT classifiers were more accurate than the CART classifier. ANN was used to eliminate the misclassification introduced by the RF, BT and CART algorithms. In this study, the prediction accuracy of ANN was 100% when certain features were used. It can be also concluded from this study that the classification based upon HRV parameters were highly accurate and reliable than that of classification based on ECG analysis. Though the number of subjects in the study was low, yet promising results were obtained. There is a need for further study with a large number of volunteers to validate the results.

REFERENCES

Adochiei, N., & David, V. (2012). *QRS time detection using Wavelet Multiresolution Analysis for determining HRV in case of ECG signals with high level noise.* Paper presented at the Electrical and Power Engineering (EPE), 2012 International Conference and Exposition on. doi:10.1109/ICEPE.2012.6463866

Aliberti, S., Tobaldini, E., Nunziata, V., Suigo, G., Giuliani, F., & D'Adda, A. et al.. (2013). Cardiac autonomic alterations impact early and late outcomes in patients with community-acquired pneumonia. *The European Respiratory Journal*, *42*(Suppl 57), 2765.

Ambrosio, R., Guevara, C., Silva, C., Heredia, A., & Moreno, M. (2014). *Electrical characterization of textile electrodes for an ECG acquisition system.* Paper presented at the Electrical Engineering, Computing Science and Automatic Control (CCE), 2014 11th International Conference on. doi:10.1109/ICEEE.2014.6978306

Arai, Y.-C. P., Ushida, T., Matsubara, T., Shimo, K., Ito, H., & Sato, Y. (2011). The influence of acupressure at extra 1 acupuncture point on the spectral entropy of the EEG and the LF/HF ratio of heart rate variability. *Evidence-Based Complementary and Alternative Medicine.* PMID:18955366

Atlaoui, D., Pichot, V., Lacoste, L., Barale, F., Lacour, J., & Chatard, J. (2007). Heart rate variability, training variation and performance in elite swimmers. *International Journal of Sports Medicine*, *28*(5), 394–400. doi:10.1055/s-2006-924490 PMID:17111320

Aubert, A., Beckers, F., & Ramaekers, D. (2001). Autonomic Cardiac Control in Athletes and Non-Athletes at Rest. *Progress in Biomedical Research*, *6*, 318–321.

Aubert, A., Ramaekers, D., Cuche, Y., Lysens, R., Ector, H., & Van de Werf, F. (1996). *Effect of long term physical training on heart rate variability.* Academic Press.

Azuaje, F., Dubitzky, W., Wu, X., Lopes, P., Black, N., Adamson, K., et al. (1997). *A neural network approach to coronary heart disease risk assessment based on short-term measurement of RR intervals.* Academic Press.

Baselli, G., Cerutti, S., Interdonato, T., Orizio, C., Perini, R., & Veicsteinas, A. (n.d.). *HRV during exercise in sedentary subjects and athletes.* Academic Press.

Blásquez, J. C. C., Font, G. R., & Ortís, L. C. (2009). Heart-rate variability and precompetitive anxiety in swimmers. *Psicothema*, (4): 531–536. PMID:19861094

Breiman, L. (1984). *Classification and regression trees.* Chapman & Hall/CRC.

Brosnan, M., La Gerche, A., Kalman, J., Lo, W., Fallon, K., MacIsaac, A., & Prior, D. L. (2014). Comparison of frequency of significant electrocardiographic abnormalities in endurance versus nonendurance athletes. *The American Journal of Cardiology*, *113*(9), 1567–1573. doi:10.1016/j.amjcard.2014.01.438 PMID:24641963

Ceylan, R., & Özbay, Y. (2007). Comparison of FCM, PCA and WT techniques for classification ECG arrhythmias using artificial neural network. *Expert Systems with Applications*, *33*(2), 286–295. doi:10.1016/j.eswa.2006.05.014

Chase, N. L., Sui, X., & Blair, S. N. (2008). Swimming and all-cause mortality risk compared with running, walking, and sedentary habits in men. *International Journal of Aquatic Research and Education*, *2*(3), 213–223.

Chen, C. M., Hsu, C. Y., Chiu, H. W., & Rau, H. H. (2011). *Prediction of survival in patients with liver cancer using artificial neural networks and classification and regression trees*. Academic Press.

Cortes, C., & Vapnik, V. (1995). Support-vector networks. *Machine Learning*, *20*(3), 273–297. doi:10.1007/BF00994018

de Abreu, L. C., Roque, A. L., de Castro, B. C., de Souza, A. C. A., Vanderlei, L. C. M., Ferreira, L. L., et al. (2014). *Responses of the geometric indices of heart rate variability to the active orthostatic test in women*. Academic Press.

de Carvalho, T. D., Pastre, C. M., Rossi, R. C., de Abreu, L., Valenti, V., & Vanderlei, L. M. (2011). Geometric index of heart rate variability in chronic obstructive pulmonary disease. *Revista Portuguesa de Pneumologia*, *17*(6), 260–265. doi:10.1016/j.rppnen.2011.10.001 PMID:21920699

DeGiorgio, C. M., Miller, P., Meymandi, S., Chin, A., Epps, J., Gordon, S., & Harper, R. M. et al. (2010). RMSSD, a measure of vagus-mediated heart rate variability, is associated with risk factors for SUDEP: The SUDEP-7 Inventory. *Epilepsy & Behavior*, *19*(1), 78–81. doi:10.1016/j.yebeh.2010.06.011 PMID:20667792

Er, M. J., Wu, S., Lu, J., & Toh, H. L. (2002). Face recognition with radial basis function (RBF) neural networks. *Neural Networks. IEEE Transactions on*, *13*(3), 697–710. PMID:18244466

Finkelstein, J. (2014). *Classification of cycling exercise status using short-term heart rate variability*. Paper presented at the Engineering in Medicine and Biology Society (EMBC), 2014 36th Annual International Conference of the IEEE.

Gavrovska, A. M., Jevtic, D. R., & Reljin, B. D. (2009). *Selection of wavelet decomposition levels in ECG filtering*. Academic Press.

Ghaffari, A., Homaeinezhad, M., Khazraee, M., & Daevaeiha, M. (2010). Segmentation of Holter ECG Waves Via Analysis of a Discrete Wavelet-Derived Multiple Skewness–Kurtosis Based Metric. *Annals of Biomedical Engineering*, *38*(4), 1497–1510. doi:10.1007/s10439-010-9919-3 PMID:20087769

Ghosh, D., Midya, B. L., Koley, C., & Purkait, P. (2005). *Wavelet aided SVM analysis of ECG signals for cardiac abnormality detection*. Academic Press.

Güler, N. F., & Koçer, S. (2005). Use of support vector machines and neural network in diagnosis of neuromuscular disorders. *Journal of Medical Systems*, *29*(3), 271–284. doi:10.1007/s10916-005-5187-4 PMID:16050082

Guzik, P., Piskorski, J., Krauze, T., Girguś, P., Wykrętowicz, A., & Wysocki, H. (2005). Numerical descriptors of Poincaré plots analysis of RR intervals are related to baroreflex sensitivity and hemodynamic parameters in healthy people. *Analysis, 1*(4), 8-9.

Ho, C. H., Brotherton, B. J., Lewis, K. E., & Uzunyan, M. Y. (2014). A High School Wrestler with Severe Bradycardia. *The Journal of Pediatrics, 165*(1), 202-202. e201.

Katona, P. G., McLean, M., Dighton, D. H., & Guz, A. (1982). Sympathetic and parasympathetic cardiac control in athletes and nonathletes at rest. *Journal of Applied Physiology*, *52*(6), 1652–1657. PMID:7107476

Kim, S. Y., Moon, S. K., Jung, D. C., Hwang, S. I., Sung, C. K., Cho, J. Y., & Lee, H. J. et al. (2011). Pre-Operative Prediction of Advanced Prostatic Cancer Using Clinical Decision Support Systems: Accuracy Comparison between Support Vector Machine and Artificial Neural Network. *Korean Journal of Radiology*, *12*(5), 588. doi:10.3348/kjr.2011.12.5.588 PMID:21927560

Lewicki, P., & Hill, T. (2006). *Statistics: methods and applications*. Tulsa, OK. Statsoft.

Lewis, R. J. (2000). *An introduction to classification and regression tree (CART) analysis*. Academic Press.

Maestri, R., Pinna, G. D., Accardo, A., Allegrini, P., Balocchi, R., D'Addio, G., & Cerutti, S. et al. (2007). Nonlinear indices of heart rate variability in chronic heart failure patients: Redundancy and comparative clinical value. *Journal of Cardiovascular Electrophysiology*, *18*(4), 425–433. doi:10.1111/j.1540-8167.2007.00728.x PMID:17284264

Mahmoodabadi, S., Ahmadian, A., Abolhasani, M., Eslami, M., & Bidgoli, J. (2006). *ECG feature extraction based on multiresolution wavelet transform*. Academic Press.

Mease, D., Wyner, A. J., & Buja, A. (2007). Boosted classification trees and class probability/quantile estimation. *Journal of Machine Learning Research*, *8*, 409–439.

Meste, O., Rix, H., Jané, R., & Caminal, P. (1991). Détection battement par battement de potentiels tardifs dans les electrocardiogrammes à haute amplification. *Innovation et technologie en biologie et médecine*, *12*(5), 517-531.

Moavenian, M., & Khorrami, H. (2010). A qualitative comparison of Artificial Neural Networks and Support Vector Machines in ECG arrhythmias classification. *Expert Systems with Applications*, *37*(4), 3088–3093. doi:10.1016/j.eswa.2009.09.021

Moody, J., & Darken, C. J. (1989). Fast learning in networks of locally-tuned processing units. *Neural Computation*, *1*(2), 281–294. doi:10.1162/neco.1989.1.2.281

Niskanen, J. P., Tarvainen, M. P., Ranta-Aho, P. O., & Karjalainen, P. A. (2004). Software for advanced HRV analysis. *Computer Methods and Programs in Biomedicine*, *76*(1), 73–81. doi:10.1016/j.cmpb.2004.03.004 PMID:15313543

Nualnim, N., Parkhurst, K., Dhindsa, M., Tarumi, T., Vavrek, J., & Tanaka, H. (2012). Effects of swimming training on blood pressure and vascular function in adults> 50 years of age. *The American Journal of Cardiology*, *109*(7), 1005–1010. doi:10.1016/j.amjcard.2011.11.029 PMID:22244035

Okano, A. H., Fontes, E. B., Montenegro, R. A., Farinatti, P. d. T. V., Cyrino, E. S., Li, L. M., et al. (2013). Brain stimulation modulates the autonomic nervous system, rating of perceived exertion and performance during maximal exercise. *British Journal of Sports Medicine*.

Ozyilmaz, L., & Yildirim, T. (2003). *Artificial neural networks for diagnosis of hepatitis disease*. Academic Press.

Pan, J., & Tompkins, W. J. (1985). A real-time QRS detection algorithm. *Biomedical Engineering, IEEE Transactions on,* (3), 230-236.

Park, J. W., Harley, R., & Venayagamoorthy, G. (2002). *Comparison of MLP and RBF neural networks using deviation signals for on-line identification of a synchronous generator*. Academic Press.

Paul, S. (2002). Addison, The illustrated wavelet transform handbook. *Institute of Physics, 1*, 117–154.

Rahman, F., Pechnik, S., Gross, D., Sewell, L., & Goldstein, D. S. (2011). Low frequency power of heart rate variability reflects baroreflex function, not cardiac sympathetic innervation. *Clinical Autonomic Research, 21*(3), 133–141. doi:10.1007/s10286-010-0098-y PMID:21279414

Richards, A., Nicholls, M., Yandle, T., Ikram, H., Espiner, E., Turner, J., & Smyth, D. W. et al. (1999). Neuroendocrine prediction of left ventricular function and heart failure after acute myocardial infarction. *Heart (British Cardiac Society), 81*(2), 114–120. doi:10.1136/hrt.81.2.114 PMID:9922344

Rodriguez, B., Jane, R., & Brooks, D. (2000). *Ventricular tachycardia risk detection using wavelet decomposition of the signal averaged ECG*. Academic Press.

Rodriguez-Galiano, V., Ghimire, B., Rogan, J., Chica-Olmo, M., & Rigol-Sanchez, J. (2012). An assessment of the effectiveness of a random forest classifier for land-cover classification. *ISPRS Journal of Photogrammetry and Remote Sensing, 67*, 93–104. doi:10.1016/j.isprsjprs.2011.11.002

Rosimini, C. (2003). Benefits of swim training for children and adolescents with asthma. *Journal of the American Academy of Nurse Practitioners, 15*(6), 247–252. doi:10.1111/j.1745-7599.2003.tb00394.x PMID:12861890

Sawane, M. V., & Gupta, S. S. (2015). Resting heart rate variability after yogic training and swimming: A prospective randomized comparative trial. *International Journal of Yoga, 8*(2), 96.

Schmitt, L., Hellard, P., Millet, G., Roels, B., Richalet, J., & Fouillot, J. (2006). Heart rate variability and performance at two different altitudes in well-trained swimmers. *International Journal of Sports Medicine, 27*(3), 226–231. doi:10.1055/s-2005-865647 PMID:16541379

Shimamoto, H., Adachi, Y., Takahashi, M., & Tanaka, K. (1998). Low impact aerobic dance as a useful exercise mode for reducing body mass in mildly obese middle-aged women. *Applied Human Science, 17*(3), 109–114. doi:10.2114/jpa.17.109 PMID:9682520

Shin, K., Minamitani, H., Onishi, S., Yamazaki, H., & Lee, M. (1993). *The power spectral analysis of heart rate variability in athletes during exercise*. Academic Press.

Singh, B. N., & Tiwari, A. K. (2006). Optimal selection of wavelet basis function applied to ECG signal denoising. *Digital Signal Processing, 16*(3), 275–287. doi:10.1016/j.dsp.2005.12.003

Sztajzel, J. (2004). Heart rate variability: A noninvasive electrocardiographic method to measure the autonomic nervous system. *Swiss Medical Weekly, 134*, 514–522. PMID:15517504

Thakor, N., Gramatikov, B., & Mita, M. (1993). *Multiresolution wavelet analysis of ECG during ischemia and reperfusion*. Academic Press.

Valentine, E., & Evans, C. (2001). The effects of solo singing, choral singing and swimming on mood and physiological indices. *The British Journal of Medical Psychology*, *74*(1), 115–120. doi:10.1348/000711201160849

Vaz de Almeida, M. D., Graça, P., Afonso, C., D'Amicis, A., Lappalainen, R., & Damkjaer, S. (1999). Physical activity levels and body weight in a nationally representative sample in the European Union. *Public Health Nutrition*, *2*(1a), 105–114. doi:10.1017/S1368980099000154 PMID:10933630

Vinet, A., Beck, L., Nottin, S., & Obert, P. (2005). Effect of intensive training on heart rate variability in prepubertal swimmers. *European Journal of Clinical Investigation*, *35*(10), 610–614. doi:10.1111/j.1365-2362.2005.01557.x PMID:16178879

Vu, T. H. N., & Park, N. (2010). *Heart rate variability pattern recognition in ambulatory environments*. Academic Press.

Winchell, R. J., & Hoyt, D. B. (1996). Spectral analysis of heart rate variability in the ICU: A measure of autonomic function. *The Journal of Surgical Research*, *63*(1), 11–16. doi:10.1006/jsre.1996.0214 PMID:8661164

Yang, Z. R. (2004). Biological applications of support vector machines. *Briefings in Bioinformatics*, *5*(4), 328–338. doi:10.1093/bib/5.4.328 PMID:15606969

Zhang, Y., de Peuter, O. R., Kamphuisen, P. W., & Karemaker, J. M. (2013). Search for HRV-parameters that detect a sympathetic shift in heart failure patients on β-blocker treatment. *Frontiers in Physiology, 4*.

KEY TERMS AND DEFINITIONS

Artificial Neural Network (ANN): An information processing model, inspired by the biological neural network, used for pattern classification, clustering, prediction, optimization and control.

Boosted Trees: Boosted trees are a class of decision trees which are used for both classification and regression problems. They generate a group of simple trees, each of which has a weak predictive accuracy. But the use of these simple trees in a rational manner significantly improves the predictive accuracy.

Classification and Regression Tree (CART): A decision-tree data mining algorithm used for data classification and regression analyses.

Electrocardiogram (ECG): The graphical representation of the electrical activity occurring within the heart is termed as ECG.

Heart Rate Variability (HRV): The variation in the time duration between consecutive heart beats is regarded as HRV.

Random Forest: Random Forest is a non-linear classification method that develops several decision trees. The algorithm uses randomly selected data and variables in order to improve the classification efficiency.

t-Test: A statistical method used to analyze the statistical significance of the means of two samples or groups. The statistical significance indicates whether the difference between the two means reflects a real difference between the populations from which the two groups were sampled.

Chapter 4

Parameter Estimation of Nonlinear Biomedical Systems Using Extended Kalman Filter Algorithm:
Development of Patient Specific Models

Kamalanand Krishnamurthy
Anna University, MIT Campus, India

ABSTRACT

Parameter estimation is a central issue in mathematical modelling of biomedical systems and for the development of patient specific models. The technique of estimating parameters helps in obtaining diagnostic information from computational models of biological systems. However, in most of the biomedical systems, the estimation of model parameters is a challenging task due to the nonlinearity of mathematical models. In this chapter, the method of estimation of nonlinear model parameters from measurements of state variables, using the extended Kalman filter, is extensively explained using an example of the three-dimensional model of the HIV/AIDS system.

INTRODUCTION

Mathematical modeling of complex biomedical systems is highly useful for analysis of the actual system under investigation. Mathematical modeling can improve our understanding of several diseases and is highly useful for diagnosis and prognosis of several diseases. In the context of modeling, doctors and engineers can work together to identify diseased states, for development of diagnostic tools and for devising proper treatment strategies (Kamalanand & Ramakrishnan, 2015).

In biology, mathematical models are often developed to mimic the physiological systems. For example, mathematical models of organs of the body such as the heart, lungs, pancreas etc, are highly useful for understanding and analyzing the normal and abnormal functionality of the organ under investigation

DOI: 10.4018/978-1-5225-0660-7.ch004

(Kamalanand & Srinivasan, 2011). Another class of biomedical models involves the modelling of cell growth and population growth of certain pathogens. These models are highly useful for analyzing the growth of cancer cells and for identification of suitable drugs for inhibiting harmful cell growth. Further, a class of models namely the predator-prey models has played an important role in modelling of biological processes. For example, the modelling of the interaction of certain pathogens with the human immune system and the modelling of co-infections (two of more infections simultaneously affecting an individual) fall under the class of predator-prey models. Such models have been proved to be highly useful for diagnosis of several infectious diseases (Mannar Jawahar & Kamalanand, 2013). Also, in recent years, the growth of computational models in the field of neurobiology has led to the improved understanding of brain functions and in development of systems based on artificial intelligence. For example, the models of biological processes developed using artificial intelligence approaches such as the artificial neural networks and support vector machines have several applications in diagnostics and pattern detection (Manickavasagam, Sutha, & Kamalanand, 2014).

The generation of a suitable mathematical model based on ordinary differential equations (ODE) or partial differential equations (PDE) is also useful for predicting the future states of the system and for analysis of the system as a whole (Filter, Xia, & Gray, 2005; Lillacci & Khammash, 2010; Arunachalam, Jacob, & Kamalanand, 2014). The development of such a model involves identification of several complex interrelationships in the system and is a time consuming task. After development of such a model which describes the actual biological system, the model must be tuned to specific cases. In other words, a mathematical model has to be patient specific so that it can be properly used for diagnosis and treatment planning applications. Hence, the important task is to tailor the model to match the measured variables of the individual patient under study (Ho & Chan, 2010, Kamalanand & Jawahar, 2015).

The patient specific mathematical models are highly useful for:

1. Predicting the progression of the disease for individual patients.
2. Predicting the health of the individual.
3. Surgery planning for a specific patient.
4. Therapy planning for a specific patient.

The process of developing a patient specific model involves estimation of the model parameters from the measured state variables of the patient. In the case of parameter estimation of ODE models, the estimation problem is considered as a linear estimation case when the model is a linear model and a nonlinear estimation problem when the model is nonlinear. Further, the estimation problem can be classified into online and offline estimation. In offline estimation, the model parameters are estimated after the state variables are measured for the specific time interval. However, in online estimation, the model parameters are updated for each and every sampling instant.

Some efficient methods for online estimation of linear model parameters are the Recursive Least Squares (RLS) algorithm and the Kalman Filter (KF) algorithm. For the nonlinear case, the Kalaman filter algorithm can be extended to obtain methods such as the Extended Kalman Filter (EKF) and Unscented Kalman Filter (UKF) algorithms which can be effectively used for model parameter estimation (La Scala & Bitmead, 1996, Ljung, 1979, Boutayeb, Rafaralahy, & Darouach, 1997, Wan & Van Der Merwe, 2000, Kamalanand & Jawahar, 2013). Further, in some cases all the state variables may not be available for measurement which makes the model parameter estimation problem even more complicated. The common problems which degrade the accuracy of the model parameter estimate are:

1. The model is highly nonlinear.
2. The model exhibits chaotic nature.
3. Few state variables are not available for measurement.
4. Measurements are corrupted by random noise.

In most cases the EKF and UKF methods provide a consistent estimate of the model parameters even though few state variables are not available for measurement and the measurements may be corrupted by random noises (Kamalanand & Jawahar, 2013).

In recent years, infectious diseases have become a major problem and have increased the mortality and morbidity of individuals. Some of the infectious diseases have spread in a pandemic manner and has been a difficult task to control such infections. The Human Immunodeficiency Virus infection / Acquired Immunodeficiency Syndrome (HIV/AIDS) is a disease of the human immune system caused by the Human Immunodeficiency Virus (HIV). AIDS has become a devastating epidemic so far and is actively spreading (Moonchai, Lenbury, & Triampo, 2010). According to the Centers for Disease Control and Prevention (CDC), approximately 50,000 people become newly infected each year (CDC, 2013). Further, the mathematical modelling of the dynamics of the HIV infection has complimented the knowledge about the infection and has further led to the development of new treatment strategies for the control of the infection. Some of the models based on ordinary differential equations have been utilized for the estimation of optimal drug dosage for antiretroviral therapy. Further, a synergetic method of treatment namely the Highly Active AntiretRoviral Therapy (HAART) has lead to the efficient treatment of the HIV infection. Several researchers have published their findings on the use of HAART based on mathematical models and computational algorithms (Joska, Gouse, Paul, Stein, & Flisher, 2010, Ge, Tian, & Lee, 2005, Kamalanand & Jawahar 2014).

In this chapter, the Extended Kalman Filter is thoroughly explained and its applicability in parameter estimation is illustrated using the three-dimensional HIV model. The adopted model consists of three state variables namely the CD4 cell population, CD8 cell population and the HIV-1 viral load and six parameters. The model accurately maps the interaction between the human immunodeficiency virus and the human immune system. Also, this model has been proved to be an efficient tool for viral load estimation and therapy planning in HIV/AIDS patients. The adopted model is highly nonlinear and chaotic. In this chapter, the usage of EKF algorithm for estimation of all six parameters of the HIV/AIDS model from measurements of the state variables has been described in detail.

BACKGROUND

In recent years, the Kalman filter and the extended Kalman filter has been widely used as a tool for state and parameter estimation, for biomedical and biological systems (Rakshit, Panigrahy, & Sahu, 2015; Roche, Lahaye, & Poline, 2004; Kim, Kim, Park, & Lee, 2001; Alacam, Yazici, Intes, & Chance, 2006, Sameni, Shamsollahi, & Jutten, 2005). A Kalman filter is an optimal estimator which estimates certain parameters of interest from indirect, inaccurate and uncertain observations. It is a recursive algorithm and hence new measurements are processed as they arrive. In other words, it is an online estimation algorithm. Further, if all noises corrupting the measurement are Gaussian in nature, then the Kalman filter minimizes the mean square error of the estimated parameters. However, if the noise corrupting the system is not Gaussian in nature, then the Kalman filter acts as a best linear estimator. The major advantage of the Kalman filter when compared to other estimators is that there is no need to invert the measurement equations. Further, the filter is easy to formulate and implement on real time systems. This filter is often used for tracking targets in the case of aircrafts and missiles (Kleeman, 1996).

Further, the process of finding the "best estimate" from noisy measurement data involves the filtering of the noise. The Kalman filter not only filters the measurements but also projects these measurements onto the estimate of the state variables. The limitation of the conventional Kalman filter is that it cannot be applied on nonlinear systems. However, many real world systems have non-linear state and measurement equations. If a Kalman filter is applied to a linearized model of a nonlinear system, then there is a loss in optimality. This problem is overcome using the modified version of the Kalman filter, known as the extended Kalman filter. The extended Kalman filter linearizes the state and measurement equations about the predicted state as an operating point. Hence at each and every sampling instant, the non-linear model is linearized by constructing the Jacobian matrix of the system (Bar-Shalom & Li, 1993; Jazwinski, 1973; Bozic, 1979; Kleeman, 1996).

Brovko et al. (1981) performed online estimation of the pulmonary blood flow using the extended Kalman Filter and have compared their results with experimental measurements using thermal dilution technique. Further, the authors have concluded that the EKF method shows promise for use in many biomedical applications, including patieat monitoring, physiological experimentation, and clinical heart function tests. Trigo et al. (2004) have proposed a method based on EKF algorithm, for estimating the conductivity/resistivity distribution in electrical impedance tomography. Alacam et al. (2006) have presented three different compartmental models of the pharmacokinetics of indocyanine green (ICG) in cancerous tumors. The authors have introduced a systematic and robust approach for modelling and analyzing ICG pharmacokinetics based on the extended Kalman filtering framework. Further, the authors have found that the proposed EKF framework effectively models multiple-compartment and multiple- measurement systems in the presence of measurement noise and uncertainties in model dynamics. Also, the authors have analyzed that the recursive nature of the Kalman filter estimator potentially allows real-time monitoring of time varying pharmacokinetic rates and concentration changes in different compartments. The authors have concluded that EKF model may provide parameters that may be useful for tumor differentiation.

McNames and Aboy (2008) have presented a state-space model of cardiovascular signals and have described how it can be used with the extended Kalman filter (EKF) to simultaneously estimate and track many cardiovascular parameters of interest. Further, the authors have demonstrated the ability of the algorithm to estimate and track several clinically relevant features of cardiovascular signals and have shown how the algorithm can be used to solve several clinically significant problems such as heart and respiratory rate estimation, artifact removal and pulse morphology characterization. Liu and He (2011) have formulated the nonlinear relationship between the 3-D activation sequence and the body surface recordings during activation and have utilized EKF to estimate the activation sequence in a recursive way.

Denis de Senneville et al. (2013) have improved the temperature measurement resolution and precision while maintaining guaranteed output accuracy in MR-Temperature imaging by combining the Measured data and a priori knowledge of 3-D data derived from a forecast based on a physical model using the extended Kalman Filter. Batmani and Khaloozadeh (2012) have used extended Kalman filter algorithm for optimal chemotherapy in cancer treatment. Cazelles and Chau (1995) have used a simple compartment model to describe the HIV/AIDS epidemic in homosexual and bisexual male, in Paris, France. Further, the authors have used EKF algorithm to efficiently estimate the parameters of the epidemic model. Also, the authors conclude that the use of Kalman filtering techniques can contribute to the better understanding and forecasting of the HIV/AIDS epidemic.

Rigatos et al. (2015) have developed a method for early diagnosis of parametric changes in intra-cellular protein synthesis models using a nonlinear Kalman Filtering approach and statistical change detection methods. The authors have demonstrated that the proposed method can provide indication within specific confidence intervals about parametric changes in the considered biological system and consequently indications about the appearance of specific diseases. Lee et al. (2015) presented a method for finding the enhanced heading and position of pedestrians using extended Kalman filter algorithm. Baker et al. (2015) have proposed a novel parameter estimation framework by combining approaches for solving identifiability issues with a filtering technique that can uniquely estimate parameters of kinetic biological models. The authors have utilized nonlinear Kalman filtering techniques for parameter estimation and have demonstrated that the adopted method can uniquely estimate parameters where conventional methods fail. Bersvendsen et al. (2016) have used a Kalman filter based state estimation approach for automated segmentation of the right ventricle in 3D echocardiography. Further, the authors have demonstrated high accuracy and less computation times using the segmentation method based on the Kalman filter technique.

PATIENT SPECIFIC MODELLING USING THE EXTENDED KALMAN FILTER

Idea behind Parameter Estimation

The goal of parameter estimation is to derive a parametric description of a physical process or an event or a system. For example, consider a mechanical system described by the mass-spring-damper equation where the model is parameterized by three parameters namely the mass of the system, the spring constant and the damping coefficient. Consider that the input to the system is a tensile of compressive force and the output of the system is the displacement of the moving end. Now the problem of parameter estimation is the estimate the three parameters of the system using measurements of input force and the output displacement. However, the estimation is complex since the measurement comes with uncertainties. In order to get a consistent estimate of the parameters, one can increase the number of independent measurements and make the system an over-determined system of equations. However, one can reduce the cost of the measurement by reducing the number of measurements and making the system an under-determined one. In both the above mentioned cases, the estimation of parameters is possible if enough prior knowledge is available about the system or if the parameters are statistically related to each other. If the mathematical model of the system is available, the parameter set can be estimated using the method of the extended Kalman filter (van der Heijden, Duin, De Ridder, & Tax, 2005).

Consider the mathematical model of a system described by ordinary differential equations of the form:

$$\left.\begin{array}{l} \dfrac{dx}{dt} = f(x(t), \theta, t) + w(t) \\ z(t) = h(x(t), t) + v(t) \end{array}\right\} \tag{1}$$

where, $x(t)$ is the state variable, θ is the model parameters to be estimated, $z(t)$ is the vector of observations and $w(t)$ and $v(t)$ are the random noises. Now, suppose if we would like to use the EKF algorithm for estimation of θ, we rewrite Equation (1) as follows:

$$\left.\begin{aligned} \frac{dx}{dt} &= f(x(t),\theta(t),t) + w(t) \\ \frac{d\theta}{dt} &= 0 + w(t) \\ z(t) &= h(x(t),t) + v(t) \end{aligned}\right\} \tag{2}$$

Now, the augmented state parameter vector is defined as $x_a^T = [x^T, \theta^T]$.

Further, a continuous differential equation can be written in discrete form using the Euler's method and the discrete EKF is then applied to estimate the parameters of the system.

Consider the continuous differential equation: $\frac{dx}{dt} = f(x(t),t)$. This equation is discretized using Euler's method as: $x_k = x_{k-1} + hf(x_{k-1}, t_{k-1})$.

Probability Theory and Gaussian Distributions

The development of probability involves three different terms namely outcomes, events and probability. Together, these three terms are called as an experiment. A trial is the act of randomly drawing a single outcome. A set Ω consists of outcomes ω_i. Each trial produces one $\omega \in \Omega$. *A* is a set of certain subsets of Ω. Each subset $\alpha \in A$ is called an event. An event is said to have occurred if the outcome ω_i of a trial is contained in α, *i.e.* $\omega \in \alpha$. $P(\alpha)$ is a real function known as the probability function, defined on *A* (van der Heijden et al., 2005; Papoulis, 1965).

A random variable $\underline{x}(\omega)$ is a mapping of Ω onto a set of numbers such as integer numbers, real numbers, complex numbers, etc. The distribution function $F_{\underline{x}}(x)$ is the probability of the event that corresponds to $\underline{x} \le x$: $F_{\underline{x}}(x) = P(\underline{x} \le x)$. The random variable $\underline{x}$ is said to be discrete if a finite number of events $x_1, x_2, x_3 \ldots$ exists for which: $P(\underline{x} = x_i) > 0$ and $\sum_i P(\underline{x} = x_i) = 1$. The random variable $\underline{x}$ is continuous if a function $P_{\underline{x}}(x)$ exists for which: $F_{\underline{x}}(x) = \int_{\xi=-\infty}^{x} P_{\underline{x}}(\xi)d\xi$. The function $P_{\underline{x}}(x)$ is called the probability density of $\underline{x}$ (van der Heijden *et al.* 2005).

The moment of order n of a random variable is defined as: $E[x^n] = \int_{x=-\infty}^{\infty} x^n P(x)dx$. The first order moment is called the expectation μ. The central moments of order n are defined as: $E[(x-\mu)^n] = \int_{x=-\infty}^{\infty} (x-\mu)^n P(x)dx$. The first central moment is always zero. The second central moment is called variance: $\mathrm{var}[x] = E[(x-\mu)^2] = E[x^2] - \mu^2$. The (standard) deviation of x denoted by σ_x is the square root of the variance: $\sigma_x = \sqrt{\mathrm{var}[x]}$ (van der Heijden et al., 2005).

A continuous random variable has a Gaussian or normal probability density: $p(x) = \frac{1}{\sigma\sqrt{2\pi}}\exp\left(\frac{-(x-\mu)^2}{2\sigma^2}\right)$. Gaussian random variables occur when the underlying process is caused by the outcomes of many independent experiments and the associated random variables add up linearly or satisfy the central limit theorem (van der Heijden *et al.* 2005). A gaussian or normal distribution of a random variable is very useful since for such cases, estimation techniques such as the least squares algorithm and the extended Kalman filters can be applied. A random variable with a Gaussian distribution is called as a normally deviate. If $\mu = 0$ and $\sigma = 1$, the distribution is called the standard normal distribution or the unit normal distribution and is denoted by *N(0,1)* (Lyon, 2014; Cohen, 1981; Reid, 1987; Shepp, 1964; Simon, 2007). In most of the practical cases such as industrial measurements, biological measurements etc., measurements from sensors are often corrupted by Gaussian random noises. The white noise is a typical example of a Gaussian noise. Such noises are also found in various fields such as economics, epidemiology, sociology etc. In a practical estimation problem such as aircraft tracking or systems corrupted by thermal noises, it is necessary to estimate the state variables and parameters of the system efficiently by filtering out the noise components of the system. Further, such Gaussian noises can affect a system through the state variables or measurement variables. In this chapter, an efficient method known as the extended Kalman filter which can estimate both the states and parameters of a system under the influence of Gaussian noises, is described in detail.

The Extended Kalman Filter

A Kalman filter that linearizes about the current mean and covariance is referred to as an Extended Kalman Filter. The EKF is used in cases where the dynamic model is nonlinear. In EKF, the estimation around the current estimate is linearized using the partial derivatives of the process and measurement functions to compute estimates. The EKF is an ad hoc state and parameter estimator that approximates the optimality of Bayes' rule by linearization (Simon, 2006, Welsh & Bishop, 2006, Krishnamurthy, 2012).

Let the state vector be $x \in \Re^n$ and the process is governed by the non-linear difference equation described by (3) and let the measurement be $z \in \Re^m$.

$$x_k = f\left(x_{k-1}, w_{k-1}\right) \tag{3}$$

$$z_k = h\left(x_k, v_k\right) \tag{4}$$

where, the random variables w_k and v_k represent the process and measurement noise. The non-linear function f in the difference Equation (3) relates the state at the previous time step *k-1* to the state at the current time step *k*.

The probability distributions of *w* and *v* are $p(w) \sim \mathrm{N}(0,\mathrm{Q})$ and $p(v) \sim \mathrm{N}(0,\mathrm{R})$. In practice, one does not know the individual values of the noise and at each time step. However, one can approximate the state and measurement vector without them as:

$$\tilde{x}_k = f\left(\hat{x}_{k-1}, 0\right) \tag{5}$$

$$\tilde{z}_k = h\left(\tilde{x}_k, 0\right) \tag{6}$$

where, $\hat{x}_k$ is a posteriori estimate of the state from a previous time step *k*. To estimate a process with non-linear relationships, new governing equations that linearize an estimate about (5) and (6), is written.

$$x_k \approx \tilde{x}_k + A\left(x_{k-1} - \hat{x}_{k-1}\right) + Ww_{k-1} \tag{7}$$

$$z_k \approx \tilde{z}_k + H\left(x_k - \tilde{x}_k\right) + Vv_k \tag{8}$$

where, x_k and z_k are the actual state and measurement vectors, $\tilde{x}_k$ and $\tilde{z}_k$ are the approximate state and measurement vectors from (5) and (6), $\hat{x}_k$ is an a posteriori estimate of the state at step *k*, the random variables w_k and v_k represent the process and measurement noise.

- *A* is the Jacobian matrix of partial derivatives of *f(.)* with respect to *x*, that is $A_{[i,j]} = \frac{\partial f_{[i]}}{\partial x_{[j]}}\left(\hat{x}_{k-1}, 0\right)$.
- *W* is the Jacobian matrix of partial derivatives of *f(.)* with respect to *w*: $W_{[i,j]} = \frac{\partial f_{[i]}}{\partial w_{[j]}}\left(\hat{x}_{k-1}, 0\right)$.
- *H* is the Jacobian matrix of partial derivatives of *h(.)* with respect to *x*: $H_{[i,j]} = \frac{\partial h_{[i]}}{\partial x_{[j]}}\left(\tilde{x}_k, 0\right)$.
- *V* is the Jacobian matrix of partial derivatives of *h(.)* with respect to *v*: $V_{[i,j]} = \frac{\partial h_{[i]}}{\partial v_{[j]}}\left(\tilde{x}_k, 0\right)$.

Now, the prediction error is defined as $\tilde{e}_{x_k} \equiv x_k - \tilde{x}_k$ and the measurement residual as $\tilde{e}_{z_k} \equiv z_k - \tilde{x}_k$. The governing equations for the error process are written as:

$$\tilde{e}_{x_k} \approx A\left(x_{k-1} - \hat{x}_{k-1}\right) + \varepsilon_k \tag{9}$$

$$\tilde{e}_{z_k} \approx H\tilde{e}_{x_k} + \eta_k \tag{10}$$

$$\hat{x}_k = \tilde{x}_k + \hat{e}_k \tag{11}$$

where, ε_k and η_k represent new independent random variables having zero mean and covariance matrices WQW^T and VRV^T. The probability distributions of the random variables are:

$$p\left(\tilde{e}_{x_k}\right) \sim \mathrm{N}\left(0, \mathrm{E}\left[\tilde{e}_{x_k} \tilde{e}_{x_k}^T\right]\right) \tag{12}$$

$$p\left(\varepsilon_k\right) \sim \mathrm{N}\left(0, \mathrm{W}\, \mathrm{Q_k} W^T\right) \tag{13}$$

$$p\left(\eta_k\right) \sim \mathrm{N}\left(0, \mathrm{V}\, \mathrm{R_k} V^T\right) \tag{14}$$

The Kalman filter equation used to estimate $\hat{e}_k$ is $\hat{e}_k = K_k \tilde{e}_{z_k}$ (Welsh & Bishop, 2006). And hence,

$$\hat{x}_k = \tilde{x}_k + K_k \tilde{e}_{z_k} \tag{15}$$

$$\hat{x}_k = \tilde{x}_k + K_k \left(z_k - \tilde{z}_k\right) \tag{16}$$

where, K_k is the Kalman gain and is obtained using the derivation of the basic Kalman filter (Welsh & Bishop, 2006). To summarize the EKF algorithm, the time and measurement update equations are given as:

Time update:

$$\hat{x}_k^- = f\left(\hat{x}_{k-1}, 0\right) \tag{17}$$

$$P_k^- = A_k P_{k-1} A_k^T + W_k Q_{k-1} W_k^T \tag{18}$$

Measurement update:

$$K_k = P_k^- H_k^T \left(H_k P_k^- H_k^T + V_k R_k V_k^T\right)^{-1} \tag{19}$$

$$\hat{x}_k = \hat{x}_k^- + K_k \left(z_k - h\left(\hat{x}_k^-, 0\right)\right) \tag{20}$$

$$P_k = \left(I - K_k H_k\right) P_k^- \tag{21}$$

The Mathematical Model of HIV/AIDS

The mathematical models used to represent various dynamical aspects of infectious disease can explain complex clinical signals and the associated symptoms. Mathematical modeling of the interaction between HIV-1 and the immune system has improved the understanding of the dynamics of the disease (de Souza, 1999). Such models that describe the interaction of HIV with the patient's immune system and the influence of drugs on the virus can be a helpful tool to decide on treatment strategies in HIV/AIDS patients (Filter et al., 2005).

A nonlinear dynamic model of HIV system was presented by de Souza in 1999. In his model, the response of the CD4 lymphocyte population, the CD8 lymphocyte population and the HIV-1 viral load is characterized by simultaneous nonlinear differential equations. Further, Ho and Ling (2010) have demonstarted that the system dynamics of this HIV model is sensitive to both the initial conditions and the system parameters. Hence, the HIV system is chaotic and exhibits a bifurcation behavior. Also, because of its chaotic nature, the system is very difficult to be controlled (Ho & Ling, 2010).

The major dynamics of the HIV infection in the human body is due to the interaction of the HIV with the T lymphocytes or T-cells of the human immune system. There are two types of T lymphocytes namely the T-helper cells (CD4+ cells) and T-cytotoxic cells (CD8+ cells). The activated T-cytotoxic cells can eliminate the host cells that are infected with virus or other bacteria (Chamberlain, 2010). The major effect of the HIV infection is the rapid depletion of CD4 cells. Due to the major role of CD4 cells in the human immune system, their depletion has a degrading effect on the functionality of the immune system (Perelson, Kirschner, & De Boer, 1993).

When HIV infects the human body, it targets the CD4 T-cells. A protein on the surface of the HIV virus has a high affinity for the CD4 protein on the surface of the T cell. Binding takes place and the contents of the HIV is injected into the host CD4 cell. After the virus has been duplicated by the host cell, it is reassembled and new virus particles emerge from the host cell (Levy, 1994; Kirschner, 1996). Further, the infected CD4 cells simulate the CD8 cells which kill the infected CD4 T-helper cells (Wang, Krueger, & Buja, 2004). This process is presented as a block diagram in Figure 1.

Figure 1. Block diagram representation of the interaction between HIV-1 and the human immune system

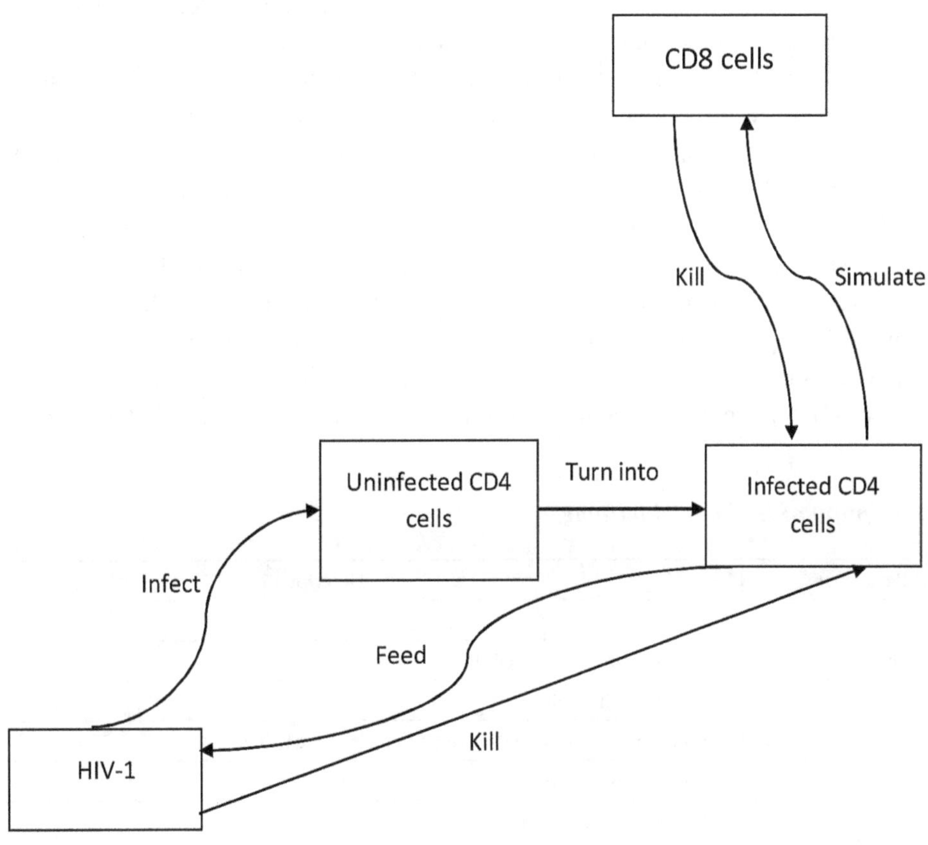

The response of the concentrations of the CD4 lymphocyte population, the CD8 lymphocyte population and the HIV-1 viral load can be characterized by the following first order nonlinear differential equation (Ho & Ling 2010; Filter et al., 2005; Iwasa, Michor, & Nowak, 2005; Dixit & Perelson, 2004, Gilchrist, Coombs, & Perelson, 2004; Barros, 2004).

$$\left.\begin{aligned} \frac{dx(t)}{dt} &= a(x_0 - x(t)) - bx(t)z(t) \\ \frac{dy(t)}{dt} &= c(y_0 - y(t)) + dy(t)z(t) \\ \frac{dz(t)}{dt} &= z(t)(ex(t) - fy(t)) \end{aligned}\right\} \tag{22}$$

where, $x(t)$, $y(t)$ and $z(t)$ are the concentrations of the CD4 lymphocyte population, the CD8 lymphocyte population and the HIV-1 viral load, respectively. x_0 and y_0 are the normal unperturbed concentrations of the CD4 and CD8 lymphocyte population. a, b, c, d, e and f are the system parameters. The human body regulates the normal levels of CD4 and CD8 cells. These normal levels are CD4N and CD8N, in the absence of the HIV-1 virus.

The parameter '*a*' represents the dynamics of this regulating mechanism for CD4 cells and the parameter '*c*' represents the dynamics of the regulating mechanism for the CD8 cells. When one individual HIV-1 copy meets a CD4 cell, the cell will be destroyed and hence these encounters decrease the growth rate of CD4 cell population. The number of those encounters is proportional to the product of the populations of HIV-1 and CD4 and the probability of one such encounter depends on this product. In this case, the constant of proportionality is the parameter '*b*'. When one CD8 cell meets an individual HIV-1 copy, it will trigger a mechanism that increases the production of CD8 cells. Hence the growth rate of CD8 cells will increase. The number of these encounters will be proportional to the product of the populations of CD8 and HIV-1 and the constant of proportionality is the parameter '*d*'. HIV-1 feeds on and kills CD4 cells and gets destroyed by CD8 cells. The killing of CD4 cells by HIV-1 depends on the encounters of HIV-1 with CD4 cells, and the destruction of HIV-1 by CD8 cells depends on the encounters of HIV-1 with CD8 cells. The parameters '*e*' and '*f*' relates to the growth rate of the HIV-1 population due to interaction with CD4 cells and destruction of HIV-1 by CD8, respectively (de Souza, 1999).

The response of the given model is shown in Figure 2 and the description of each parameter is provided in Table 1. This model has been proved to be an efficient tool for viral load estimation and therapy planning in HIV/AIDS patients (Kamalanand & Jawahar, 2014; Kamalanand & Jawahar, 2013).

Table 1. Description of HIV model parameters

Model Parameter	Description
a	Death rate of CD4 cells
b	Rate of infection of CD4 cells by virus
c	Death rate of CD8 cells
d	Rate of increase of CD8 cells in response to increased viral load
e	Rate of increase of viral load
f	Rate of decrease of viral load

Figure 2. Variation of (a) CD4 cell population, (b) CD8 cell population and (c) viral load shown as a function of sampling instants

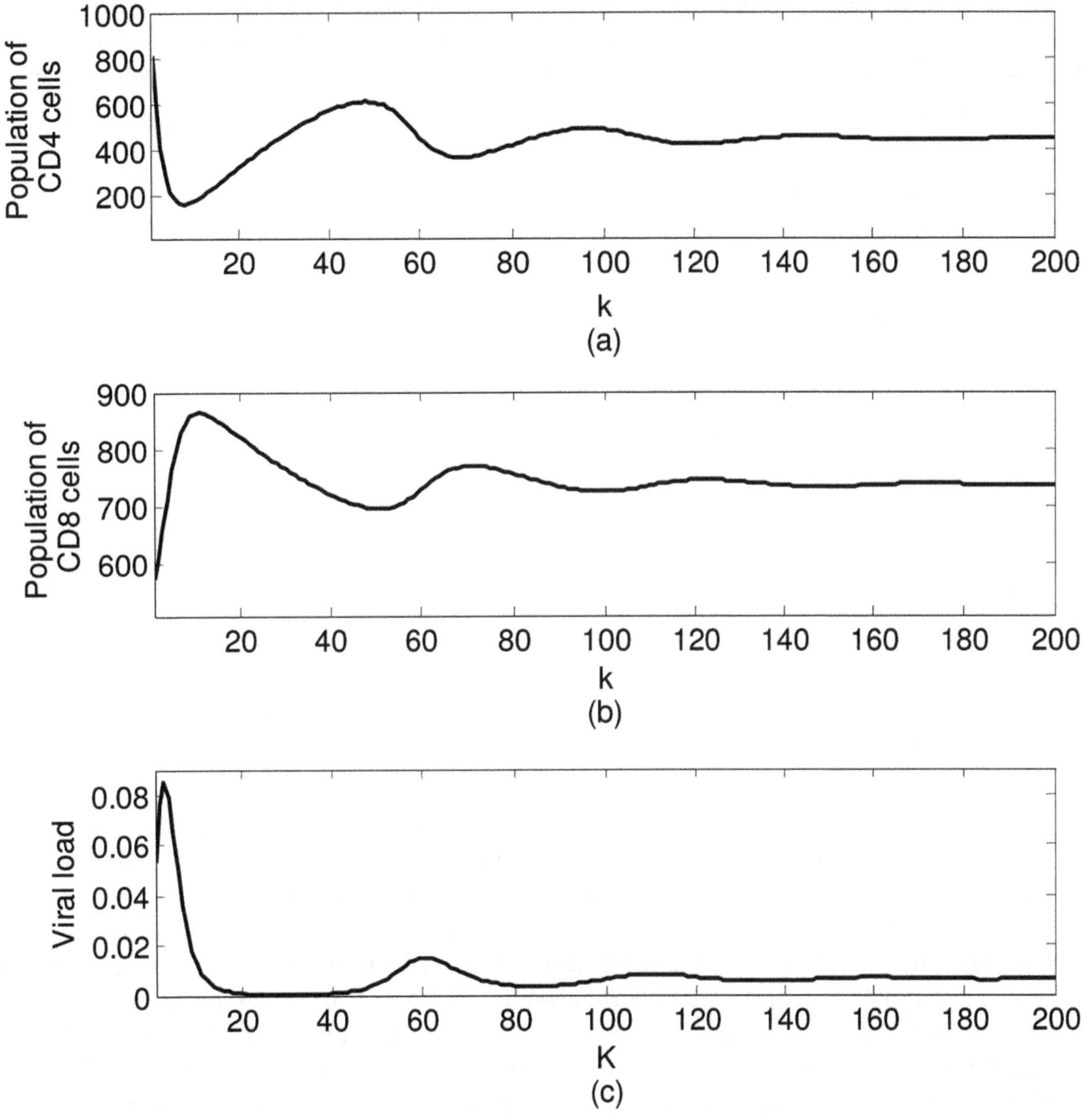

Estimation of HIV Model Parameters Using Extended Kalman Filter

To use the HIV model as a tool for treatment decisions, the model parameters must be determined from measurements that are acquired on equipment that is accessible to local health services (Filter et al., 2005). Even though there are general observations that can be made from the model and its structure, it is only when the model is tailored to each patient's individual parameters that clear benefits in the treatment strategy arise (Filter & Xia, 2003).

As described in Equation (2), the estimation of the model parameters of the given set of nonlinear differential equations requires the equations to be rewritten by considering the parameters of the system as the states of the system. Since the parameters of the model should not change as a function of time, the rate of change of the parameters is equated to zero. In this way, the estimation of the *a, b, c, d, e* and *f* parameters of the HIV model using extended Kalman filter algorithm, requires the estimation problem to be formulated as follows:

$$\left.\begin{aligned}
\frac{dx(t)}{dt} &= a(t)(x_0 - x(t)) - b(t)x(t)z(t)\\
\frac{dy(t)}{dt} &= c(t)(y_0 - y(t)) + d(t)y(t)z(t)\\
\frac{dz(t)}{dt} &= z(t)(e(t)x(t) - f(t)y(t))\\
\frac{da}{dt} &= 0\\
\frac{db}{dt} &= 0\\
\frac{dc}{dt} &= 0\\
\frac{dd}{dt} &= 0\\
\frac{de}{dt} &= 0\\
\frac{df}{dt} &= 0
\end{aligned}\right\} \tag{23}$$

Hence, all the six parameters of the model are estimated as states of the system. The convergence plots for the values of parameters *a, b, c, d, e* and *f* estimated using the extended Kalman filter are presented in Figures 3 to 8 respectively. The time taken for completing hundred iterations was found to be 6.96 seconds. Figure 3 shows the convergence of estimated value of parameter '*a*' namely the death rate of CD4 cells, with the actual value as a function of iteration number. It is seen that the estimated value converges to the true value within thirty iterations of the EKF algorithm. Initial oscillations in the estimated value are also found to be minimal. The Convergence of estimated value of parameter '*b*', namely the rate of infection of CD4 cells by virus, with actual value is shown as a function of iteration number in Figure 4. It is found that the convergence of estimated value with true value of parameter '*b*' is achieved within sixty iterations. Initially, the deviation of estimated value with actual value appears to be high and the error decreases gradually until convergence occurs.

Similarly, Figure 5 shows the convergence of estimated value of parameter '*c*' namely the death rate of CD8 cells, with the actual value as a function of iteration number. It appears that the estimated value converges with the true value within thirty iterations. Before convergence, the deviation of the estimated value from the actual value appears to be similar to the deviation observed in the case of parameter '*a*'. The Convergence of estimated value of parameter '*d*' namely the rate of increase of CD8 cells in response to increased viral load, with actual value is shown as a function of iteration number in Figure

Figure 3. Convergence of estimated value of parameter 'a' with actual value shown as a function of iteration number

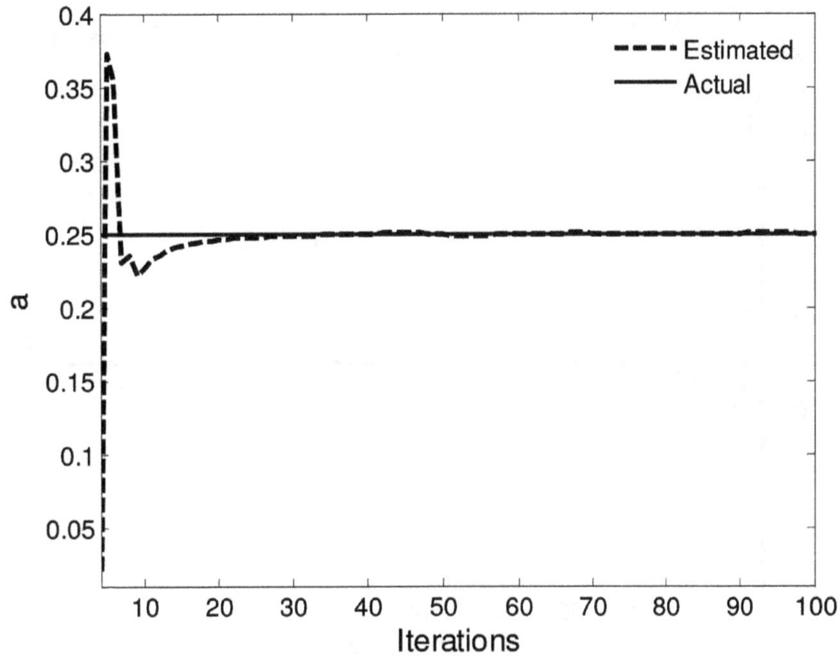

Figure 4. Convergence of estimated value of parameter 'b' with actual value shown as a function of iteration number

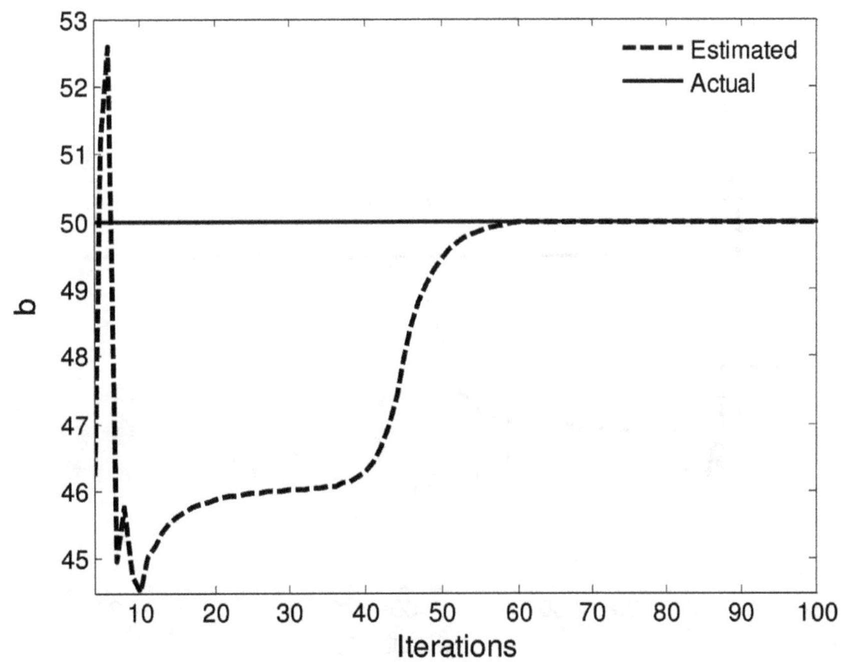

Figure 5. Convergence of estimated value of parameter 'c' with actual value shown as a function of iteration number

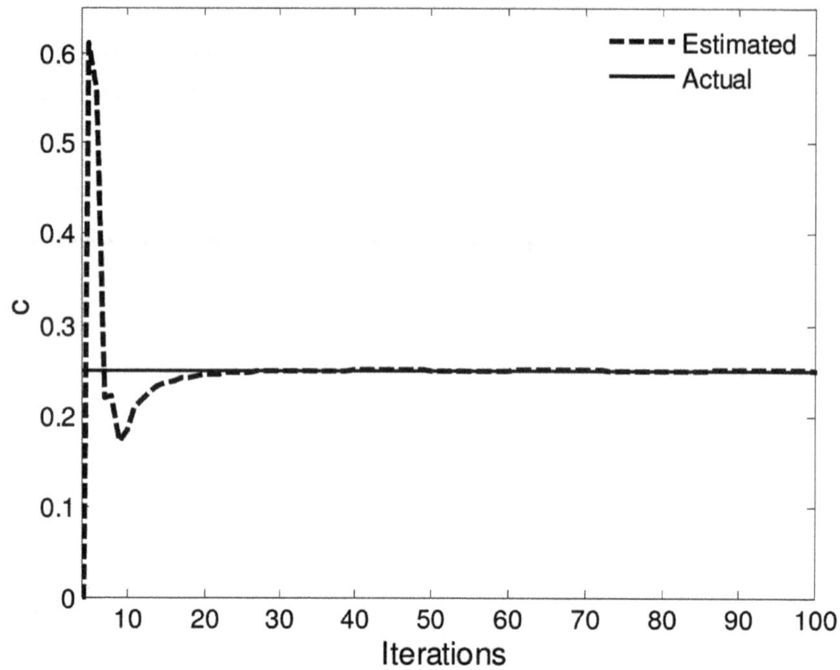

Figure 6. Convergence of estimated value of parameter 'd' with actual value shown as a function of iteration number

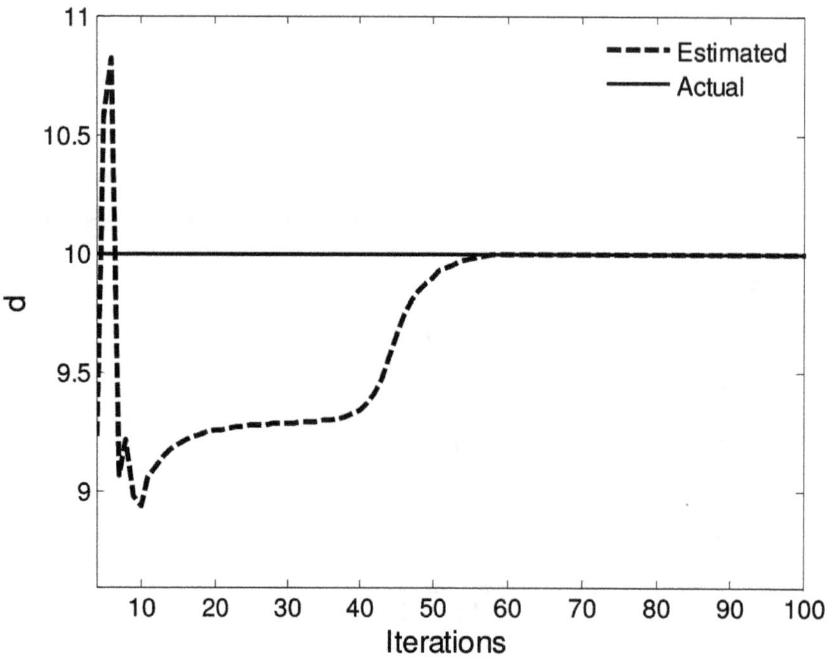

Figure 7. Convergence of estimated value of parameter 'e' with actual value shown as a function of iteration number

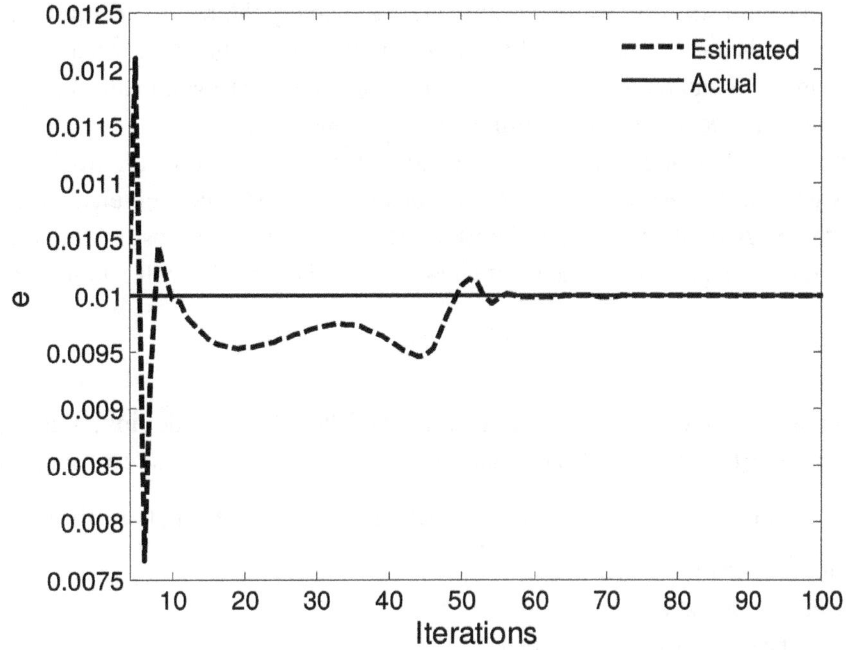

Figure 8. Convergence of estimated value of parameter 'f' with actual value shown as a function of iteration number

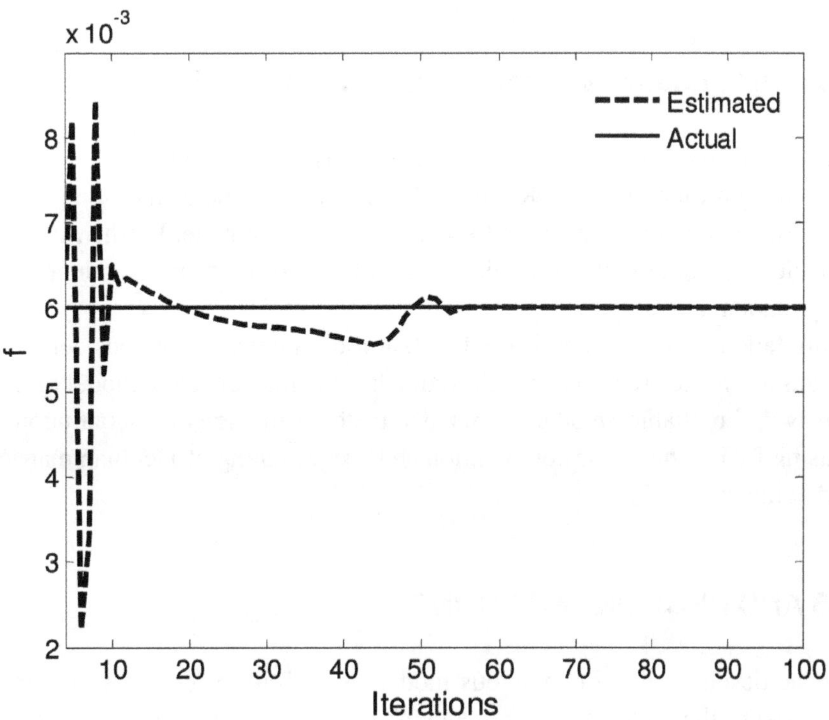

6. The convergence plot for estimation of parameter '*d*' appears to be similar to that of parameter '*b*'. Also, convergence is achieved within sixty iterations.

The Convergence of estimated value of parameter '*e*' namely the rate of increase of viral load and parameter '*f*' namely the rate of decrease of viral load, with actual value is shown as a function of iteration number in Figures 7 and 8 respectively. In both the cases, the estimated values oscillate around the true value and convergence is achieved within sixty iterations.

Results demonstrate that the estimated value of parameters '*a*' and '*c*' converge to the true value within thirty iterations whereas twice the number of iterations is required for convergence of other parameters with their true values. Also, it appears that the EKF method is efficient for estimating the all the parameters of the HIV model using measurements of CD4 cell population, CD8 cell population and viral load.

EKF Summary

Step 1: Consider a suitable continuous dynamic model of the process under investigation.
Step 2: Rewrite the differential equation by taking all the parameters as state variables of the system, (ie. $\frac{d\theta}{dt} = 0$) and acquire the measured values at each sampling instant from the real world process.
Step 3: Perform the time update step:
- Project the state ahead.
- Project the error covariance ahead.

Step 4: Perform the measurement update step:
- Compute the Kalman Gain.
- Update the estimate.
- Update the error covariance.

Step 5: End.

Advantages and Limitations of the Extended Kalman Filter

The main advantage of the EKF algorithm is that it is easy to use and works very well in practical estimation problems. Further, extended Kalman filter is almost same as the basic Kalman filter, This method is also computationally efficient and provides a stable estimate. Further, it works well even if some state variables are not available for measurement and also if the measurement of state variables are corrupted by random noises.

The major limitation of this method is the fact that it does not work in considerable nonlinearities. Further, only Gaussian noise processes are allowed. Also, the mathematical model of the process needs to be continuously differentiable. In other words, parameter estimation of discontinuous models cannot be performed using EKF. Finally, the computation and programming of Jacobian matrices can be quite error prone and complex.

SOLUTIONS AND RECOMMENDATIONS

In cases where the development of continuous models is difficult or not possible, one can develop a discontinuous model of the biological system and efficiently use the Unscented Kalman Filter (UKF) algorithm for parameter estimation. The unscented Kalman filter uses the unscented transformation for state and parameter estimation. In this method, the Jacobian matrices are not computed and hence UKF is computationally simpler when compared to the EKF method.

FUTURE RESEARCH DIRECTIONS

In recent years, patient specific models have been utilized efficiently for biomedical applications such as diagnosis, therapy planning and drug dosage estimation. In the context of the HIV/AIDS epidemic, several researchers have reported their findings on the estimation of key parameters of the HIV system using model based approaches (Ciupe, Bivort, Bortz, & Nelson, 2006; Huang, Liu, & Wu, 2006; Liang, Miao, & Wu, 2010; Ouattara, 2005, Putter, Heisterkamp, Lange, & De Wolf, 2002; Wu, Ding, & De Gruttola, 1998; Wu, Zhu, Miao, & Perelson, 2008; Xia, 2003). The extended Kalman filter serves as an efficient tool for development of such patient specific models and the methods described in this chapter can be extended to other infectious diseases such as malaria, H1N1, etc., for efficient diagnostics and planning treatment strategies.

CONCLUSION

Parameter estimation is an important task for development of patient specific models of physiological and biological processes. However, the online estimation of model parameters in biomedical systems is a challenging task due to the nonlinear and chaotic nature of such systems. Further, the measurements obtained from biomedical systems such as biosignals are often corrupted by random noises and artifacts. In such cases, the extended Kalman filter served as an useful and efficient tool for parameter estimation. The EKF algorithm is used in cases where the dynamic model is nonlinear. This algorithm can be effectively used for parameter estimation of nonlinear system from the measurements of state variables. Further, this method provides a consistent estimate of the model parameters even though few state variables are not available for measurement and the measurements may be corrupted by random noises (Brignell & White, 1996; Regtien, Van Der Heijden, Korsten, & Otthius, 2004; van der Heijden et al., 2005). In this chapter, the method of parameter estimation of nonlinear systems using the EKF algorithm has been explained in detail. The three dimensional mathematical model of the HIV/AIDS system has been used as an illustrative example for explaining the usage of EKF algorithm for parameter estimation. The adopted model consists of three state variables namely the CD4 cell population, CD8 cell population and the HIV-1 viral load and six parameters. The model accurately maps the interaction between the human immunodeficiency virus and the human immune system. Also, this model has been proved to be an efficient tool for viral load estimation and therapy planning in HIV/AIDS patients. Further, the adopted model is highly nonlinear and chaotic. Results demonstrate that the extended Kalman filter technique is efficient for online estimation of all the six parameters of the HIV/AIDS system. This study appears to be of high clinical relevance since the estimation of HIV/AIDS parameters is useful for proper diagnosis and staging of the disease and also for therapy planning in HIV/AIDS patients.

REFERENCES

Alacam, B., Yazici, B., Intes, X., & Chance, B. (2006). Extended Kalman filtering for the modeling and analysis of ICG pharmacokinetics in cancerous tumors using NIR optical methods. *Biomedical Engineering. IEEE Transactions on, 53*(10), 1861–1871.

Arunachalam, K., Jacob, L. V., & Kamalanand, K. (2014). Design and analysis of finite element based sensors for diagnosis of liver disorders using biocompatible metals. *Technology and Health Care: Official Journal of the European Society for Engineering and Medicine, 22*(6), 867-875.

Baker, S. M., Poskar, C. H., Schreiber, F., & Junker, B. H. (2015). A unified framework for estimating parameters of kinetic biological models. *BMC Bioinformatics, 16*(1), 104. doi:10.1186/s12859-015-0500-9 PMID:25886743

Bar-Shalom, Y., & Li, X. R. (1998). Estimation and Tracking: Principles, Techniques, and Software. Artech House.

Barros, L. C. (2004, June). Fuzzy set-based model to compute the life expectancy of HIV infected populations. In *Fuzzy Information, 2004. Processing NAFIPS'04. IEEE Annual Meeting of the* (Vol. 1, pp. 314-318). IEEE.

Batmani, Y., & Khaloozadeh, H. (2013). Optimal chemotherapy in cancer treatment: State dependent Riccati equation control and extended Kalman filter. *Optimal Control Applications and Methods, 34*(5), 562–577. doi:10.1002/oca.2039

Bersvendsen, J., Orderud, F., Massey, R., Fossa, K., Gerard, O., Urheim, S., & Samset, E. (2016). Automated Segmentation of the Right Ventricle in 3D Echocardiography: A Kalman Filter State Estimation Approach. *IEEE Transactions on Medical Imaging, 35*(1), 42–51. doi:10.1109/TMI.2015.2453551 PMID:26168434

Boutayeb, M., Rafaralahy, H., & Darouach, M. (1997). Convergence analysis of the extended Kalman filter used as an observer for nonlinear deterministic discrete-time systems. *Automatic Control. IEEE Transactions on, 42*(4), 581–586.

Bozic, S. M. (1979). *Digital and Kalman filtering*. London: Edward Arnold.

Brignell, J. E., & White, N. M. (1996). *Intelligent Sensor Systems: 2nd*. Institute of Physics Publishing.

Brovko, O., Wiberg, D. M., Arena, L., & Bellville, J. W. (1981). The extended Kalman filter as a pulmonary blood flow estimator. *Automatica, 17*(1), 213–220. doi:10.1016/0005-1098(81)90096-0

Cazelles, B., & Chau, N. (1995). Adaptive dynamic modelling of HIV/AIDS epidemic using extended Kalman filter. *Journal of Biological System, 3*(03), 759–768. doi:10.1142/S0218339095000691

Centers for Disease Control and Prevention (CDC). (2013). *Today's HIV/AIDS epidemic*. Author.

Chamberlain, N. R. (2010). *HIV Infections and AIDS*. Available from: http://www.atsu.edu/faculty/chamberlain/Website/lectures/lecture/aids.htm

Ciupe, M. S., Bivort, B. L., Bortz, D. M., & Nelson, P. W. (2006). Estimating kinetic parameters from HIV primary infection data through the eyes of three different mathematical models. *Mathematical Biosciences*, *200*(1), 1–27. doi:10.1016/j.mbs.2005.12.006 PMID:16469337

Cohen, E. A. Jr. (1981). A note on normal functions of normal random variables. *Computers & Mathematics with Applications (Oxford, England)*, *7*(5), 395–400. doi:10.1016/0898-1221(81)90124-3

De Senneville, B. D., Roujol, S., Hey, S., Moonen, C., & Ries, M. (2013). Extended Kalman filtering for continuous volumetric MR-temperature imaging. *Medical Imaging. IEEE Transactions on*, *32*(4), 711–718.

de Souza, F. M. C. (1999). Modeling the dynamics of HIV-1 and CD4 and CD8 lymphocytes. *Engineering in Medicine and Biology Magazine, IEEE*, *18*(1), 21–24. doi:10.1109/51.740960 PMID:9934596

Dixit, N. M., & Perelson, A. S. (2004). Complex patterns of viral load decay under antiretroviral therapy: Influence of pharmacokinetics and intracellular delay. *Journal of Theoretical Biology*, *226*(1), 95–109. doi:10.1016/j.jtbi.2003.09.002 PMID:14637059

Filter, R. A., & Xia, X. (2003). Computer based HIV/AIDS parameter estimation for practitioners and patients. In *Proceedings of the First African Control Conference*.

Filter, R. A., Xia, X., & Gray, C. M. (2005). Dynamic HIV/AIDS parameter estimation with application to a vaccine readiness study in Southern Africa. *Biomedical Engineering. IEEE Transactions on*, *52*(5), 784–791.

Ge, S. S., Tian, Z., & Lee, T. H. (2005). Nonlinear control of a dynamic model of HIV-1. *Biomedical Engineering. IEEE Transactions on*, *52*(3), 353–361.

Gilchrist, M. A., Coombs, D., & Perelson, A. S. (2004). Optimizing within-host viral fitness: Infected cell lifespan and virion production rate. *Journal of Theoretical Biology*, *229*(2), 281–288. doi:10.1016/j.jtbi.2004.04.015 PMID:15207481

Ho, C. Y. F., & Ling, B. W. K. (2010). Initiation of HIV therapy. *International Journal of Bifurcation and Chaos in Applied Sciences and Engineering*, *20*(04), 1279–1292. doi:10.1142/S0218127410026484 PMID:20543654

Ho, W. H., & Chan, A. L. F. (2010). Hybrid Taguchi-differential evolution algorithm for parameter estimation of differential equation models with application to HIV dynamics. *Mathematical Problems in Engineering*.

Huang, Y., Liu, D., & Wu, H. (2006). Hierarchical Bayesian methods for estimation of parameters in a longitudinal HIV dynamic system. *Biometrics*, *62*(2), 413–423. doi:10.1111/j.1541-0420.2005.00447.x PMID:16918905

Iwasa, Y., Michor, F., & Nowak, M. A. (2005). Virus evolution within patients increases pathogenicity. *Journal of Theoretical Biology*, *232*(1), 17–26. doi:10.1016/j.jtbi.2004.07.016 PMID:15498589

Jazwinski, A. H. (1970). *Stochastic Processes and Filtering Theory*. Academic Press.

Joska, J. A., Gouse, H., Paul, R. H., Stein, D. J., & Flisher, A. J. (2010). Does highly active antiretroviral therapy improve neurocognitive function? A systematic review. *Journal of Neurovirology*, *16*(2), 101–114. doi:10.3109/13550281003682513 PMID:20345318

Kamalanand, K., & Jawahar, P. M. (2013). Reconstructed bifurcation diagrams of CD4 cells and HIV-1 viral load dynamics under the effect of antiretroviral drugs. *Network Modeling Analysis in Health Informatics and Bioinformatics*, *2*(4), 303–305. doi:10.1007/s13721-013-0047-5

Kamalanand, K., & Jawahar, P. M. (2014). Hybrid BFPSO algorithm based estimation of optimal drug dosage for antiretroviral therapy in HIV-1 infected patients. *BMC Infectious Diseases*, *14*(Suppl 3), E14. doi:10.1186/1471-2334-14-S3-E14

Kamalanand, K., & Jawahar, P. M. (2015). Prediction of Human Immunodeficiency Virus-1 Viral Load from CD4 Cell Count Using Artificial Neural Networks. *Journal of Medical Imaging and Health Informatics*, *5*(3), 641–646. doi:10.1166/jmihi.2015.1430

Kamalanand, K., & Jawahar, P. M. (n.d.). Unscented Transformation for Estimating the Lyapunov Exponents of Chaotic Time Series Corrupted by Random Noise. International Journal of Mathematical Sciences, 7(4), 1–6.

Kamalanand, K., & Ramakrishnan, S. (2015). Effect of gadolinium concentration on segmentation of vasculature in cardiopulmonary magnetic resonance angiograms. *Journal of Medical Imaging and Health Informatics*, *5*(1), 147–151. doi:10.1166/jmihi.2015.1370

Kamalanand, K., & Srinivasan, S. (2011). Modelling and analysis of normal and atherosclerotic blood vessel mechanics using 3D finite element models. *ICTACT Journal on Soft Computing, special issue on Fuzzy in Industrial and Process Automation, 2*(1), 261-264.

Kim, H. C., Kim, K. Y., Park, J. W., & Lee, H. J. (2001). Electrical impedance tomography reconstruction algorithm using extended Kalman filter. In *Industrial Electronics, 2001. Proceedings. ISIE 2001. IEEE International Symposium on* (Vol. 3, pp. 1677-1681). IEEE. doi:10.1109/ISIE.2001.931960

Kirschner, D. (1996). Using mathematics to understand HIV immune dynamics. *AMS Notices, 43*(2).

Kleeman, L. (1996, January). Understanding and applying Kalman filtering. In *Proceedings of the Second Workshop on Perceptive Systems*. Curtin University of Technology.

Krishnamurthy, K. (2012). A Method for Estimating the Lyapunov Exponents of Chaotic Time Series Corrupted by Random Noise Using Extended Kalman Filter. In *Mathematical Modelling and Scientific Computation* (pp. 237–244). Springer Berlin Heidelberg.

La Scala, B. F., & Bitmead, R. R. (1996). Design of an extended Kalman filter frequency tracer. *IEEE Transactions on Signal Processing*, *44*(3), 739–742. doi:10.1109/78.489052

Lee, M. S., Ju, H., Song, J. W., & Park, C. G. (2015). Kinematic model-based pedestrian dead reckoning for heading correction and lower body motion tracking. *Sensors (Basel, Switzerland)*, *15*(11), 28129–28153. doi:10.3390/s151128129 PMID:26561814

Levy, J. A. (1994). Long-term survivors of HIV infection. *Hospital Practice (Office Ed.)*, *29*(10), 41–44. doi:10.1080/21548331.1994.11443088 PMID:7929674

Liang, H., Miao, H., & Wu, H. (2010). Estimation of constant and time-varying dynamic parameters of HIV infection in a nonlinear differential equation model. *The Annals of Applied Statistics*, *4*(1), 460–483. doi:10.1214/09-AOAS290 PMID:20556240

Lillacci, G., & Khammash, M. (2010). Parameter Identification of Biological Networks Using Extended Kalman Filtering and X2 Criteria.*49th IEEE Conference on Decision and Control*. doi:10.1109/CDC.2010.5717460

Liu, C., & He, B. (2011). Noninvasive estimation of global activation sequence using the extended Kalman filter. *Biomedical Engineering. IEEE Transactions on*, *58*(3), 541–549.

Ljung, L. (1979). Asymptotic behavior of the extended Kalman filter as a parameter estimator for linear systems. *Automatic Control. IEEE Transactions on*, *24*(1), 36–50.

Lyon, A. (2014). Why are Normal Distributions Normal? *The British Journal for the Philosophy of Science*, *65*(3), 621–649. doi:10.1093/bjps/axs046

Manickavasagam, K., Sutha, S., & Kamalanand, K. (2014). Development of Systems for Classification of Different Plasmodium Species in Thin Blood Smear Microscopic Images. *Journal of Advanced Microscopy Research*, *9*(2), 86–92. doi:10.1166/jamr.2014.1194

Mannar Jawahar, P., & Kamalanand, K. (2013). Computational Techniques for Infectious Diseases and Clinical Research. *European Journal for Biomedical Informatics*, *9*(2), 1-2.

McNames, J., & Aboy, M. (2008). Statistical modeling of cardiovascular signals and parameter estimation based on the extended Kalman filter. *Biomedical Engineering. IEEE Transactions on*, *55*(1), 119–129.

Moonchai, S., Lenbury, Y., & Triampo, W. (2010). Cellular automata simulation modeling of HIV infection in lymph node and peripheral blood compartments. *International Journal of Mathematics and Computers in Simulation*, *4*, 124.

Ouattara, D. A. (2005, September). Mathematical analysis of the HIV-1 infection: Parameter estimation, therapies effectiveness, and therapeutical failures. In *27th Annual International Conference of the IEEE Engineering in Medicine and Biology Society, Shanghai, China*. doi:10.1109/IEMBS.2005.1616541

Papoulis, A. (1965). Probability, random variables and stochastic processes. New York: McGraw-Hill.

Perelson, A. S., Kirschner, D. E., & De Boer, R. (1993). Dynamics of HIV infection of CD4+ T cells. *Mathematical Biosciences*, *114*(1), 81–125. doi:10.1016/0025-5564(93)90043-A PMID:8096155

Putter, H., Heisterkamp, S. H., Lange, J. M. A., & De Wolf, F. (2002). A Bayesian approach to parameter estimation in HIV dynamical models. *Statistics in Medicine*, *21*(15), 2199–2214. doi:10.1002/sim.1211 PMID:12210633

Rakshit, M., Panigrahy, D., & Sahu, P. K. (2015). EKF with PSO Technique for Delineation of P And T Wave In Electrocardiogram (ECG) Signal.*2nd International Conference Signal Processing and Integrated Networks (SPIN)*. doi:10.1109/SPIN.2015.7095293

Regtien, P., Van Der Heijden, F., Korsten, M. J., & Otthius, W. (2004). *Measurement science for engineers*. Elsevier.

Reid, J. G. (1987). Normal functions of normal random variables. *Computers & Mathematics with Applications (Oxford, England)*, *14*(3), 157–160. doi:10.1016/0898-1221(87)90147-7

Rigatos, G. G., Rigatou, E. G., & Djida, J. D. (2015). Change detection in the dynamics of an intracellular protein synthesis model using nonlinear Kalman filtering. *Mathematical Biosciences and Engineering*, *12*(5), 1017–1035. doi:10.3934/mbe.2015.12.1017 PMID:26280184

Roche, A., Lahaye, P. J., & Poline, J. B. (2004, April). Incremental activation detection in fMRI series using kalman filtering. In *Biomedical Imaging: Nano to Macro, 2004. IEEE International Symposium on* (pp. 376-379). IEEE. doi:10.1109/ISBI.2004.1398553

Sameni, R., Shamsollahi, M. B., & Jutten, C. (2005). Filtering electrocardiogram signals using the extended Kalman filter. In *Engineering in Medicine and Biology Society, 2005. IEEE-EMBS 2005. 27th Annual International Conference of the* (pp. 5639-5642). IEEE. doi:10.1109/IEMBS.2005.1615765

Shepp, L. (1964). Normal functions of normal random variables. *SIAM Review*, *6*(4), 459–460. doi:10.1137/1006100

Simon, D. (2006). *Optimal state estimation: Kalman, H infinity, and nonlinear approaches*. John Wiley & Sons. doi:10.1002/0470045345

Simon, M. K. (2007). *Probability distributions involving Gaussian random variables: A handbook for engineers and scientists*. Springer Science & Business Media.

Trigo, F. C., Gonzalez-Lima, R., & Amato, M. B. P. (2004). Electrical impedance tomography using the extended Kalman filter. *Biomedical Engineering. IEEE Transactions on*, *51*(1), 72–81.

Van Der Heijden, F., Duin, R., De Ridder, D., & Tax, D. M. (2005). *Classification, parameter estimation and state estimation: an engineering approach using MATLAB*. John Wiley & Sons.

Wan, E., & Van Der Merwe, R. (2000). The unscented Kalman filter for nonlinear estimation. In *Adaptive Systems for Signal Processing, Communications, and Control Symposium 2000. AS-SPCC. The IEEE 2000* (pp. 153-158). IEEE. doi:10.1109/ASSPCC.2000.882463

Wang, G., Krueger, G. R., & Buja, L. M. (2004). A simple model to simulate cellular changes in the T cell system following HIV-1 infection. *Anticancer Research*, *24*(3A), 1689–1698. PMID:15274342

Welch, G., & Bishop, G. (2006). *An introduction to the kalman filter. 2006*. Chapel Hill, NC: University of North Carolina.

Wu, H., Ding, A. A., & De Gruttola, V. (1998). Estimation of HIV dynamic parameters. *Statistics in Medicine*, *17*(21), 2463–2485. doi:10.1002/(SICI)1097-0258(19981115)17:21<2463::AID-SIM939>3.0.CO;2-A PMID:9819839

Wu, H., Zhu, H., Miao, H., & Perelson, A. S. (2008). Parameter identifiability and estimation of HIV/AIDS dynamic models. *Bulletin of Mathematical Biology*, *70*(3), 785–799. doi:10.1007/s11538-007-9279-9 PMID:18247096

Xia, X. (2003). Estimation of HIV/AIDS parameters. *Automatica*, *39*(11), 1983–1988. doi:10.1016/S0005-1098(03)00220-6

KEY TERMS AND DEFINITIONS

AIDS: Acquired Immune Deficiency Syndrome (AIDS) is the spectrum of conditions caused by infection with the human immunodeficiency virus (HIV).

CD4: (Cluster of Differentiation 4) is a glycoprotein which is present on the surface of immune cells namely the T- helper cells, monocytes, macrophages, and dendritic cells.

CD8: (Cluster of differentiation 8) is a trans-membrane glycoprotein which serves as a co-receptor for the T cell receptor.

HIV-1: The most widespread type of HIV strain.

Measurement Noise: The noise that corrupts the state variables while they are measured using a sensor.

Offline Parameter Estimation: Technique of logging data from a process and estimating model parameters after data collection.

Online Parameter Estimation: Technique of estimating model parameters while the process is under operation.

Patient Specific Model: A model tailored for a specific patient.

State Variable: State variables are a set of variables that are used to describe the mathematical state of a dynamical system.

Chapter 5
Two-Directional Two-Dimensional Principal Component Analysis Based on Wavelet Decomposition for High-Dimensional Biomedical Signals Classification

Hong-Bo Xie
Queensland University of Technology, Australia

Tianruo Guo
The University of New South Wales, Australia

ABSTRACT

Here, we present a multi-scale two-directional two-dimensional principal component analysis (MS2D²PCA) method for the efficient and effective extraction of essential feature information from signals. Time-invariant multi-scale matrices are constructed in the first step. The two-directional two-dimensional principal component analysis then operates on the multi-scale matrices to reduce the dimension, rather than vectors in conventional PCA. Results are presented from an experiment to classify twenty hand motions using 89-channel EMG signals recorded in stroke survivors, which illustrates the efficiency and effectiveness of the proposed method for biomedical signal analysis. With this multi-scale two-directional two-dimensional principal component analysis for high-dimensional signal classification, spatial-time-frequency discriminant information from high-dimensional EMG electrode array can be effectively extracted and reduced using the proposed method. Compared with the time domain feature extraction in conjunction with PCA, MS2D²PCA performed better with higher classification accuracy and less PCs in EMG classification. The efficiency and effectiveness of the method can be further validated by using high-dimensional EEG, MEG, fMRI signals. Although the present study focuses on high-dimensional signal pattern classification, based on the PCs obtained at multiple scales, it is relatively straightforward to expand MS2D²PCA for high-dimensional signal compression, denoising, component extraction, and other related tasks.

DOI: 10.4018/978-1-5225-0660-7.ch005

INTRODUCTION AND BACKGROUND

Most biomedical signals are typically non-linear and non-stationary. Time-frequency (TF) analysis including the wavelet transform (WT), offers simultaneous interpretation of the biomedical signal in both the time and frequency domains, allowing the elucidation of local, transient or intermittent components at various scales (Xie, Zheng, & Guo, 2009). However, there are typically a large amount of wavelet coefficients generated from such a two-dimensional analysis. In addition, noise artifacts as well as redundant information may be present in these time-frequency coefficients. Principal component analysis (PCA) decomposes the covariant structure of the dependent variables into orthogonal components by calculating the eigenvalues and eigenvectors of the data covariance matrix. It linearly projects the original data from a high-dimensional space to a set of uncorrelated components in a low-dimensional feature space, while simultaneously preserving the most original information. Therefore, WT combined with PCA (WT-PCA) has been one of the most powerful approaches for simultaneously extracting discriminative features and reducing the dimension for biosignals classification tasks. The basic algorithm for this hybrid method consists of decomposing biomedical signals into the time-frequency plane, re-arranging the time-frequency elements into a row vector, and reducing the dimension using PCA. Examples of application of this algorithm in the area of electromyographic (EMG) signal analysis include Englehart et al. (Chan, Englehart, Hudgins, & Lovely, 2001; Engelhart, Hudgins, Parker, & Stevenson, 1999), who decomposed four channels of transient EMG signals using short-time Fourier transform (STFT), WT, and wavelet packet transform (WPT) methods to discriminate six hand motions for prosthetic hand control. They compared the performance of PCA feature reduction against the Euclidean distance class separability (CS) criterion. The results indicated TF-PCA was vastly superior to TF-CS in classification accuracy, as well as a significant improvement of all TF-based methods compared to time domain feature extraction when using a linear discriminant analysis (LDA) classifier. The study of Khezri and Jahed (Khezri & Jahed, 2007) using adaptive neuro-fuzzy inference system further confirmed the superiority of TF-PCA hybridization in EMG-based hand motion pattern recognition. Chan et al. (Chan et al., 2001) performed a comparative study to identify acoustic words from 'one' to 'nine' from facial EMG signals. They found similar effectiveness and applicability of TF-PCA methods in speech recognition, especially WT-PCA. Chu et al. (Chu, Moon, & Mun, 2006) improved the TF-PCA technique by employing a self-organizing feature map (SOFM) to transform PCA-reduced TF features into a new feature space with high class separability. Kiatpanichagij and Afzulpurkar (Kiatpanichagij & Afzulpurkar, 2009) inserted an entropy-based supervised discretization procedure between the WPT and PCA steps to improve EMG classifier generalization and training speed on overlapping segmented signals. Qi et al. (Qi, Wakeling, Green, Lambrecht, & Ferguson-Pell, 2011) utilized the principal components of EMG intensity spectra obtained from non-linearly-scaled wavelets to compare motor unit recruitment patterns during isometric ramp and step muscle contractions, as well as dynamic concentric and eccentric contractions of the human biceps brachii. The same WT-PCA scheme was also employed to discriminate between fast and slow muscle fibers (Von Tscharner & Goepfert, 2006), investigate motor unit recruitment patterns between and within muscles of the triceps muscles (J. M. Wakeling, Uehli, & Rozitis, 2006), as well as quantify dynamic muscle dysfunction in children and young adults with cerebral palsy (J. Wakeling, Delaney, & Dudkiewicz, 2007). Weiderpass et al. (Weiderpass et al., 2013) investigated the alternations of thigh and calf muscles recruitment strategies during gait among non-diabetic and diabetic neuropathic patients by using an adaptive optimal kernel time-frequency representation and discrete WT followed by PCA.

For electrocardiographic (ECG) analysis, Martis et al. (Martis et al., 2012) developed an approach for discriminating arrhythmia from normal sinus rhythm based on feature extraction using discrete Daubechies-4 wavelet transform as well as feature reduction using PCA. Korurek and Nizam (Korurek & Nizam, 2010) employed the PCA compressed discrete Daubechies-5 wavelet coefficients to classify normal heart beats and five types of arrhythmia for the diagnosis of cardiovascular disease. Ghorbanian et al. (Ghorbanian, Jalali, Ghaffari, & Nataraj, 2012) conducted a similar study to analyse five symptoms of heart failure using a continuous Haar wavelet transform followed by PCA reduction and multi-layered perceptron neural network classification. They evaluated the proposed algorithm using the MIT-BIH database, resulting in 99.5% sensitivity, 99.66% positive predictive accuracy, and 99.17% total accuracy. More recently, Martis et al. (Giri et al., 2013) further compared the effects of wavelet coefficient reduction by PCA, independent component analysis (ICA), and linear discriminant analysis (LDA) for automated diagnosis of five types of arrhythmia. Giri et al. (Giri et al., 2013) carried out a similar comparative study for the automatic detection of coronary artery disease using PCA, ICA, and LDA to reduce the number of discrete WT coefficients extracted from particular ECG signal sub-bands. A similar WT-PCA approach was also applied to automatically detect electroencephalographic (EEG) analysis epileptic activity (Acharya, Sree, Alvin, & Suri, 2012) and classify right and left hand movement (Azar, Balas, & Olariu, 2014) for brain-machine interface control. Furthermore, atherosclerosis and four types of brain blood vessel disease were diagnosed by WT-PCA from Doppler ultrasound signals by Dirgenali and Uguz (Uguz, 2012).

Although the TF-PCA algorithm, particularly WT-PCA, has achieved great success in the analysis of various biomedical signals, most of these applications have been based on single site or multiple channel (typically <10) recordings. More recently, with the improvements in physiological measurement equipment for EMG, EEG, and magnetoencephalography (MEG), new technology permits registration of up to 256 channels using high-density multi-electrode arrays. Such arrays with small electrode sizes and inter-electrode spacing can cover large areas of the tissue, providing extra spatial information which is largely independent of any "classical" temporal information. A question naturally arising is whether TF-PCA continues to be superior for the analysis of high-dimensional biomedical signals analysis. In TF-PCA, the time-frequency elements must be transformed into a 1D array row by row. If the scheme of TF-PCA is duplicated directly to high-dimensional data, concatenating the huge number of TF coefficients into a 1D array leads to a high-dimensional vector space, where it is difficult to evaluate the covariance matrix accurately due to its large size as well as the relatively small number of training samples. Besides the 'curse of dimensionality' dilemma and 'small sample size' problem, computing the eigenvectors of a large covariance matrix is computationally expensive. Furthermore, there are other issues such as numerical instability in the subsequent pattern recognition as well as lowering down the computational complexity and storage requirements, among others.

From the point of view of biomedical application, sub-band signals have different physiological meanings. For example, EEG α, β, γ waves relate to particular brain function, whilst the 5-40 Hz EMG band reflects the firing rate of motor units, with higher than 40 Hz relates to the form of motor unit action potentials (Karlsson, Roeleveld, Gronlund, Holtermann, & Ostlund, 2009). If we arrange all the time-frequency coefficients for different sub-bands into a 1D array to perform PCA, any physiological or physical meaning of the obtained PCs is lost. Local principal component analysis (LPCA) advocates dividing a complex high dimensional data set into multiple subsets with specific characteristics (Einbeck, Evers, & Bailer-Jones, 2008). The original data set is then presented by multiple PCA subset representations. This subspace segmentation not only fits the original data set with lower error, but also ensures that the PCs of subsets have corresponding physical meaning.

In fact, a two-dimensional time-frequency plane can be regarded as an image. It is thus feasible to apply image processing techniques to indicate time-frequency matrix (TFM) characteristics. Two-dimensional principal component analysis (2DPCA) developed by Yang et al. (Yang, Zhang, Frangi, & Yang, 2004) is a 2D image representation and reduction technique, in which an image matrix does not need to be transformed into a 1D array. Many experimental results have indicated that 2DPCA is computationally more efficient than PCA in the extraction of image features (Mashhoori & Jahromi, 2013). Although 2DPCA is typically able to obtain a higher recognition accuracy than PCA, a vital unresolved problem is that 2DPCA needs many more coefficients for image or TF matrix representation than PCA (D. Q. Zhang & Zhou, 2005). If 2DPCA is applied to the time-frequency matrix of high-dimensional biomedical signals, a similar dilemma to that of PCA remains. Zhang and Zhou (D. Q. Zhang & Zhou, 2005) indicated that 2DPCA essentially operates along the row direction of the image matrix and, thus, proposed an alternative 2DPCA operating along the column direction. By simultaneously considering the row and column directions, they developed the two-directional two-dimensional principal component analysis ($2D^2PCA$) for a more efficient image representation and recognition. Inspired by LPCA and $2D^2PCA$ in imaging processing, the purpose of this study is to develop an efficient and effective time-frequency feature extraction method for fully exploiting the spatial-time-frequency (STF) information of high-dimensional biomedical signals. The key idea is that the high-dimensional signals in the same sub-band have similar physiological characteristics and range of values. It is, therefore, natural to divide the time-frequency representation of such high-dimensional signals into multi-scale matrices, which consider both the spatial correlation and the physiological characteristics of sub-band signals between channels. $2D^2PCA$ is then performed to reduce the dimension of multi-scale matrices in a highly efficient manner for pattern classification. The method is, therefore, termed as multi-scale two-directional two-dimensional principal component analysis ($MS2D^2PCA$). To illustrate the efficiency and effectiveness of the proposed method, results are presented on the recognition of 20 hand movements from 89-channel EMG signals recorded in stroke survivors.

METHODS

Principal Component Analysis (PCA)

Principal component analysis has been called one of the most valuable results from applied linear algebra. PCA is used abundantly in all forms of analysis - from biomedical signals to medical images - because it is a simple, non-parametric method of extracting relevant information from confusing data sets. With minimal additional effort PCA provides a roadmap for how to reduce a complex data set to a lower dimension to reveal the sometimes hidden, simplified dynamics that often underlie it.

The derivation of principal components is based on the assumption that the signal **x** is a zero-mean random process being characterized by the correlation $R_x = E[\mathbf{x}\mathbf{x}^T]$. The principal components of **x** result from applying an orthonormal linear transformation $\Psi = [\psi_1, \psi_2, \cdots, \psi_p]$ to **x**,

$$\mathbf{w} = \Psi^T \mathbf{x}, \tag{1}$$

so that the elements of the principal component vector $\mathbf{w} = [w_1, w_2, \cdots, w_p]^T$ become mutually uncorrelated. The first principal component is obtained as a scalar product $w_1 = \psi_1^T \mathbf{x}$, where the vector ψ_1 is chosen so that the variance of w_1,

$$E[w_1^2] = E[\psi_1^T \mathbf{x}\mathbf{x}^T \psi_1] = \psi_1^T \mathrm{R}_x \psi_1 \tag{2}$$

is maximized subject to the constraint that $\psi_1^T \psi_1 = 1$. The maximal variance is obtained when ψ_1 is chosen as the normalized eigenvector corresponding to the largest eigenvalue of R_x, as denoted λ_1 ; the resulting variance is

$$E[w_1^2] = \psi_1^T \mathrm{R}_x \psi_1 = \lambda_1 \psi_1^T \psi_1 = \lambda. \tag{3}$$

Subject to the constraint that w_1 and the second principal component w_2 should be uncorrelated, w_2 is obtained by choosing ψ_2 as the eigenvector corresponding to the second largest eigenvalue of R_x, and so on until the variance of **x** is completely represented by $\mathbf{w}$. Accordingly, to obtain the whole set of *p* different principal components, the eigenvector equation for R_x needs to be solved,

$$R_x \Psi = \Psi \Lambda, \tag{4}$$

where Λ denotes a diagonal matrix with the eigenvalues $\lambda_1, \lambda_2, \cdots, \lambda_p$. Since R_x is rarely known in practice, the $p \times p$ sample correlation matrix, defined by

$$\hat{R}_x = \frac{1}{M} \mathbf{X}\mathbf{X}^T, \tag{5}$$

replaces R_x when the eigenvectors are calculated in Equation (4).

Two-Directional Two-Dimensional Principal Component Analysis (2D²PCA)

Figure 1 shows a schematic diagram of 2D²PCA, in this case using an example input TFM obtained from multichannel EMG recordings (refer to Section 2.4 for details of the EMG protocol). Without loss of generality, we consider an *m* by *n* time-frequency matrix $\mathbf{A}$ obtained from any time-frequency decomposition. Let $\mathbf{X} \in \Re^{n \times q}$ and $\mathbf{Y} \in \Re^{m \times p}$ be matrices having orthonormal columns $n \times q$ and $m \times p$, respectively. We can simultaneously project **A** onto $\mathbf{X}$ to yield the $m \times q$ matrix $\mathbf{B} = \mathbf{AX}$, and onto $\mathbf{Y}$ to yield the $p \times n$ matrix $\mathbf{C} = \mathbf{Y}^T \mathbf{A}$. In contrast to conventional PCA for one-dimensional array applications, 2D²PCA operates on a matrix in both horizontal and vertical directions. The total scatter of the projected samples, a measure of the discriminatory power of a projection matrix, can be characterized by its trace of the covariance matrix of the projected matrix. From this point of view, maximisation of the generalized total scatter is the criterion adopted to find the optimal projection matrices $\mathbf{X}$ and $\mathbf{Y}$ for row and column directions, respectively:

Figure 1. Schematic diagram of two-directional two-dimensional principal component analysis to obtain the reduced time-frequency matrix F (right) from an input time-frequency matrix A (left)

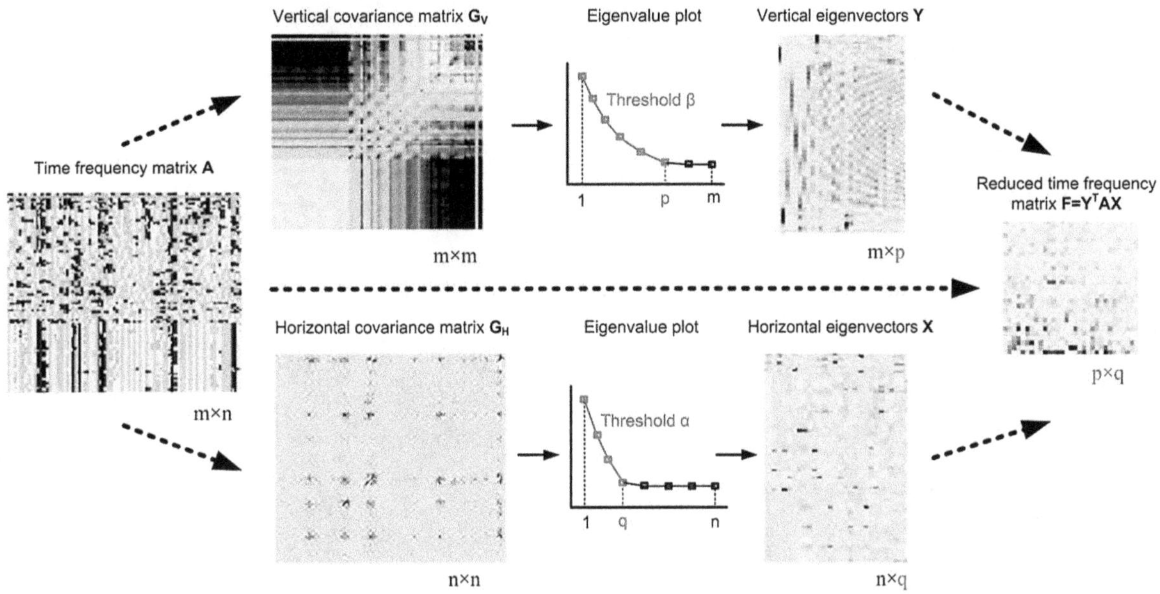

$$
\begin{aligned}
J(\mathbf{X}) &= tr\{E[(\mathbf{B}-E(\mathbf{B}))(\mathbf{B}-E(\mathbf{B}))^T]\} \\
&= tr\{E[(\mathbf{AX}-E(\mathbf{AX}))(\mathbf{AX}-E(\mathbf{AX}))^T]\} \\
&= tr\{\mathbf{X}^T E[(\mathbf{A}-E(\mathbf{A}))^T(\mathbf{A}-E(\mathbf{A})]\mathbf{X}\},
\end{aligned} \tag{6}
$$

$$
\begin{aligned}
J(\mathbf{Y}) &= tr\{E[(\mathbf{C}-E(\mathbf{C}))(\mathbf{C}-E(\mathbf{C}))^T]\} \\
&= tr\{E[(\mathbf{Y}^T\mathbf{A}-E(\mathbf{Y}^T\mathbf{A}))(\mathbf{Y}^T\mathbf{A}-E(\mathbf{Y}^T\mathbf{A}))^T]\} \\
&= tr\{\mathbf{Y}^T E[(\mathbf{A}-E(\mathbf{A}))(\mathbf{A}-E(\mathbf{A}))^T]\mathbf{Y}\},
\end{aligned} \tag{7}
$$

where $tr\{\bullet\}$ is the trace.

Considering the $m \times q$ matrix $\mathbf{B} = \mathbf{AX}$ obtained by projecting $\mathbf{A}$ onto $\mathbf{X}$ in Equation (6), the horizontal covariance matrix is denoted by

$$
\mathbf{G}_h = E[(\mathbf{A}-E(\mathbf{A}))^T(\mathbf{A}-E(\mathbf{A}))], \tag{8}
$$

which is an $n \times n$ positive semi-definite matrix.

Suppose that the training feature set is $\boldsymbol{\Omega} = (\mathbf{A}_1, \mathbf{A}_2, \cdots, \mathbf{A}_\mathrm{N})$, where each $\mathbf{A}_i (i = 1, 2, \cdots, \mathrm{N})$ denotes the *i*th $m \times n$ time-frequency matrix and $\mathbf{N}$ is the number of training samples. The average TFM is given by

$$
\bar{\mathbf{A}} = \frac{1}{N}\sum_{i=1}^{N} \mathbf{A}_i \tag{9}
$$

Denoting the *k*th row vectors of $\mathbf{A}_i$ and $\bar{\mathbf{A}}$ by $\mathbf{A}_i^k$ and $\bar{\mathbf{A}}_h^k$, respectively, these TFMs can be represented by

$$\mathbf{A}_i = [(\mathbf{A}_i^1)^T, (\mathbf{A}_i^2)^T, \cdots, (\mathbf{A}_i^m)^T]^T, \tag{10}$$

and

$$\bar{\mathbf{A}} = [(\bar{\mathbf{A}}_h^1)^T, (\bar{\mathbf{A}}_h^2)^T, \cdots, (\bar{\mathbf{A}}_h^m)^T]^T. \tag{11}$$

The horizontal covariance matrix can then be obtained from the outer product of these TFM row vectors:

$$\begin{aligned}\mathbf{G}_h &= \frac{1}{N}\sum_{i=1}^{N}\left(\mathbf{A}_i - \bar{\mathbf{A}}\right)^T\left(\mathbf{A}_i - \bar{\mathbf{A}}\right)\\ &= \frac{1}{N}\sum_{i=1}^{N}\sum_{k=1}^{m}\left(\mathbf{A}_i^k - \bar{\mathbf{A}}_h^k\right)^T\left(\mathbf{A}_i^k - \bar{\mathbf{A}}_h^k\right)\end{aligned} \tag{12}$$

Similarly, for the $p \times n$ matrix $\mathbf{C} = \mathbf{Y}^T\mathbf{A}$ obtained by projecting $\mathbf{A}$ onto $\mathbf{Y}$ in Equation (7), the vertical covariance matrix can be denoted by

$$\mathbf{G}_v = E[(\mathbf{A} - E(\mathbf{A}))(\mathbf{A} - E(\mathbf{A}))^T], \tag{13}$$

which is $m \times m$ positive semi-definite matrix.

TMFs and their average are now denoted by column vectors:

$$\mathbf{A}_i = [(\mathbf{A}_i^1)^T, (\mathbf{A}_i^2)^T, \cdots, (\mathbf{A}_i^n)], \tag{14}$$

$$\bar{\mathbf{A}} = [(\bar{\mathbf{A}}_v^1)^T, (\bar{\mathbf{A}}_v^2)^T, \cdots, (\bar{\mathbf{A}}_v^n)]. \tag{15}$$

where $\mathbf{A}_i^j$ and $\bar{\mathbf{A}}_v^j$ denote the *j*th column vectors of $\mathbf{A}_i$ and $\bar{\mathbf{A}}$, respectively.

Now, the vertical covariance matrix of Equation (13) can be constructed from the outer products of column vectors:

$$\begin{aligned}\mathbf{G}_v &= \frac{1}{N}\sum_{i=1}^{N}(\mathbf{A}_i - \bar{\mathbf{A}}_h)(\mathbf{A}_i - \bar{\mathbf{A}}_h)^T\\ &= \frac{1}{N}\sum_{i=1}^{N}\sum_{j=1}^{n}(\mathbf{A}_i^j - \bar{\mathbf{A}}_v^j)(\mathbf{A}_i^j - \bar{\mathbf{A}}_v^j)^T\end{aligned} \tag{16}$$

Zhang and Zhou (D. Q. Zhang & Zhou, 2005) demonstrated that the optimal projection matrices $\mathbf{X}$ and $\mathbf{Y}$ are composed of the orthonormal eigenvectors $\mathbf{X}_1, \mathbf{X}_2, \cdots, \mathbf{X}_q$ of $\mathbf{G}_h$ corresponding to the *q* largest eigenvalues and $\mathbf{Y}_1, \mathbf{Y}_2, \cdots, \mathbf{Y}_p$ of $\mathbf{G}_v$ corresponding to the p largest eigenvalues, respectively. The value of p or q can be controlled by simple threshold settings as follows:

$$\frac{\sum_{k=1}^{q} \lambda_k}{\sum_{k=1}^{n} \lambda_k} \geq \alpha \tag{17}$$

$$\frac{\sum_{j=1}^{p} \lambda_j}{\sum_{j=1}^{m} \lambda_j} \geq \beta \tag{18}$$

where $\lambda_1, \lambda_2, \cdots \lambda_q$ (λ_p) are the q (p) largest eigenvalues of $\mathbf{G}_h$ ($\mathbf{G}_v$) and α and β are pre-set thresholds. In practice, we set a ratio γ of total energy preserved as in PCA (for example >85%) and then set $\alpha = \beta$, each corresponding to the energy conservation rate.

After obtaining the projection matrices $\mathbf{X}$ and $\mathbf{Y}$, 2D^{2}PCA projects the m by n TFM $\mathbf{A}$ onto $\mathbf{X}$ and $\mathbf{Y}$ simultaneously, yielding the reduced p by q matrix

$$\mathbf{F} = \mathbf{Y}^T \mathbf{A} \mathbf{X}. \tag{19}$$

Using the above procedure, an $m \times n$ dimensional feature matrix $\mathbf{A}$ is projected into a $p \times q$ dimensional feature matrix $\mathbf{F}$.

Robust Covariance Matrix Estimation

A characteristic property of most biomedical signals is that they often contain outliers. For example, EMG signals are typically contaminated by the ECG, crosstalk, motion artefact, random amplifier noise, as well as power line interference and its harmonics. The 2D^{2}PCA algorithm involves the estimation of covariance matrices in two directions, each of which may be affected by outliers which alter the variances and the correlation. Moreover, their condition number may be substantially increased due to outliers. As a result, the orientation of eigenvectors and the subspace spanned by the principal components are thus significantly distorted. Such perturbation in the eigenvectors leads to skewed projection directions estimated by the 2D^{2}PCA. Several methods have been proposed for robustly estimating the covariance matrix, including the minimum covariance determinant (MCD), S-estimator, as well as the use of memberships to control the effect of each data point on the covariance matrix (Heo, Gader, & Frigui, 2009). However, most of these methods are not computationally efficient, and we have proposed the use of time-frequency soft threshold method to denoise the TFM prior to estimation of the covariance matrix in order to eliminate outlier interference (Han, Liu, Xi, & Guo, 2007). The soft threshold is defined by

$$\lambda = \sigma \sqrt{2 \ln P}, \tag{20}$$

where $\sigma = Q/0.6745$ is a rough estimate of the signal variance. Q is the median absolute deviation of wavelet coefficients, and P is the total number of points at the corresponding decomposition level.

Time-Frequency Analysis

Most biomedical signals are characterized by time-varying signal properties, i.e. from the statistical perspective, they are non-stationary. Therefore, time-variant signal processing methods have been part of the standard repertoire in biomedical signal analysis. Both the frequency distribution and time-frequency characteristics of transient signal components are particularly useful for biomedical signal detection, classification, and prediction, leading to more frequently applications of time-variant analysis methods. Transient, spindle-like oscillations are almost always synonymous with transient signal components in EEG/MEG analysis. Therefore, brain computer interface and epileptic seizure prediction research are inconceivable without the use of time-frequency processing techniques (da Silva, 2013). Another example is the time-variant analysis of the cardiorespiratory system, where the main goal is the quantification of short-term and long-term variations of ongoing oscillations (respiratory movements, blood pressure waves) (Addison, 2005). EMG signal is an integrated part of motor control and gait balance analyses in which all recordings are time-variant (Xie & Wang, 2006). There could be many more examples like these. Signal components with time-variant properties may occur at different frequencies. Therefore, time-variant, frequency-selective approaches are required for their "time-frequency" analysis. The algorithms which make time-frequency analysis possible are called time-frequency techniques. The best-known and most frequently applied techniques in biomedical engineering are the short-time Fourier transform, wavelet transform, wavelet packet transform (Addison, 2005; da Silva, 2013; Wacker & Witte, 2013; Xie & Wang, 2006). In this Chapter, we focus on develop the 2D^{2}PCA based on discrete wavelet transform, thus, only a brief introduction of discrete wavelet transform is provided. Readers may refer to other publications for details of time-frequency analysis and its applications in biomedical signal processing.

The procedure of discrete wavelet decomposition of a signal $x[n]$ is schematically shown in Figure 2. Each stage of this scheme consists of two digital filters and two downsamplers by 2. The first filter, $g[\bullet]$ is the discrete mother wavelet, high-pass in nature, and the second, $h[\bullet]$ is its mirror version, low-pass in nature. The downsampled outputs of first high-pass and low-pass filters provide the detail, D_1 and the approximation, A_1, respectively. The first approximation A_1 is further decomposed and this process is continued as shown in Figure 2.

Figure 2. The procedure of discrete wavelet decomposition of a signal x[n]

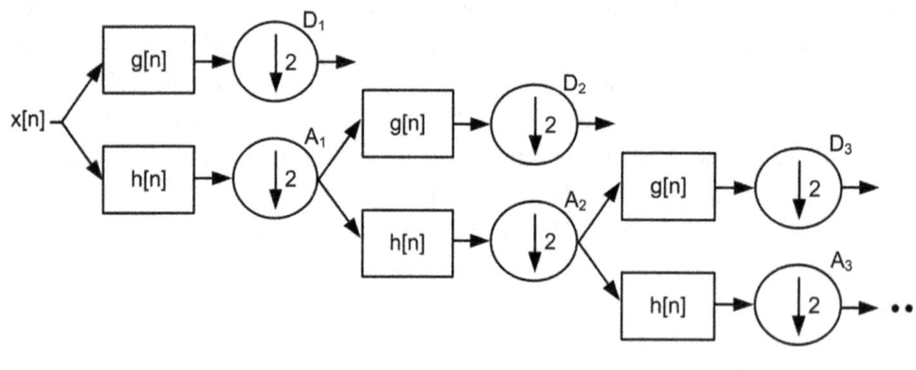

All wavelet transforms can be specified in terms of a low-pass filter *h*, which satisfies the standard quadrature mirror filter condition,

$$H(z)H(z^{-1}) + H(-z)H(-z^{-1}) = 1, \tag{21}$$

where $H(z)$ denotes the *z*-transform of filter *h*. Its complementary high-pass filter can be defined as

$$G(z) = zH(-z^{-1}). \tag{22}$$

A sequence of filters with increasing length (indexed by *i*) can be obtained:

$$\begin{aligned} H_{i+1}(z) &= H(z^{2^i})H_i(z) \\ G_{i+1}(z) &= G(z^{2^i})H_i(z) \end{aligned}, \tag{23}$$

where $i = 0, 1, \cdots, I-1$ and the initial condition $H_0(z) = 1$. It is expressed as a two-scale relation in time domain

$$\begin{aligned} h_{i+1}(k) &= [h]_{\uparrow 2^i} * h_i(k) \\ g_{i+1}(k) &= [g]_{\uparrow 2^i} * h_i(k) \end{aligned}, \tag{24}$$

where the subscript $[\bullet]_{\uparrow m}$ indicates the up-sampling by a factor of *m* and *k* is the equally sampled discrete time.

The normalised wavelet and scale basis function $\varphi_{i,l}(k)$, $\xi_{i,l}(k)$ can be defined as

$$\begin{aligned} \varphi_{i,l}(k) &= 2^{i/2} h_i(k - 2^i l) \\ \xi_{i,l}(k) &= 2^{i/2} g_i(k - 2^i l) \end{aligned}, \tag{25}$$

where the factor $2^{i/2}$ is an inner product normalisation, I and l are the scale and translation parameter, respectively. The discrete wavelet transform can thus be described as

$$\begin{aligned} a_{(i)}(l) &= x(k) * \varphi_{i,l}(k) \\ d_{(i)}(l) &= x(k) * \xi_{i,l}(k) \end{aligned}, \tag{26}$$

where $a_{(i)}(l)$ and $d_{(i)}(l)$ are the approximation and detail coefficients at resolution *i*, respectively.

Multi-Scale Two Directional Two-Dimensional Principal Component Analysis (MS2D²PCA)

In this section, we describe the multi-scale two directional two-dimensional principal component analysis algorithm based on the construction of multi-scale spatial-time-frequency matrices, as well as the use of the method to extract discriminant feature information from these matrices. Figure 3 illustrates the proposed algorithm, which can be described as follows:

Figure 3. Multi-scale two-directional two-dimensional principal component analysis method for high-dimensional biomedical signal classification. S is the number of channels, the D_{ij} represents discrete wavelet detail coefficients vector for channel i at scale j and the A_{iL} denotes the corresponding approximation coefficients vector for channel i

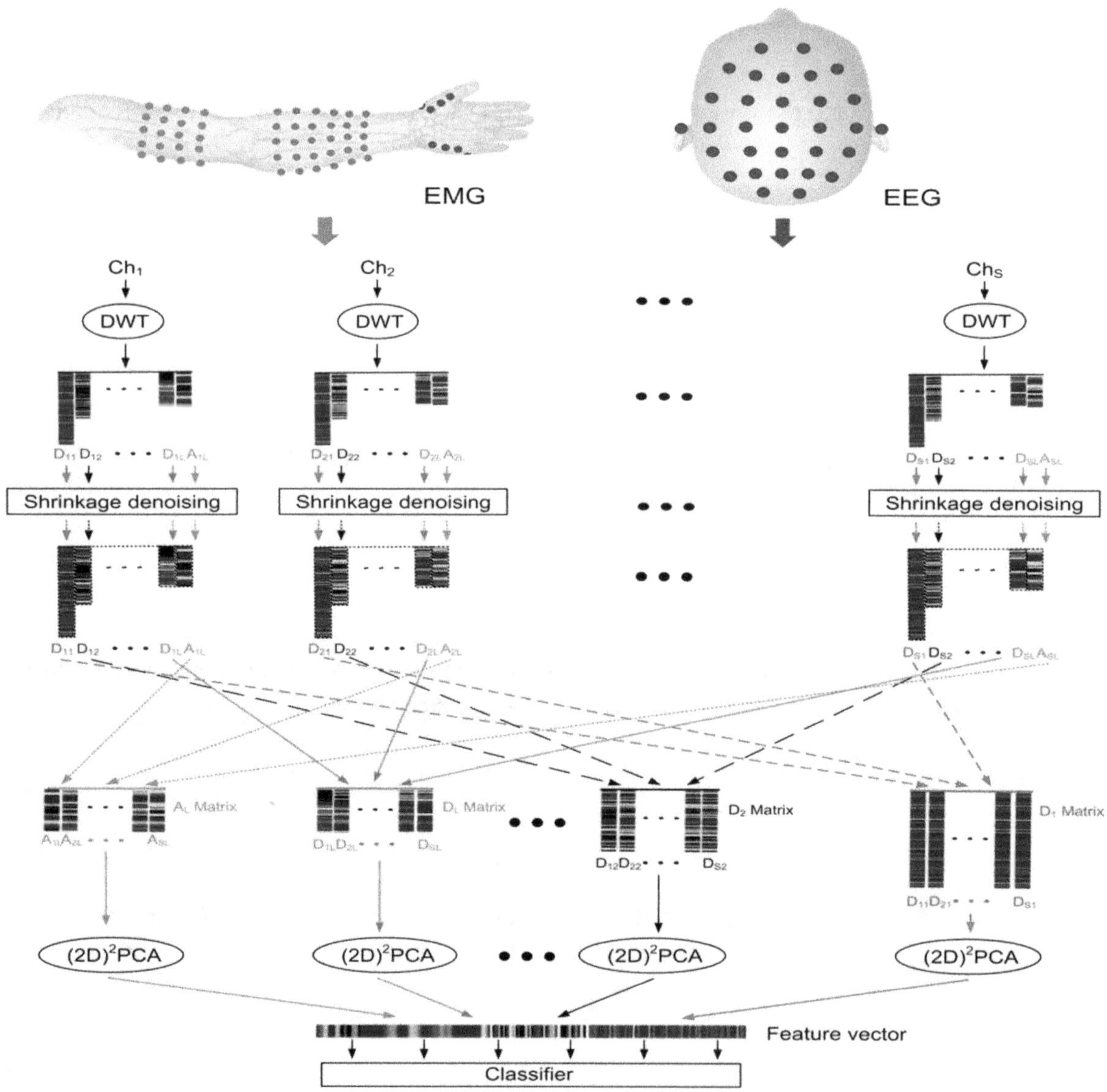

1. High-dimensional signals in channels 1 to S are first segmented by a moving window. Choose an appropriate time-frequency decomposition method. That is, specify the mother wavelet function and decomposition depth. The discrete wavelet transform is then employed to decompose each time-segment of individual channels into details $D_1, D_2, \cdots, D_L$ and approximate A_L under the same decomposition level L.
2. The Wavelet shrinkage soft threshold method (Han et al., 2007) is then employed to denoise the coefficients at each scale.
3. The multi-scale matrices are constructed: The wavelet approximation coefficients A_L from each of the S decompositions are collected into one matrix $\mathbf{A}_L$, where the gth ($g = 1, 2, \cdots, S$) row of $\mathbf{A}_L$ consists of the approximation coefficients of channel g. Similarly, the wavelet details D_1 to D_L for each of the S decompositions are collected into L matrices $\mathbf{D}_1$ to $\mathbf{D}_L$, where the gth row of D_h $(h = 1, 2, \cdots, L)$ consists of the detail coefficients of channel g at scale h. It should be noted that the sizes of matrices $\mathbf{A}_L$ and $\mathbf{D}_L$ are equal, whilst the sizes of $\mathbf{D}_1$ to $\mathbf{D}_L$ vary. A total of $(L+1)$ matrices is formed, each containing the spatial-time-frequency correlation information within the signal channels at the corresponding scale.
4. $2D^2$PCA is subsequently carried out on each of the $(L+1)$ matrices to extract the most informative features, as well as reduce the dimension based on the user-specified threshold of total energy preserved.
5. The reduced feature matrices are sequenced into a vector.
6. Since the discriminant abilities of principal components (PCs) at various scales are different, a simple distance-based technique is applied to re-order all PCs (Xie, Zheng, & Guo, 2009).
7. Only those PCs with high discriminant ability are retained and others are discarded.
8. Finally, the performance of the algorithm can be evaluated by feeding the vector of optimal PCs obtained into a classifier.

Note that the wavelet transform in step (1) can be replaced by other time-frequency representation methods, such as short time Fourier transform, continuous wavelet transform, wavelet packet transform, S transform, multivariate empirical mode decomposition, and symplctic geometry spectrum analysis, among others (Xie & Dokos, 2013a, 2013b; Xie, Guo, Sivakumar, Liew, & Dokos, 2014; Xie & Wang, 2006; Xie, Zheng, & Guo, 2009). However, the manner to construct the multi-scale matrices is the same, arranging those coefficients at the same scale or sub-band into one matrix.

Classifier Scheme

Three typical EMG classifiers, support vector machine (SVM) (Xie, Zheng, Guo, Chen, & Shi, 2009), extreme learning machine (ELM) (Huang, Zhou, Ding, & Zhang, 2012), and Gaussian mixture model (GMM) (X. Zhang & Zhou, 2012), were employed to evaluate the classification performance of the proposed algorithm. SVM constructs the optimal hyperplane with largest margin for separating data between two groups. For two-dimensional data, single hyperplane is enough to separate the data into two groups such as +1 or -1. Two hyperplanes are needed to separate the data points for three-dimensional data. For the multi-classification problem in this study, one against one technique is employed to extend the binary classifier for multiple hand motion recognition. ELM which is a Single-hidden Layer Feed forward Neural network (SLFN) with at most L hidden nodes and with almost any nonlinear activation function can exactly learn L distinct observations. ELM can be considered as a linear system after the input weights and the hidden layer biases are chosen randomly. The output weights (linking the hidden layer to the output layer) of ELM can be analytically determined through simple generalized inverse operation of the hidden layer output matrices. ELM can approximate any target continuous function and classify any disjoint regions. The GMM is a parametric probability density function represented as a weighted sum of Gaussian component densities. It assumes that the features are normally distributed, and each class is characterized by its mean and covariance matrix. GMM is commonly used as a parametric model of the probability distribution of continuous measurements or features in a biometric system, such as vocal-tract related spectral features in the speaker recognition system. GMM parameters are estimated from training data using the iterative expectation-maximization (EM) algorithm or maximum A-posteriori (MAP) estimation from a well-trained prior model.

Experimental Protocol and Performance Evaluation

Data used to validate the proposed algorithm are 89-channel high-density EMG signals recorded from 12 stroke subjects on the affected side of the upper arm, forearm and hand. The initial purpose of this data collection was to recognise arm and hand movements for robot-aided stroke rehabilitation to improve upper limb function (X. Zhang & Zhou, 2012). The experimental protocol for each subject consisted of 20 functional finger, hand, wrist, and elbow movements. Details relating to electrode placements and 20 arm/hand movements are described in Zhang and Zhou (X. Zhang & Zhou, 2012). Each experimental trial contained five repetitions of one movement. The surface EMG signals were sampled at 2000 Hz per channel, filtered with a fourth-order Butterworth band-pass filter (30–500 Hz) to remove movement artifacts and high-frequency noise. For each movement, the recorded EMG data was composed of five active segments corresponding to five repetitions of muscle contraction. For each active segment, the 89-channel EMG data were further segmented into a series of overlapping windows (window length: 256 ms, overlap step: 128 ms). Low decomposition level often leads to information loss whilst large decomposition level increases the computational cost without performance improvement. A mother wavelet was employed to simultaneously decompose 89-channel signals over five levels. The remaining procedures for $MS2D^2PCA$ described in Section 2.3 were employed to extract the multi-scale PCs. SVM, ELM, and GMM were employed to evaluate the classification performance of the proposed algorithm. The accuracy for each test was the percentage of correctly classified windows over all the testing windows including all the movements. Since the recorded EMG data consisted of five active segments for each movement, for each subject, the performance was evaluated as the averaged accuracy across the five-folds. In five-fold cross-validation, the original EMG data is partitioned into five equal sized subsamples. Of the five subsamples, a single subsample is retained to test the classification performance, and the remaining four subsamples are used as training data. The cross-validation process is then repeated five times (the *folds*), with each of the five subsamples used exactly once as the test data. The five results from the folds were then averaged. An overall performance was then evaluated as the mean and standard (SD) of classification accuracies across all the subjects.

RESULTS

Spatial Multi-Scale Muscle Activity Patterns

Using the proposed multi-scale spatial matrix technique, the spatial EMG activity at each scale was obtained. Since approximate coefficients at level 5 contained considerable low-frequency artifact, whilst the detail coefficients for level 1 corresponded to high-frequency components greater than 500 Hz, both of these were discarded in the analysis. Figure 4 shows the typical contour plots obtained for the twenty movements for subject 5 at scales D2-D5 of Coiflet 4 mother wavelet. The five panels from left to right in the first row corresponded to the spatial-time-frequency activities of intended movements corresponding to ulnar wrist up, fingers 3-5 flexion, index-finger flexion, thumb extension, and wrist extension. With each intended movement, a significant difference between the intensity of the surface EMG signals at D2 over the upper limb muscles can be readily discerned in these contour plots. The second row of Figure 4 indicates the STF distributions of hand open, elbow flexion, wrist supination, index-finger extension, and wrist pronation at scale D3. The third row displays EMG activities corresponding to wrist flexion, elbow extension, hand closing, tip pinch, thumb flexion at scale D4. The final row of Figure 4 displays the specific characteristics of the five remaining movements, namely fingers 3-5 extension, lateral pinch, fine pinch, gun posture, and ulnar wrist down. Similar to the panels in the top row, there was significant discrepancy in the intensity distributions of the remaining contour plots, indicating useful discriminant information in the multi-scale matrices.

Figure 4. Contour plots of multi-scale matrices for 89-channel EMG traces of 20 hand movements obtained from subject 5

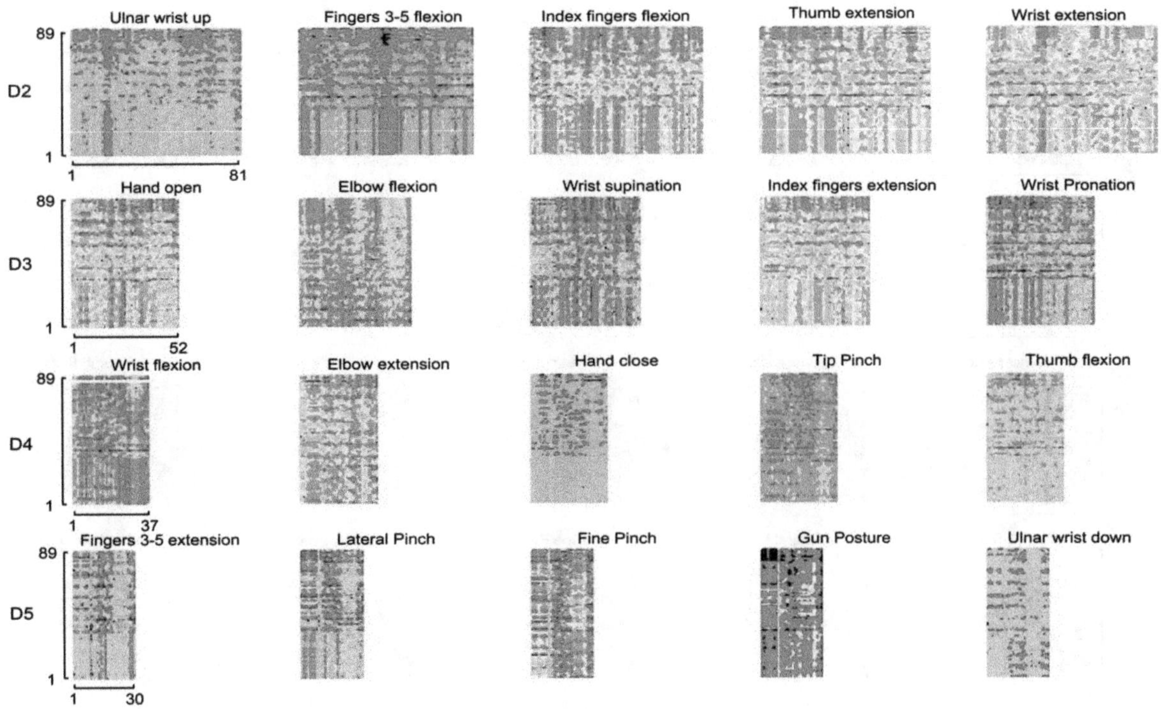

The proposed two-directional two-dimensional principal component analysis was then used to reduce the dimension of each matrix. Figure 5 shows the contour plots of each matrix in Figure 3 following dimension reduction using 2D²PCA when the energy conservation rate and total energy preserved were 98% and 88% respectively. Compared with Figure 4, the intensity difference between certain sub-panels in Figure 4 is further enhanced, including, for example, those in the first row. On the other hand, the matrix size at each scale (row) was significantly decreased. Table I summarise the matrix sizes at all scales before and after 2D²PCA for 93%, 88%, and 83% total energy conserved for subject 5. If conventional PCA was used with all time-frequency coefficients arranged into a 1D array, the size of the covariance matrix would be 17800×17800, i.e., $(89 \times (81 + 52 + 37 + 30))^2$. It would be obviously problematic to compute such a high dimensional covariance matrix containing more than 3×10^8 elements. However, the use of multi-scale matrices followed by 2D²PCA resulted in the size of all covariance matrices being less than 100×100, avoiding the curse of dimensionality and small sample issue as well as improving the numerical stability.

Effect of Mother Wavelet and Number of PCs

Though various mother wavelet functions have been applied in multi-channel EMG analysis for various purposes, little is known about the performance of mother wavelet function on high-density EMG classification. In this study, we first decomposed EMG signals using broad wavelet families, including Haar, Daubechies, Coiflet, Morlet, and Meyer wavelet. After obtaining PCs at various scales, they were re-ordered based on a distance criterion implying their discriminant ability (Xie, Zheng, & Guo, 2009).

Figure 5. The contour plots of multi-scale matrices reduced using 2D²PCA for 89-channel EMG signals of 20 hand movements obtained from subject 5

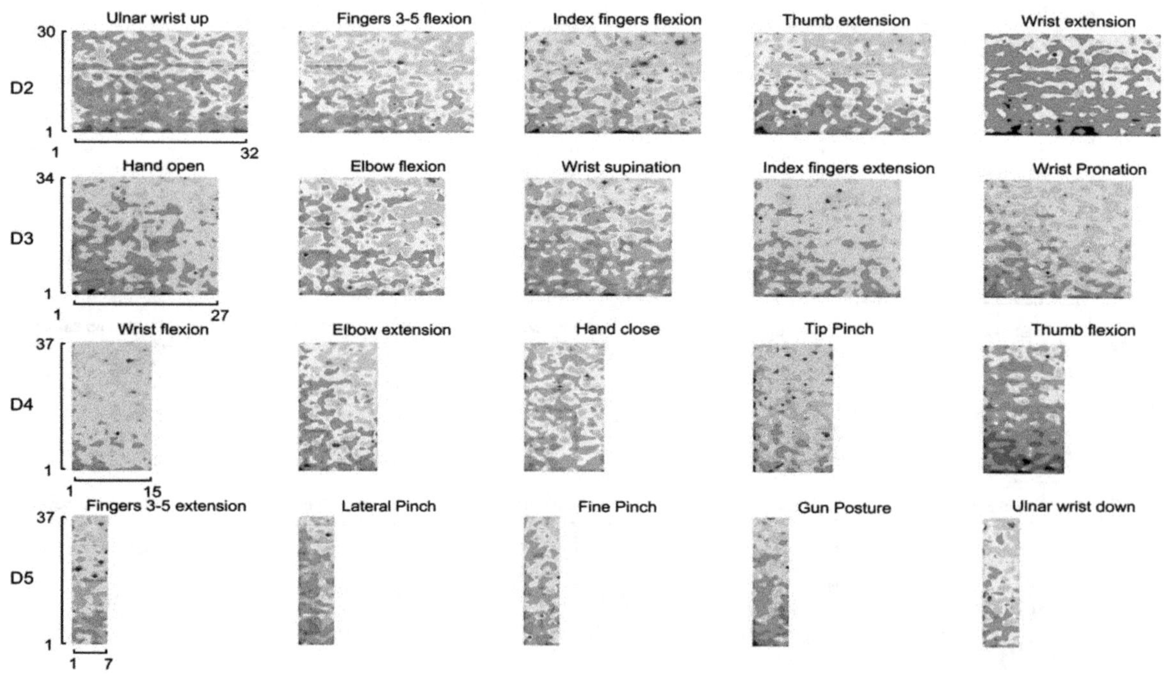

We first evaluated the effects of mother wavelet and total PC number on the classification accuracy using three classifiers. The Coiflet 4 mother wavelet consistently yielded the lowest classification error and it was employed in the analysis thereafter. Figure 6 illustrates the average accuracy against total PC number across the 12 subjects when the total energy conserved was 88% and the energy conservation rate was 98%. With the increasing number of PCs, the accuracy of all three classifiers initially increased and then entered a relatively flat range with moderate fluctuations. The total number of PCs achieving the highest accuracy for all three classifiers is less than 90. In a previous study (X. Zhang & Zhou, 2012), with PCA reduction of the time domain feature set for the same EMG dataset, the optimal number of PCs was found to be over 150. The $MS2D^2PCA$ method outperformed the PCA for similar classification accuracy with considerably less PCs. However, there was a slight decrease in GMM accuracy after it reached its peak accuracy, with these accuracies being significant inferior to the two other classifiers ($p < 0.05$). Beyond that, therefore, we only evaluated the performance of the SVM and ELM.

Effect of Energy Conservation Rate

Energy conservation rate is the ratio of energy before and after feature reduction in each iteration. A large energy conservation rate results in more information loss, whilst a low rate increases the computational burden. To reach a trade-off between these two factors, three energy conservation rates of 97%, 98% and 99%, were employed to assess its effect on classification accuracy. Figure 7 shows the average accuracy across all 12 subjects at these energy conservation rates for the SVM and ELM classifiers. For both classifiers, there was no significant difference among these energy conservation rates ($p<0.01$). However, similar to the previous results, the optimal PCs to achieve the highest SVM accuracy were all in the range of 40 to 60, whilst the optimal PCs for ELM were all around 80. The general concept underlying SVM is to map the original input space to a higher-dimensional feature space where the training set is separable. In contrast, ELM consists of single hidden layer feed-forward neural networks (SLFNs), which randomly selects the original input feature weights and analytically determines the SLFN output weights. This is why the optimal number of SVM PCs was consistently lower than ELM. However, SVM translation of the training set into a higher-dimensional space incurs both computational and learning-theoretic costs. On the other hand, ELM tends to provide the best generalization performance at extremely fast learning speed. Therefore, the ELM training was much faster than SVM, even though more PCs were required.

Figure 6. The effect of number of PCs on the high-dimensional EMG signals classification for $MS2D^2PCA$ method

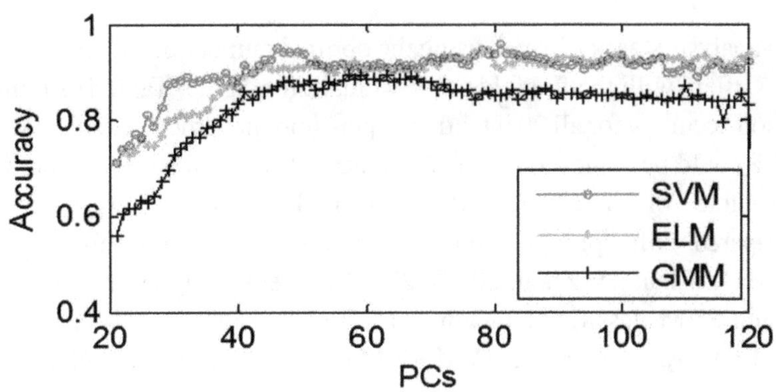

Figure 7. The effect of energy conservation rate for MS2D²PCA on high-dimensional EMG signal classification for SVM (upper panel) and ELM (lower panel)

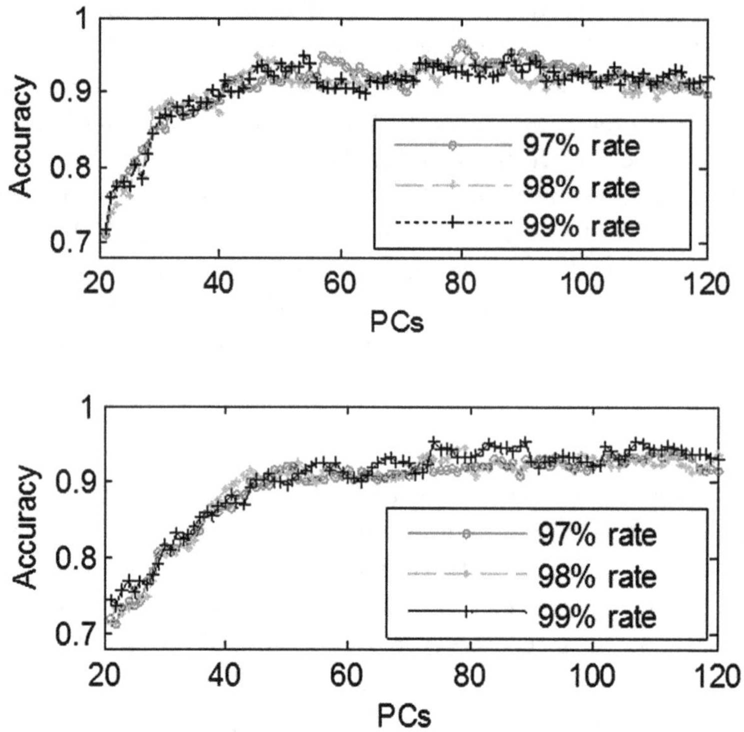

Effect of Total Energy Conserved

For PCA analysis, a typical recommendation is to set the threshold of total energy conserved between 0.8 and 0.95. Figure 8 shows the classification accuracy for SVM and ELM for three threshold values of total energy conserved, i.e., 93%, 88%, and 83%. With a reduction in threshold, there was a decrease in the ELM accuracy. However, there was no significant difference in the accuracy for SVM. The insensitivity of SVM to the total energy preserved may be due to its adaptive ability to map input features to high-dimensional feature space.

Recognition of Intended Movements

Pattern recognition analysis was performed using the optimal number of PCs previously determined and SVM and ELM classifiers with the fivefold cross-validation scheme. Table II summarizes the subject-specific classification accuracy for all 20 intended upper-limb movements. A high average classification accuracy above 95% could be achieved for most subjects. Across all subjects, there was no significant difference in the accuracy of SVM and ELM (p>0.05), although the average accuracy for ELM was slightly lower. Compared with a previous study on the same EMG dataset using PCA reduction in the time domain feature (X. Zhang & Zhou, 2012), 2D²PCA yielded higher average accuracy with much fewer PCs for the same SVM classifier, indicating the efficiency and effectiveness of 2D²PCA. Although the PCs needed for ELM was higher than SVM, ELM exhibited better computational efficiency due to

Figure 8. The effect of total energy conserved for MS2D²PCA on high-dimensional EMG signal classification for SVM (upper panel) and ELM (lower panel)

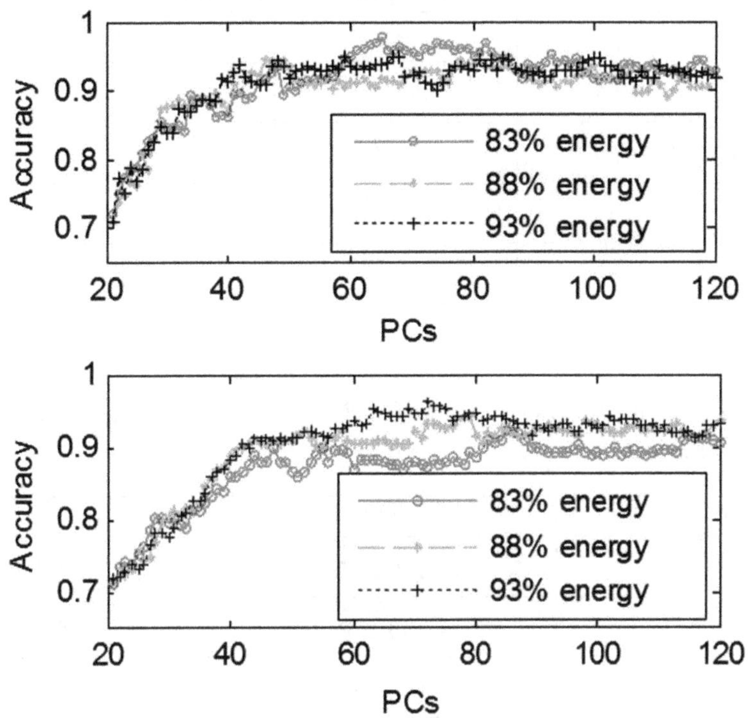

its unique learning scheme. In addition, the average accuracy of MS2D²PCA-ELM was also higher than GMM, LDA, and SVM classifiers used in conjunction with PCA in (X. Zhang & Zhou, 2012). This further suggested that MS2D²PCA was more effective than PCA for high-dimensional EMG classification. It should be emphasized, however, that EMG activity is subject-dependent for both healthy subjects and stroke survivors. Therefore, the structure and information distribution in the multi-scale matrices varied between subjects, which led to different reduced sizes with MS2D²PCA. Ultimately, this subject-specific spatial- time-frequency distribution of EMG feature information led to inconsistent classification errors among different stroke subjects. The subject-specific EMG activity and classification performance suggested that optimal myoelectric pattern-recognition control system parameters should be individually customized for stroke survivors.

CONCLUSION AND FUTURE RESEARCH DIRECTIONS

Multi-channel bio-signals recorded using large arrays exhibit specific spatial and temporal characteristics in multiple frequency bands. However, most existing methods work in time, frequency, time-frequency, or spatial-temporal domains. Time-frequency algorithms that simultaneously utilize spatial domain information are still relatively new and few in number, probably due to the complexity of data attributes in 3D feature space. In essence, PCA aims to find the single best (in the sense of least-square error) subspace for a given dimension. Since biomedical signals at various scales (sub-bands) possess different physical

Table 1. Multi-scale matrix size at various threshold values of total energy conserved for subject 5

Size	Total Energy Conserved (%)			
Scale	100%	93%	88%	83%
D2	89×81	33×32	30×32	25×29
D3	89×52	35×27	34×27	29×25
D4	89×37	43×16	37×15	32×14
D5	89×30	43×8	37×7	30×4

Table 2. Pattern recognition results (mean ± sd) of 89-channel emg for 12 subjects, averaged across fivefold tests for each subject (unit: %)

Subject	SVM	ELM
1	93.04 ± 5.26	94.13 ± 7.34
2	87.39 ± 13.27	86.24 ± 10.89
3	97.49 ± 1.23	96.93 ± 1.42
4	92.26 ± 7.37	91.40 ± 5.25
5	96.30 ± 3.46	95.75 ± 3.38
6	97.64 ± 1.88	96.96 ± 2.31
7	99.81 ± 0.21	99.46 ± 0.16
8	99.90 ± 0.15	99.34 ± 0.92
9	95.68 ± 3.57	95.25 ± 2.86
10	98.55 ± 1.44	98.89 ± 0.98
11	99.48 ± 0.27	99.13 ± 0.37
12	99.45 ± 0.71	98.87 ± 1.02
Average	96.41 ± 3.81	96.02 ± 3.95

and physiological relevance, we have proposed to divide the original high dimensional time-frequency matrix dataset into multiple matrices. Such subspace segmentation renders the data set better fitted by multiple separate models at each scale.

In conventional array-based PCA, a 2D time-frequency feature matrix is usually transformed into a 1D vector and modelled as a point in a high-dimensional vector space. However, this approach leads to several issues, such as the "curse of dimensionality" dilemma and the small sample size problem, leading to numerical instability, as well as high computational complexity and storage requirements in classification. Aimed at the problem of high volume feature space, a novel multi-scale two-directional two-dimensional principal component analysis has been proposed in this study, which used $2D^2PCA$ instead of PCA to find the optimal subspace at each scale. The size of individual row or column vectors in a matrix is much smaller than that of a single long vector transformed from the matrix, circumventing the high dimensionality. Furthermore, as the input feature vectors to be analysed are actually the rows or columns of the matrix, the feature set is significantly enlarged, avoiding the small sample size problem.

In order to test this approach, $MS2D^2PCA$ was used to extract and classify specific STF patterns in 89-channel EMG signals from the stroke subjects for identification of 20 hand movements. The multi-scale spatial matrix technique revealed subtle STF pattern differences between movements, whilst $2D^2PCA$ effectively solved the dilemma of high dimensionality in the subsequent classification. The segmented subspace and enlarged feature set are the major reasons for the optimal dimension of the proposed method (less than 90) being much lower than PCA on the same data set (about 150) (X. Zhang & Zhou, 2012). In addition, the 3D spatial-time-frequency information is well preserved by using the multi-scale matrices rather than reshaping these to a long vector. Finally, each row of the vertical or horizontal scatter matrices captures the local information contained in the corresponding rows of the training matrix, characterizing the overall scatter of the corresponding local region for all training samples. Therefore, $2D^2PCA$ is a feature extraction method combining local and global information simultaneously. This is why $MS2D^2PCA$ achieved slightly higher accuracy using much fewer PCs.

For the general purpose of robust covariance estimation, approaches based on subset selection, outlier rejection, and fuzzy weight have been proposed with successful applications in, for example, the common spatial pattern filter (Heo et al., 2009). In real world applications, however, large amounts of training samples are not always available for biomedical signals, whilst the fuzzy weight method needs to cluster the training data set into a pre-defined number of clusters. Each data point weight is calculated as a function of the cluster membership values, significantly increasing the computational burden. In $MS2D^2PCA$, in order to alleviate the computational complexity for limited samples, a wavelet soft threshold method was employed to denoise the multi-scale matrices, which can be regarded as an alternative outlier rejection method for covariance estimation. In future, it will be necessary to develop fast robust covariance estimation algorithms to improve the performance of $MS2D^2PCA$.

A novel multi-scale two-directional two-dimensional principal component analysis for high-dimensional signal classification has been proposed and examined in this study. Spatial-time- frequency discriminant information from high-dimensional EMG electrode array can be effectively extracted and reduced using the proposed method. Compared with the time domain feature extraction in conjunction with PCA, $MS2D^2PCA$ performed better with higher classification accuracy and less PCs in EMG classification. The efficiency and effectiveness of the method can be further validated by using high-dimensional EEG, MEG, fMRI signals. Although the present study focuses on high-dimensional signal pattern classification, based on the PCs obtained at multiple scales, it is relatively straightforward to expand $MS2D^2PCA$ for high-dimensional signal compression, denoising, component extraction, and other related tasks.

REFERENCES

Acharya, U. R., Sree, S. V., Alvin, A. P. C., & Suri, J. S. (2012). Use of principal component analysis for automatic classification of epileptic EEG activities in wavelet framework. *Expert Systems with Applications*, *39*(10), 9072–9078. doi:10.1016/j.eswa.2012.02.040

Addison, P. S. (2005). Wavelet transforms and the ECG: A review. *Physiological Measurement*, *26*(5), R155–R199. doi:10.1088/0967-3334/26/5/R01 PMID:16088052

Azar, A., Balas, V., & Olariu, T. (2014). Classification of EEG-Based Brain–Computer Interfaces. In B. Iantovics & R. Kountchev (Eds.), *Advanced Intelligent Computational Technologies and Decision Support Systems* (Vol. 486, pp. 97–106). Springer International Publishing. doi:10.1007/978-3-319-00467-9_9

Chan, A. D. C., Englehart, K., Hudgins, B., & Lovely, D. F. (2001). Myo-electric signals to augment speech recognition. *Medical & Biological Engineering & Computing*, *39*(4), 500–504. doi:10.1007/BF02345373 PMID:11523740

Chu, J. U., Moon, I., & Mun, M. S. (2006). A real-time EMG pattern recognition system based on linear-nonlinear feature projection for a multifunction myoelectric hand. *IEEE Transactions on Bio-Medical Engineering*, *53*(11), 2232–2239. doi:10.1109/TBME.2006.883695 PMID:17073328

da Silva, F. L. (2013). EEG and MEG: Relevance to Neuroscience. *Neuron*, *80*(5), 1112–1128. doi:10.1016/j.neuron.2013.10.017 PMID:24314724

Einbeck, J., Evers, L., & Bailer-Jones, C. (2008). Representing Complex Data Using Localized Principal Components with Application to Astronomical Data. In A. Gorban, B. Kégl, D. Wunsch, & A. Zinovyev (Eds.), *Principal Manifolds for Data Visualization and Dimension Reduction* (Vol. 58, pp. 178–201). Springer Berlin Heidelberg. doi:10.1007/978-3-540-73750-6_7

Engelhart, K., Hudgins, B., Parker, P. A., & Stevenson, M. (1999). Classification of the myoelectric signal using time-frequency based representations. *Medical Engineering & Physics*, *21*(6-7), 431–438. doi:10.1016/S1350-4533(99)00066-1 PMID:10624739

Ghorbanian, P., Jalali, A., Ghaffari, A., & Nataraj, C. (2012). An improved procedure for detection of heart arrhythmias with novel pre-processing techniques. *Expert Systems: International Journal of Knowledge Engineering and Neural Networks*, *29*(5), 478–491. doi:10.1111/j.1468-0394.2011.00606.x

Giri, D., Acharya, U. R., Martis, R. J., Sree, S. V., Lim, T. C., Ahamed, T., & Suri, J. S. (2013). Automated diagnosis of Coronary Artery Disease affected patients using LDA, PCA, ICA and Discrete Wavelet Transform. *Knowledge-Based Systems*, *37*, 274–282. doi:10.1016/j.knosys.2012.08.011

Han, M., Liu, Y. H., Xi, J. H., & Guo, W. (2007). Noise smoothing for nonlinear time series using wavelet soft threshold. *IEEE Signal Processing Letters*, *14*(1), 62–65. doi:10.1109/LSP.2006.881518

Heo, G., Gader, P., & Frigui, H. (2009). RKF-PCA: Robust kernel fuzzy PCA. *Neural Networks*, *22*(5-6), 642–650. doi:10.1016/j.neunet.2009.06.013 PMID:19592217

Huang, G. B., Zhou, H. M., Ding, X. J., & Zhang, R. (2012). Extreme Learning Machine for Regression and Multiclass Classification. *IEEE Transactions on Systems, Man, and Cybernetics. Part B, Cybernetics, 42*(2), 513–529. doi:10.1109/TSMCB.2011.2168604 PMID:21984515

Karlsson, J. S., Roeleveld, K., Gronlund, C., Holtermann, A., & Ostlund, N. (2009). Signal processing of the surface electromyogram to gain insight into neuromuscular physiology. *Philosophical Transactions of the Royal Society a-Mathematical Physical and Engineering Sciences, 367*(1887), 337-356. doi: DOI 10.1098/rsta.2008.0214

Khezri, M., & Jahed, M. (2007). Real-time intelligent pattern recognition algorithm for surface EMG signals. *Biomedical Engineering Online*, *6*(1), 45. doi:10.1186/1475-925X-6-45 PMID:18053184

Kiatpanichagij, K., & Afzulpurkar, N. (2009). Use of supervised discretization with PCA in wavelet packet transformation-based surface electromyrogram classification. *Biomedical Signal Processing and Control*, *4*(2), 127–138. doi:10.1016/j.bspc.2009.02.004

Korurek, M., & Nizam, A. (2010). Clustering MIT-BIH arrhythmias with Ant Colony Optimization using time domain and PCA compressed wavelet coefficients. *Digital Signal Processing*, *20*(4), 1050–1060. doi:10.1016/j.dsp.2009.10.019

Martis, R. J., Krishnan, M. M. R., Chakraborty, C., Pal, S., Sarkar, D., Mandana, K. M., & Ray, A. K. (2012). Automated Screening of Arrhythmia Using Wavelet Based Machine Learning Techniques. *Journal of Medical Systems*, *36*(2), 677–688. doi:10.1007/s10916-010-9535-7 PMID:20703662

Mashhoori, A., & Jahromi, M. Z. (2013). Block-wise two-directional 2DPCA with ensemble learning for face recognition. *Neurocomputing*, *108*, 111–117. doi:10.1016/j.neucom.2012.12.005

Qi, L. P., Wakeling, J. M., Green, A., Lambrecht, K., & Ferguson-Pell, M. (2011). Spectral properties of electromyographic and mechanomyographic signals during isometric ramp and step contractions in biceps brachii. *Journal of Electromyography and Kinesiology*, *21*(1), 128–135. doi:10.1016/j.jelekin.2010.09.006 PMID:21067944

Uguz, H. (2012). A hybrid system based on information gain and principal component analysis for the classification of transcranial Doppler signals. *Computer Methods and Programs in Biomedicine*, *107*(3), 598–609. doi:10.1016/j.cmpb.2011.03.013 PMID:21524813

Von Tscharner, V., & Goepfert, B. (2006). Estimation of the interplay between groups of fast and slow muscle fibers of the tibialis anterior and gastrocnemius muscle while running. *Journal of Electromyography and Kinesiology*, *16*(2), 188–197. doi:10.1016/j.jelekin.2005.07.004 PMID:16139523

Wacker, M., & Witte, H. (2013). Time-frequency Techniques in Biomedical Signal Analysis A Tutorial Review of Similarities and Differences. *Methods of Information in Medicine*, *52*(4), 279–296. doi:10.3414/ME12-01-0083 PMID:23703538

Wakeling, J., Delaney, R., & Dudkiewicz, I. (2007). A method for quantifying dynamic muscle dysfunction in children and young adults with cerebral palsy. *Gait & Posture*, *25*(4), 580–589. doi:10.1016/j.gaitpost.2006.06.009 PMID:16876416

Wakeling, J. M., Uehli, K., & Rozitis, A. I. (2006). Muscle fibre recruitment can respond to the mechanics of the muscle contraction. *Journal of the Royal Society, Interface*, *3*(9), 533–544. doi:10.1098/rsif.2006.0113 PMID:16849250

Weiderpass, H. A., Pachi, C. G. F., Yamamoto, J. F., Hamamoto, A., Onodera, A. N., & Sacco, I. C. N. (2013). Time-frequency analysis methods for detecting effects of diabetic neuropathy. *International Journal for Numerical Methods in Biomedical Engineering*, *29*(9), 1000–1010. doi:10.1002/cnm.2545 PMID:23620093

Xie, H. B., & Dokos, S. (2013a). A hybrid symplectic principal component analysis and central tendency measure method for detection of determinism in noisy time series with application to mechanomyography. *Chaos, 23*(2). doi. *Artn, 023131*. doi:10.1063/1.4812287

Xie, H. B., & Dokos, S. (2013b). A symplectic geometry-based method for nonlinear time series decomposition and prediction. *Applied Physics Letters, 103*(5). doi:10.1063/1.4817181

Xie, H. B., Guo, T. R., Sivakumar, B., Liew, A. W. C., & Dokos, S. (2014). Symplectic geometry spectrum analysis of nonlinear time series. *Proceedings of the Royal Society a-Mathematical Physical and Engineering Sciences, 470*(2170). doi:10.1098/rspa.2014.0409

Xie, H. B., & Wang, Z. Z. (2006). Mean frequency derived via Hilbert-Huang transform with application to fatigue EMG signal analysis. *Computer Methods and Programs in Biomedicine*, *82*(2), 114–120. doi:10.1016/j.cmpb.2006.02.009 PMID:16616796

Xie, H. B., Zheng, Y. P., & Guo, J. Y. (2009). Classification of the mechanomyogram signal using a wavelet packet transform and singular value decomposition for multifunction prosthesis control. *Physiological Measurement*, *30*(5), 441–457. doi:10.1088/0967-3334/30/5/002 PMID:19349648

Xie, H. B., Zheng, Y. P., Guo, J. Y., Chen, X., & Shi, J. (2009). Estimation of wrist angle from sonomyography using support vector machine and artificial neural network models. *Medical Engineering & Physics*, *31*(3), 384–391. doi:10.1016/j.medengphy.2008.05.005 PMID:18586548

Yang, J., Zhang, D., Frangi, A. F., & Yang, J. Y. (2004). Two-dimensional PCA: A new approach to appearance-based face representation and recognition. *IEEE Transactions on Pattern Analysis and Machine Intelligence*, *26*(1), 131–137. doi:10.1109/TPAMI.2004.1261097 PMID:15382693

Zhang, D. Q., & Zhou, Z. H. (2005). (2D)(2)PCA: Two-directional two-dimensional PCA for efficient face representation and recognition. *Neurocomputing*, *69*(1-3), 224–231. doi:10.1016/j.neucom.2005.06.004

Zhang, X., & Zhou, P. (2012). High-Density Myoelectric Pattern Recognition Toward Improved Stroke Rehabilitation. *IEEE Transactions on Bio-Medical Engineering*, *59*(6), 1649–1657. doi:10.1109/TBME.2012.2191551 PMID:22453603

Chapter 6
Medical Image Enhancement Using Edge Information–Based Methods

S. Anand
Mepco Schlenk Engineering College, India

ABSTRACT

Medical image enhancement improves the quality and facilitates diagnosis. This chapter investigates three methods of medical image enhancement by exploiting useful edge information. Since edges have higher perceptual importance, the edge information based enhancement process is always of interest. But determination of edge information is not an easy job. The edge information is obtained from various approaches such as differential hyperbolic function, Haar filters and morphological functions. The effectively determined edge information is used for enhancement process. The retinal image enhancement method given in this chapter improves the visual quality of the vessels in the optic region. X-ray image enhancement method presented here is to increase the visibility of the bones. These algorithms are used to enhance the computer tomography, chest x-ray, retinal, and mammogram images. These images are obtained from standard datasets and experimented. The performance of these enhancement methods are quantitatively evaluated.

INTRODUCTION

Medical Image Processing is an important sub-discipline of biomedical engineering and it enables quantitative analysis and visualization of medical images of numerous modalities. Medical imaging technology allows the people to see the interior portions of the body without really opening too much of the body. The processing of medical images includes advantages such as:

1. It can be reproduced any number of times and retains the originality of the data
2. Powerful tool to display the images
3. Enhancement of images to make them easier for the Physician to interpret

DOI: 10.4018/978-1-5225-0660-7.ch006

4. Quantifying changes over time and
5. Quick comparison of images, etc.

The images can be acquired from any of the modalities e.g. radiography, magnetic resonance imaging, nuclear medicine, ultrasound, elastography, tactile imaging, photoacoustic imaging, thermography, conventional tomography, computer-assisted tomography, echocardiography, functional near-infrared spectroscopy, etc. Each image acquired from any modality have their own merits and demerits and sometimes these images are poor in quality. These distortions in the images cause inadequate presentation of interested objects / region, which can result in inaccurate analysis. The main contributions of this chapter includes:

1. Using differential hyperbolic tangent function based edge enhancement in CT, retinal, and mammogram images,
2. Edge enhancement of x-ray Image by Haar Filters,
3. Enhancement of vasculature in optic disc region based on edge information along with morphological operators.

This chapter is organized as follows. The background section reviews various research in the edge detection and image enhancement. It also describes various researches in the enhancement of retinal, mammogram and x-ray images. First section analyzes the hyperbolic filter based CT, retinal and mammogram enhancement algorithm. It also describes an unsharp filter for retinal image enhancement. Second section analyzes the edge enhancement of chest x-ray image by Haar filters. Third section analyzes the enhancement of vasculature in optic disc region based on edge information along with morphological operators. This chapter ends with future research directions of this research and conclusion.

BACKGROUND

Enhancement techniques have been widely used in the field of medical image processing, where the subjective quality of images is important for human interpretation and diagnosis. Image enhancement plays an important role in making important decision based on the image information. The techniques of medical image enhancement are to improve some useful information present in an image, or / and remove or reduce some unwanted information. Various enhancement algorithms have been developed apply on medical images. Image enhancement is a process, so that the enhanced image is more suitable than the original image for a specific application (Gonzalez, & Woods, 2009). Medical image enhancement is necessary if the original is not a good candidate for subsequent processing (Yang, Su, & Sun, 2010; Li, Yanmei, & Hailun, 2010). In many cases, enhancement improves the quality of the image and facilitates diagnosis (Anand, & Gayathri 2015; Anand, & Shantha Selva Kumari, 2013, 2014; Anand, Shantha Selva Kumari, Jeeva, & Thivya, 2013a; 2013b; Sundaram, Ramar, Arumugam, & Prabin, 2011; Li, 2010; Tay, Garson, Acton, & Hossack, 2010; Peng, Yingjun, Biao, Wei, & Deling, 2007).

Image enhancement is the process to improve an image, so that it looks subjectively better (Yu, Kuo, Guei, & Chyou, 2012). However, subjective quality of an image depends largely on the sharpness and explicitness of edges. The lack of sharpness is due to wrong focus of imaging equipment, motion blur, etc. Sharpness is directly related to human sight properties and visibility. Emphasizing the edges there by enhancing sharpness provide better visibility. Since edges are higher perceptual importance, the primary objective of this Chapter is to focus on edge information based methods to enhance the medical images like retinal image, x-ray image etc. Among various techniques, edge information based enhancement methods are successful due to their promising results (Karen, Yicong, Agaian, & Hongwei, 2011; Bhutada, Anand G. G, & Saxena, 2011; Zhiguo, & Yi, 2011; Eltoukhy, Faye, &Samir, 2010; Phan et al., 2009; Akram et al., 2009; Peng et.al, 2007). However, determination of reliable edge information is not an easy task due to two important reasons:

1. Noise sensitivity,
2. Illumination dependent.

While detecting edges, noise also pronounces. Therefore, successful determination of edge information in an image and using it for efficient enhancement process leads to better-quality images.

Conventional edge determination algorithms are very sensitive to fine structure of edges and suffer in distinguishing the weak edge from noise. To combat with noise, pre-smoothing algorithms are devised and they combine Gaussian smoothing while estimating gradients. They are more effective in higher noise conditions at the cost of dislocated and suppressed weak edges (Olivier, & Truchetet, 2010; Rakesh, Probal, & Murthy, 2004; Mitra, 2002). Thus, there is a need for tradeoff between the level of smoothing and the accuracy of estimated edge location. Difference of Gaussian (DoG) kernels ensure optimal tradeoff as in canny edge detection (Canny, 1986), but the tradeoff is sensitive to category of edge (sharp or smooth) and signals to noise ratio. Hyperbolic tangent (HBT) function also provides good tradeoff and has the advantage of better localization than DoG (Saravanakumar, Sim, Surendra, & Fook, 2006). In particular, when the smoothing parameter is greater than one, the localization and detection performances of DoG are degraded, but HBT perform well. This chapter intends to use Differential HBT (DHBT) function in edge determination purpose.

Good local contrast gives natural look to an image. Increasing the contrast of the interested structures is one of the main approaches in the enhancement algorithm. Local contrast enhancement algorithm such as unsharp masking (USM) attempts to increase the appearance of large-scale light-dark transitions and small-scale edges. Classical USM brings out the information along with the noise. USM is a common image sharpening method in which the filter has the effect of masking edges and fine detail in the image crisper. Laplacian of Gaussian (LoG) based USM is a widely used image sharpening enhancement algorithm. Image sharpening improves the contrast by adding the scaled edge information near the boundaries of objects (Konstantinos, Vasudev, & Giordano, 1999). Kim and Cho (2008) presented statistical method based on feature noise adaptive USM for local enhancement. Sharpening is an important process in images to increase the contrast between bright and dark regions to bring out boundary features and lead to a better-looking image. Sharpening enhancement can be interpreted as addition of missing higher frequency components in the frequency domain. It only enhances the details already present and improves the steepness of edges. USM is an image manipulation technique, often available in all digital image-processing software. USM processed image has greater visual acuity than the original and it is a filter that amplifies high-frequency components already present. Digital USM is a flexible and powerful way to increase sharpness, especially in scanned images. However, it creates unwanted and conspicuous edge effects, or increase image noise due to high pass characteristics. Undesired effects are reduced by applying this to desired regions of images. USM can increase either sharpness or (local) contrast because these are both forms of increasing differences between values. Sharpness refers to very small-scale (high frequency) differences and contrast referring to larger scale (low frequency) differences. Similar to USM, deconvolution increases the apparent sharpness of an image. For deconvolution to be effective, all variables in the image scene and capturing device need to be modeled, including aperture, focal length, distance to subject, lens and media refractive indices and geometries. Applying deconvolution successfully to general-purpose camera images is usually not feasible. In this context low cost, easily available USM techniques may be preferred and therefore all image processing software have USM.

Zhiguo (2011), discusses a fuzzy logic based image-sharpening algorithm. Image smoothing and sharpening based on nonlinear diffusion equation also an interested work presented by Dai et.al (2008). Though these methods improve the contrast by sharpening process, they are influenced by the noise (Kim, 2008). Undesirable distortions in uniform areas and consequently, some artifacts appear in the output image due to the usage of linear high pass filter. Approaches are available to control the noise effect by smoothing operation at the cost of loss/unreliable edge information. Even though sharpening methods are simple and have many applications, they still have problems (Karen et al., 2011). A new USM scheme, called nonlinear USM (NLUSM) introduced by Karen (2011), offers flexibility to users. NLUSM aims to embed different types of filters into the nonlinear filtering operator, and to choose different linear or nonlinear operations for the fusion processes that combine the enhanced filtered portion of the image with the original image. It allows the NLUSM parameter selection to be performed manually. Leveraging on the advantages of these two techniques, nonlinear filtering and USM techniques, the new scheme can enhance the contrast of specific regions, objects and details to achieve better visibility. Therefore, increase in contrast near the interested structures and without (or) reduced noise effect is still in ongoing research.

Uneven illumination is one of the critical issue in edge information determination process. Compensating the uneven illumination present in an image and determining the edges is an important need for enhancement algorithms. This will aid the automatic image screening for detection and recognition. It helps diagnosing and managing a large number of diseases either automatically/semi automatically or manually. In order to extract the edge information from non-uniform weak illumination images, different algorithms were proposed (Anand et al., 2014; Arandiga, Cohen, Donat, & Matei, 2010; Wanpeng, Rensheng, & Dong, 2008; Saravanakumar et al., 2006; Desolneux, Moisan, & Morel, 2001). The ability to resolve edge detail is of paramount importance in medical imaging systems especially in chest x-ray images (Ming, Youfu, Qinghao, Ting, & Jian, 2012).

Histogram equalization (HE) is an image processing method to adjust the contrast. It is useful in images with backgrounds and foregrounds that are both bright or both dark. HE often produces unrealistic effects in photographs. Adaptive Histogram Equalization (AHE) differs from ordinary HE in respect that the adaptive method computes several histograms, each corresponding to a distinct section of the image and uses them to redistribute the intensity values of the image. It is therefore suitable for improving the local contrast of an image and bringing out more detail. However, AHE has a tendency to amplify noise in relatively homogeneous regions. A variant of adaptive histogram equalization called contrast limited adaptive histogram equalization (CLAHE) introduced by Zuiderveld (1994), has given very good results by limiting the amplification in the case of image contrast enhancement. It is advantageous not to discard the part of the histogram that exceeds the clip limit but to redistribute equally among all histogram bins. But it is not suitable for biomedical images containing fine details.

CT is one of the important radiological diagnosis method which allows better visualization of specifically different structured soft-tissues (Li, Yanmei, & Hailun, 2010). They are subject to a variety of imperfections due to various effects. In a CT image the distribution of gray levels reduces the overall contrast. Moreover, the selection of reconstruction kernels determines the tradeoff between image sharpness and pixel noise. In order to achieve good quality images and complete proper diagnoses, radiologists use image pre-processing algorithms. So, resolving the high frequency in low contrast structures is one of the most common tasks performed by those interpreting CT.

The retina is the unique region of the human body where the vascular conditions are observed directly. Optic fundus photography technique has become a common procedure to diagnose vascular and nonvascular pathology and duly indicate many eye diseases (Jian et al., 2008). The assessment of the characteristics of the vessels plays an important role in a variety of medical diagnoses and treatment. Automatic analysis techniques instead of manual observation/measurements have been widely used (Bock, Meier, Nyul, & Michelson, 2010). However, it is difficult to extract the vessels automatically because of its low contrast. One of the difficulties in image capture of the ocular fundus is image quality, which is affected by factors such as medial opacities, defocus, or presence of artifact.

Analyzing the retinal images plays important role in detection of some diseases in early stages. Retinal blood vessels act as the detecting tool for many diseases in early or later stage, there is a wide range of vessels widths in retinal images, from less than one pixel to more than ten pixels. The small vessels, which are of less than two pixels widths, are generally low contrast. Enhancement of vessel's contrast before extraction greatly improves the performance of vessel extraction algorithm. Retinal images play an important role in diagnosing many eye diseases. However, images are often noisy, uneven illumination and low contrast. Techniques improve to contrast, sharpness and reducing noise are therefore required to aid the human interpretation or automatic analysis of the retinal images. Joshi, & Jayanthi Sivaswamy, (2008), Peng et al. (2007), Grisan, Giani, Ceseracciu, & Ruggeri, (2006), and Foracchia, Grisan, & Ruggeri, (2005), signify retinal image enhancement and its applications. Histogram equalization has been shown to be inappropriate for retinal images (Peng et al., 2007).

Unsharp masking-based enhancement is partly effective but is not capable of handling uneven illumination (Joshi et al., 2008). A local normalisation of each pixel to zero mean and unit variance aims to compensate lighting variation and enhancing local contrast but also introduces artifacts due to amplification of noise (Peng et al., 2007). Early detection is the primary solution for improving breast cancer prognosis. Although x-ray mammogram is an effective method for screening the breast cancer, interpretation of such mammograms requires skill and experienced radiologist. Thus, computer aided analysis can act as a second reader before the final decision. Image processing algorithms plays an important role in mammogram analysis, especially in abnormal areas of mammogram. Mammogram image enhancement improves the appearance of images, to accentuate certain features in an image (Eltoukhy et al, 2010). Film mammography has limited detection capability for low contrast lesions in dense breasts. Although, varieties of contrast enhancement algorithms are present in the literature dealing with images having fine details such as mammogram is still a research issue (Anand et al., 2013; Sundaram et al., 2011; Kim, Park, Song, & Park, 1997). Similarly, the ability to resolve fine picture detail, low/high contrast, non-uniform luminance is paramount importance in chest x-ray images for viewing bone structure is still research issue.

DIFFERENTIAL HYPERBOLIC TANGENT (DHBT) FILTER BASED ENHANCEMENT

Image enhancement technique is simple, appealing and powerful tool in medical image processing and the main purpose is to bring out hidden detail in an image and help diagnosing. Enhancing contrast, edges etc. are some common image pre-processing algorithms used by physicians to visualize the medical images for diagnosis. This section aims to analyze the algorithms focus on the effective detection of edge information and uses it suitably for image enhancement process. The first part of this section describes the DHBT function and its significance in edge enhancement on CT, retinal and mammogram images. The second part of this section explains sharpening of retinal image enhancement based on DHBT. DHBT filter function has a narrower spatial window profile than Gaussian filter and indicates better edge localization with less smoothing effect. Similar to Gaussian function, the new one dimensional DHBT filter function is defined as

$$f'\left(x\right) = 0.5\sigma\left\{\sigma - \sigma\tanh\left(\sigma x\right)^{2}\right\} \tag{1}$$

Equation 1 satisfies edge detection criteria like detection, localization and suppression of false edge responses. The DHBT based edge determination is capable of detecting edges in various medical images such as CT, retinal image (fundus), and mammogram. The effectiveness of the DHBT is demonstrated on the images obtained from BrighamRAD, DRIVE (Digital Retinal Images for Vessel Extraction), STARE (STructured Analysis of the Retina) and MIAS (Mammographic Image Analysis Society). They are evaluated both qualitatively and quantitatively. The common problem of Gaussian (excess amount of smoothness dislocate the edge information) is illustrated on these images. While operating the DoG filter with smoothing parameter $\sigma > 1$, some of the edge information are lost or dislocated. The example illustration of CT images, retinal images and mammogram images are given Figure 1, Figure 2 and Figure 3. Figure 1 illustrates the results of edge determination of DHBT on CT images. Figure 2 and Figure 3 illustrate the results of edge determination of DHBT on retinal images and mammogram image respectively. First column of these figures have the originals. In the second column edges determined from DoG method is shown. In the third column edges determined from DHBT method by Equation 1 is presented. When the smoothing level is $\sigma = 1$, the DoG's edge information in the form of gradients are wider and has poor localization than the DHBT. The DHBT based differentiation provides thin and well-localized edge information. While Gaussian function's 'σ' i.e. smoothness increases, the noise influence decreases conversely, edge feature's localization losses. In DoG, the smoothing provides better noise control, but the edge width increases and hence leads to poor localization of edge features. From the Figure 1 to 3 the DHBT base edge information are well localized and smoothing effect is under control therefore fine details that are very useful for enhancement process are preserved.

- **Performance Comparison:** The algorithms' performance is evaluated on selective images taken from their corresponding image databases. Edge determination performances are evaluated by reconstruction estimation measure through MSE (Agaian, Panetta, Nercessian, & Danahy, 2010; Pellegrino, Vanzella, &Torre, 2004; Agaian, Panetta, & Grigoryan, 2001; Elder, 1999; Carlsson, 1988). For twenty CT images, which are obtained from BrighamRAD, the MSE is computed and

Figure 1. Edge detection on CT images from left to right: Original, DoG filter, and DHBT filter

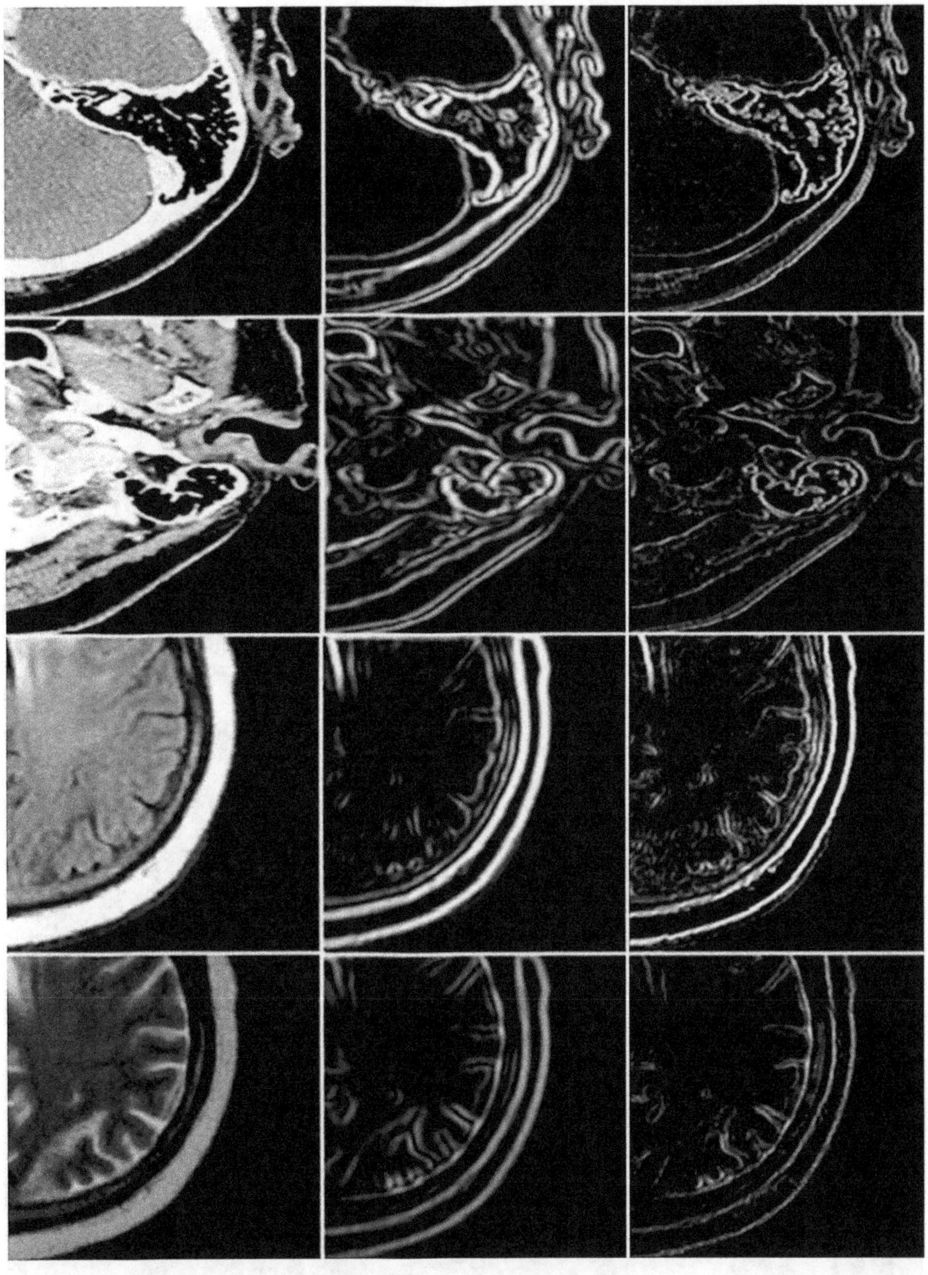

their values are tabulated in Table 1. In Table 2, the calculated MSE for mammogram images from MIAS is presented. Twenty images from MIAS database are considered in this experiment. In both CT and mammogram cases, the MSE is lower in DHBT based method and points out that DHBT algorithm has improved performance in edge detection. The testing can be extended for retinal images obtained from DRIVE that have the manually drawn ground truth vessel facility (Staal, Abramoff, Niemeijer, Viergever, & Ginneken, 2004). Also, the effectiveness of this algo-

Figure 2. Edge detection on retinal images from left to right: Original, DoG filter, and DHBT filter

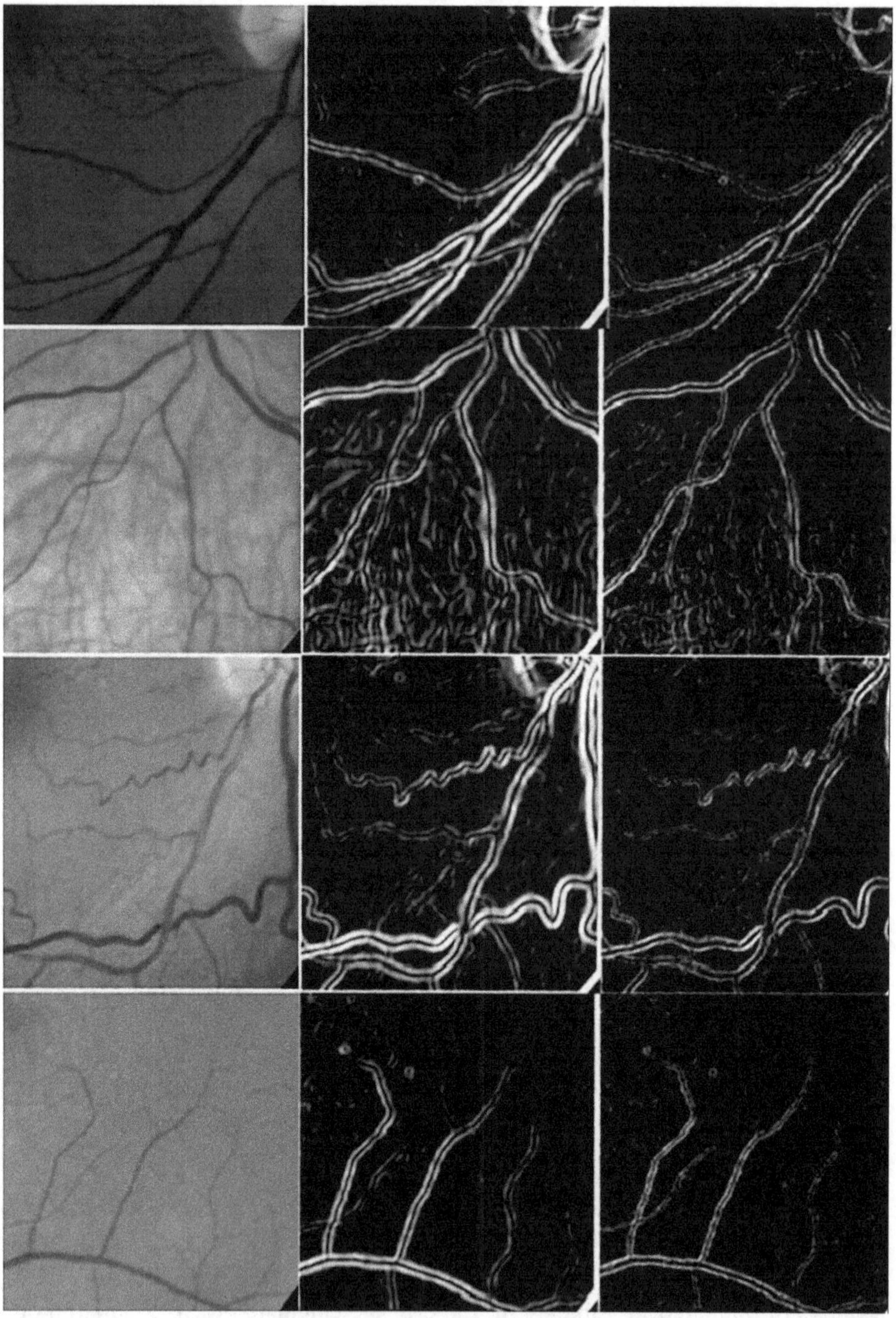

rithm is evaluated by Pratt's Figure of Merit (F) (Pratt, 2007). In this case, 'F' metric is used to evaluate the detection and localization performance of edge detection. Seventeen images from DRIVE images are considered to compare canny. All cases shown in Table 3, 'F' improves in DHBT based method.

Figure 3. Edge detection on mammogram Images from left to right: Original, DoG filter, and DHBT filter

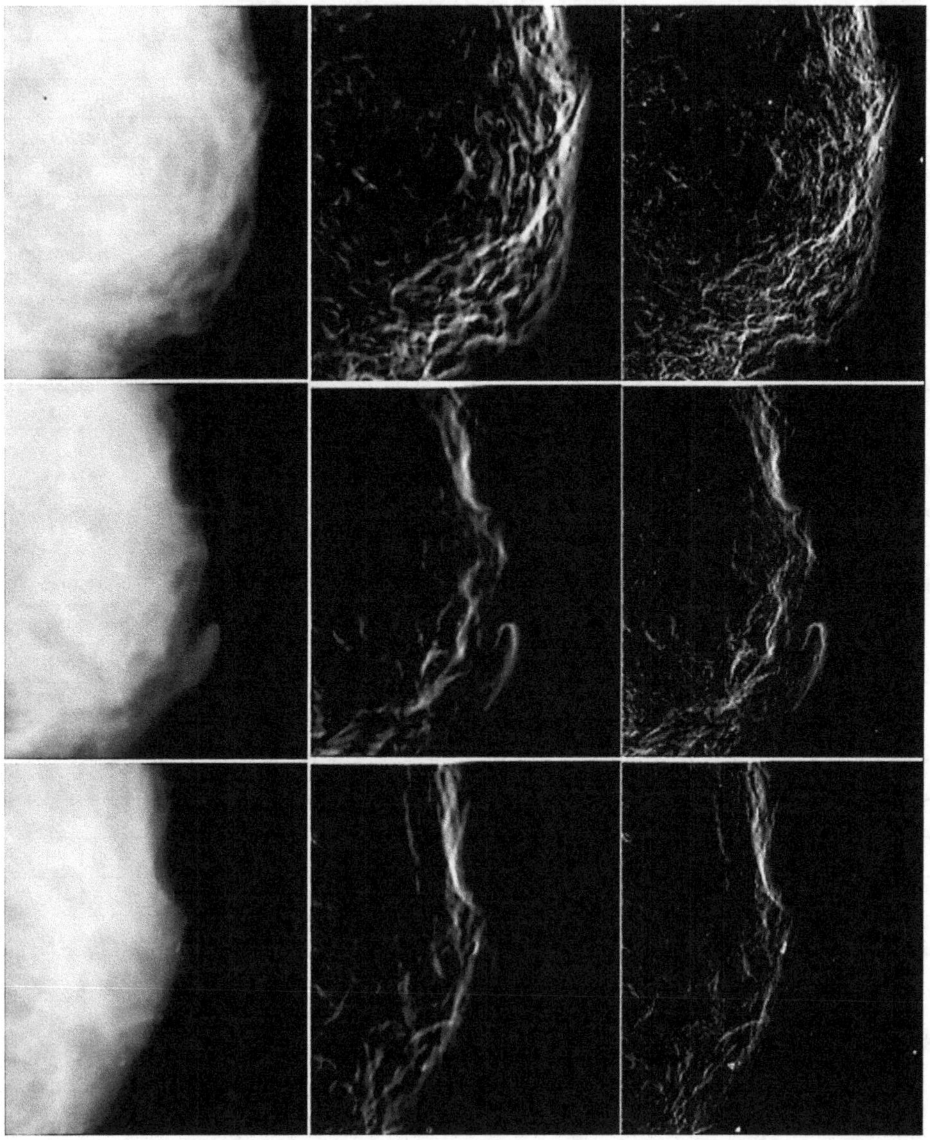

Since this algorithm makes use of the DHBT, the computation time also get reduced. (i.e.). Computing time is reduced from 0.148734 seconds to 0.12613 seconds while running the DoG based detection and the DHBT filter algorithm for an image size 512 × 512, by Pentium 4 processor 2.4 GHz.

- **Retinal Image Enhancement:** Image sharpening in Retinal Images is a classic problem in the field of medical image enhancement. The primary objective of image sharpening is to highlight fine details or to enhance the blurred regions. This sharpening filter has the 'high emphasis' character in frequency domain. The blurred regions are either in error or as an effect of image acquisition. Image sharpening applications are ranging from document and medical imaging to industrial inspection and autonomous guidance in military systems. In order to sharp an image, improving

Table 1. Performance comparison of edge detection MSE reconstruction estimation: CT image

Image	Sobel	Canny	DHBT	Image	Sobel	Canny	DHBT
1	0.4668	0.4325	0.4181	11	0.0713	0.0694	0.0624
2	0.2887	0.2453	0.2270	12	0.0771	0.0748	0.0668
3	0.2499	0.2083	0.1925	13	0.0986	0.0947	0.0863
4	0.1222	0.1177	0.1073	14	0.1031	0.0997	0.0905
5	0.1061	0.1019	0.0913	15	0.2741	0.2336	0.2144
6	0.1180	0.1150	0.1023	16	0.4651	0.3780	0.3350
7	0.1791	0.1712	0.1610	17	0.1607	0.1510	0.1370
8	0.0601	0.0711	0.0713	18	0.3737	0.3314	0.3026
9	0.0645	0.0631	0.0590	19	0.1295	0.1231	0.1141
10	0.1818	0.1740	0.1633	20	0.2162	0.1993	0.1794

Table 2. Performance comparison of edge detection MSE reconstruction estimation: MIAS image

Image	Sobel	Canny	DHBT	Image	Sobel	Canny	DHBT
mdb209	0.1871	0.1657	0.1355	mdb227	0.2320	0.2069	0.1755
mdb211	0.2344	0.1953	0.1549	mdb231	0.1724	0.1481	0.1210
mdb213	0.1453	0.1312	0.1044	mdb233	0.2417	0.2139	0.1654
mdb216	0.2735	0.2351	0.1827	mdb236	0.1873	0.1628	0.1314
mdb218	0.2277	0.1922	0.1524	mdb238	0.3136	0.2547	0.1945
mdb219	0.2992	0.2584	0.2075	mdb239	0.3149	0.2518	0.1942
mdb222	0.1939	0.1682	0.1337	mdb240	0.1701	0.1586	0.1231
mdb223	0.1261	0.1196	0.0965	mdb241	0.1590	0.1441	0.1152
mdb226	0.1302	0.1245	0.0993	mdb245	0.2189	0.1916	0.1583

Table 3. Performance comparison of edge detection figure of merit (F): DRIVE image

Image	Canny	DHBT	Image	Canny	DHBT
im0001	0.20238	0.264522	Im0010	0.199444	0.268728
Im0002	0.19857	0.270272	im0011	0.201483	0.273627
im0003	0.178733	0.24855	Im0012	0.203267	0.273876
Im0004	0.206219	0.283835	im0013	0.226447	0.286023
im0005	0.20292	0.265183	Im0014	0.213397	0.288617
Im0006	0.191799	0.262796	im0015	0.224543	0.29044
im0007	0.209926	0.270424	Im0016	0.214689	0.28529
Im0008	0.21141	0.278549	im0017	0.201505	0.273589
im0009	0.221457	0.283229			

the contrast near the edges is the common approach. For that, the scaled edge information is added near the boundaries of objects in an image (Konstantinos et al., 1999). In order to emphasize the high frequency components, the original image frequency is added with its high frequency to obtain the sharpened image. DHBT filter provides better tradeoff between smoothing parameter and edge feature and has effective noise treatment, avoids unwanted frequency boosting near the boundaries. Image sharpening improves the contrast around the edges of objects to increase the image's definition and is applied to a retinal image to bring out image detail. It emphasizes the edges and makes the image appearance sharper.

In order to prove the ability of the DHBT function in image sharpening, it is tested on various retinal images. The results are compared with LoG based image sharpening. The enhanced retinal images are presented in Figure 4 and Figure 5. First column of Figure 4 and Figure 5 refer to the original and second column, third column correspond to DHBT, LoG based sharpened images. The low contrast thin vessels are sharpened in a better way in DHBT method than the LoG based method. These images are obtained from STARE database (Adam, Valentina, & Michael, 2000). The robustness in the noise environment is the important characteristics of DHBT filter. It is verified by adding various levels of Gaussian noise to the original image and DHBT and LoG are tested. The performance is measured with Structural SIMilarity (SSIM) (Wang, Bovik, Sheikh, & Simon celli, 2004). The SSIM index is a method for measuring the similarity between two images. The SSIM index is a quality measure of one of the images being compared with the other image, which is regarded as of perfect quality. It is an improved version of the universal image quality index. The SSIM index provides a metric based upon local measures of luminance and contrast. The SSIM index compares the local structural similarity of an image against an ideal image, which is free of noise and distortion. The SSIM index varies between -1 and +1, where -1 indicates the worst local similarity to the ideal image and +1 indicates the best local similarity to the ideal image SSIM decreases with increase in noise levels (Gaussian noise variance from $\sigma^2 = 1$ to 30) for both cases, but in LoG, the SSIM more rapidly decreases than the DHBT. Therefore, the distortion in LoG due to inclusion of noise is higher than the DHBT. Figure 6shows the plot between the noise level and average SSIM for 20 DRIVE images. From the Figure 6, it is known that DHBT is more robust than LoG in noise environment. Table 4 shows the performance comparison of DHBT with LoG USM STARE retinal images using SSIM. SSIM is used to evaluate the enhancement (Bhutada et al., 2011; Tay et al., 2010; Gupta et al., 2007).

EDGE ENHANCEMENT OF X-RAY IMAGE BY HAAR FILTERS

For medical applications, x-ray images are usually generated by passing the resulting radiation through the patient's body on to a photographic plate to produce a radiograph. x-ray image often suffers from poor illumination due to factors related to the light path. This poor illumination seriously affects the subsequent processing steps that depends on it. Therefore, there is a need for enhancement step. In particular, efficient and reliable edges have key role in chest x-ray. Therefore, exact edge feature detection in the x-ray image is the precondition of successful diagnostic completion.

Edge is defined as a sharp intensity change in a gray image and edge detection is a process of detecting the presence and location of these intensity transitions. Moreover, the edge detection algorithms are sensitive to contrast, noise and uneven (or) bad illumination, thus correct edge detection is difficult.

Figure 4. Sharpening of retinal cropped images from left to right: originals, DHBT base and LoG base

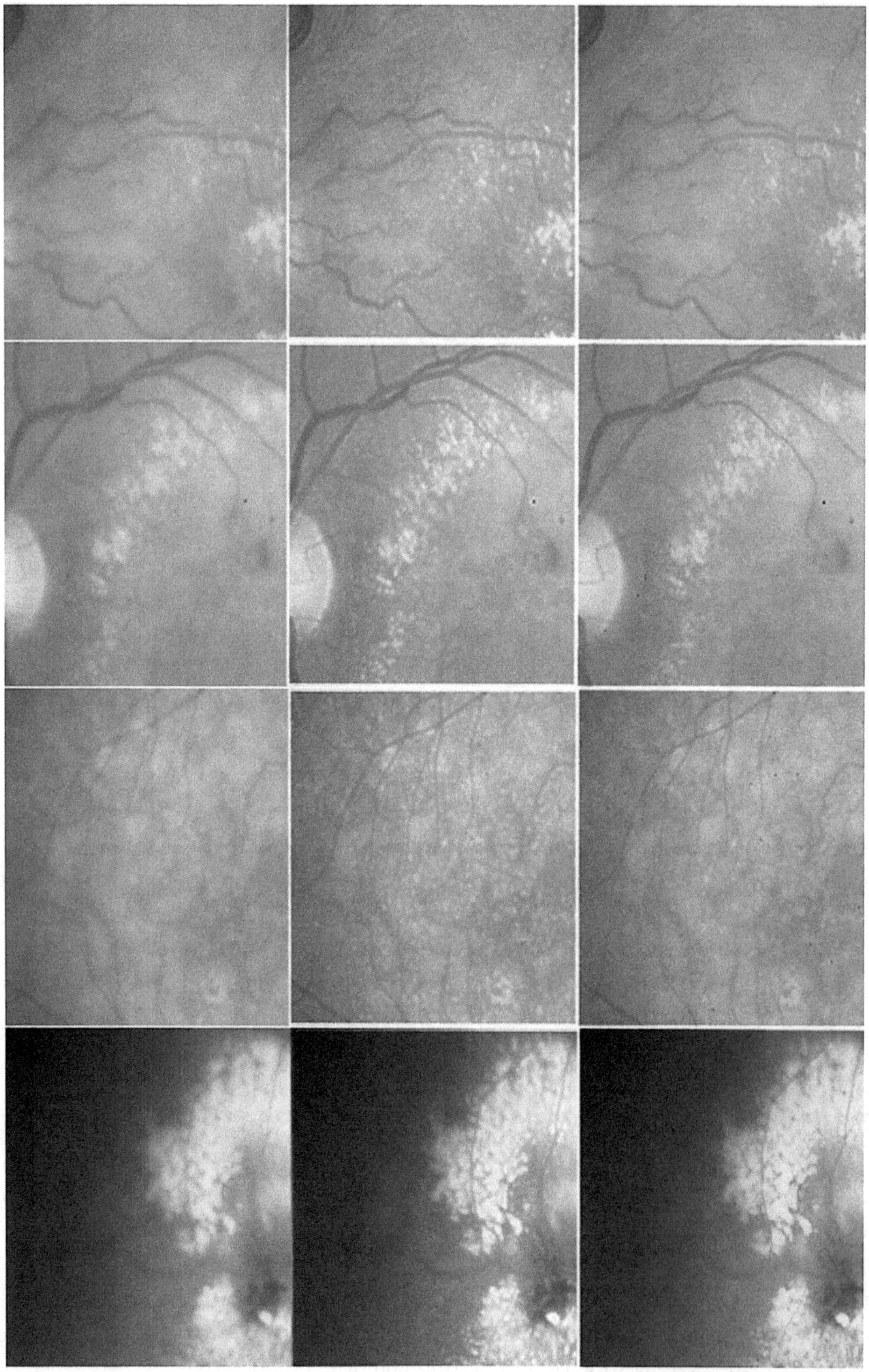

Figure 5. Sharpening of retinal cropped images from left to right: originals, DHBT base and LoG base

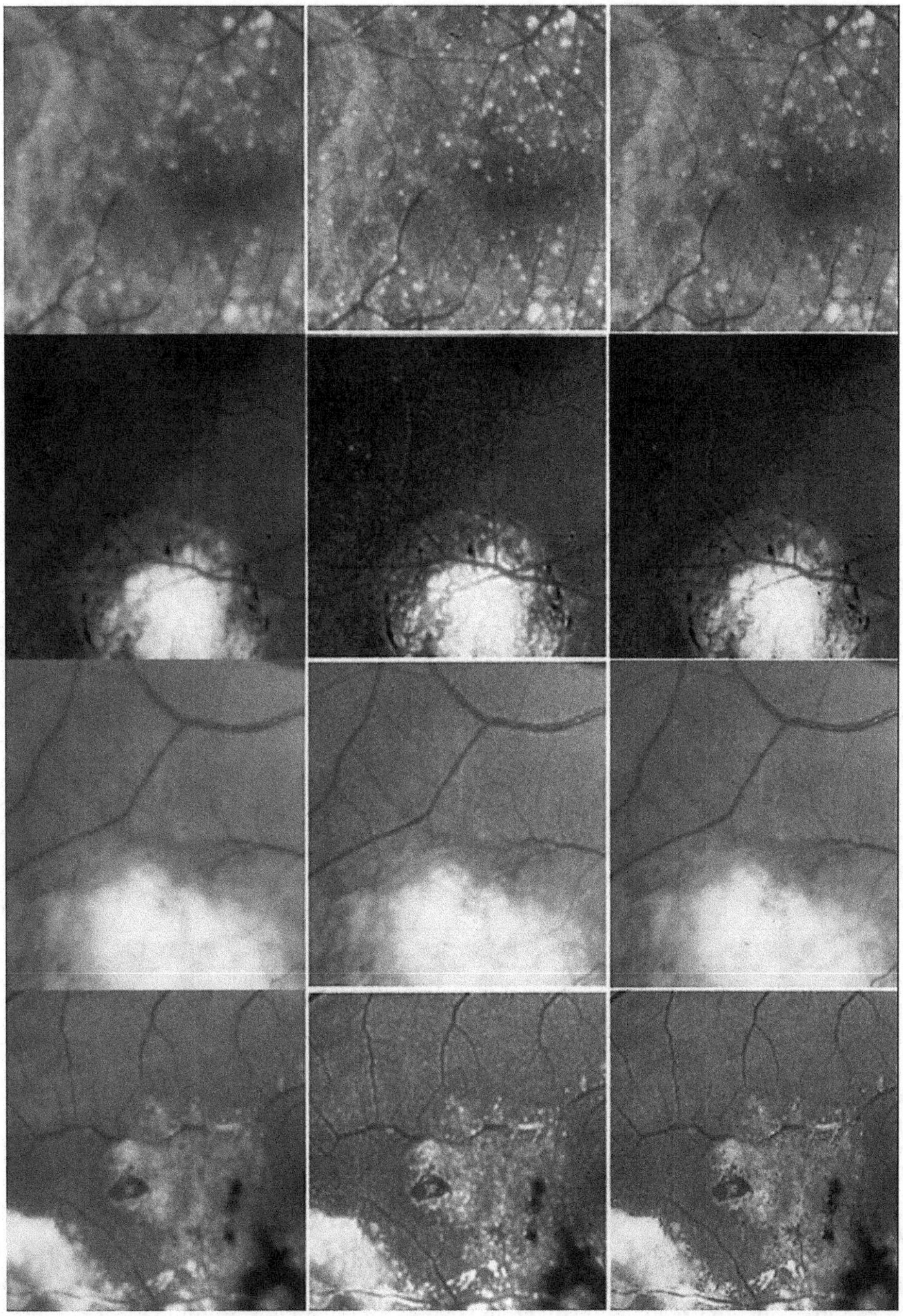

Figure 6. Performance comparisons of DHBT and LoG USM in noise environment for retinal images

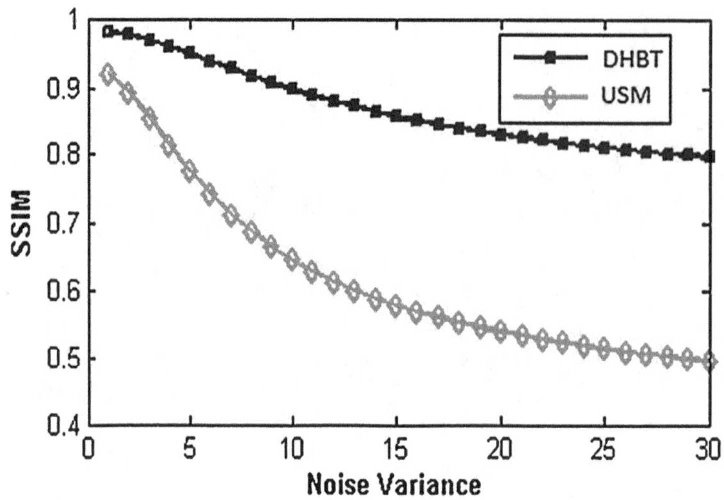

Table 4. Performance comparison of DHBT and LoG USM in STARE retinal images

Image	SSIM		Image	SSIM	
	DHBT	LoG		DHBT	LoG
im0001	0.971248	0.908277	im0011	0.973198	0.906199
im0002	0.969199	0.899390	im0012	0.968588	0.861951
im0003	0.970773	0.912116	im0013	0.976635	0.925057
im0004	0.973711	0.923420	im0014	0.969868	0.888689
im0005	0.962885	0.876790	im0015	0.968841	0.888177
im0006	0.978102	0.941239	im0016	0.972420	0.906482
im0007	0.974807	0.930067	im0017	0.976679	0.927938
im0008	0.977000	0.946637	im0018	0.970613	0.901781
im0009	0.972150	0.888485	im0019	0.973331	0.931273
im0010	0.975929	0.931816	im0020	0.979679	0.930567

Especially for the non-uniform, weak illumination and low contrast images (i.e.) x-ray image, the gray level differences between the object (i.e.) bone and background will possibly be low in some place of the image and variant in the whole image.

Since the Haar filters 'ψ' are high pass in nature, it acts as an edge filter and their responses are equal to edge information. Haar filters computes the similarity between the normalized Haar function and neighborhood pixels. In practice, 2D discrete Haar of an image is computed by separable implementation. Haar filter splits images into sub bands. 2D version of the Haar filter banks contains low pass and high pass filter. In the 2D case, the 1D analysis Haar filters first applied to the columns of the image and two sub band images are obtained. After applying, the 1D analysis Haar filter to each row of the two sub band images, four sub band images, one approximation sub band and three detail sub bands obtained. The vertical, horizontal and diagonal detail sub bands contain edges and specify the directional similarity. This similarity measure is computed as

$$S = \left(b_i - \frac{3\sigma_i}{4} \hat{b}_i + w_i \cdot MAD \right) * \psi . \tag{2}$$

In Equation 2 where $*$ de notes the convolution operation. The details of edge enhancement based on the above similarity measure are as follows: Divide the image into sub blocks having b_i neighborhood pixels. For each block, the index 'i' varies with the block size $L \times L$, i.e.) $i = 1,2,\ldots L$. Subtract the local mean $\hat{b}_i$ and local variance σ_i to remove the undesirable dependency on the average luminance. MAD is the mean absolute deviation that measures the data dispersion and it is sensitive to outliers. The value of MAD computed by

$$MAD = \frac{median\left(Y : 1 \le t \le M \times N\right)}{0.6745}.$$

where

$$Y = \left[\frac{1}{L^2} \sum_{q=1}^{L^2} \left[b_q\left(q\right) - \bar{b}_i \right]^2 \right]^{\frac{1}{2}}.$$

for the image size $M \times N$ of the L^2 neighborhoods. Edge regions have larger Y compared to smooth neighborhood regions. The suitable w_i weights are typically inversely proportional to the local variance 'σ_i'. This method uses conventional separable extension from 1D Haar wavelet filter operated on 2D image both row and column wise. As a result, the illumination corrected horizontal, vertical and diagonal direction sub bands are obtained and they imply the similarity measure in the corresponding direction. Combination of all sub bands at various scales provide S. This method is tested on chest x-ray images to prove the wide scope of this algorithm. Figure 7 and Figure 8 show the enhanced results of chest x-ray image using Haar based edge similarity measure (HSM). HSM has more distinct, sharper and well localized edges than Edge based Similarity (ESM). The common problem of low illumination x-ray is enhanced. The first column of the

Figure 7 and Figure 8 is presented with eight original x-ray images obtained from PHIL image data base and web source. They are enhanced by this algorithm and presented in the second column. While comparing second column results with third column which refer to method described in Saravanakumar et al. (2006), it is easy to recognize that Haar based method provides well distinct edges. The visually good results which are presented in Figure 7 and Figure 8 qualitatively compared through SSIM and tabulated in Table 5.

Figure 7. Enhancement of chest X ray images from left to right: original, HSM method, ESM method

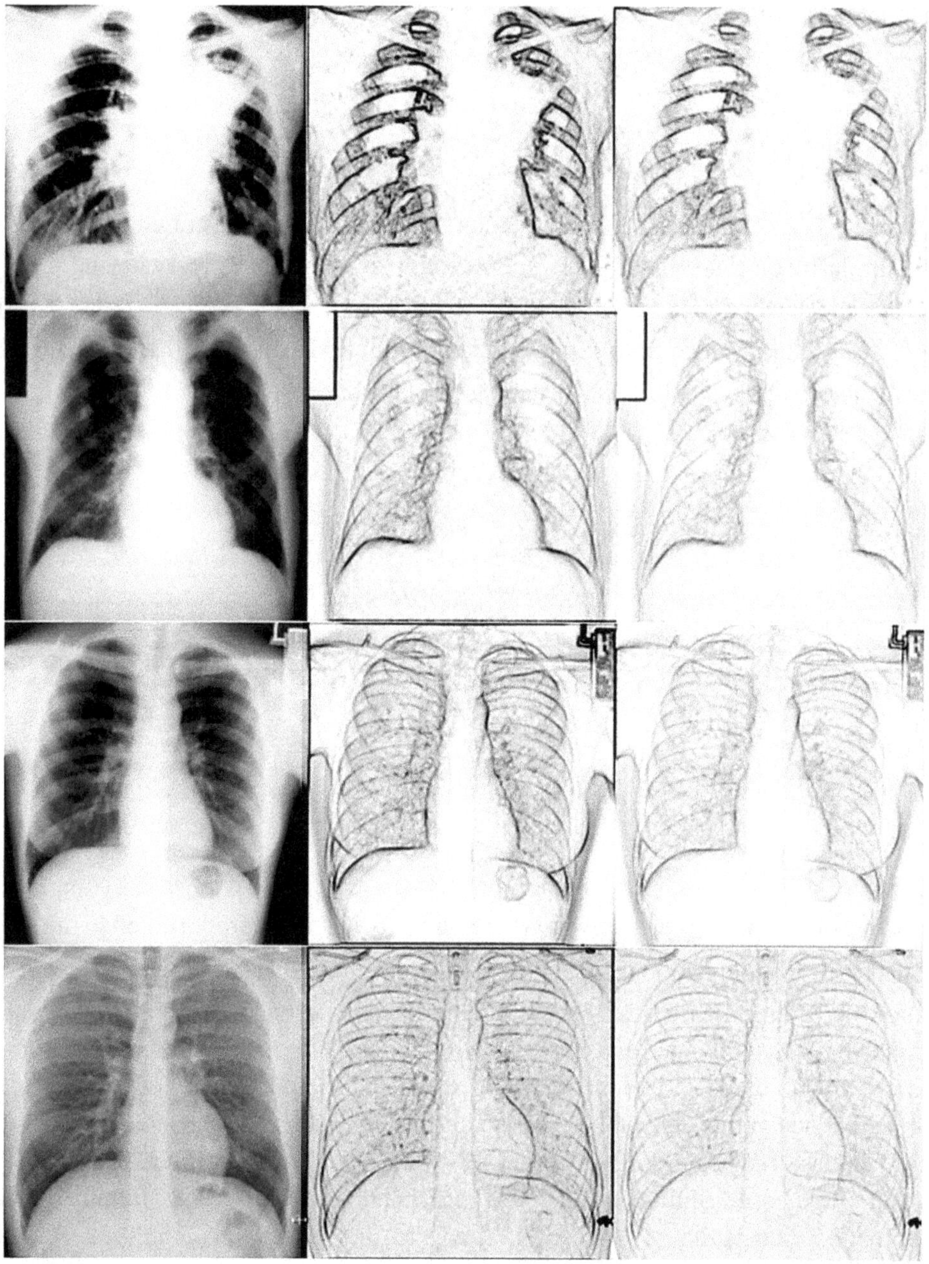

ENHANCEMENT OF VASCULATURE IN OPTIC DISC REGION

Analyzing the Optic Disc (OD) and its region in the digital fundus images is essential since it serves as the screening tool for examining the existence of many retinal diseases. The OD region is the major gateway of vision and changes in the rim of retinal OD, deformation of OD boundary, dilated pupil, nerve damage and retinal blood vessels act as the detecting tool for diseases in early or later stage. Vasculature

Figure 8. Enhancement of chest X ray images from left to right: original, HSM method, ESM method

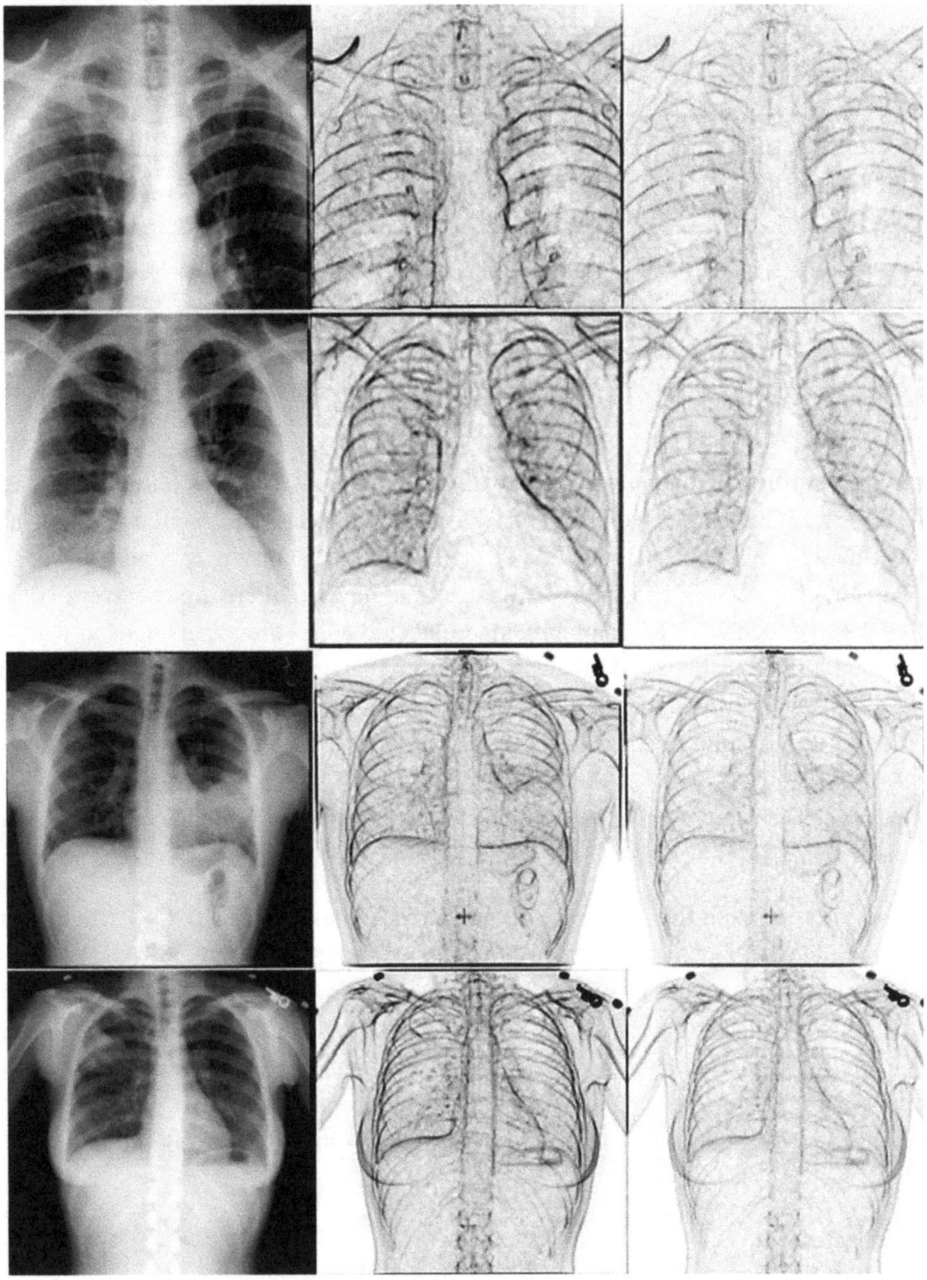

within the OD region is the one of the clinically interested part and enhancing the details of the retinal vasculature is indispensable (Foracchia, Grisan, & Ruggeri, 2004). In order to enhance the vascular tree emerging from the OD region, OD boundary must be traced, for which the center point of the OD acts as the seed point. The vessels within the OD are enhanced by the method uses edge information along with morphological operators (EDSMF).

Table 5. SSIM comparison chest x-ray image edge enhancement

Image	SSIM	
	ESM	HSM
1	0.97928	0.982903
2	0.966719	0.970454
3	0.962385	0.968072
4	0.97497	0.978625
5	0.97497	0.978625
6	0.982495	0.98651
7	0.962513	0.969837
8	0.981385	0.986638

- **Retinal Vasculature Enhancement:** The advances in digital retinal photography and imaging techniques have allowed precise characterization of subtle retinal vascular changes and offering an easy accessible to study the health and disease (Abramoff, Garvin, & Sonka,2010; Arturo, et al. 2010; Aliaam et al., 2008). In EDSMF enhancement method, there are two steps (i) superimposing of edges (ii) flood fill. The complemented detected edges are superimposed with the original image. Flood fill, also called seed fill, is an algorithm that determines the area connected to a given node in a multi-dimensional array. The flood fill algorithm takes three parameters: a start node, a target color and a replacement color. The average pixel value of the retinal blood vessels found within the OD region is taken as the replacement color. The start and the end node is taken from the retinal edges detected by means of edge detection technique. Replacement color selected is the filling element within the edges of superimposed image and the vessels are enhanced.

This method is tested with the three sets of standard databases MESSIDOR (Methods to evaluate segmentation and indexing techniques in the field of retinal ophthalmology), STARE and DRIVE. The retinal blood vessels enhancement is essential for detection of retinal diseases. Enhancement of blood vasculature is found within the OD region by the EDSMF, hold their importance. Vasculature enhanced images are shown in Figure 9, and Figure 10 respectively. In Figure 9 the original retinal image is shown, the algorithms are applied on green band of the color retinal image.

Additional enhanced results are presented in Figure 11. It illustrates the complete image processing steps:

1. OD center detection,
2. OD boundary tracing,
3. Enhanced images (EDSMF).

The enhancement of cropped OD region for vasulature is evaluated using enhancement measure (EME) (Agaian et al., 2010). It is a quantitative measure of image enhancement that is related with concepts of the Webers Law of the human visual system, argued that the human visual detection depends on the ratio, rather than difference. The Weber definition of contrast is used to measure the local contrast of a single object. EME of various OD regions cropped from DRIVE and MESSIDOR database images and enhanced images are presented in Table 6 and Table 7. They are compared with EME of standard

Figure 9. OD region enhancement from left to right original, green band of original, EDSMF method

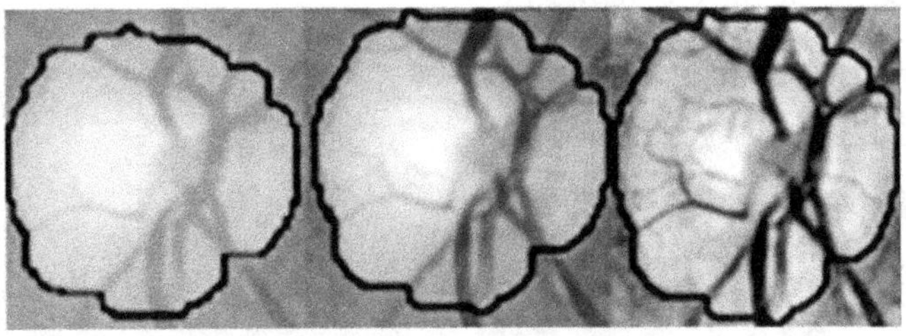

Figure 10. OD region enhancement from left to right: green band of original, EDSMF method

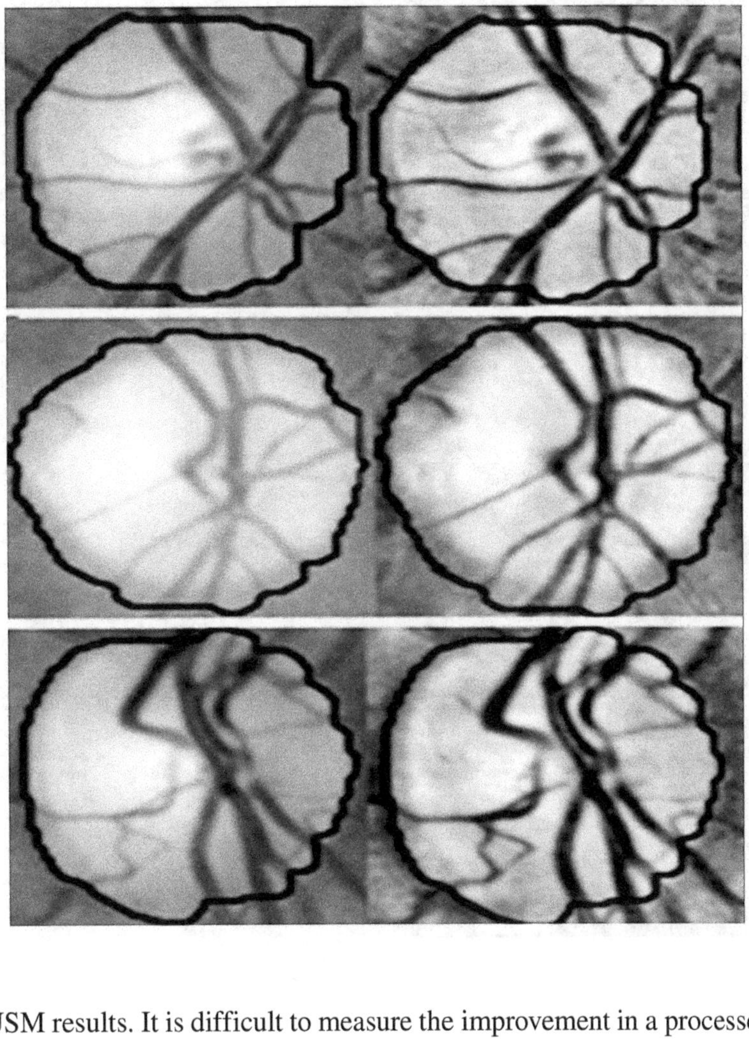

CLAHE and NLUSM results. It is difficult to measure the improvement in a processed image. It is said to be enhanced than original image if the desirable information is perceived in a better way. The high value of EME indicates the enhancement in the output image, and low value of EME indicates hidden information is not enhanced. From the experimental results, it is clear that EDSMF gives better level of enhancement without compromising the edge information. Although the proposed technique provides stronger contrast enhancement while preserving more edge information, the quality of the original do not affect.

Figure 11. Retinal image OD region analysis from left to right: center detection, boundary detection, cropped OD nearby region, EDSMF enhancement

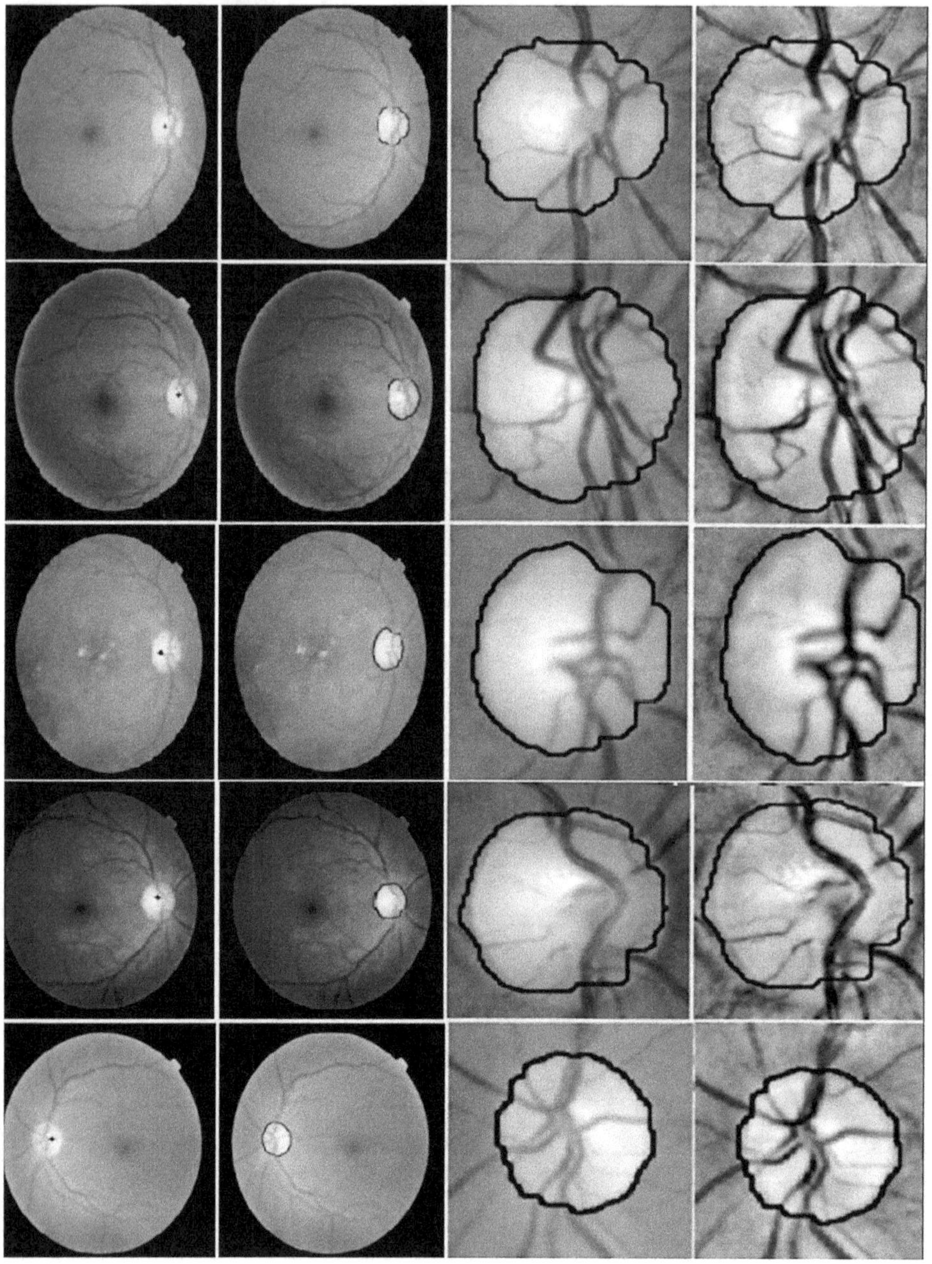

Table 6. EME comparison of OD region enhancement: DRIVE images

Image	Original	EDSMF	CLAHE	NLUSM
1_test	5.29	10.17	5.29	9.06
10_test	4.33	7.72	4.45	11.68
12_test	5.00	12.58	6.38	9.95
13_test	3.35	31.04	21.01	8.82
14_test	3.96	5.73	3.05	10.18
16_test	3.36	4.95	2.72	8.77
17_test	3.88	27.06	22.40	9.74
19_test	6.35	18.45	9.68	13.89
2_test	4.10	7.48	3.25	10.16
20_test	5.80	12.44	6.79	9.95
3_test	6.53	17.45	7.28	10.51
4_test	5.62	21.79	8.89	12.12
6_test	3.33	6.22	2.22	8.46
9_test	2.75	4.71	2.32	7.19

Table 7. EME comparison of OD region enhancement: MESSIDOR images

Image	Original	EDSMF	CLAHE	NLUSM
10	6.52	28.56	22.13	13.80
11	6.92	20.33	11.72	14.23
12	3.86	4.95	3.44	8.75
13	4.48	10.78	5.66	8.99
14	11.63	32.78	27.45	22.43
15	5.36	20.42	8.13	17.65
16	9.41	32.78	22.49	25.91
3	3.94	8.56	2.95	12.51
4	7.24	22.58	12.88	15.28
5	5.63	21.70	9.52	15.70
6	5.82	24.75	11.76	15.14
7	6.85	27.00	14.58	16.78
8	7.64	34.56	25.40	22.12
9	6.25	24.18	9.94	18.39

FUTURE RESEARCH DIRECTIONS

In the growth of contrast enhancement and edge enhancement algorithms, still there are some issues need to be addressed in future. Since the enhancement is the subjective process, automatic selection of adjustable parameter setting is crucial. There are very limited number of research in the literature which efficiently incorporate the human visual parameters along with enhancement algorithms. Enhancement process differ from one imaging modality to another imaging modality, one image type to another image type, one application to another application, global enhancement technique which is image independent is very challenging. Moreover, incorporating histogram information in the local spatial domain is another potential area to work in image enhancement.

CONCLUSION

This chapter described the hyperbolic filter based CT, retinal and mammogram enhancement algorithm. It also analyzed a hyperbolic filter based unsharp filter for retinal image enhancement, edge enhancement of chest x-ray image by Haar filters and the enhancement of vasculature in optic disc region based on edge information along with morphological operators. The tests are performed on images obtained from standard database. In many cases, enhancement improves the quality of the image and facilitates diagnosis. Enhancement measure (EME), structural similarity measure (SSIM), mean squared error (MSE) and figure of merit (F) are used as performance evaluation parameters.

REFERENCES

Abramoff, M. D., Garvin, M. K., & Sonka, M. (2010). Retinal imaging and image analysis. *IEEE. Reviews in Biomedical Engineering*, *3*, 169–208. doi:10.1109/RBME.2010.2084567 PMID:22275207

Adam, H., Valentina, K., & Michael, G. (2000). Locating Blood Vessels in Retinal Images by Piecewise Threshold Probing of a Matched Filter Response. *IEEE Transactions on Medical Imaging*, *19*(3), 203–210. doi:10.1109/42.845178 PMID:10875704

Agaian, S. S., Panetta, K. A., & Grigoryan, A. M. (2001). Transform based image enhancement algorithms with performance measure. *IEEE Transactions on Image Processing*, *10*(3), 367–382. doi:10.1109/83.908502 PMID:18249627

Agaian, S. S., Panetta, K. A., Nercessian, S. C., & Danahy, E. E. (2010). Boolean derivatives with application to edge detection for imaging systems. *IEEE Transactions on Systems, Man, and Cybernetics. Part B, Cybernetics*, *40*(2), 371–382. doi:10.1109/TSMCB.2009.2024771 PMID:19884097

Akram, M. U., Atzaz, A., Aneeque, S. F., & Khan, S. A. (2009). Blood vessel enhancement and segmentation using wavelet transform.*IEEE International Conference on Digital Image Processing*. doi:10.1109/ICDIP.2009.70

Aliaam, A. H., Abdel, R. Y., Atef, Z. G., Amr, A. S., & Ghoneim, A. R. (2008). Optic disc detection from normalized digital fundus images by means of vessels direction matched filter. *IEEE Transactions on Medical Imaging*, *27*(1), 11–18. doi:10.1109/TMI.2007.900326 PMID:18270057

Anand, S., ShanthaSelvaKumari, R., Jeeva, S., & Thivya, T. (2013). Contourlet transform based sharpening enhancement of retinal images and vessel extraction application. *Biomedizinische Technik. Biomedical Engineering*, *58*, 87–96. PMID:23314502

Anand, S., & Gayathri, S. (2015). Mammogram image enhancement by two stage adaptive histogram equalization. *Optik-International Journal of Light and Electron Optics*, *126*(21), 3150–3152. doi:10.1016/j.ijleo.2015.07.069

Anand, S., Kumari, R. S. S., Jeeva, S., & Thivya, T. (2013). Directionlet transform based sharpening and enhancement of mammographic x-ray images. *Biomedical Signal Processing and Control*, *8*(4), 391–399. doi:10.1016/j.bspc.2013.02.001

Anand, S., & Shantha Selva Kumari, R. (2013). Sharpening enhancement of computed tomography (CT) images using hyperbolic secant square filter. *Optik-International Journal for Light and Electron Optics*, *124*(15), 2121–2124. doi:10.1016/j.ijleo.2012.06.026

Anand, S., Shantha Selva Kumari, R., Thivya, T., Jeeva, S. (2013). Sharpening enhancement of ultrasound images using contourlet transform. *Optik-International Journal for Light and Electron Optics*, *124*, 4789–4792.

Arandiga, F., Cohen, A., Donat, R., & Matei, B. (2010). Edge detection insensitive to changes of illumination in the image. *Image and Vision Computing*, *28*(4), 553–562. doi:10.1016/j.imavis.2009.09.002

Arturo, A., Manuel, E. G., & Diego, M. (2010). Detecting the optic disc boundary in digital fundus images using morphological, edge detection and feature extraction techniques. *IEEE Transactions on Medical Imaging*, *29*(11), 1860–186. doi:10.1109/TMI.2010.2053042 PMID:20562037

Bhutada, G. G., Anand, R. S., & Saxena, S. C. (2011). Edge preserved image enhancement using adaptive fusion of Images Denoised by Wavelet and Curvelet Transform. *Digital Signal Processing*, *21*(1), 118–130. doi:10.1016/j.dsp.2010.09.002

Bock, R., Meier, J., Nyul, L. G., & Michelson, G. (2010). Glaucoma risk index: Automated glaucoma detection from color fundus images. *Medical Image Analysis*, *14*(3), 471–481. doi:10.1016/j.media.2009.12.006 PMID:20117959

Brigham, R. A. D. (2013). *Department of Radiology, Brigham and Women's Hospital*. Harvard Medical School. Retrieved from http://brighamrad.harvard. edu/Cases/bwh/hcache/group0-index.html

Canny, J. (1986). A Computational Approach to Edge Detection. *IEEE Transactions on Pattern Analysis and Machine Intelligence*, *8*(6), 679–698. doi:10.1109/TPAMI.1986.4767851 PMID:21869365

Carlsson, S. (1988). Sketch Based Coding of Gray Level Images. *Signal Processing*, *15*(1), 57–83. doi:10.1016/0165-1684(88)90028-X

Dai, F., Zheng, N., & Xue, J. (2008). Image smoothing and sharpening based on nonlinear diffusion equation. *Signal Processing*, *88*(11), 2850–2855. doi:10.1016/j.sigpro.2008.05.008

Desolneux, A., Moisan, L., & Morel, J. M. (2001). Edge Detection by Helmholtz Principle. *Journal of Mathematical Imaging and Vision*, *14*(3), 271–284. doi:10.1023/A:1011290230196

DRIVE. (2013). *Digital Retinal Images for Vessel Extraction*. Retrieved from http://www.isi.uu.nl/Research/Databases/DRIVE/

Elder, J. (1991). Are edges incomplete. *International Journal of Computer Vision*, *34*(2/3), 97–122. doi:10.1023/A:1008183703117

Eltoukhy, M. M., Faye, I., & Samir, B. B. (2010). Breast cancer diagnosis in digital mammogram using multiscalecurvelet transforms. *Computerized Medical Imaging and Graphics*, *34*(4), 269–276. doi:10.1016/j.compmedimag.2009.11.002 PMID:20004076

Foracchia, M., Grisan, E., & Ruggeri, A. (2004). Detection of optic disc in retinal images by means of a geometrical model of vessel structure. *IEEE Transactions on Medical Imaging*, *23*(10), 1189–1195. doi:10.1109/TMI.2004.829331 PMID:15493687

Foracchia, M., Grisan, E., & Ruggeri, A. (2005). Luminosity and contrast normalization in retinal images. *Medical Image Analysis*, *3*(3), 179–190. doi:10.1016/j.media.2004.07.001 PMID:15854840

Gonzalez, & Woods. (2009). *Digital Image Processing*. Prentice Hall.

Grisan, E., Giani, A., Ceseracciu, E., & Ruggeri, A. (2006). Model based illumination correction in retinal images.*IEEE Int. Symposium Biomedical Imaging, Nano to Macro*. doi:10.1109/ISBI.2006.1625085

Gupta, S., Kaur, L., Chauhan, R. C., & Saxena, S. C. (2007). A versatile technique for visual enhancement of medical ultrasound images. *Digital Signal Processing*, *17*(3), 542–560. doi:10.1016/j.dsp.2006.12.001

Jian, C., Jie, T. B., Zichun, T., Jian, X., Yakang, D., & Jian, Z. (2008). Retinal vessel enhancement and extraction based on directional field. *Journal of X-Ray Science and Technology*, *16*, 189–201.

Joshi, G. D., & Sivaswamy, J. (2008). Colour Retinal Image Enhancement based on Domain Knowledge. *Sixth Indian Conference on Computer Vision, Graphics and Image Processing*. doi:10.1109/ICVGIP.2008.70

Karen, F. P., Yicong, Z., Agaian, S., & Hongwei, J. (2011). Nonlinear unsharp masking for mammogram enhancement. *IEEE Transactions on Information Technology in Biomedicine*, *15*(6), 918–928. doi:10.1109/TITB.2011.2164259 PMID:21843996

Kim, J. K., Park, J. M., Song, K. S., & Park, H. W. (1997). Adaptive mammographic image enhancement using first derivative and local statistics. *IEEE Transactions on Medical Imaging*, *16*(5), 495–502. doi:10.1109/42.640739 PMID:9368105

Kim, Y. H., & Cho, Y. J. (2008). Feature and noise adaptive unsharp masking based on statistical hypotheses test. *IEEE Transactions on Consumer Electronics*, *54*(2), 823–830. doi:10.1109/TCE.2008.4560166

Konstantinos, K., Vasudev, B., & Giordano, B. (1999). Image sharpening in the JPEG domain. *IEEE Transactions on Image Processing*, *8*(6), 874–878. doi:10.1109/83.766864 PMID:18267500

Li, Y, Yanmei, L., Hailun, F. (2010). Study on the methods of image enhancement for liver CT images. *Optik - International Journal for Light and Electron Optics, 121*, 1752-1755.

MESSIDOR. (2013). *Methods to evaluate segmentation and indexing techniques in the field of retinal ophthalmology*. Retrieved from http://messidor.crihan.fr/

MIAS. (2013). *Mammographic Image Analysis Society*. Retrieved from http://peipa.essex. ac.uk/info/mias.html

Ming, Z., Youfu, L., Qinghao, M., Ting, Y., & Jian, L. (2012). Improving histogram-based image contrast enhancement using gray-level information histogram with application to X-ray images. *Optik-International Journal for Light and Electron Optics, 123*(6), 511–520. doi:10.1016/j.ijleo.2011.05.017

Mitra, B. (2002). Gaussian based edge-detection methods: A survey. *IEEE Transactions on Systems, Man and Cybernetics. Part C, Applications and Reviews, 32*(3), 252–260. doi:10.1109/TSMCC.2002.804448

Olivier, L., & Truchetet, F. (2010). A nonlinear derivative scheme applied to edge detection. *IEEE Transactions on Pattern Analysis and Machine Intelligence, 32*(2), 242–257. doi:10.1109/TPAMI.2008.282 PMID:20075456

Pellegrino, F., Vanzella, W., & Torre, V. (2004). Edge detection revisited. *IEEE Transactions on Systems, Man, and Cybernetics. Part B, Cybernetics, 34*(3), 1500–1518. doi:10.1109/TSMCB.2004.824147 PMID:15484920

Peng, F., Yingjun, P., Biao, W., Wei, J., & Deling, M. (2007). Enhancing retinal image by the contourlet transform. *Pattern Recognition Letters, 28*(4), 516–522. doi:10.1016/j.patrec.2006.09.007

Phan, T. H. (2009). Vessel enhancement filter using directional filter bank. *Computer Vision and Image Understanding, 113*(1), 101–112. doi:10.1016/j.cviu.2008.07.009

PHIL. (2012). *Public Health Image Library*. Retrieved from http://phil.cdc.gov/phil

Pratt, W. K. (2004). *Digital Image Processing*. New York: John Wiley and Sons.

Rakesh, R. R., Probal, C., & Murthy, C. A. (2004). Thresholding in edge detection: A statistical approach. *IEEE Transactions on Image Processing, 13*(7), 927–936. doi:10.1109/TIP.2004.828404 PMID:15648859

Saravanakumar, S. (2006). A Luminance- and contrast-invariant edge-similarity measure. *IEEE Transactions on Pattern Analysis and Machine Intelligence, 28*(12), 2042–2048. doi:10.1109/TPAMI.2006.236 PMID:17108378

Staal, J. J., Abramoff, M. D., Niemeijer, M., Viergever, M. A., & Ginneken, B. (2004). Ridge based vessel segmentation in color images of the retina. *IEEE Transactions on Medical Imaging, 23*(4), 501–509. doi:10.1109/TMI.2004.825627 PMID:15084075

STARE. (2013). *STructured Analysis of the Retina project.* Retrieved from http://www.ces.clemson.edu/~ahoover/stare/

Sundaram, M., Ramar, K., Arumugam, N., & Prabin, G. (2011). Histogram Modified Local Contrast Enhancement for mammogram images. *Applied Soft Computing, 11*(8), 5809–5816. doi:10.1016/j.asoc.2011.05.003

Tay, P. C., Garson, C. D., Acton, S. T., & Hossack, J. A. (2010). Ultrasound despeckling for contrast enhancement. *IEEE Transactions on Image Processing, 19*(7), 1847–1860. doi:10.1109/TIP.2010.2044962 PMID:20227984

Wang, Z., Bovik, A. C., Sheikh, H. R., & Simoncelli, E. P. (2004). Image quality assessment: From error measurement to structural similarity. *IEEE Transactions on Image Processing, 13*(4), 600–612. doi:10.1109/TIP.2003.819861 PMID:15376593

Wanpeng, C., Rensheng, C., & Dong, Y. (2008). An illumination-independent edge detection and fuzzy enhancement algorithm based on wavelet transform for non-uniform weak illumination images. *Pattern Recognition Letters*, *29*(3), 192–199. doi:10.1016/j.patrec.2007.09.012

Yang, Y., Su, Z., & Sun, L. (2010). Medical image enhancement algorithm based on wavelet transform. *IET Electronics Letters*, *46*(2), 120–121. doi:10.1049/el.2010.2063

Yu, R. L., Kuo, L. C., Guei, Y. L., & Chyou, H. C. (2012). Gaussian mixture modelling of histograms for contrast enhancement. *Expert Systems with Applications*, *39*(8), 6720–6728. doi:10.1016/j.eswa.2011.12.018

Zhiguo, G., & Yi, L. (2011). An image sharpening algorithm based on fuzzy logic. *International Journal for Light and Electron Optics*, *122*(8), 697–702. doi:10.1016/j.ijleo.2010.05.010

Zuiderveld, K. (1994). Contrast Limited Adaptive Histogram Equalization. Cambridge, MA: Academic Press. doi:10.1016/B978-0-12-336156-1.50061-6

KEY TERMS AND DEFINITIONS

Chest X-Ray: A chest x-ray produces images of the heart, lungs, airways, blood vessels and the bones of the spine and chest.

Computed Tomography: CT is an imaging procedure that uses special equipment to create detailed pictures of areas inside the body.

Edge Information: A set of points in a digital image at which the image brightness changes sharply typically organized into a curved line segments termed edges.

Image Enhancement: Image Enhancement process to improve visual information for a specific application.

Mammogram Image: A mammogram is an x-ray image to examine the breast tissue for any suspicious.

Medical Imaging: Medical Imaging is the technique of creating visual representations of the interior of a body for clinical analysis and medical intervention.

Retinal Fundus Image: The fundus of the eye is the interior surface of the eye opposite the lens and includes the retina, optic disc, macula, and fovea.

Chapter 7
Success Dimensions of ICTs in Healthcare

Pankaj Deep Kaur
G.N.D.U. Regional Campus, India

Pallavi Sharma
G.N.D.U. Regional Campus, India

ABSTRACT

During the last decades, the call for Information and Communication Technologies (ICTs) in healthcare has been augmented to endow with healthcare services at a global scale and to trim down medical errors that cost human lives. Enriched with explosive computing and high communicating power, ICTs like Internet, mobile telephony, and other enabled gadgets plays a prominent role in our day-to-day activities. With the potential to provide access to service for patients in difficult-to reach areas and facilitating medical record keeping and information sharing are the main considerations of leveraging ICTs in realm of clinical care. The insurgence of these innovating technologies into healthcare sectors is not only blurring the boundaries for the emergence of other new technologies but also causing a paradigm shift in providing acute and preventative care in public health. The main goal of this chapter is to offer readers an insight into how the emergence of ICTs have transformed healthcare sector by delivering cost-efficient and quality of care to patients.

INTRODUCTION

In the era of information age and globalization, Information and Communication Technologies (ICTs) are considered to have a catalyzing effect in delivering efficient, timeliness and quality of healthcare services (Lindberg, Nilsson, Zotterman, Soderberg, & Skar, 2013). Being referred to as a 'key instrument' in healthcare, ICTs facilitates an effective electronic means for communicating, processing and transformation of information with the intent to improve human health. Since, more and more patients are seeking and prioritizing quality of healthcare in their lives, innovations in and use of emerging ICTs in healthcare sectors has considerably increased over the last ten years. Active patient involvement, care process management and remote care are some of the notable benefits from these innovations in public health.

DOI: 10.4018/978-1-5225-0660-7.ch007

Prospective applications of digital technologies in healthcare sector cannot be undervalued. Concerted efforts have been made worldwide to kindle the use of ICTs in healthcare. With the increase in the number of patients suffering from chronic diseases (such as diabetes mellitus, cardio-respiratory diseases), modern healthcare services are over-powered with high annual expenses. Addressing to these financial issues, ICTs allocate cost-effective patient treatment and health promotion. From clinical data digitalization to appointment reminders by SMS alerts, the use of ICTs is increasingly mounting around the world with intend to reduce health expenditure and to raise patients and lay personnel involvement. Although the implementation of ICTs in healthcare is an expensive measure, but possesses a high cost-saving potential benefits in the long run.

BACKROUND

Effective communication and reliable information can be well thought-out as essential elements in area of public health. According to (World Health Organization [WHO], 2004) technology forms the backbone of any organization's services to diagnose, prevent and treat illness. Healthcare organization in the vein to maintain healthy lifestyles and healthy minds seek for more optimal solutions and strategies to increase their medical services. As more and more patients are prioritizing the quality of care in their lives, healthcare industries are persistently placed under giant demands to enhance both infrastructure and information- handling abilities.

With the widespread increase in chronic diseases such as chronic obstructive pulmonary disease, cardiovascular disease (mainly ischemic heart disease), diabetes mellitus, certain cancers (stomach, primarily lung and breast cancer) in various developed countries; healthcare organizations attributed sedentary lifestyle and genetic predisposition of the population to strictly linked with the health damaging behaviors of modern age. Traditional medical approaches focused on the treatment of diseases, however when referred to primary prevention in the modern age the concepts are renewed. In primary prevention, innovation focuses firstly on modifying risk factors that includes accidents; family history; work environmental factors etc and are highly dependent on individual behaviors and lifestyle management (WHO, 2008). Following the similar vein of primary prevention, there are different emerging models that made a big splash towards changing trends in Healthcare Information Technology [HIT].

Technological change is crucial for incessant modernization of healthcare field. The main healthcare drivers in the era of 1960s were Medicaid and Medicare. Since the mainframes and storage were so bulky and costly, health organizations typically have a shared mainframe environment and shared accounting systems. During 1970s there prompted a need to slighter the communication gap among health organizations and to set up isolated departmental systems such as pharmacy, clinical labs etc. Smaller computers were installed in single departments with improved terminals and connectivity, thus proliferating different departmental systems. The era of 1980s was heavily driven by emerging networking solutions (e.g. DRGs) and non-traditional software applications that had entered the market. As a result of this driven, Information Technology (IT) in healthcare hospitals started incorporating diverse software applications so that clinical and financial systems could converse to each other in some restricted way. In the decade of 1990s, hospitals driven by IT perspective now had ease of access to distributed, broad computing systems and Integrated Delivery Network (IDN) for data integrating and reporting. The era of 2000s was driven by much advanced integrated technology. Diverse clinical applications were installed alongside the bedside in hospitals to make a staid run towards real-time decision support systems such as Electronic Medical

Records (EMRs), Electronic Health Records (EHRs), Personal Health Records (PHRs), Content Based Image Retrieval Systems (CBIRs) etc. With the intent to achieve more personalized health record the period from 2010 till now is witnessing IT driven change in healthcare with the foreword of "eHealth" or more distinctively "Smart eHealth". Supported by electronic process and communication, eHealth encompasses diverse range of systems or services that are collaboration of healthcare, medicine and Information Technology (IT). The evolution of health information technologies is as shown in Figure 1.

Healthcare systems are at risk due to spiraling costs, increasing demands, inconsistent quality of data and poor coordinated care-processes. In this scenario, investment in Information and Communication Technologies (ICTs) can be viewed as an emergent solution in providing higher and safer quality of care processes that are more responsive to patient's needs. However, while introducing ICTs; healthcare service organizations have to face many challenges towards the implementation and adoption of ICTs as well as organizational support to recruit and employ top quality employees to make best usage of ICT tools. Given the supportive organization culture, right policies, and resources; ICTs can be considered as a powerful tool in the hands of caregivers (WHO, 2004). In this state-of-art, use of information technologies for searching, collecting, and extracting meaningful data from large repositories could prove as an efficient method to determine and analyze different medical conditions.

MAIN FOCUS OF THE CHAPTER: INTRODUCTION TO DIFFERENT TECHNOLOGICAL ASPECTS IN HEALTHCARE

Cloud Computing

With the increase in the levels of life expectancy, many developed countries intend at stretching resources (for example, community care, healthcare professional and financial resources) to provide more quality of care in real time. Therefore, to provide more cost-effective and innovative solutions to this growing

Figure 1. Evolution of health information technologies

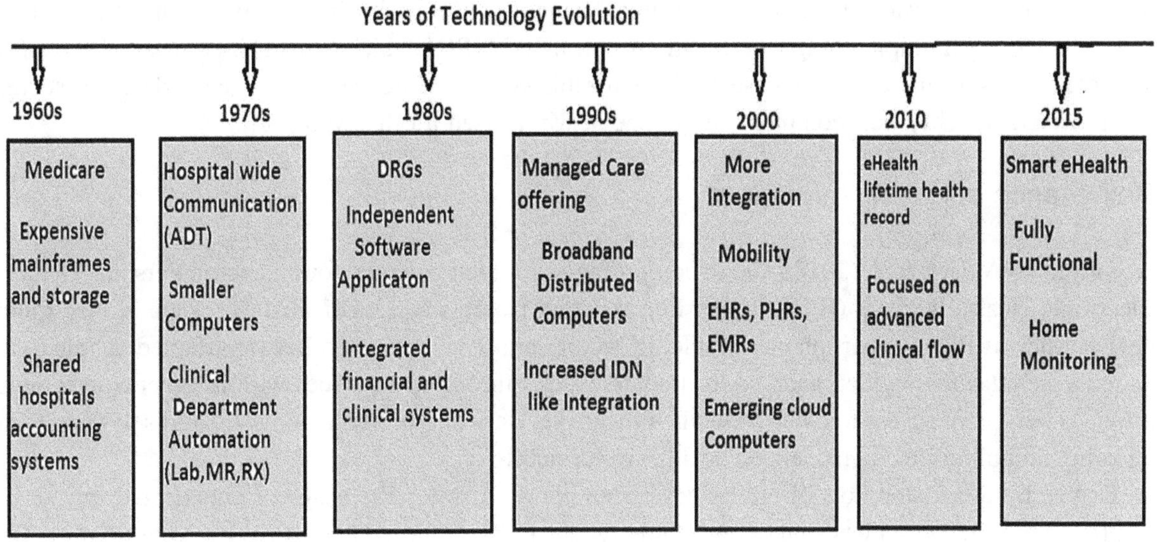

problem, the concept of cloud computing has been proposed in healthcare (Kaur & Chana, 2014). As a new model to deliver range of ICT services in remote areas, cloud computing has emerged as a new computing paradigm to deliver for more scalable, convenience and "pay-as-you-go" services for the end users (Barrow, 2011). The efforts of proposing cloud computing in healthcare can be categorized into three categories as follows:

1. Storage and Manipulation of Healthcare Data,
2. Deliverance of e-health services.

Storage and Manipulation of Healthcare Data

To shift the burden of healthcare providers for maintaining and managing the complex healthcare data, researchers have proposed many cloud-based-architecture solutions to exploit the computing and storage facilities provided by the cloud. Considering the massive volume of medical images, a cloud-based intelligent hospital file management system was proposed in 2010 (Guo, Chen, Chen, & Tang, 2010) that was implemented using Picture Archiving and Communication System (PACS) and Hadoop Distributed File System (HDFS) to solve problems of storing, sharing and exchanging of medical images across the boundaries between hospitals.

In 2012(Pandeya et al., 2012), addresses the design characteristics of an automatic cloud-based system architecture that could collect patient health records and store them into cloud repository using certain software services available in cloud. This proposed prototype system could be used as testbed for analysis of Electrocardiogram (ECG) data.

In 2013 (Venkatesh, Premkumar, & Sivaguru, 2013) authors proposed another cloud based platform architecture consisting of six independent layers. This architecture uses message queue as a cloud engine that can support access to high volume of structured and semi-structured medical data. Since in this system each layer works in a loosely coupled communication environment it can satisfy massive service requests concurrently, thus supporting ubiquitous healthcare services.

In 2014, another cloud-based architecture has been proposed in which all the medical images are processed only in one-write -many-read schema (read-only mode) (Arka & Chellappan, 2014). That is, the images that are pushed into cloud-environment cannot be altered by client users. Further, this system can contain many multiple storage centers simultaneously. MySQL which is an open-source and powerful application, has been used as database platform for this system. Moreover, to bridge the database server and browser, Apache, most commonly used web-server is used for this web-portal.

Deliverance of E-Health Services

According to Alagoz et al. (2010), Cloud computing has a great potential for managing Personal Health/ Electronic Health Records ([PHR/EHR). For assisting patients and medical staff, usage of electronic devices such as PDAs, smart phones, Tablet PCs etc promises a sense of relief for affected people (e.g. patients, healthcare providers) and on healthcare expenditure. These devices with Internet connections provides persistent access to cloud based healthcare services and promote domestic and self care; thus allowing ubiquitous and personalized healthcare services.

Driven by this vision, lots of efforts have been put on to study the usage of Cloud platform for e-health service delivery. For instance, Accenture and AT &T proposed a Medical Imaging Solution for assisting the medical professionals in reviewing medical images such as Magnetic Resonance Imaging (MRI), CT scans and X-rays in a remote way. In 2010, a cloud based emergency medical service system was proposed (Koufi, Malamateniou, & Vassilacopoulos, 2010) for the patient monitoring, accurate safety alerts etc. All the activities in this system are done through PHRs from the call to an ambulance service till patient's discharge from the hospital. Another cloud based system in 2010 was proposed (Rolim et al., 2010) for automatic collecting patients' data through a network of sensors connected to medical devices. This system provides 24/7 real time data and allows to deliver the patient's vital data to medical center's "cloud" for further processing storage and distribution. Figure 2 illustrates how data flow takes place through cloud based environment. It is a two-way data-sharing process in which after patient monitoring via medical devices, the data gathered is stored in medical center's cloud and a replicate copy of data is stored at its data center. The data is further processed in cloud-based environment and could be accessible easily amongst healthcare professionals and patients.

Rising Concerns in Cloud-Based Environment

According to Erdogmus (2009), the main drivers of cloud computing are simplification, economics and convenience with which cloud-based services are being delivered. According to one view, by providing IT services in the cloud much of the expense is being shifted to pay-as-you-go model, hence freeing the IT organizations from the hassle of installing and maintaining applications locally. However, users are also concerned with issues related to governance, security and integration issues. In accordance with the survey conducted by IDC (International Data Corporation) in 2008, 75% of IT executives rated security as main cloud-computing issue while 64% of respondents rated availability and performance as the next two issues (Cisco, 2009). According to another survey conducted by EDUCAUSE (a nonprofit association that endeavor to advance higher education through the use of information technology) reported that 69% of respondents considered data security and privacy issues as prime barriers to prevail over (Goldstein, 2009). Additionally, breakdown of a cloud provider that hosts client's data in their data centers can cause stern aftermaths for those who shared their personal data with such provider.

Figure 2. Data flow through cloud based environment

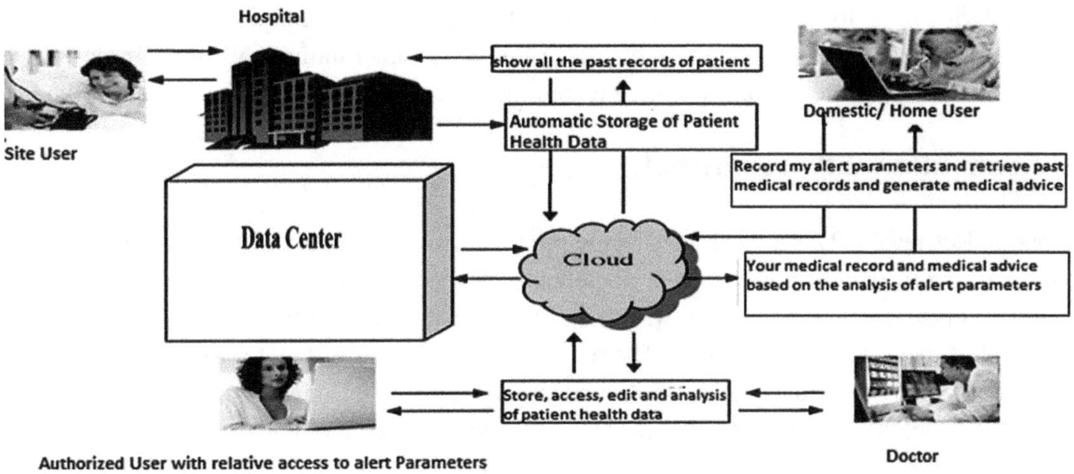

According to ISO/IEC 27001: 2013(Fernandez-Aleman & Lozoya, 2013) security has many different aspects; but with regards to healthcare the security requirements are broader, that is, users want adequate level of Quality of Service (QoS). QoS apart from different aspects of security also includes 'adaptability' feature, which can be defined as the quickness towards change. This feature can be implemented in modular design systems by the application of international standards so as to avoid expensive maintenance and modifications. According to Kaufman (2009), in Internet-based computing paradigm since the data on the cloud resides in a shared milieu and users are not aware of the exact location of their data, therefore users have to accept the fundamental premise of trust (Zissis & Lekkas, 2012). As a result of such privacy related problems the cloud-based platforms have limited adoption in healthcare realm. Reliability is also a major issue for cloud users. For example, in year 2012 (also called as leap year bug) Azure (Microsoft's cloud platform) had to suffer a worldwide, extensive outage for more than 24 hours. Consequently, due to some "misconfigured network device" in West Europe sub-region Azure customers had to undergo loss of service. In the same year on 15 June, another power outage of Amazon Web Services (AWS) that lasted for six hours, affected Amazon Relational Database Service, Elastic Compute Cloud (EC2) and AWS Elastic Beanstalk that are made to run from Amazon's data centers in Northern Virginia. On 26 October 2012, Google App Engine which is responsible for hosting Web application slows down due to some errors for about four hours causing 55% of App Engine requests to fail (McCarthy, 2012). If such similar outages persistently affect cloud-based healthcare solutions, its effect on the working of healthcare providers could be more dramatic.

BIG DATA ANALYTICS IN HEALTHCARE

Digitization of healthcare has accumulated massive volume of data at an unprecedented rate. Healthcare data gathered from diverse data sources such as laboratory, medication, narrative and imaging data has much greater potential to deliver best patient-centric, evidence-based, and accountable care. With the expansion of large and bulky clinical data repositories, healthcare organizations are progressively using diverse data analytical techniques to scrutinize and exploit the relationships and patterns found in datasets so as to enhance medical decisions. Big data analytics deal with the proper utilization of medical data using information retrieval and data mining techniques (Murdoch, & Detsky, 2013). These technologies have much greater prospective for healthcare improvement and can be used to obtain information about specific individuals or for generic use. For example, finding the "medical pathways" for an individual from large unrelated data and using the same data as input for other individuals with similar pathways. Different data analytics technologies applied to healthcare databases can be explained as follows:

Healthcare Information Retrieval

Information Retrieval (IR) can be defined as the process of searching for the most relevant information to a user's query from large collections of documents. IR techniques intend to retrieve the information as accurate as possible and in the same way as stored in the database.IR techniques generally deal with the retrieval of medical text and images. The main challenge in medical text retrieval is with the ambiguity and complexity of medical queries and records (Babashzadeh, Huang, & Daoud, 2013). However, to tackle the problem of ambiguity, diverse standard medical terminologies such as Unified Medical Language System (UMLS), International Classification of Disease (ICD), Medical Subject Headings

(MeSH) etc have been widely used in healthcare domain. Further to improve the search quality of query retrieval and to fill up semantic gap among the queries, reformulation and query expansion techniques have been used (Jain, Thao, & Zhao 2012).

Medical image retrieval can be addressed in two ways: -

1. Content based approach,
2. Text-based approach.

Content Based Image Retrieval

For the content based image retrieval, visual features of the images are being employed. In this search process, user provides the sample of the medical image and the retrieval is achieved by comparing image descriptors (which are numerical by nature and can be represented in vector form) of the query image with all the set of images in the health database. Although colour is an important visual feature of an image, it is not used because most of the medical images are grayscale. The other two main visual features used in medical image search are shape and texture (Hwang, Lee, & Choi, 2012). Shape of an image is determined by applying edge detection or segmentation to an image. After this step, rotation and scaling can be applied to each segment of an image in order to describe shape features of an image. Texture of an image reflects the pixel values or intensities about colour of an image. To match the texture of query image with all those set of images in database, edge detection (determining the edge pixels within defined area of an image) and co-occurrence matrices (comparing grey-tones of an image in spatial matrices to capture similarity numerical value of an image) approaches are used widely in medical domain.

Text Based Image Retrieval

Text based image retrieval approach is based on the content of an image that includes the modality of an image, present body part, disease or abnormity described etc. Yale Image Finder (Xu, McCusker, & Krauthammer, 2008), BioText (Wooldridge, et al., 2007), ARRS Goldminer (Kahn & Thao, 2007) are some of the typical text-based image retrieval systems. Further, researchers presented use of UMLS and MeSH medical ontologies to improve the quality search of medical images. However, text-based image retrieval method is not as effective as content based approach due to the fact that text based approach involves manual annotation which is often subjective and time consuming by nature.

Healthcare Data Mining

Data mining can be defined as the process of extracting previously implicit information from large datasets. Data mining is essentially a data driven approach that has the prospective to answer unknown medical/health related questions to enhance the merit of healthcare delivery. It is a pertinent approach to "discover" patterns from large datasets under observation to assist caregivers in better decision making (Bellazzi & Zupan, 2008). Data mining offers many opportunities in the domain of medical informatics, bio-informatics, and health informatics such as discovering previously unidentified facts (e.g. finding relationship between a medicine and its associated side effects), predicting different future scenarios (e.g. what are the consequences of clinical trials on public health) etc. The typical unidentified health related questions (for e.g. what is the association between patient's profile and drug dosage? Or what

Figure 3. Healthcare data mining techniques

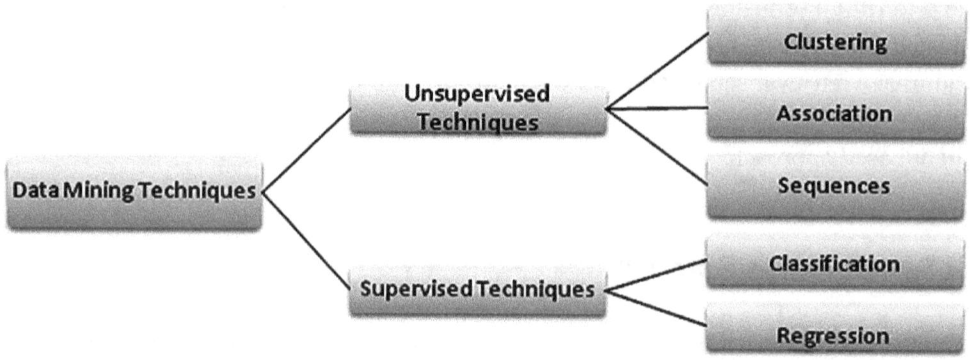

side-effects do a particular drug have on patient's health etc) are solvable using data mining techniques such as unsupervised(descriptive) techniques (for e.g. sequences, clustering and associations) and supervised (predictive) techniques (for e.g. regression and classification techniques) as shown in Figure 3.

Unsupervised or Descriptive Techniques

Data mining techniques based on the serendipitously identification of unknown or inherit medical or health patterns that already pre-exist in healthcare datasets. The three main techniques under unsupervised data mining can be defined as:

Clustering Technique

1. The data *clustering technique* is based on grouping of medical/health records under study into clusters or segments by measuring the similarity characteristics between objects (Belciug, 2009). For instance, clustering technique can be followed to find discrete symptoms of disease with alike characteristics. The objective of clustering approach is to discover a new set of categories among data instances and their evaluation is intrinsic. Clustering groups datasets into different subsets in such a fashion that similar datasets are grouped together in one subset, while different datasets belong to different groups. Some of the applications of clustering in healthcare (Haraty, Dimishkieh, & Masud, 2015) can be discussed as below:
2. K-means clustering algorithm has been used with statistical analysis to analyze cancer disease in each subset of genes.
3. Hierarchical clustering can be used to categorize patients into different groups based on their time length of stay in hospitals so as to provide better utilization of resources.
4. To analyze protein-protein functional interactions by considering genomic data.
5. Clustering method has been used to identify healthcare fraud detection when no historical labeled data exists.
6. Clustering Based Approach can be used to identify recurrence of breast Cancer.
7. k-Means Clustering Algorithm is used for Pattern Discovery in Healthcare Data Association Technique.

Association Technique

The *association* technique is used to identify type of association or relationships that exist among the medical records of single transactions. Association technique has the potential to discover what types of diseases have a tendency to form group (for e.g. bacterial or viral), support pandemic/epidemic surveillance (Ilayaraja & Meyyappan, 2013). Association technique is one of the most essential approaches used to find out frequent patterns among a set of data instances in data repository. In healthcare, this approach has been used to analyze health state, relationships among diseases and symptoms. Currently, this approach is used by researchers to determine associations linking diseases and their prescribed drugs. In addition, this approach has been used by various healthcare insurance companies to settle on the fraud and abuse. Applications of association technique in healthcare (Kai et al., 2014) can be listed as below:

1. Association technique is used for the identification of occurrence of diseases in particular geographical area at particular time.
2. Associate rule technique can be used in order to build clinical decision support system in order to identify the non-communicable diseases in non-reachable areas.
3. Association technique has been used to generate rules for heart disease patients (Nahar et al., 2013).
4. This approach has been used to classify diabetes-2 affected patients with equal width interval.

Sequencing Technique

The *sequencin*g pattern approach discovers the type of association that exists among the medical records of sequential transactions (Bellazzi & Zupan, 2008). To provide personalized patient care and to analyze outpatients' admission from time to time health organizations follows sequential pattern.

Supervised or Predictive Techniques

To forecast numerical or categorical value of any health record (e.g. drug pricing, finest dosage of drug) supervised or predictive data mining techniques are employed. Supervised data mining techniques can be defined as:

Classification Technique

The *classification* technique is used to predict one or more discrete value based on already predefined set of attributes or categories. For instance, it can forecast whether a given clinical treatment will harm, cure, or have no outcome on patient's health. It divides data instances into target classes. With the help of classification technique, a risk factor can be allied to patients by scrutinizing their patterns of diseases. There are two methods of classification, namely, Binary and multilevel. In binary classification, only two achievable classes such as, "low" or "high" risk patients may exist while in multilevel, more than two target classes exist for example, "low", "medium" and "high" risk patients. Some of the applications of classification technique (Luk et al., 2007) are as below:

1. Classification techniques can be used to predict the treatment cost of healthcare services.
2. Decision trees are used in order to forecast the survivability of breast cancer patient.

3. Classification and Regression Tree (CART) and Artificial Neural Networks (ANN) algorithms have been applied for the detection and treatment of tumors and to scrutinize experimental trials of cancer vaccination.
4. Similarly, using classification data mining technique has proved advantageous for the identification of heart diseases and its associated risk factors.

Regression Technique

The *regression* technique is used to forecast one or more numerical variables such as pass or fail on a continuous scale, for instance, calculating the number of admissions expected in a year in each hospital. Regression examples in healthcare (Xie et al., 2015) are discussed as below:

1. Regression technique can be used to estimate the relative risk level of various diseases such as, Angina, Diabetes stroke, etc.
2. This technique is widely used to provide continuous monitoring to patients, to estimate number of hospitalization days and for effective utilization of hospital resources.

In the modern age, data mining can be considered as a vital tool with the potential of performing predictive and descriptive analysis in healthcare management. Regardless of numerous benefits of data mining in healthcare realm, Shillabeer and Roddick (2007) in their studies have indicated a few intrinsic conflicts such as security and privacy of patient's health record when it is stored, processed, and shared. Therefore, before getting on applying data mining techniques, health organizations must impose some policy measures with its stakeholders and partner agencies.

ISSUES AND CHALLENGES IN IMPLEMENTING BIG DATA ANALYTICS

Big data technology plays a prominent role in delivering timely, cost-effective and patient –centered care. However, the adoption rate of these technologies remains low, in spite of its decreasing costs, increasing ubiquity, and impending benefits in clinical decision-making. The issues and challenges that come across in the way of successful implementation of big data analytics in healthcare province can be detailed as below:

Data Access and Sharing of Information

In order to craft effective and accurate decision-making in healthcare, it is necessary that data gathered by Healthcare Information Systems [HIS] is available in complete, accurate and timely manner. This inflict the governance and the data management agencies to make the data open and manage it in standardized manner using metadata and formats, standardized Application Programming Interfaces (APIs) etc. Although, this standardization and sharing of information about organization's operations assists in business intelligence and better decision making but on the other hand, culture of competitiveness and secrecy is also threatened.

Heterogeneous Data

Unstructured data comprises data being produced during social media interactions, data stored in fax transfers, PDF documents, emails and many more. To work with this kind of data is often costly and cumbersome too. In addition, it is not feasible to convert all data into structured one. Structured data, on the other hand, is well integrated in a manageable way unlike unstructured data which is completely unprocessed and unorganized.

Scalability

In healthcare sector, the medical devices often endeavor to work in association with other devices to increase performance and work in large clusters. Information sharing requires sharing of resources which has escort towards the problem of scalability and workload balancing. Also, to handle the problem of system failure in large clusters is a difficult task. In concern with the above scenarios, there has been a gigantic shift in the use of underlying technologies. For example, solid state Drives are being used instead of Hard Disk Drives (HDD) for performing data transfers. Therefore, what kind of devices should be used for data storage and data transfer is a big question before data management agencies.

Data Management Issues

Resolving issues of data access, updating, utilization, and governance have demonstrated to be tentative blocks in using Big Data analytics. There are diverse sources of data that are varied by its format, size, and method of compilation. During data gathering, to ensure data validity and data accuracy various protocols have been often followed. However, due to massive volume of data, it is impractical to ensure validity of every data item. Therefore, there is need to find out new approaches for data validation and data qualification. Thus, there is no ideal solution to data management problems.

Privacy and Security

The large number of users, devices and generated traffic all merge to create massive volume of data. Apart from consumers, this intelligence based information is valuable to hackers also. Mingling of personal information of patients with external data sets, results in inference of new specifics of that person that are needed to be kept secretive. As a result, health organizations are searching ways to utilize, protect and gain insights from "big data". With the data being available through mobile devices, Internet, and the cloud just having a firewall is not an efficient solution for data security. In order to defense against unintelligible actions of hackers, there is need by health organizations to adopt new security paradigms. Organizations need the ability to aggregate data into intellectual form, so that data altering and data reporting could be done in real time. To establish this, there must be complete visibility in datasets so that any access to that particular data could be monitored. However, success results of this visibility approach are still not confirmed yet. Hence, security and privacy issues pose a major challenge towards adoption of big data analytics technique in healthcare data management.

MOBILE COMPUTING

The advent of mobile ICTs in healthcare has made healthcare professionals highly mobile and autonomous in nature, thus enabling them to solve troubles at the point of action (Sherry & Salvador, 2001). With the purpose to provide access to indispensable resources and information "anytime, anywhere" mobile ICTs are making its way in healthcare at a swift pace. The usage of "*mHealth*" or mobile health to transform the relationship between patients and caregivers is escalating more rapidly as compared to access to Internet. Henceforth, role of mobile/wireless solutions in supporting healthcare cannot be held in low esteem. Mobile ICTs have lessened the paperwork for physicians, community healthcare practitioners, nurses and other community workers by providing diverse applications that could access patient's health records or mobile chronically ailing patients such as diabetes. The generalized mHealth architecture is shown in Figure 4.

1. The person having health problem uses various WSN (Wireless Sensor Networks) devices such as Pedometers, Blood glucose monitoring applications etc. to scrutinize different health parameters such as liver, heart etc.
2. Data hub (usually a PDA or cellphone) acts as a mini-gateway, which aggregates data from WSN devices using wireless solutions (such as Machine to Machine (M2M) Communication Protocol, Bluetooth, Zigbee etc.) and examines the vital signs of the person and transmits data to medical network via Internet.
3. The medical network receives the information related to patient's medical status which can be easily accessed by physicians. The medical network is usually operated by a clinic, hospital or a telemedicine center.
4. The most crucial function of medical network is to handle multiple users and to protect all personal data. If any intimidating medical condition is detected, the systems can trigger a treatment procedure to user through feedback system.

Figure 4. Generalized mHealth architecture

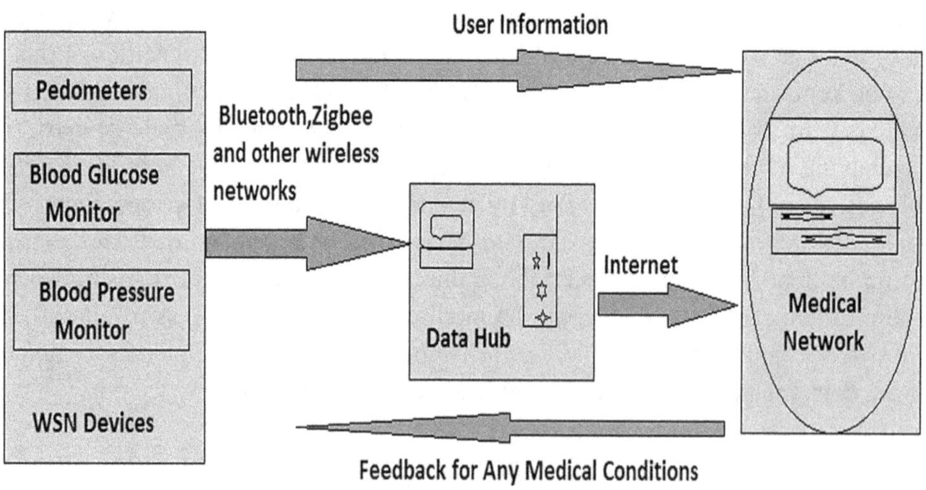

Figure 5. Working dimensions for mobile solutions

		Place: Same	Place: Different
Time	Same	**1. Same Time, Same Place** Tasks that can be done in same time and at same place. Example: Support for members meeting	**2. Same Time, Different Place** Tasks that can be done at same time but at different place. Example: Video Conferencing
	Different	**3. Different Time, Same Place** Tasks that must be done at same place but at different time. Example: Support for shift work	**4. Different time, Different Place** Tasks that are done at different time and different place. Example: e-mail

Mobility has different aspects in different environments. The extent to which mobility affects an individual depends on his nature of work (relaxing, working, travelling etc); amount of time involved; his preferences etc. By enabling individuals to carry devices that help out to stay in communication with their friends, organizations, and family, the mobile solutions establish to have an emergent impact on their lifestyle. This may engross direct communication by telephone, paging, teleconferencing, using voice or data messages, storage, access and retrieval of documents or database etc. To determine the value of mobile solutions two dimensions have been proposed: time and place. With the work being either independent or dependent of one or both dimensions; mobile applications could work in any one of the four quadrants: at any time and a particular place and same place; anytime and anywhere; a particular time and particular place; a particular time and anyplace as shown in Figure 5

Healthcare organizations are constantly choosing wireless solutions to remain connected with their outbound workforce inside a corporate atmosphere. For instance, mobile solutions assist healthcare practitioners, workers and patients whenever healthcare providers are away from their office or home. Mobile or monitoring applications could also be adopted by ambulatory care needed patients to use services provided by mobile healthcare providers. Consequently, mobile devices allow flexible employment hours that are extended beyond those actual hours spent in clinics or offices including break time, travelling to meetings, evenings, travelling to and from work. Thus flexibility and mobility are the major drivers of wireless solutions adopted by many companies and institutions.

Issues Impinging the Potential of Mobile Solutions

There are number of issues that could affect the potential of mobile solutions for e-health accomplishment. These issues engross adoption, usability, change management, interoperability, privacy, return on investment and security. These issues can be considered as detailed below:

Adoption

Supporting technological changes by user population depends on both functionalities of mobile solutions and excellence of user interface. The main questions of concern related with the adoption of wireless/ mobile solutions are (Zhu, Nah, & Zhao, 2003)

1. Does the design of interface and mobile devices affect user adoption?
2. What factors are responsible for the adoption of mobile solutions by users?
3. To what extent do enjoyment and trust (in using mobile devices) participate in adoption of mobile computing?

Zhu et al. (2003) proposed various factors that actually influence the exploit and intentions of using mobile devices that includes perceived effectiveness (degree of mobility, service offerings, coverage, compatibility and reliability), perceived user-friendliness (navigation, input and output modalities, bandwidth), enjoyment (focused attention, congruence of skills and challenges, perceived ease of use, interactivity, perceived usefulness).

Usability

To leverage all the benefits associated with mobile applications, it is required that these applications are confirmed to be useful from human perspective. As mobile applications develop and provide more diverse functionalities, they become inevitably more complex. Thus, it prompted need to balance ease of use and complexity with higher usability. Quality of system determines the adoption and usability of any information system. Factors such as interface design, mobile device design, ease of use, ease of learning, user satisfaction etc. tend to have critical impact on the usability of a device. Although wireless /mobile solutions have substantial potential, yet consumers' adoption relies on their usability. Usability testing is one of the standard evaluation approaches to identify the problems encountered by users and promising method to evaluate wireless applications (Sehgal et al., 2011)

Interoperability

Degeneration of any existing systems characteristics must be avoided that could plague healthcare IT field. Therefore, interoperability of new technology with the existing systems or databases is required. Interoperability can be defined as the capability of diverse systems to collaborate or inter-operate with one another. Interoperability means enabling the organizations and individuals to extensively adopt mobile computing technology and its related services in such a manner that multiple mobile platforms can exchange information in a cohesive manner and eventually works together impeccably (Shiraz, Gani, Khokhar, & Buyya, 2013). For example, solutions running on various dissimilar Mobile Cloud instances and use of resources in other varied Cloud instances. To realize this Interoperability solutions, standards such as, infrastructure, application, platform, data, service, and management are required at all levels. However, issues such as confidentiality, privacy, regulatory and legal concerns must be considered while mapping any software or healthcare record information with particular database.

Health Literacy

According to World Health Organization (WHO), health literacy represents the social and cognitive skills to gain access and motivate other individuals to utilize information for maintaining good health. Health literacy presents a major challenge for healthcare sector. Without having enough health literacy skills among individuals, health conditions may go unchecked or worsen, ill-informed decisions may be taken, and questions may go unasked or remain unanswered. Hence limited health literacy is prone to worse health outcomes and low health statues. Therefore, healthcare systems that are specifically designed for consumer benefits are unusual because no or limited healthcare experiences (Sehgal et al., 2011). Consequently, to optimize the use of mobile solutions, it is essential that users' health literacy level must align with the increasing consumers' demands for Mobile personal health records (mPHRs).

Privacy and Security

Issues such as confidentiality and privacy of health record are strictly regulated according to government guidelines. In order to maintain security and privacy by encoded database and communications every mobile application must hold on to these guidelines. Reliability is another consideration that a system must ensure so that user services are not interrupted and loss of information could be prevented. Parallel testing during testing phase is one way to ensure system reliability and confidence (Mikkelsen & Aasly, 2001).

Return on Investment (ROI)

Despite of providing healthcare services to underserved populations through mobile computing, the relative value of the Mobile Health Clinic (MHC) model has not been explicated. In this scenario, return on investment (ROI) algorithm has been considered to answer this question: can the face value of the services provided by mobile health programs be computed in terms of quality of life years saved and anticipated emergency department expenditures evaded?

ROI on any new technology could be calculated by considering costs such as hardware/software costs, maintenance, installation, research and development etc. Mobile solutions signify a higher investment than just the purchase costs (Holtshousen & Smit, 2007). ROI for any MHC can be calculated as

$$\begin{aligned}&Relative\ value\ of\ Mobile\ Health\ Clinic\left(MHC\right)services\\&= annual\ estimated\ emergency\ department\ costs\ shunned\\&+value\ of\ life\ years\ saved\end{aligned}$$

$$ROI\ Ratio = \frac{Relative\ value\ of\ the\ mobile\ health\ clinic\ services}{Annual\ cost\ to\ run\ the\ mobile\ health\ clinic}.$$

To achieve the real benefit of mobile solutions it is necessary that process and technology should be assembled about a plan that clinches mobility. As mobile computing unfolds, healthcare organizations must access its value and technical propositions to find out the real value it offers in terms of lower cost and quality of life preservation as compared to existing systems.

INTERNET OF THINGS (IOT) AND SENSOR TECHNOLOGIES

In medical environment, human agent is frequently considered as being both the perpetrator and supervisor of actions thus depending on their cognition, perception and decision-making abilities. According to (Ball, Garets, & Handler, 2003), this relying on human loop and lacking of reliable and independent actions, facts and information is the main cause of medical errors. However, the advent of newer technologies like Internet of Things in healthcare has promised to provide cheap, small and ubiquitous sensors attached to smart logic actuators that could offer diverse opportunities to support historical and appropriate information, care-control and self-determining decision-making at the time of need. Despite of increased scarcity and cost of clinical skills in health organizations, Internet of Things has augmented human agent potential to enhance patient care. The word 'thing' in IoT refers to 'virtual and real entities that have the capability of being recognized' and used in human milieu (De Saint-Exupery, 2009). These entities or 'things' are capable of being converted from submissive objects that cannot move or sense their surroundings to active objects with actuators or sensors and can communicate with the environment using any communication hub such as web.

With the development of care models and technology in healthcare realm, sensing is persistently mounting with the adoption in home-care applications by all those who are in need to manage their wellness and health proactively. Use of sensors could now be found in diverse counter of healthcare applications for instance, allergy detection, home testing pregnancy or AIDS etc. Recently, uses of biosensors have been found in environmental related applications to detect pesticides, bacteria and other hazardous metal in water test samples. Smart intelligent sensor technologies are profusely providing delivery of wireless data stream and digital processing of signals. The growth of use of sensors in healthcare domain and integration with ICTs can be illustrated as shown in Figure 6(McAdams et al., 2012).

IoT technology enables machines to directly communicate and control the command of physical actuators to support full motion of robotics i.e. all actions are independent of any human interface (Patel et al., 2011). The ubiquitous usage of mobile solutions and miniaturization of sensors and processes has enabled the development of smart sensors that could be placed or worn in the interior of human body to sense cardiac events, blood pressure and pulse. The usage of smart watches, glasses and wristbands that facilitate monitoring of specialized diseases, body activity by the use of accelerometers, walking motions, heart rate and many more are the applications of sensor technologies in healthcare. Figure 7 shows the progress of healthcare programs using ICT technologies.

Figure 6. Growing use of sensors in healthcare domain

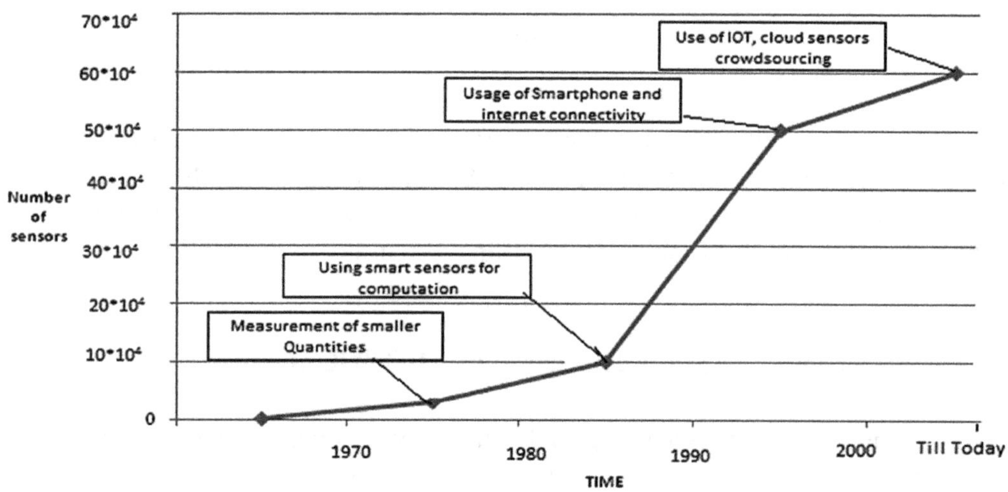

Figure 7. Progression of healthcare programs using ICT technologies

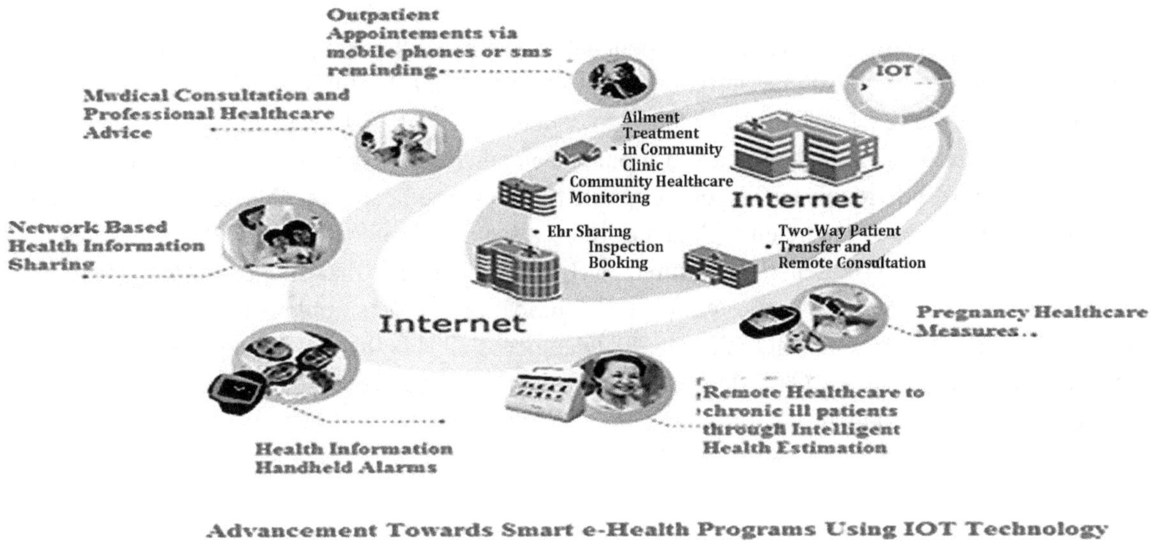

The role of sustainable activities plays an important role in the healthcare kingdom. Apart from diagnostic clinical applications, it is eventually the individual's decision how they are willing to use ICTs technologies for modifying their lifestyles and behaviors. IoT technology has the prospective to revolutionize patient's health by supporting decision-making capabilities and to act independently in specific cases that are self-regulating. Driven by close amalgamation with ICT technology capabilities, IoT and sensor technology will keep on becoming smarter. IoT has the potential to facilitate a pace change towards patient's safety by augmenting passive entities with smarter sensor technology downward to nano-scale. This combination of ICT and sensor technology will make available an exhilarating platform for the prospect of innovative products and services.

Issues Influencing the Adoption of IoTs in Healthcare

To minimize long term impact, maximize efficacy and to keep medical costs minimum, it is necessary that evolution of these newer technologies will reach rising level of competence. In spite of all the above positive scenarios aligned with the use of IoT and sensor technologies in healthcare sectors, there persists certain challenges towards its adoption and can be detailed as below:

Standardization of Connectivity Devices

Connecting different communication hubs with different medical devices developed for different tasks can pose a considerable problem. In addition, lack of communication protocol standards amongst medical devices permit manufactures to device their own solutions. Consequently, not all the device solutions will be able to communicate with hospital's PHRs or EHRs systems more effectively. This lack of standardization of connecting devices emerges as an obstacle to any effort for expanding large scale connectivity in healthcare province. Therefore, there prompted a need to identify standards before using any medical device for seamlessly transfer of medical records.

Reliability

In healthcare sector, there is often a fear of patient data breaches. If 'hacking' of medical data takes place, it eventually leads to backlash that are going to be so substantial. In this scenario, it is necessary that medical devices developed are reliable enough to counteract the actual occurring of 'hacking' events. As more and more medical technologies turn out to be connected with medical devices, an increasing attempt is made by individuals to find-out loophole to access medical data. Hence, manufactures must ensure that their device is secure enough and develop a security protocol to ensure data security on its ongoing way. Reliability is generally ensured by QoS mechanisms that supports acknowledgments. Many standardized solutions to main reliable communication consists implementation of the Message Queuing Telemetry Transport (MQTT) protocol (Zang et al., 2011) that has been proposed by OASIS, open standards consortium. MQTT supports one-to -many message-passing distributions employed by publish/subscribe mechanisms.

Data Security

Security and privacy issues can occur at various levels in IoT. To ensure data security, the entire IoT system must confirm to sequence of properties, such as integrity, confidentiality, authorization, authentication, availability, privacy and non-repudiation (Jiang et al., 2015). Conversely, to achieve these properties in IoT perspective is extremely challenging. Firstly, Short-range low-data protocols and scarcity of object resources greatly limits the packet size and transmission operations, thereby affecting the security protocols. Secondly, Heterogeneity of medical devices could cause minimum set of functionalities to be implemented by all communication hubs so as to support interpretability amongst different devices. In this scenario, many encryption-decryption techniques are often implemented to accomplish authenticity, confidentiality, and integrity. However, in set of connections with constrained devices, node's complexity increases to share keys and decrypting incoming messages becomes difficult. An alternative solution in this situation is to make use of homomorphic encryption design which can directly aggregate encrypted data, avoiding the need of unnecessary intermediate decryptions. In addition, for persistence to memory data on-chip One-Time-Programmable (OTP) technology, on-chip ROM memory and off-chip flash memory could also be used.

Device Management

Managing the objects in IoT environmental characteristics is of supreme importance. IoT communication environment consists of connected devices through which communication takes place as well as applications that are need to be remotely managed. During transmission of data, different complex management processes such as configuring the device/network, switching on/off the device, updating firmware/software, monitoring the device/network, recovering from errors, connectivity statistics, and gathering data etc takes place. Solutions to effectively manage these processes must consider the heterogeneity of devices connected. Standard device management solution encompasses of SNMP (Harrington, Presuhn, & Wijnen, 2002), TR-069, and NETCONF protocols and appliances such as switches, routers and smart phones (Sehgal, et al., 2012). Newer solutions like Open Mobile Alliance (OMA) Device Management (DM) (OMA-DM), protocol could also be used to effectively manage targeting devices such as mobile phones and PDAs. Recently, successor of OMA-DM protocol, OMA LWM2M (Lightweight Machine to

Machine) management protocol has been proposed (Klas et al., 2014) targeting mobile devices in which apart from SMSs being used for wakeup operations, it could be used to manage management operations such as, PUT, GET, POST.

OPPORTUNITIES, BENEFITS, ISSUES, AND CONTROVERSIES

Healthcare can be considered as the best ever growing sectors as compared to other sectors in all economics. The main objective of information technologies in healthcare is to improve the overall health outcomes by providing diverse functionalities such as online prescription refills, online billing, appointment scheduling, improved patient-provider communications, online medical records, and online pharmacies, physician directories etc. These applications highlight the impending and prospective view of ICTs in healthcare industry. The major opportunities and benefits of ICT technologies are outlined below:

1. Improved patient safety.
2. Greater efficiency of operation.
3. Low-cost technologies for clinical video case conferencing.
4. Use of hand-held technologies such as PDAs (personal digital assistants) to improve the timeliness and effectiveness of systems.
5. Use of mobile phone technology (mHealth) for disease surveillance.
6. Development of routine health information systems (RHIS) as an open source technology to examine health conditions of patients.
7. To optimize hospital bed-days, clinicians and other resources.
8. Use of electronic decision support systems for ordering and interpretation of pathology tests.

The primary benefits of using ICTs in healthcare can be summarized as shown in Figure 8.

Figure 8. Primary benefits of ICT technologies in healthcare

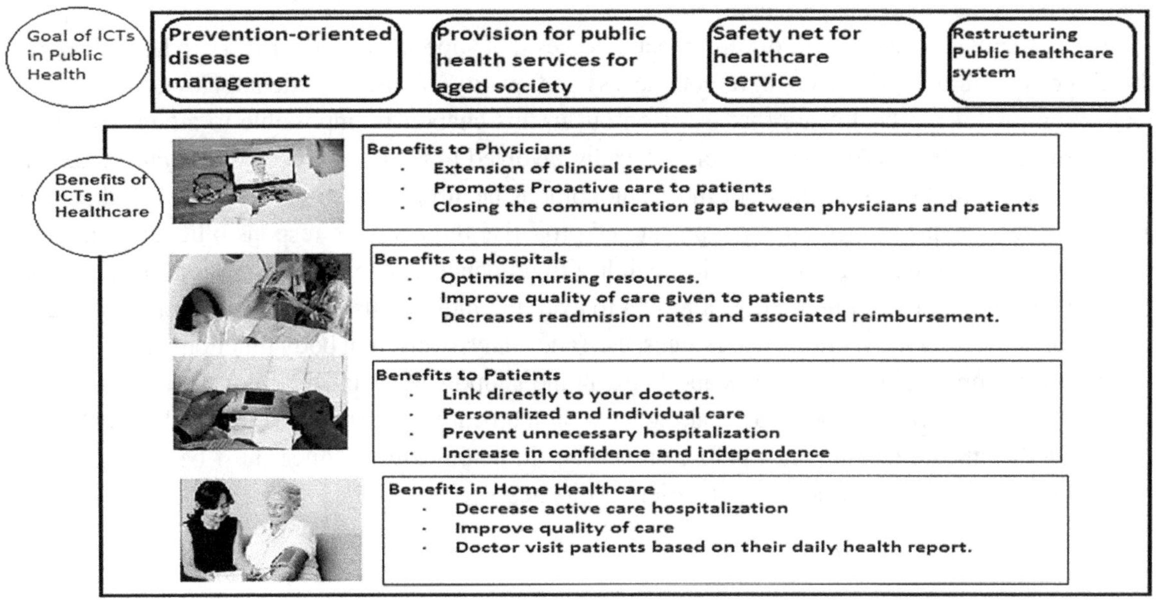

Use of ICTs in healthcare can assist healthcare providers to target multiple issues to maximize healthy outcomes. Undoubtedly, ICTs has played a noteworthy role in healthcare organizations and will keep on playing a better role in endeavoring quality of healthcare services. As an integral part of organization's strategies, ICTs are responsible for the assimilation of information across the entire healthcare sectors. Despite of such positive impact, the reasons for the slow adoption of ICTs in healthcare sector are as follows:

1. Lack of Engagement of Clinicians and other end users.
2. Inadequate resources and lack of skilled and experienced employees.
3. Accessibility and Usability Issues.
4. High Cost involved in ICTs investment.
5. Lack of Senior Management Sponsorships.
6. Limited Health Literacy and inadequate understanding of health domain by IT companies.
7. Data and Presentation materials are subject to idiosyncratic differences.
8. Privacy Concerns
9. Lack of a universal standard for formatting electronic records.

FUTURE RESEARCH DIRECTIONS

The promotion of ICTs in healthcare for the prevention of chronic diseases is already up-and –coming but it also encompasses sturdy challenges such as endowing time and money towards its adoption as a solution for maintaining healthy status. Support of ICTs in healthcare has augmented much in the last few decades and is persistently budding from hospitals to patient's homes via eHealth practices. From the estimated reports as previously mentioned in the chapter, it can be accomplished that role of ICTs is not just limited for elderly or chronic patients but it also lends a hand in inducing lifestyle modification in healthy individuals. Therefore, role of ICTs is not just limited to the value of maintaining "a longer and healthier life", but should offer users with more direct rewards that may include, social-acceptance being trendy, cross-modal experiences, etc.

In this chapter, we thrash out different technologies that support the use of ICTs in healthcare with the aim of providing cost-effective, remote-access and quality of care to patients. However, the actual realization of ICTs in healthcare that is vision out in this chapter is impossible to attain without the involvement of policy makers that are unreservedly involved in healthcare ecosystem. Future research direction points to the development of more autonomous health guidance systems that could augment and motivate patient's decision making power and proactive them to take responsibility in maintaining healthy lifestyle. In the envisage scenario, such health guidance systems with the support of users and pervasive technologies can be used as a model to examine individuals' profile (health behaviors, risk factors, preferences, intervention goals, values, etc.) and analyze different body functions. These systems when used in combination with EHRs and PHRs could support personalized information of users that could be further utilized for decision-making and communicating amongst professionals. Lastly, these persuasive healthcare technologies before embarking in healthcare province must be evaluated from ethical outlook to promote wellbeing of patients at its best.

CONCLUSION

In this chapter, diverse technologies such as cloud-computing, big data analytics, mobile computing, IoT and sensor technologies that support ICTs emergence in healthcare realm have been discussed and their potential to deliver timely, cost-effective, remote access and quality of healthcare services to patients has been explored. In addition, some of the opportunities and controversies regarding ICTs development along with the future research directions were laid out. Although, ICTs currently plays a noteworthy role in healthcare organizations and will keep on playing a better role in endeavoring quality of healthcare services but still it entails more focus on the effectiveness and adoption in consumer healthcare applications. Usability is critical for ICTs and for successfully leveraging its benefits in our day-to-day life activities; ICTs adoption should be quick and effortless. This would result in capitalizing the inherent benefits of ICTs. ICTs and its supporting technologies are bound to embrace more functions and competence so as to dispense their users a trendy, streamlined and healthy lifestyle experience.

REFERENCES

Alagoz, F., Valdez, A. C., Wilkowska, W., Ziefle, M., Dorner, S., & Holzinger, A. (2010). From cloud computing to mobile internet from user focus to culture and hedonism: The crucible of mobile health care and wellness applications. In 5th *International Conference on Pervasive Computing and Applications(ICPCA'10)*. IEEEComputerSociety. doi:10.1109/ICPCA.2010.5704072

Arka, H.I., & Chellappan, K. (2014). Collaborative compressed I-cloud medical image storage with decompress viewer. In *Proceedings of Medical and Rehabilitation Robotics and Instrumentation* (MRRI '13). doi:10.1016/j.procs.2014.11.041

Babashzadeh, A., Huang, J., & Daoud, M. (2013). Exploiting semantics for improving clinical information retrieval. In *Proceedings of the 36th International ACM Conference on Research and Development in Information Retrieval.* Association For Computer Machinery. doi:10.1145/2484028.2484167

Ball, M. J., Garets, D. E., & Handler, T. J. (2003). Leveraging information technology towards enhancing patient care and a culture of safety in the US. *Methods of Information in Medicine*, *42*(5), 503–508. PMID:14654884

Barrow, M. (2011, December 23). Patients get right to see medical records online. *The Times.* Retrieved from http://www.thetimes.co.uk/tto/health/news/article3266823.ece

Belciug, S. (2009). Patients length of stay grouping using the hierarchical clustering algorithm. *Annals of the University of Craiova, 36*(2), 79-84.

Bellazzi, R., & Zupan, B. (2008). Predictive data mining in clinical medicine: Current issues and guidelines. *International Journal of Medical Informatics*, *77*(2), 81–97. doi:10.1016/j.ijmedinf.2006.11.006 PMID:17188928

Cisco. (2009). *The Cisco powered network cloud: An exciting managed ser-vices opportunity.* Available at http://www.cisco.com/en/US/solutions/collateral/ns341/ns525/ns537/whitepaper c11-532553.html

De Saint-Exupery, A. (2009). *Internet of Things: Strategic research roadmap*. Retrieved from http://www.sintef.no/upload/IKT/9022/CERP-IoT%20SRA_IoT_v11_pdf.pdf

Erdogmus, H. (2009). Cloud computing: Does nirvana hide behind the nebula? *IEEE Software*, *26*(2), 4–6. doi:10.1109/MS.2009.31

Fernandez-Aleman, J. L., & Lozoya, P. A. A. (2013). To evaluate, Security and privacy in electronic health records: A systematic literature review. *Journal of Biomedical Informatics*, *46*(3), 541–562. doi:10.1016/j.jbi.2012.12.003 PMID:23305810

Goldstein, P. (2009). *Alternative IT sourcing strategies: from the campus to the cloud*. EDUCAUSE Center for Applied Research. Available at: https://net.educause.edu/ir/library/pdf/EKF/EKF0905.pdf

Guo, L., Chen, F., Chen, L., & Tang, X. (2010). The building of cloud computing environment for e-health. In *Proceedings of the International Conference on e-Health Networking, Digital Ecosystems and Technologies* (EDT'10). Shenzhen, China: IEEE Computer Society. doi:10.1109/EDT.2010.5496512

Haraty, R. A., Dimishkieh, M., & Masud, M. (2015). An Enhanced k-Means Clustering Algorithm for Pattern Discovery in Healthcare Data. *International Journal of Distributed Sensor Networks*, *2015*, 1–11. doi:10.1155/2015/615740

Harrington, D., Presuhn, R., & Wijnen, B. (2002). *An Architecture for Describing Simple Network Management Protocol (SNMP) Management Frameworks*. Standard(STD) 62, RFC 3411.

Holtshousen WS, & Smit A. (2007). A cost-efficiency analysis of a mobile dental clinic in the public *services. South African Dental Association, 62*(8), 336-338.

Hwang, K. H., Lee, H., & Choi, D. (2012). Medical image retrieval: Past and present. *Journal of Healthcare Informatics Research*, *18*(1), 3–9. doi:10.4258/hir.2012.18.1.3 PMID:22509468

Ilayaraja, M., & Meyyappan, T. (2013). Mining Medical Data to Identify Frequent Diseases using Apriori Algorithm. In *Proceedings of the 2013 International Conference on Pattern Recognition, Informatics and Mobile Engineering* (PRIME'13). doi:10.1109/ICPRIME.2013.6496471

Jain, H.K., Thao, C., & Zhao, H. (2012). Enhancing electronic medical record retrieval through semantic query expansion. *Journal of Information Systems and e-Business Management, 10*(2), 165–181. doi:10.1007/s10257-010-0133-5

Jiang, H., Shen, F., Chen, S., Li, K. C., & Jeong, Y. S. (2015). A secure and scalable storage system for aggregate data in IoT. *Journal of Future Generation Computer Systems.*, *49*, 133–141. doi:10.1016/j.future.2014.11.009

Kahn, C. H. Jr, & Thao, C. (2007). GoldMiner: A radiology image search engine. *AJR. American Journal of Roentgenology*, *188*(6), 1475–1478. doi:10.2214/AJR.06.1740 PMID:17515364

Kai, E., Rebeiro-Hargrave, A., Inoue, S., Nohara, Y., Maruf, R. I., Nakashima, N., & Ahmed, A. (2014). Empowering the healthcare worker using the Portable Health Clinic. In *28th International Conference on Advanced Information Networking and Applications (AINA'14)*. doi:10.1109/AINA.2014.108

Kaufman, L. M. (2009). Data security in the world of cloud computing. *IEEE Security and Privacy*, *7*(4), 61–64. doi:10.1109/MSP.2009.87

Kaur, P.D., & Chana, I. (2014). Cloud based intelligent system for delivering health care as a service. *Journal of Computer Methods and Programs in Biomedicine*, *113*(1), 346-359. doi:10.1016/j.cmpb.2013.09.013

Klas, G., Rodermund, V. F., Shelby, V. Z., Akhouri, S., & Holler, E. J. (2014). *"Lightweight M2M": Enabling Device Management and Applications for the Internet of Things*. Retrieved from http://archive.ericsson.net/service/internet/picov/get?DocNo=1/28701-FGB101973

Koufi, V., Malamateniou, F., & Vassilacopoulos, G. (2010).Ubiquitous access to cloud emergency medical services.*IEEE International Conference on Information Technology and Applications in Biomedicine*. doi:10.1109/ITAB.2010.5687702

Lindberg, B., Nilsson, C., Zotterman, D., Soderberg, S., & Skar, L. (2013). Using Information and Communication Technology in home care for communication between patients, family members, and healthcare professionals: A systematic review. *International Journal of Telemedicine and Applications*, *2013*, 1–31. doi:10.1155/2013/461829 PMID:23690763

Luk, J. M., Lam, B. Y., Lee, N. P. Y., Ho, D. W., Sham, P. C., Chen, L., & Fan, S.-T. et al. (2007). Artificial neural networks and decision tree model analysis of liver cancer proteomes. *Journal of Biochemical and Biophysical Research Communications*, *361*(1), 68–73. doi:10.1016/j.bbrc.2007.06.172 PMID:17644064

McAdams, E., Gehin, C., Massot, B., & McLaughlin, J. (2012). The challenges Facing Wearable Sensor Systems.*International Conference on Wearable Micro and Nano Technologies for Personalized Health*.

McCarthy, J. (2012). *Down for the count: 9 high-profile cloud outages*. Available at: http://www.crn.com/slide-shows/cloud/240012554/down-for-the-count-9-high-profilecloud outages. htm?pgno=4

Mikkelsen, G., & Aasly, J. (2001). Concordance of information in parallel electronic and paper based patient records. *International Journal of Medical Informatics*, *63*(3), 123–131. doi:10.1016/S1386-5056(01)00152-6 PMID:11502428

Murdoch, T. B., & Detsky, A. S. (2013). The inevitable application of big data to health care. *Journal of the American Medical Association*, *309*(13), 1351–1352. doi:10.1001/jama.2013.393 PMID:23549579

Nahar, J., Imam, T., Tickle, K. S., & Chen, Y. P. (2013). Association rule mining to detect factors which contribute to heart disease in males and females. *Expert Systems with Applications*, *40*(4), 1086–1093. doi:10.1016/j.eswa.2012.08.028

Pandeya, S., Voorsluys, W., Niua, S., Khandokerb, A., & Buyyaa, R. (2012). An autonomic cloud environment for hosting ECG data analysis services. *Future Generation Computer Systems*, *28*(1), 147–154. doi:10.1016/j.future.2011.04.022

Patel, P., Pathak, A., Texeira, T., & Issarny, V. (2011). Towards application development for the Internet of Things. In *Proceedings of the 8th Middleware Doctoral Symposium (MDS '11)*. ACM. doi:10.1145/2093190.2093195

Rolim, C. O., Koch, F. L., Westphall, C. B., Werner, J., Fracalossi, A., & Salvador, G. S. (2010). A Cloud Computing Solution for Patient's Data Collection in Health Care Institutions. In *Proceedings of 2ndInternational Conference on eHealth, Telemedicine and social Medicine* (ETRLEMED'10). IEEE Computer Society. doi:10.1109/eTELEMED.2010.19

Sehgal, A., Perelman, V., Kuryla, S., & Schonwalder, J. (2012). Management of Resource Constrained Devices in the Internet of Things. *IEEE Communications Magazine*, *50*(12), 144–149. doi:10.1109/MCOM.2012.6384464

Sherry, J., & Salvador, T. (2001). Running and grimacing: the struggle for balance in mobile work. In B. Brown, N. Green, & R. Harper (Eds.), *Wireless World: Social and Interactional Aspects of the Mobile Age* (pp. 108–120). Berlin, Germany: Springer.

Shillabeer, A., & Roddick, J. (2007). Establishing a lineage for medical knowledge discovery. In *Proceedings of the 6th Australasian Conference of Data Mining and Analytics (AusDM '07)*. Darlinghurst, Australia: Australian Computer Society.

Shiraz, M., Gani, A., Khokhar, R. H., & Buyya, R. K. (2013). A Review on Distributed Application Processing Frameworks in Smart Mobile Devices for Mobile Cloud Computing. *IEEE Communications Society*, *15*(3), 1294–1313. doi:10.1109/SURV.2012.111412.00045

Venkatesh, T., Premkumar, N., & Sivaguru, G. (2013). Efficient cloud platform providing an omnipresent healthcare services. *International Journal of Innovative Research in Computer and communication Engineering, 1*(2), 193-199. Retrieved from http://www.rroij.com/open-access/efficient-cloud-platform-providing-anomnipresent-healthcare-services.pdf

WHO. (2004). *eHealth for Health-care Delivery: Strategy 2004-2007*. Geneva, Switzerland: WHO. Retrieved from http://www.who.int/eht/en/eHealth_HCD.pdf

WHO. (2008). *Report on the global tobacco epidemic*. Retrieved from http://www.who.int/tobacco/mpower/mpower_report_full_2008.pdf

Wooldridge, L., Lissina, A., Vernazza, J., Gostick, E., Laugel, B., Hutchinson, S. L., & Sewell, A. K. et al. (2007). Enhanced immunogenicity of CTL antigens through mutation of the CD8 binding MHC class I invariant region. *European Journal of Immunology*, *37*(5), 1323–1333. doi:10.1002/eji.200636765 PMID:17429845

Xie, Y., Schreier, G., Chang, D.C., Neubauer, S., Liu, Y., Redmond, S.J., & Lovell, N.H. (2015). Predicting Days in Hospital Using Health Insurance Claims. *IEEE Journal of Biomedical and Health Informatics, 19*(4), 1224-1233. doi:10. d109/JBHI.2015.2402692

Xu, S., & McCusker, J. (1968-70). Yale Image Finder (YIF): A new search engine for retrieving biomedical images. *Journal of Bioinformatics*, *24*(17). doi:10.1093/bioinformatics/btn340

Zhang, Y., Yu, R., Xie, S., Yao, W., Xiao, Y., & Guizani, M. (2011). Home M2M networks: Architectures, standards, and QoS improvement. *IEEE Communications Magazine*, *49*(4), 44–52. doi:10.1109/MCOM.2011.5741145

Zhu, W., Nah, F. F. H., & Zhao, F. (2003). Factors influencing user adoption of mobile computing. In J. Mariga (Ed.), Managing e-commerce and mobile computing technologies (pp. 260-271). Hershey, PA: Iron Mountain Incorporated (IRM) Press. doi:10.4018/978-1-93177-746-9.ch018

Zissis, D., & Lekkas, D. (2012). Addressing cloud computing security issues. *Journal of Future Generation Computer Systems*, *28*(3), 583–592. doi:10.1016/j.future.2010.12.006

KEY TERMS AND DEFINITIONS

Big Data Analytics: The process of collecting, organizing and analyzing large data sets (big data) to uncover unknown correlations, hidden patterns, customer preferences, market trends and other useful business information.

Cloud Computing: Cloud computing is based on sharing of computer resources to achieve economy of scale. It is a type of Internet based computing in which resources; information and other services are delivered to organization's devices via Internet.

eHealth: The term used in healthcare practice, usually supported by electronic process and communications. Various forms of eHealth include Electronic Health Records (EHRs), clinical decision support systems, healthcare information system, etc.

Information and Communication Technologies (ICTs): The term that includes wireless networks, the Internet, cell phones, computer and network hardware and software, and other communication mediums that have endow society with an immense array of communication capabilities such as videoconferencing, instant messaging, distance learning, etc.

Internet of Things (IoTs): A network of physical devices that are embedded with other electronic or sensor devices and have the capability to collect and exchange data over network without requiring any direct integration between the physical world and computer-based systems.

mHealth: One of the form of eHealth in which mobile phones are used for real-time monitoring of patient's health and providing information to healthcare practitioners.

Mobile Computing: Technology that allows users to access Internet or transmit data, video and voice via any wireless solutions (without having any fixed physical link) from anywhere in the world.

Chapter 8
Non-Invasive Cuffless Blood Pressure Monitoring System

Harinderjit Singh
Panjab University, India

Dilip Kumar
Sant Longowal Institute of Engineering and Technology, India

ABSTRACT

These days most of the Blood Pressure (BP) measuring devices are having inflatable cuff that is needed to be occluded on the patient's arm for measuring blood pressure. This technique is not suitable in cases where continuous measurement of BP is required. Therefore, this work is aimed at designing of non-invasive and continuously monitors the blood pressure by using Pulse Transit Time (PTT) technique. For taking out PTT both of the signals are extracted from the body of the patient with the help of bio sensors i.e. Electrocardiogram (ECG) sensor and Photoplethysmogram (PPG) sensor. PTT was measured by taking the peak to peak time difference of ECG signal and PPG signal and this PTT is indirectly correlated with blood pressure, based on which Systolic Blood Pressure (SBP) and Diastolic Blood Pressure (DBP) is calculated.

INTRODUCTION

Stressful lifestyle is the main reason for degrading a person's health (Hey et al., 2012), which may lead to some critical diseases like asthma, diabetes, heart attack, obesity, headache and premature deaths (Fiala et al., 2010). Over the last couple of decades, hypertension or high BP is the main reason for heart attack and other cardiovascular diseases. Experts estimated that the number of patients in India with high BP is likely to rise from 140 million in 2008 to nearly 215 million by 2030 (Kumar et al., 2014). The key problem of BP is rarely accompanied by any symptoms. Normally, the BP changes very frequently in a day. Therefore, only one measurement of high BP is not the correct method of analyzing high BP patients. Mostly the BP measuring electronic devices is having inflatable cuff that is needed to be occluded on the patient's arm for measuring the BP. This indirect technique is continuous and it has no doubt for its truthfulness, but has increased hazard, the cuff is safe but un-reliable and occasional. The cuff based

DOI: 10.4018/978-1-5225-0660-7.ch008

technique is not suitable in cases where continuous monitoring of BP is required by the doctor about the patients. Therefore, a non-invasive and continuous method of blood pressure monitoring is required (da Silva & P. M. P., 2013), with the help of this method proper treatment can be provided immediately for reducing the chances of serious cardiovascular problems. The blood pressure is mainly classified into six groups i.e. Hypotensive, normal, pre-hypertension, High blood pressure- Stage-1, High blood pressure- Stage-2 and Hypertensive with systolic and diastolic blood pressure. This measurement of SBP/DBP can be performed with direct and indirect techniques.

There are various methods available for blood pressure measurement, but these are cannot be applied for continuous monitoring of blood pressure. As in case of invasive method, it is continuous but there is a need to insert catheter in the artery, which is not possible for a long time. This method of BP measurement provides continuous and much accurate measurement about the absolute cardiovascular pressure from probes or transducers inserted directly into bloodstream. But this accuracy is obtained at the cost of increased disturbance to the patient and pain due to the catheter. This type of technique is only applied to the patient where a sudden change in pressure is needed to be captured and monitor patient during critical care. This type of measurement is required where intensive care is required. Its application is limited because of its invasiveness; therefore it is given to seriously ill patients.

There are different cuff based devices have been developed to measure blood pressure, specially an e-health systems is developed from a desktop platform for wireless mobile monitoring of blood pressure shows the disadvantages of conventional blood pressure meter that limits its application in home monitoring only. These conventional blood pressure meters are very bulky, complex and the capability of these instruments for taking several readings is inconvenient. Indeed, the invention of cuff-less technology in the medical system with different approach to measure blood pressure is the basic motivation of the present work. In case of non-invasive conventional cuff type blood pressure measurement, it is also not suitable for continuous measurement because in this case cuff is applied on the arm to occlude the blood, then the pressure is released to measure blood pressure so it causes an unpleasant feeling for the users. So, the method chosen for finding the Blood pressure must be continuous.

The pulse transit time approach is a continuous measurement technique due to this reason my major task was to calculate pulse transit time by using two sensors i.e. PPG and ECG sensor. This developed device will be a huge gap between automatic blood pressure monitoring devices that can be used while walking. It is a convenient approach; there is no need of inflatable cuffs. It dispenses with Photoplethysmogram sensor that is applied on the finger, and dispenses with an electrocardiogram sensor in which electrodes are applied on the extremities of the body. After this work, it will be very much helpful for medical as well as home monitoring application as it gives continuous outputs.

The major requirement behind the initiation of this work is to overcome the limitations of all available methods by designing Cuff-less BP monitoring product that could be used to measure blood pressure non-invasively and continuously. It could be easy to use and be a cost effective personal blood pressure monitoring device. Continuous monitoring is necessary because hypertension patients are presently increasing these days because of this we need a system which can easily monitor blood pressure. There are many devices available in the market. One of them widely used for cuff based blood pressure machine as existing devices.

In this chapter a focus is put on how to develop a Pulse Transit Time (PTT) technique based non-invasive continuous blood pressure monitoring device. This chapter includes Electrocardiogram (ECG) and Photoplethysmogram (PPG) sensors and their interfacing with the PIC microcontroller. An ECG sensor consists of three types of electrodes i.e., Right arm, left arm electrodes for taking potential difference between arms and right leg as a reference electrode. Photoplethysmogram sensor consists of an infrared transmitter and a light receiver. When the heart pumps, the receiver signal varies and it generates the pulsating waveform. The output obtained from ECG and PPG sensors is fed to PIC microcontroller for processing. The microcontroller detects the peak value of PPG and ECG sensors and then calculates PTT, termed as the time difference between the generation of ECG R-wave and inclination of PPG signal. This PTT is indirectly related to BP and correlate well to it. At the end the calculated Systolic/Diastolic blood pressure is displayed on the LCD. The continuous monitoring data of BP can also be stored in the memory of the PIC controller for further investigations. The developed device is tested on various age group subjects and the observed results are compared with the existing calibrated BP apparatus. The main objectives of this chapter are as follows:

To Design a Heart Beat Monitor Using Photoplethysmogram (PPG) Sensor

This first objective was obtained by taking a signal of heart beat pulse with the help of photoplethysmogram sensor. This sensor is based on the principle of IR photo transmitter and receiver, photo transmitter emits infrared light that is of wavelength 630nm. It is transmitted through the index finger. Some part of this infrared light got absorbed by finger and some part is detected by the light receiver. When the blood pulse circulates from the heart to the extremity position, each instant of time there some light is absorbed by pulse of blood according to the there are changes in output signal these signals are used to monitor the heart beats.

To Design Electrocardiogram (ECG) Generator Using Electrocardiogram (ECG) Sensor

The second objective is to generate ECG waveform and its peak value detection. The ECG sensor used for generating ECG signal consisting of low power amplifier circuit, i.e. INA122P to obtain electrocardiogram signal from the body. Using this sensor ECG waveforms are generated for further processing.

To Develop Software that Can Analyze the Electrocardiogram (ECG) and Photoplethysmogram (PPG) Signals Acquired from the Body

The third objective is to develop software that can measure blood pressure using ECG and PPG signal. As once both ECG and PPG signals are obtained from the body with the help of sensors. This work was based on pulse transit time to calculate blood pressure, where PTT is the time required by the blood pulse to circulate from heart to the extremity or the peak to peak time difference between ECG signal and PPG signal. This time is calculated by developing C-language software for the PIC microcontroller.

ECG signal extracted from the ECG sensor is an analog output in nature, so this signal output is connected as input to analog channel of microcontroller, PIC microcontroller is consisting of 10-bit ADC for conversion. Initially we can set this ECG peak value so that the timer should start from that level. Photoplethysmogram sensor output is interfaced with the interrupt of the PIC microcontroller, gives digital output that is in the form high and low, as once this pin detects high signal (i.e. Pulse) from PPG sensor the timer turns off and PTT is displayed on the LCD

To Design a Non-Invasive Cuff-Less Blood Pressure Meter Based on Pulse Transit Time (PTT)

The fourth objective is to monitor cuff-less blood pressure. PTT value obtained from the timer is used in the relation to calculate blood pressure. This relationship was developed by using the LMS algorithm to few parameters and then these parameters are used to calculate blood pressure values. This developed system is able to measure blood pressure without using any cuff and displaying systolic/ Diastolic blood pressure. This system will be a challenge to all cuff based devices.

To Design a System to Access the Daily Body Condition of the Subject at Home or Outdoor

The fifth objective is to design a system that is able to measure continuous blood pressure, without causing any problem to the patient. It can be applied anywhere home or hospital. This designed product can be minimized and can be used wirelessly and the data collected from this can be transmitted anywhere.

PREVIOUS METHODS

In the old days, there are many methods developed for measuring blood pressure. Initially, the BP measuring system was discovered by Stephen Hales in 1733 with the insertion of tubes directly into the animal's artery (Booth, 1977) and it is correlated with millimetres of mercury (i.e., mm hg) then the calculated result is 176 mm hg of blood pressure for persons around 7.5 feet height. A few years later an experiment performed by a French surgeon in which, a pipe was inserted directly to patient's artery for the measurement of blood pressure and the calculated result of BP value is approximately 120 mm Hg. After these experiments, there various BP measuring systems are invented, the Von Basch Sphygmomanometer system was invented in 1876, (Booth, 1977). This device consists of a balloon and a pressure manometer is connected along with it. This balloon fixed on the wrist and it is compressed until no pulse is observed. The manometer connected with balloon used to detect the pressure in the artery.

The methods which are invented up to this time are only experimental analysis and so far these approaches cannot be properly executed. In 1896 an Italian physician, Riva Rocci discovered a technique in which a cuff based mercury sphygmomanometer is used to measure blood pressure and this technique was very easy to perform. This ordinary cuff was connected along with a mercury manometer and it can be used to measure systolic blood pressure (SBP).

A few years later, a new approach was developed by Nicolai Korotkoff in 1904. In this new approach a stethoscope is applied along with the cuff compressed on the patient's artery, the stethoscope was used to hear korotkoff sound at systolic blood pressure (when heart pumps) and also at low pressure, i.e. Diastolic blood pressure (when the heart relaxes). This technique gives a new approach for measuring both systolic and diastolic blood pressures. This technique is very accurate due to which even after hundred years there had been very minor changes are made with this technique but the base method is still same.

According to Chan, K. et al., (2001), the blood pressure is carried out with the help of pulse wave velocity is inversely proportional to pulse transit time. This paper purposed that data can then be relayed to the Internet for analysis and viewing. The wireless application protocol (WAP) is used for displaying the information on portable wireless devices. The subjects' cardiovascular condition can thus be obtained for monitoring or pre-diagnostic purposes

The work suggested by Deb, S (2007) is based on pre ejection period. This pre ejection period was calculated by using pulse transit time and pulse arrival time relation. Three different types of measurement are taken, i.e. during resting, exercise and recovering. By using this data for different objects a relationship was developed between pre-ejection and blood pressure and calibration procedure is performed by using digital blood pressure measuring machine, linear regression model is developed to calculate systolic blood pressure only. For the calculation of diastolic blood pressure further improvement in system is required.

According to Fiala, J (2010) the main concentration is on continuous measurement of the blood pressure of the individual's body. This work purposed that an implantable device is designed for continuous measurement of blood pressure. This implantable device comes into the category of invasive because it needs to operate on patient to implant this sensor on the patient's artery for continuous measurement, it also can measure other parameters like blood oxygen level and haemoglobin level in blood. This technique isn't reliable for cuff-less technique.

According to Kim, Y (2010) a wrist-worn band type system is developed for measuring various parameters. This is designed for measuring parameters like PPG, skin temperature, fall detector, systolic blood pressure. All these parameters can be wirelessly transmitted using zigbee communication to any phone. A drawback of this system is that its measurement is limited because of its limited contact with the body as for continuous measurement continuous contact with body is required. Along with this, this work also proposes the idea that this device can also be designed in the shape of wearable device which can be used as continuous blood pressure monitoring system.

Manimegalai, P et al., (2012), suggested a wavelet approach is developed for monitoring ECG and PPG signal. A discrete wavelet approach is developed in LabVIEW software for calculating pulse rate. It is also used for calculating PTT by using parameters, i.e. ECG and PPG signals that indicate the change of BP. A de-noising circuit is also developed to remove the noise in ECG and PPG signal, So this wavelet based approach promises to measure BP continuously by using Pulse Transit Time. This technique was used for regularly monitoring the cardiac health of patients. This technique is used to monitor different parameters like pulse rate, pulse transit time and blood pressure. This technique requires more research for accuracy in blood pressure value.

A new method is developed by Goli & Jayanthi (2014) to measure blood pressure, this method is on pulse wave velocity and this pulse wave velocity is correlated with pulse transit time. Firstly the pulse wave velocity is calculated with the help of velocity, distance and time relationship. To measure blood pressure a mathematical relation is developed between blood pressure and pulse wave velocity. This relationship consists of two uncelebrated constants and these constants are celebrated with the help of least mean square algorithm. After this, the difference between both SBP/DBP values is calculated and then the comparison is performed with the blood pressure calculated by using cuff.

According to Younessi, H. et al., (2014) a relationship between pulse transit time and pulse wave velocity is developed. This pulse wave velocity is used to calculate blood pressure. This work gives an approach to measure continuously monitor blood pressure. But the relationship developed to calculate blood pressure needs very complex calculation by once taking the number of readings for calculating few parameters such as blood density and stiffness of arterial wall, and then it can be used to calculate BP. This method does not require accurate calculation of coefficient in critical situation. The most important application of this system is in operating rooms during high-risk condition and general anaesthesia. Its accuracy depends on the initial calibration of parameters. Continuous measurement of blood pressure depends on present method can be suggested for observing blood pressure changes during surgery and crisis conditions.

TECHNIQUES FOR BLOOD PRESSURE MEASUREMENT

Invasive Technique of Blood Pressure Monitoring

This invasive technique is the basic measurement technique for Blood pressure. This method have proved the "high end of accuracy" to measure BP at very low values of pressure. This method consists of a pressure transducer which is coupled along with a catheter and it is inserted directly in the artery of the patient. This method was not suitable, as it requires a needle to be inserted into an artery for such a long time while measuring BP, this technique is hurtful and it may also be a cause of the epidemic.

Non-Invasive Method for Blood Pressure Measurement

Nowadays, Blood pressure is most frequently measured with the help of a sphygmomanometer. It is consisting of occluding cuff and inflating bulb which consists of a valve to release pressure and a manometer. A manometer is a device which is connected to mercury filled tube. Historically, it has been used to measure the height of mercury in tube to reflect the circulating pressure. Sphygmomanometer was the instrument which is used by doctors from last 100 of years. It has become the "gold standard" in non-invasive measurement. Today blood pressure values are measured in millimeters of mercury (mmHg), although electronic devices have already eliminated the use of mercury. In future, invention of nanotechnology promises a better innovation in medical instrumentation which optimistically sustains human healthiness. Steps to measure Blood pressure using cuff are shown below:

Step 1: Select the appropriate size cuff.

Step 2: Palpate for the brachial artery along the inner upper arm.

Step 3: Now cover the cuff evenly and comfortably around the arm, centring the bladder over the brachial artery. Don't rely on cuff marking; find the centre ahead of time by time folding the bladder in half. The lower cuff edge should be 2.5 cm above the anti-cubital space. Tell the patient not to talk.

Step 4: Determine the level of the maximum inflation by rapidly inflating the cuff while watching for the point where you no longer feel the pulse. To that reading add 30 mm/hg.

Step 5: Deflate the cuff rapidly and steadily, then wait 15 to 30 sec and insert the stethoscope earpiece, making sure they point forward, apply the bell head lightly but with complete contact over the palpated artery.

Step 6: Inflate the cuff rapidly and steadily to the level of maximum inflation.

Step 7: Release the air so the pressure falls at 2 to 3 mm/hg per second.

Step 8: Listen the korotkoff sound at two points at starting of sound it is systolic pressure and at last sound it is diastolic pressure.

This measurement technique is having the drawback that it cannot be applied for continuous measurement because most of the BP measurements do not require continuous measurement. Therefore, non-invasive measurement technique is used for comfort and safety of the patient.

There are so many non-invasive techniques used to measure blood pressure. BP is basically measured in millimeters of mercury (mm Hg). The devices used for indirect measurement are hand-operated type, which are based on auscultatory techniques, Semiautomatic type, which is based on oscillatory techniques and automatic devices, which are also based on oscillatory techniques. Various blood pressure measurement techniques used for non-invasive measurement (Ward & Langton, 2007) are discussed below:

- **Palpation Technique:** Palpation was a very common method used to measure BP and it is basically applied in critical situations. It was used to take rough idea for measuring only systolic BP, i.e. >70 mm Hg, but in this method diastolic BP cannot be measured. This technique was not a suitable method for measuring BP as it gives only an estimated value of SBP.
- **Doppler Technique:** Doppler method for measuring BP was also similar to palpation technique as it is also limited only for SBP measurements. In this method the fundamental function is executed with Doppler probe, because with the circulation of blood either runs away or towards it, a sound wave is produced and is recognized by it and this was done by implementing the concept of switching frequency.
- **Auscultation Technique:** In this type of techniques a stethoscope is used along with the cuff, this technique was developed by Russian Surgeon, Nikolai Korotkoff in 1905. It is produced with the formation of bubble in the blood, disturbance in the vessel or instant expansion of vessel wall and combination of all these circumstances.
- This sound was produced due to the flow of blood through the artery where cuff was placed, with respect to this Korotkoff sound both systolic and diastolic blood pressures can be easily measured.
- **Oscillatory Technique:** The oscillatory method requires two cuffs and two bellows and these are coupled with the measurement gauge. There are two types of cuff, one is occluding cuff and the other is sensing cuff which are overlapped with each other. Both of the bellows present the value of pressure detected from both the cuffs with the help of a single measuring gauge which is on the other side connected to a lever. By using this type of arrangement SBP/DBP values are measured accurately.
- **Liquid Manometers Method:** In this method as the air pressure rises in cuff it forces the liquid up to the manometer. It consists of mainly two types of manometers i.e. open manometer (it is generally employed in sphygmomanometer to monitor pressure of the gauge) and on the other hand, closed manometer (it is basically used to measure absolute pressure and it is generally employed in mercury type barometers). Therefore, closed type manometers are used for measuring blood pressure.
- **Aneroid Gauge Method:** As in case of mercury manometer there is problem of toxicity, to overcome this problem aneroid gauge method is used in place of mercury manometer. In this method when pressure rises the below connected to the gauge is expanding and this change in pressure is indicated on the scale. But the main drawback of this method is that it requires a proper calibration otherwise it may lead to an error in measurement.
- **Automatic Systems:** In this method the position of the diaphragm is taken care, as the air pressure changes, it is recognized and displayed on LCD. The accuracy of this system depends on the

number of compressible components used in the system. With the help of this system SBP/DBP can be measured by single gauge.

- **Pulse Transit Time Technique:** This method is totally different and advanced technique in which cuff is removed and only electrocardiogram and photoplethysmogram sensors are used to measure blood pressure, in this method the peak to peak time difference between ECG and PPG signal was taken and this time is known as pulse transit time (PTT) in other words this is the time taken by our blood to circulate from the heart to any extremity (Kim & Lee, 2010) of the body. This PTT is used to calculate both SBP and DBP.

METHODOLOGY

Pulse Transit Time Technique

Every day this world is updating with latest and advanced technologies in biomedical engineering there are various advanced machines have been developed for blood pressure monitoring. Because it became a basic need for a cardiac patient to check their cardiac health. In the past few years only three types of non-invasive and cuffless devices have been developed, i.e. Pulse Wave Velocity, Pulse Transit Time and Photoplethysmogram. This type of methods is only developed to measure regularly without creating any disturbance to the patient. This system can be directly installed on patients in hospital. This method consists of Electrocardiogram (ECG) and Photoplethysmogram (PPG) signals which are directly applied for blood pressure monitoring. Figure 1 represents the time difference is calculated with the help of peak to peak difference in R-wave of electrocardiogram signal and rising edge of the photoplethysmogram signal (Shriram et al., 2010)

Figure 1. The time difference electrocardiogram and photoplethysmogram signals are taken to calculate pulse transit time

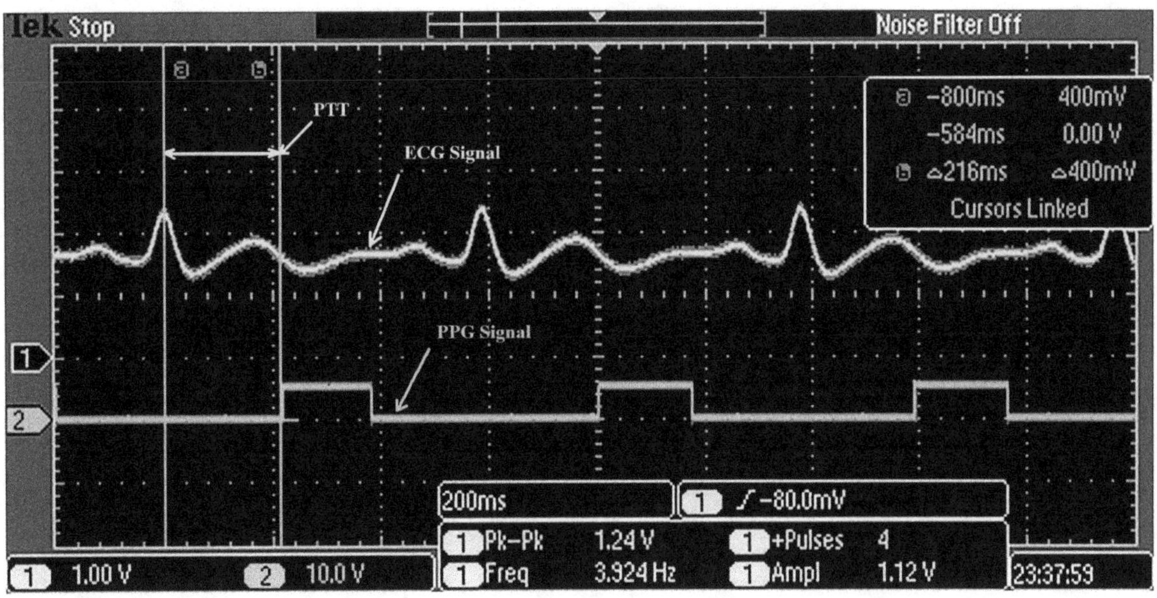

The pulse transit time is generally a time in which the blood circulates from the heart to any extremity position of the body (Deb et al., 2007), by using this time we can calculate pulse wave velocity (McCarthy et al., 2011) and it is a velocity of blood by which it circulates from the heart to any extremity of the body. It has been found that as the velocity of blood in vessel rises, there is a rise in blood pressure and as the velocity of blood is declined, there is a declination in blood pressure (Xu et al. 2012), by observing these changes, the outcome of this shows that there is some direct relation among pulse wave velocity and blood pressure, one more thing is that the time and velocity are having indirect relation therefore the outcome of this relation shows that Blood pressure is also having indirect relation with pulse transit. Figure 2 shows the basic block diagram of this method.

Electrocardiogram Sensor

Electrocardiogram sensor employed here with ECG electrodes on the body of the patient for detecting the electrical signals produced by the heart. These signals are produced due to depolarization and repolarization, which occurs due to every beat of the heart. There are of three types of main electrodes used for taking out electrical signals from the i.e. Lead 1 (it is between right arm and left arm electrodes), Lead 1 (it is between right arm and left leg electrodes) and Lead 3 (it is between left arm and left leg electrodes). After connecting these leads the potential difference between these three leads are taken. In all three cases, one remains an act as positive and other is the negative terminal. Figure 3 represents the hardware interfacing of an ECG sensor.

Photoplethysmogram Sensor

PPG sensor is based on the principle of IR photo transmitter and receiver, photo transmitter emits infrared light that is of wavelength 630nm. When PPG sensor is placed on the finger of the patient, the IR light transmitter transmits the light through the index finger. Some part of this infrared light got absorbed during the change in volume of blood in the finger and some part is detected by the light receiver. When the blood circulates from heart to an extreme position of the body, then at every instant there is some light absorbed by pulse of blood accordingly there is some change occurs in output signal and these signals are used to monitor the heart beats. Figure 4 represents the hardware interfacing of PPG sensor on the finger of the patient.

Figure 2. Block diagram of pulse transit time based blood pressure monitoring system

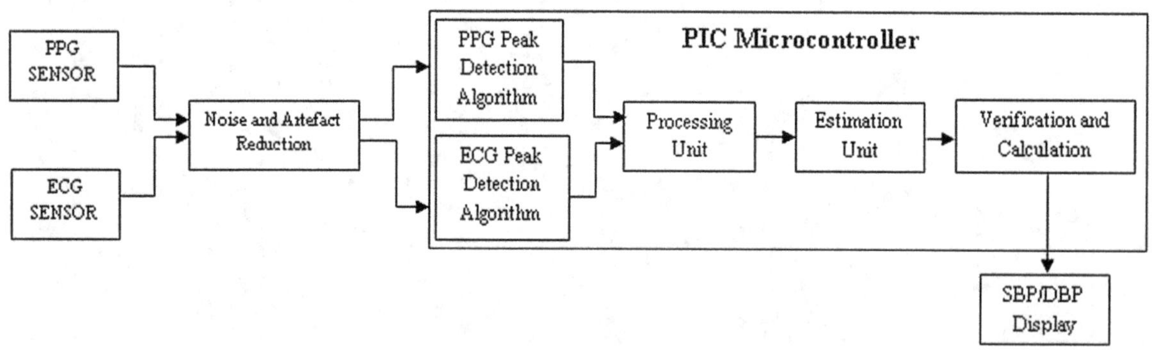

Figure 3. Electrocardiogram sensor

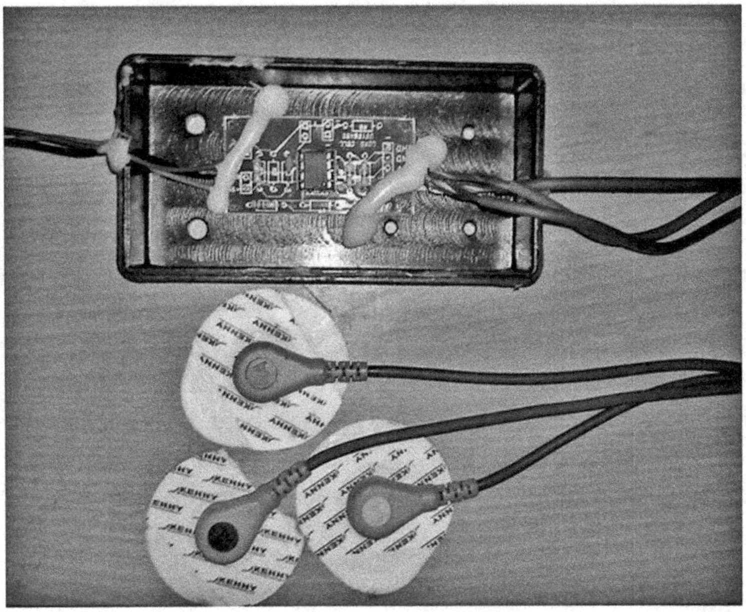

Figure 4. Photoplethysmogram sensor

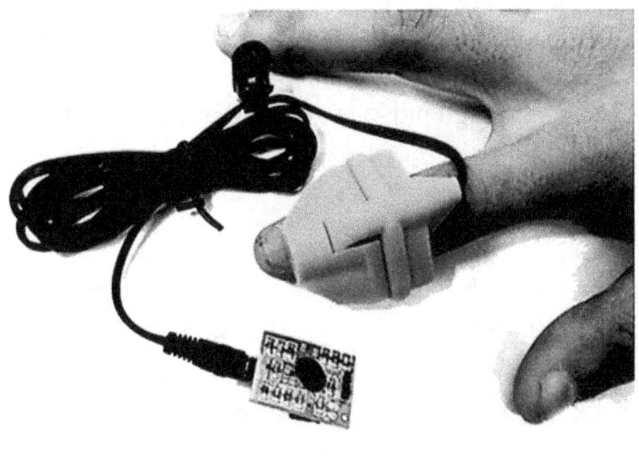

Motion Artifact Reduction

Any type of disturbance in output signal due to the motion of the sensor is known as the motion artifact. The artifacts in PPG sensor output occurs due to the movement of the body while taking measurements, this is basically due to poor reception of light at the IR receiver of the sensor. To reduce these types of errors in measurements the PPG sensor must be manufactured in a way that there must be no loss in signal occur and this can only be possible if the IR transmitter and receiver, both are placed in some covered material, by placing opposite each other. By taking care of these factors we can obtain pure and lossless PPG signal output from the sensor. The problem of motion artifact also occurs in case of ECG signal because, while taking measurements if the patient keep moving then there may be chances if false readings. For removing this type of error, we the electrodes must be of good quality. There are generally two electrodes can be applied for taking ECG signal output, i.e. right arm and left arm. But this output is not of a good quality, so one thing should be done for taking out a pure ECG signal is that a reference electrode must be connected.

R-Peak Detection

In case of the PIC microcontroller, it consists of a 10 bit ADC. So, the signal received from the ECG sensor is analog in nature and this analog signal must be converted to digital for further processing. Therefore, its output is fed into the analog channel. The digital output from the ADC shows the peak level of each individual and accordingly we can select the peak level by using buttons and the ECG peak is detected. This R-wave peak varies from person to person due to this an option is provided to increase or decrease this level manually by using switches. Electrocardiogram sensor interfaced with PIC microcontroller gives analog outputs in the voltage range of 2.7-5.5V and frequency range of 3.5 Hz. This analog signal must be converted in digital signal for further processing. As once the peak is detected in range of 2.24V or more then the timer of PIC microcontroller starts.

PPG Peak Detection

To detect the PPG peak, it has been interfaced with the interrupt input of the PIC microcontroller. This pin keeps on check the status of the input received from the sensor, as the blood pulse comes, the PPG peak is detected. Photoplethysmogram sensor gives digital output of the range of 5V and having operating current range of 100mA. The PPG output signal received from the sensor is connected to interrupt input of a microcontroller. When the high pulse is detected at this pin interrupt goes to high due to this timer stops.

Pulse Transit Time Calculation

After analog to digital conversion both the signals are fed into the microcontroller. In this unit pulse transit time is calculated by initially selecting a pre-scaled value of ECG peak level, as the peak level of ECG is selected the controller start monitoring the ECG peaks as the selected value is detected the timer starts and then it goes to check interrupt from PPG sensor, once the peak of PPG is detected the timers stops and the timer value is in hexadecimal, then it is to be converted into decimal with the help of code then the converted value is displayed on screen and also used for further calculation of SBP and DBP.

Pulse Wave Velocity Calculation

Pulse wave velocity (PWV) is calculated by using the relation between velocity and time (Hennig & Patzak, 2013), Equation (1) represents the relationship between PWV and PTT

$$Pulse\,Wave\ Velocity, PWV = \frac{\left(Distance\ between\ heart\ and\ fingertip, D\right)}{(Pulse\ Transit\ Time)} \tag{1}$$

The distance between the heart and finger is calculated by using a relation as shown in eq. (2)

$$D = BCF \times height\left(in\ cm\right) \tag{2}$$

where, BCF is a Body correlation factor. For adults, it is 0.6, based upon the survey on different subjects it is found that the length of the artery from heart to finger is approximately 60% of an individual's height. From (1) and (2), It can be simplified to (Gesche et al., 2012)

$$PWV = \frac{BCF \times height\left(cm\right)}{PTT\left(in\ ms\right)} \tag{3}$$

Blood Pressure Calculation

Now, the relation between pulse transit time and pulse wave velocity is used to relate blood pressure with respect to pulse wave velocity. This shows an indirect relation of BP with PWV (Cattivelli & Garudadri, 2009), eq. (4) and (5) showing the systolic blood pressure (SBP) and diastolic blood pressure (DBP) relationship with PWV i.e.,

$$SBP = a_{Sys} \times pwv + b_{Sys} \tag{4}$$

where, a_{Sys} and b_{Sys} are constant coefficient parameters for systolic blood pressure, these parameters are calculated with the help of least mean square algorithm.

$$DBP = a_{Dia} \times pwv + b_{Dia} \tag{5}$$

where, a_{Dia} and b_{Dia} are constant coefficient parameters for diastolic blood pressure, these parameters are calculated with the help of least mean square algorithm.

Hardware Description

The interfacing of the ECG and the PPG sensor are done with PIC microcontroller (PIC18F452). This microcontroller is chosen because of the analog signals received from the ECG sensor and this microcontroller comes with 10 bit ADC and 8 channels which mean it can process 8 analog signals at one time. So, this makes pulse transit time calculation easier. Designed hardware of the prototype is depicted in Figure 5.

Four input switches are also interfaced with the hardware. Where, switch 1 is for increment the value of ECG step size and height of the subject, switch 2 is used to decrement the value of ECG step size and height of the subject, switch 3 for entering selected ECG and PPG values and switch 4 is for reset.

Software Description

Figure 6 shows the flow chart of pulse transit time, pulse wave velocity and SBP/DBP calculation. The following steps are followed in software program for calculation of blood pressure (Ward & Langton, 2007)

Figure 5. Controller part of the hardware

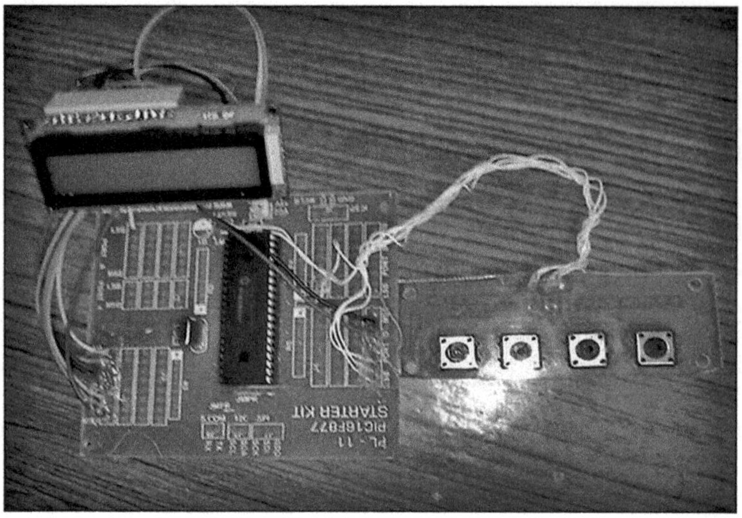

Figure 6. Flowchart

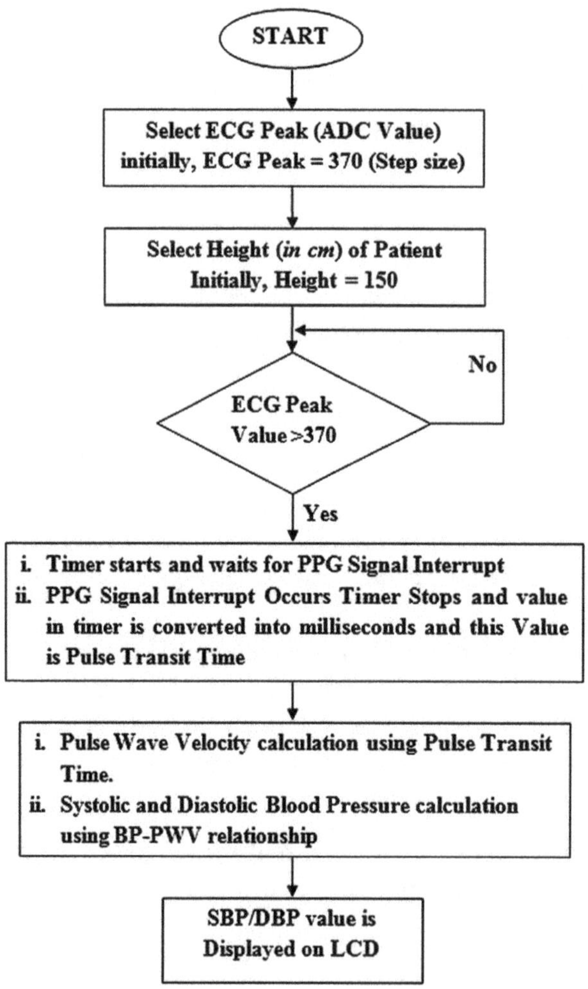

Step 1: Initializing the system, after connecting ECG electrodes on the body.

Step 2: Set the ECG step size value by using an increment and decrement switches (sw1 and sw2) and switch 3 for entering the final ECG step size.

Step 3: Set the height of the subject by using an increment and decrement switches (sw1 and sw2) and switch 3 for entering the final height in centimetres.

Step 4: After entering both ECG peak step size and height of the subject, it keeps monitoring the ECG peak (ADC step size) value, if it is below the selected ADC (Analog to digital converter) value, it will keep on monitoring, once the selected point or greater peak comes the timer of microcontroller turns on.

Step 5: Once the timer is turned on then it will wait for the interrupt signal from the PPG sensor, on reception of interrupt signal, the timer turns off and the value in timer is converted into decimal to display it on the Liquid Crystal Display (LCD) and this value is the PTT.

Step 6: This Pulse Transit Time value is applied for calculating the Pulse Wave Velocity (Sola et al. 2013) by using mathematical relationship that is expressed in equation (3).

Step 7: PWV calculated in step (6) is used for calculating blood pressure, i.e., SBP/DBP and this value are also displayed on the LCD. The LCD screen is used here to display Systolic and Diastolic blood pressure. However, only alphanumeric characters are displayed on LCD for which ASCII numbers are sent on the data pins of LCD by the microcontroller.

EXPERIMENTAL RESULTS

The developed system was tested on different subjects in different health conditions, in which whole setup was used for different subjects at different time for calculation of pulse transit time and pulse wave velocity was too computed. Table 1 shows, these are *Pulse wave velocity* (PWV) value calculations by using PTT for male and female subjects of different age and sex groups.

By using these readings, a graph is plotted between PWV and PTT. Figure 7 shows that "PWV" is inversely related to "PTT" i.e., with an increase in PTT, PWV decreases.

Later on the calculation of pulse wave velocity, least mean square algorithm (i.e., equation (6)) is employed (Cattivelli & Garudadri, 2009) for calculating constant parameters viz., a_{Sys}, b_{Sys}, a_{Dia} and b_{Dia}. These constant coefficients are derived using Least Mean Square algorithm in which initially these coefficients are calibrated by using BP value measured by cuff based machine and PWV measured by PTT method and after some time these coefficients are updated according to the previous inputs (He et al., 2013) the results shows that initially 10 to 15 BP values are required for calibrating coefficients

$$Y_K = a \times X_K + b \tag{6}$$

where, $Y_K = \begin{bmatrix} BP1 \\ \vdots \\ BPn \end{bmatrix}$ and $X_K = \begin{bmatrix} PWV1 \\ \vdots \\ PWVn \end{bmatrix}$ (7)

Table 1. Pulse wave velocity calculation using Pulse Transit Time

Subjects	Age	M/F	Height (cm)	PTT (ms)	PWV (cm/sec)
Subject 1	23	M	173	236	439
Subject 2	25	F	155	212	438
Subject 3	30	M	185	255	435
Subject 4	28	M	180	270	400
Subject 5	27	F	165	218	454
Subject 6	25	M	176	224	471
Subject 7	24	F	170	219	465
Subject 8	40	M	175	155	677
Subject 9	42	M	178	172	619
Subject 10	45	M	185	190	582
Subject 11	58	M	167	210	477
Subject 12	74	M	171	294	348
Subject 13	61	F	160	280	342
Subject 14	47	F	155	246	378
Subject 15	39	F	168	301	334

Then number of observation are collected in matrices form i.e. BP(k) and PWV(k) where, k is an integer. The complete apparatus is setup up along with PPG sensor, ECG electrodes and OMRON BP monitoring machine are attached on body is shown in Figure 8.

The calculated parameters are applied to the BP-PWV relationship to determine SBP and DBP. These values are calculated for different subjects and these are compared with reference values calculated with cuff based OMRON BP machine as shown in Figure 9 and error is also calculated between them that are shown in Table 2.

Error percentage is calculated by equation 8 between the measured value and the true value obtained from cuff based BP monitoring existing device.

$$Percentage\ Error = \frac{Measured\ value - True\ Value}{True\ Value} \times 100 \tag{8}$$

Figure 10 represents the graphical comparison between the measured readings of an OMRON blood pressure monitoring machine and pulse transit time based BP measuring machine.

FUTURE SCOPE

In the coming future this is the new version of technology, which is having endless scope. This is due to the basic techniques which we are using till now are all based on occluding cuff dependent machines. As

Figure 7. Graphical representation between pulse wave velocity and pulse transit time

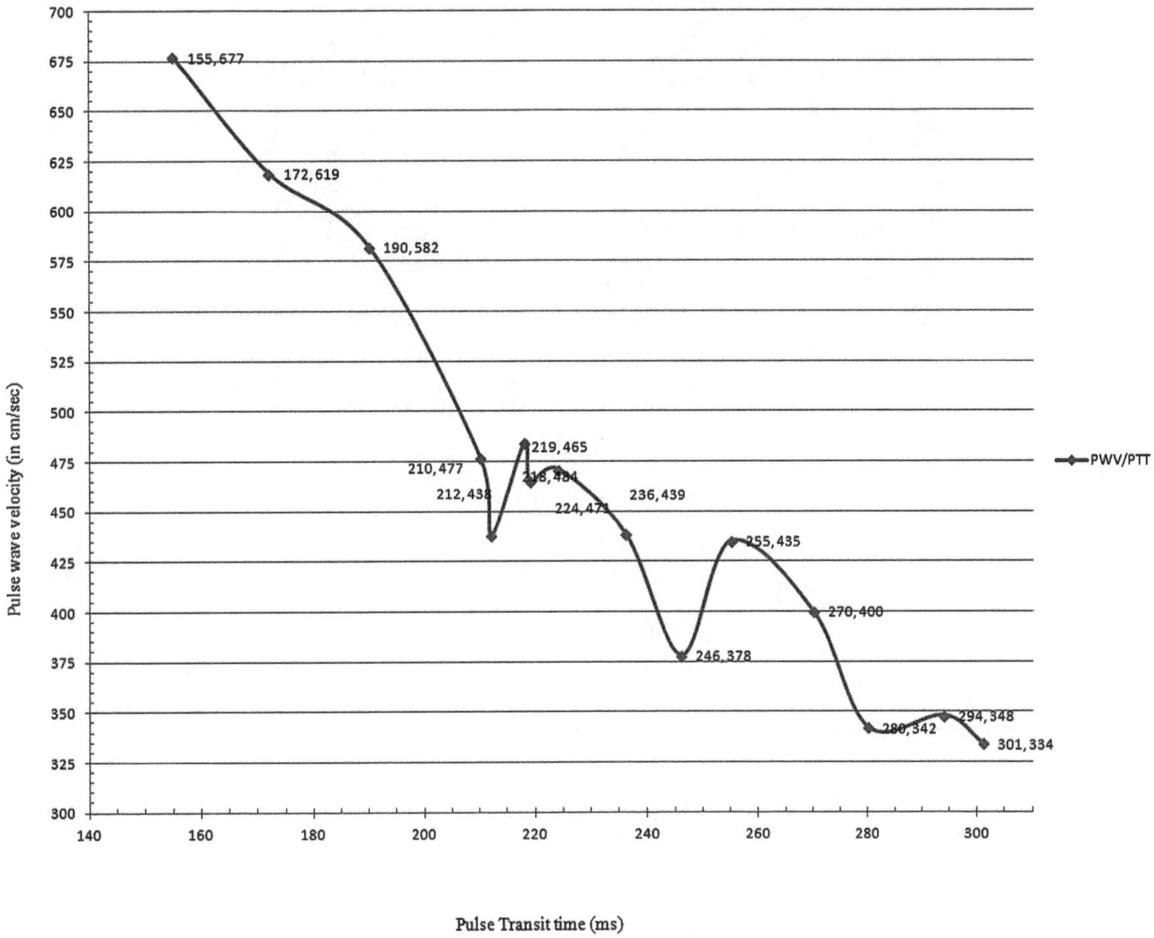

Figure 8. Complete hardware setup along with OMRON blood pressure machine

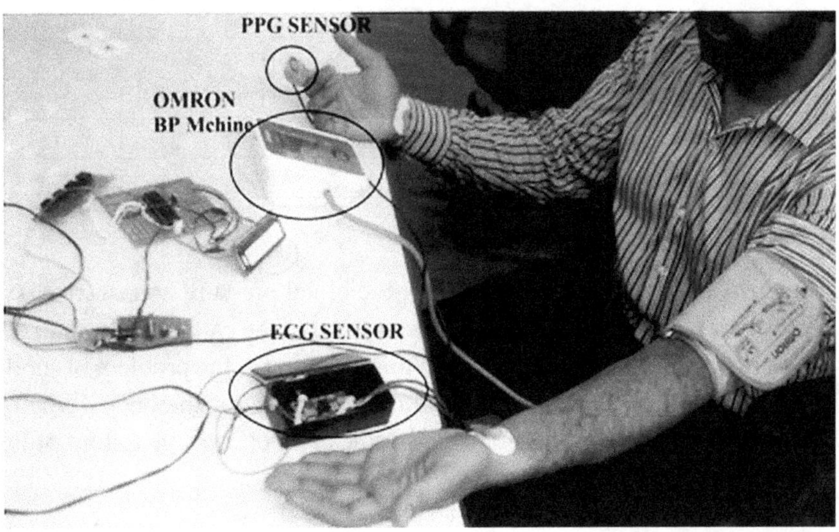

Figure 9. Systolic blood pressure/diastolic blood pressure reading on both machines on same time

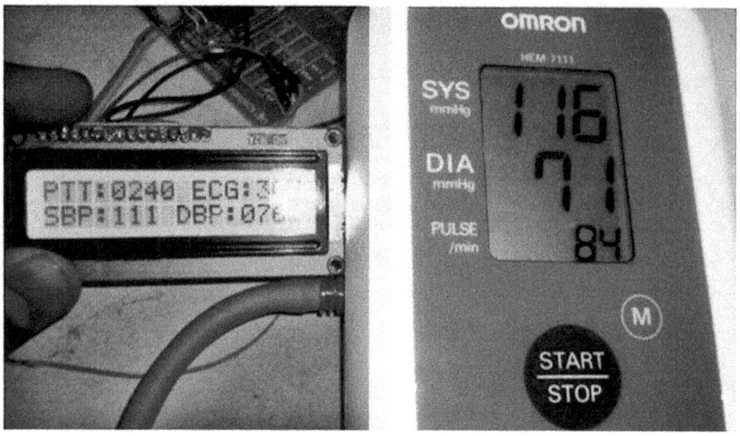

Table 2. Comparison between Cuff based BP device and PTT based BP monitoring system

Subjects	SBP/DBP (in mm hg)			SBP % Error	DBP % Error
	Using PPT Method	Using Cuff Machine	Using Sphygmomanometer		
Subject 1	112/77	116/71	116/71	3.4	8.4
Subject 2	112/76	117/73	116/73	4.2	4.1
Subject 3	111/75	112/72	111/72	0.89	4.1
Subject 4	106/70	108/73	109/72	1.8	4.1
Subject 5	114/78	119/80	119/81	4.2	2.5
Subject 6	116/81	120/83	122/82	3.3	2.4
Subject 7	115/80	118/76	118/76	2.5	5.2
Subject 8	145/90	147/93	147/92	2.7	3.2
Subject 9	137/85	143/87	144/88	4.1	2.2
Subject 10	132/84	135/82	136/83	2.2	2.4
Subject 11	127/88	130/87	131/87	2.3	1.1
Subject 12	109/69	110/72	111/73	0.9	4.1
Subject 13	108/68	112/65	113/66	3.5	4.6
Subject 14	113/73	111/70	111/71	1.8	4.2
Subject 15	107/66	108/68	109/68	0.9	2.9

now we have developed a system which can monitor the blood pressure non- invasively. But this technique requires a proper calibration of coefficients because all of the calculation work is dependent on it.

There are few improvements that are required in this system, i.e. the problem of motion artifacts has to be reduced. This artifact basically occurs due to the movement of the body while taking measurements, because in case of Photoplethysmogram sensor the error occurs due to loss of light reception in

Figure 10. Graphical representation to compare SBP/DBP readings of cuff and PTT based systems

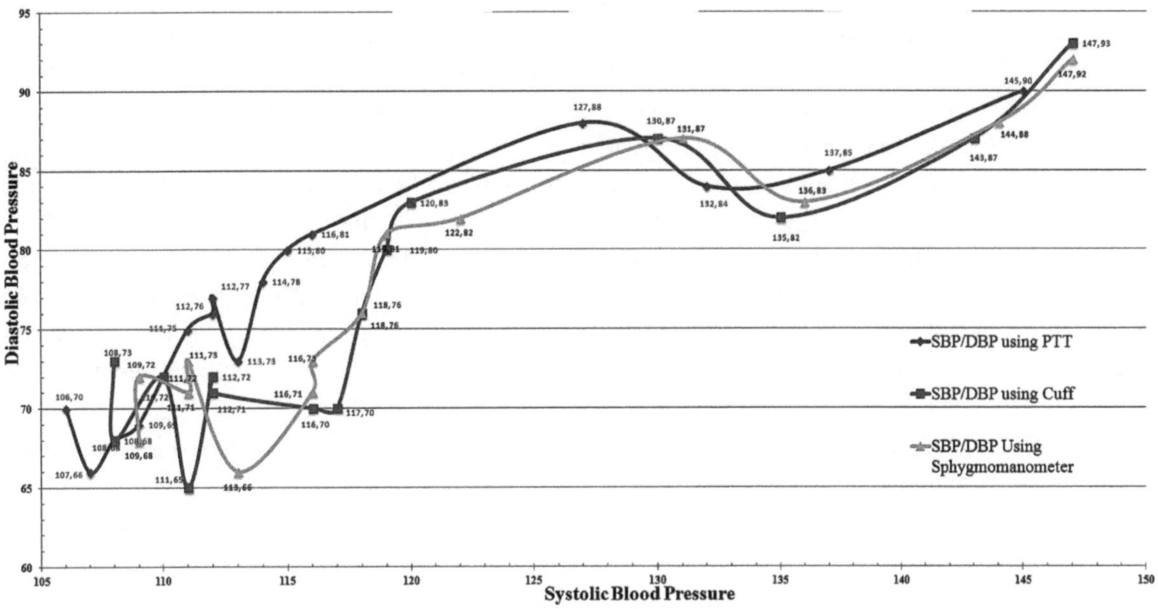

IR receiver of the sensor. In this system an accelerometer sensor can be interfaced along with a PPG sensor to reduce the artifacts due to the motion of the body.

This product can be developed by using Surface Mounted Devices (SMD) components. The product size can be reduced so that it can be designed wearable and battery operated after that we can also use Bluetooth and Zigbee for wireless transmission of the data for online estimation of the subjects. This data can be directly transmitted to doctors so that he can provide the best medication even he is not near to the subject.

CONCLUSION

This chapter presents a method to develop an automated blood pressure monitoring system, which can measure BP indirectly and without the use of any cuff. By comparing different techniques for blood pressure estimation we found that the pulse wave velocity is new and advance technique for continuous monitoring blood pressure, we can also say that Pulse transit time is the best approach for finding blood pressure non-invasively and without using cuff. The results of this technique show an error of -5 mm Hg to +2 mm Hg in systolic BP and -6 mm hg to +5 mm Hg in Diastolic BP.

This device can be easily applied clinically because this device does not require any needle to be inserted or does not require any type of device which causes any type of problem to patient in hospital as we are using very familiar devices (Electrocardiogram sensors and a PPG sensor which is similar to an spO2 sensor) but the only difference is that we are not using any cuff for this method. The most important clinical advantage of this technique is that it provides real time blood pressure monitoring of patient it is helpful especially for critical patients.

As this is a new technique for measuring blood pressure indirectly, but still, this method requires some advancement like the problem of motion artifact has to be removed and the other problem is the proper calibration of the constant parameters is required. In this system we are using two sensors, i.e. PPG and ECG sensors. By using output waveforms of these two sensors pulse transit time is calculated. The other issue with this device is that every person's heart produces different level of electrical pulse which is detected by ECG sensor so we have to take care of the peak limit of each person. For reducing this type of errors, this device is having flexible input values of ECG peak levels and hence it can be used for anyone. Experimental results demonstrate that the accuracy of the developed system is 5%.

The ECG sensor used here is producing an analog output so this analog signal must be converted into digital signals. From analog to digital conversion, ECG sensor is interfaced with the analog channel of PIC18F452. PIC18 microcontroller is used because it consists of a 10 bit analog to digital converter, which can be easily used for further processing. PPG sensor is connected with interrupt input of a microcontroller

After the development of this product testing was done with respect to cuff based blood pressure measurement machine and the error is produced. This system is tested in various conditions like in resting position, during exercise. There occurs a change in blood pressure because during exercise our blood pressure is increased.

REFERENCES

Booth, J. (1977). A short history of blood pressure measurement. *Proceedings of the Royal Society of Medicine, 70*(11), 793–799.

Cattivelli, F. S., & Garudadri, H. (2009, June). Noninvasive cuffless estimation of blood pressure from pulse arrival time and heart rate with adaptive calibration. In *Wearable and Implantable Body Sensor Networks, 2009. BSN 2009. Sixth International Workshop on* (pp. 114-119). IEEE. doi:10.1109/BSN.2009.35

Chan, K. W., Hung, K., & Zhang, Y. T. (2001). Noninvasive and cuffless measurements of blood pressure for telemedicine. In *Engineering in Medicine and Biology Society, 2001.Proceedings of the 23rd Annual International Conference of the IEEE* (*Vol. 4*, pp. 3592-3593). IEEE. doi:10.1109/IEMBS.2001.1019611

Da Silva, P. M. P. (2013). *A pervasive system for real-time blood pressure monitoring*. Academic Press.

Deb, S., Nanda, C., Goswami, D., Mukhopadhyay, J., & Chakrabarti, S. (2007, November). Cuff-less estimation of blood pressure using pulse transit time and pre-ejection period. In *Convergence Information Technology, 2007. International Conference on* (pp. 941-944). IEEE. doi:10.1109/ICCIT.2007.206

Fiala, J., Bingger, P., Foerster, K., Heilmann, C., Beyersdorf, F., Zappe, H., & Seifert, A. (2010, November). Implantable sensor for blood pressure determination via pulse transit time. In Sensors, 2010 IEEE (pp. 1226-1229). IEEE. doi:10.1109/ICSENS.2010.5690619

Gesche, H., Grosskurth, D., Küchler, G., & Patzak, A. (2012). Continuous blood pressure measurement by using the pulse transit time: Comparison to a cuff-based method. *European Journal of Applied Physiology, 112*(1), 309–315. doi:10.1007/s00421-011-1983-3 PMID:21556814

Goli, S., & Jayanthi, T. (2014, January). Cuff less Non-Invasive Blood Pressure Measurement Using Pulse Transit Time measurement. *International Journal of Recent Development in Engineering and Technology*, *2*(1), 2347–6435.

He, X., Goubran, R. A., & Liu, X. P. (2013, May). Evaluation of the correlation between blood pressure and pulse transit time. In *Medical Measurements and Applications Proceedings (MeMeA), 2013 IEEE International Symposium on* (pp. 17-20). IEEE. doi:10.1109/MeMeA.2013.6549697

Hennig, A., & Patzak, A. (2013). Continuous blood pressure measurement using pulse transit time. *Somnologie-Schlafforschung und Schlafmedizin*, *17*(2), 104–110. doi:10.1007/s11818-013-0617-x

Hey, S., Gharbi, A., von Haaren, B., Walter, K., Konig, N., & Loffler, S. (2009, February). Continuous noninvasive pulse transit time measurement for psycho-physiological stress monitoring. In *eHealth, Telemedicine, and Social Medicine, 2009. eTELEMED'09. International Conference on* (pp. 113-116). IEEE.

Kim, Y., & Lee, J. (2010, August). Cuffless and non-invasive estimation of a continuous blood pressure based on ptt. In *Information Technology Convergence and Services (ITCS), 2010 2nd International Conference on* (pp. 1-4). IEEE. doi:10.1109/ITCS.2010.5581266

Kumar, K. S., Bhowmik, D., & Duraivel, S. (2014). Hypertension Epidemic in India-A Comprehensive Review of Clinical Features, Management and Remedies. Academic Press.

Manimegalai, J., & Thanushkodi. (2012). Estimation of cardiovascular parameters from ECG and PPG signals. *Bioengineering Conference (NEBEC), 2012 38th Annual Northeast*. IEEE. doi:10.1109/eTELEMED.2009.35

Manimegalai, P., Jacob, D., & Thanushkodi, K. (2012, March). Estimation of cardiovascular parameters from ECG and PPG signals. In *Bioengineering Conference (NEBEC), 2012 38th Annual Northeast* (pp. 237-238). IEEE. doi:10.1109/NEBC.2012.6207051

McCarthy, B. M., O'Flynn, B., & Mathewson, A. (2011, August). An investigation of pulse transit time as a non-invasive blood pressure measurement method. Journal of Physics, 307(1). doi:10.1088/1742-6596/307/1/012060

Shriram, R., Wakankar, A., Daimiwal, N., & Ramdasi, D. (2010, April). Continuous cuffless blood pressure monitoring based on PTT. In *Bioinformatics and Biomedical Technology (ICBBT), 2010 International Conference on* (pp. 51-55). IEEE. doi:10.1109/ICBBT.2010.5479013

Sola, J., Proenca, M., Ferrario, D., Porchet, J. A., Falhi, A., Grossenbacher, O., & Sartori, C. et al. (2013). Noninvasive and nonocclusive blood pressure estimation via a chest sensor. *Biomedical Engineering. IEEE Transactions on*, *60*(12), 3505–3513. doi:10.1109/TBME.2013.2272699

Ward, M., & Langton, J. A. (2007). Blood pressure measurement. *Continuing Education in Anaesthesia Critical Care & Pain*, *7*(4), 122–126. doi:10.1093/bjaceaccp/mkm022

Xu, L., Guo, X., Yang, F., Yin, S., Zhang, X., & Meng, M. Q. H. (2012, June). Implementation of cuffless continuous blood pressure measurement system based on Android. In *Information and Automation (ICIA), 2012 International Conference on* (pp. 552-556). IEEE. doi:10.1109/ICInfA.2012.6246866

Younessi, H. M., Khalilzadeh, M. A., & Joharinia, S. (2014). Continuous and Cuffless Blood Pressure Monitoring Based on ECG and SpO2 Signals ByUsing Microsoft Visual C Sharp. *Journal of Biomedical Physics & Engineering*, *4*(1), 27–32. PMID:25505765

Chapter 9
Electromyogram and Inertial Sensor Signal Processing in Locomotion and Transition Classification

Deepak Joshi
Indian Institute of Technology (IIT) Delhi, India

Michael E. Hahn
University of Oregon, USA

ABSTRACT

Signal processing in biomedical engineering is essentially required for classification while serving mainly two aims. The first is noise removal and the second is signal representation. Signal representation deals with transforming the signal in such a way that the signal is most informative in that particular domain for the application at hand. This chapter will describe signal processing methods like spectrogram with specific applications to locomotion and transition classification using Electromyography (EMG) data. A wavelet analysis application on foot acceleration signals for automatic identification of toe off in locomotion and the ramp transition is also shown. Finally, the performance of EMG and accelerometer performance across different time windows of a gait cycle in locomotion and transition classification is presented with an emphasis on fusing the data from both sensors for better classification.

INTRODUCTION

A signal is a single-valued representation, real or complex, of information as a function of an independent variable recorded from some sensing device. Physically, it is a form of energy being produced by a process. Various types of signals exist and the method of signal processing needed to process a signal heavily depends on the type of the signal. Broadly, there are four types of signals:

DOI: 10.4018/978-1-5225-0660-7.ch009

1. Deterministic,
2. Stochastic,
3. Chaotic, and
4. Fractal.

Deterministic signals can be represented mathematically using certain parameters and hence prediction of deterministic signal in future, based on past values, is possible. Stochastic signals are random in nature with no closed loop mathematical expression and hence are not predictable in future. Fractal signals have interesting property of scale-invariance i.e. at any level of magnification the signal looks similar in structure. Chaotic signals lie somewhere between deterministic and stochastic signals. They deemed to be deterministic in a very sensitive sense and hence are not predictable in future with reasonable accuracy. Biomedical signals are generally stochastic in nature and need signal processing methods for various applications. Biomedical signal processing in various applications serves mainly two aims. The first is noise removal and the second is signal representation. The main source of noise in biomedical signals is noise in electronic instrumentation. Other sources consist of electromagnetic interference and skin motion or physiological artifacts. For example, while recording electromyogram (EMG) nearby the chest one can observe the artifacts of electrocardiogram (ECG) in the EMG profile. There have been many provisions in hardware and experimental protocols to remove such noise and artifacts, however complete removal is not possible without using signal processing tools. Signal representation deals with transforming the signal in such a way that the signal is most informative in that particular domain for the application at hand. One such application is classification of locomotion and transitions in assistive devices where noise removal and signal representation are critical for successful, rapid and safe classification.

Locomotion classification is crucial in lower limb prosthesis control. Powered lower limb prosthesis provides sufficient torque and stability to the amputee so that they can negotiate in different terrains with reduced energy consumption. The key component for powered prosthesis to be facilitated with such features is accurate locomotion classification. Based on the classified locomotion, the artificial limb changes the damping profile to provide with net required torque output. For seamless transition in a powered prosthesis it is critical to classify the upcoming locomotion ahead of time (ideally before toe off of the transitional gait cycle) to ensure safe transition. Hence the selection of required data is critical and depends on the application at hand. For example, if someone is interested in analyzing the offline data of a cerebral palsy patient then the full gait cycle (heel strike to heel strike) may be available. However, for the application of real time actuation in prosthesis and orthosis control, the data available is limited. Hence, within this framework of classification the selection of sensors is critical. EMG represents the muscular activity and has been used widely for various applications like prosthetic control, gait analysis, disease diagnosis, and neuro-muscular coordination (Gea Drost et.al. 2006; Anjana Goen and D. C. Tiwari 2013). With the advancement in technology, miniaturized inertial sensors like accelerometers have shown promise in locomotion classification and other clinical gait analysis applications. Ambulatory monitoring of daily activities is the other area where accelerometer is of great importance as a sensing device.

EMG is the summation of electrical activity, action potential, of all the motor units recorded by the electrode. EMG signals are recorded by placing electrodes in, on, or near a muscle and amplifying the electric potential between two electrodes, that results from the generation and propagation of action potentials along muscle fibers. These muscle fibers are innervated by motor neurons from the spinal cord. The electrodes used are generally made of silver/silver chloride (Ag/AgCl) with some application of conductive gel at the skin-electrode interface. The electrodes serve as a transducer which converts the ionic activity of cells inside the body into the electric current outside the body. To reduce the effect of common mode electromagnetic noise the electrodes are used in differential mode. Such a differential mode also offers to measure localized activity within the muscle. After removing the noise from the EMG signal it is required to represent the EMG signal for the application in hand. Signal representation of EMG signal for various applications essentially consists of representing the signal in 1) time domain, 2) frequency domain, and 3) time-frequency domain. Time domain processing may include autocorrelation, whitening, normalization, etc. Autocorrelation gives a measure of matching the signal to itself while shifting the signal, known as lag, in past and future. Therefore, the autocorrelation is a function of lag. Whitening temporally decorrelates the value of signal at various instant of time thereby increasing the statistical degree of freedom. Normalization involves scaling the time and amplitude axis of the signal with respect to a reference value. Frequency domain processing may include filtering, coherence, etc. Filtering involves removing the unwanted frequency from the signals while coherence evaluates the frequencies in synchronization between two signals. The time-frequency domain processing consists of simultaneous time-frequency representation, including Spectrogram, wavelet decomposition, etc. Spectrogram is a fixed resolution time-frequency representation while wavelet offers a choice of multi-resolution. The present chapter will describe these signal processing tools like spectrogram with specific applications to EMG.

The popularity of using tri-axial accelerometers in locomotion classification has increased in recent years for clinicians and researchers. Accelerometers directly measure acceleration and hence avoid any error of calculating acceleration by integrating velocity and displacement. Accelerometers for human movement quantification generally utilize sensors like strain gauge, piezoresistive, capacitive and piezoelectric. A tri-axial accelerometer simultaneously records the acceleration in all the directions. The signal processing tools for EMG are equally applicable to accelerometers as both of them represents the movement information; however, care must be taken for low frequency and gravity biased signal from an accelerometer while selecting a signal representation method. For example, approximate entropy and fractal analysis have been considered as important time domain signal processing tools for quantification of human movement via accelerometry. Apart from locomotion classification, accelerometry has been especially advantageous in the identification of gait events like heel strike and toe off. A particular wavelet application on acceleration signals of the foot for automatic identification of toe off in locomotion and the ramp transition is presented.

In recent years, multisensory fusion and integration has shown several benefits over single sensor data for biomedical systems. In a particular case of locomotion and transition classification, the sensor fusion approach provides better classification accuracy and robust performance. In this chapter, the EMG and accelerometer performance across different time window of a gait cycle in locomotion and transition classification is presented.

This chapter presents a brief review of approaches for the EMG and accelerometer signal processing in locomotion and transition classification. It is organized in the following sections: Locomotion and transition classification, where some popular methods in use will be briefly described; Spectrogram approach for EMG signal representation, where basic principles of spectrogram approach presented; wavelet analysis of foot acceleration for gait event detection; and finally, a comparison of acceleration and EMG across gait cycle in locomotion classification is presented with an insight on sensor fusion.

LOCOMOTION AND TRANSITION CLASSIFICATION

The estimated number of lower limb amputations every year in the United States is 120,000 leading to limited involvement of the individual in various physical activities (T. R. Dillingham et.al. 2002). Lower limb prostheses are designed to partially restore function in the lower limb. Passive prostheses allow for level over ground walking but do not provide net torque for walking over varied terrain. Advancements in embedded system technology have facilitated the introduction of powered prostheses which allow desired impedance for terrain walking (Au. S. et. al. 2008; F. Sup et. al. 2008). Hence, it becomes critical to accurately classify the locomotion in current powered prosthesis. Moreover, an ideal powered prosthesis must also provide the seamless transition while switching between the locomotion modes which requires to accurately identify the movement intention of amputee. While the classification problem needs to know what the amputee is currently doing; the seamless transition is an anticipation problem and therefore needs to know that what the amputee is about to do. A ramp transition is schematically shown in Figure 1.

Current powered prostheses lack in such anticipation and requires some "cueing" in the form of either manual intervention or compensatory movements which add cognitive load to the amputee resulting in non-effective use of the prosthesis. As mentioned, the seamless transition is an anticipation problem and hence becomes challenging as the future data is not available in the real time scenario. This leads to a broadened scope to investigate choice of sensors, methods in signal processing and signal representation, and various classification algorithms to solve this anticipation problem.

SENSORS

Various choices of sensors have been explored in past few decades for locomotion and transition classification. The primary criterion to select a sensor modality is the richness of information – the other criteria being the relative ease of placement (i.e. donning and doffing), the cosmesis and social acceptance (R Kobetic et. al. 2009). A detailed review of sensors for locomotion and transition classification can be found elsewhere (Michael R Tucker et. al. 2015). As EMG represents the true physiological represen-

Figure 1. Ramp ascent and descent transition from overground walking

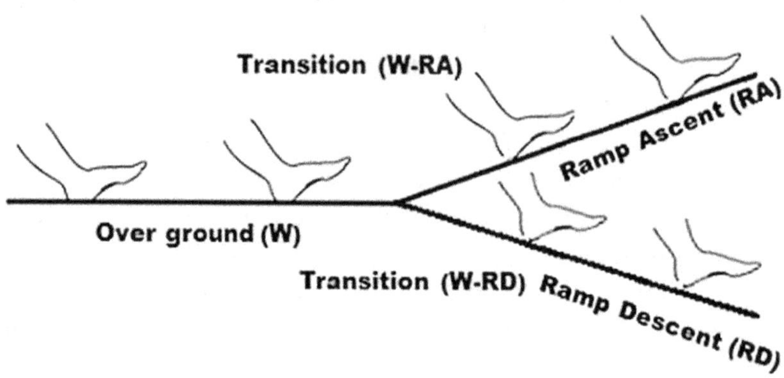

tation of muscle contraction, it is perhaps the most promising source of information for decoding the motion intention, and potentially other application of classification. However, due to the non-stationary nature of locomotion and EMG signal being highly susceptible to noise – due to artifacts and sweating, it requires extensive signal processing, followed by signal presentation, before being fed into the classifier. Particular to application in motion classification, EMG signal has shown respectable accuracy in respective applications (R. H. Chowdhary et.al. 2013; D. Graupe et. al. 1982; D. Graupe et. al. 1985; Y Huang et.al. 2005; X Zhang et. al. 2012). Due to the miniaturized sensing technology, the body mounted sensors have been used extensively in the last decade for various applications.

Specific to locomotion classification the accelerometer has been the preferred choice. A range of classifiers – including Simple threshold, Hierarchical scheme, Decision Trees, k-nearest neighborhood, Artificial Neural Network (ANN), Support Vector Machine (SVM), Naïve Bayes and Gaussian Mixture Model (GMM), Fuzzy Logic, and Markov Models (Culhane et.al. 2004; Ermes et. al. 2008; Maurer et. al. 2006; Parkka et. al. 2006; Doukas and Maglogiannis 2008; Wu et. al. 2007; Allen at. al. 2006; Salarian et. al. 2007; Pober et. al. 2006), have been used for activity classification using features from accelerometer data. A detailed review can be found elsewhere (Stephen J. Preece et.al. 2009). Subjects worn with EMG and accelerometer are shown in Figure 2.

SPECTROGRAM APPROACH FOR EMG

Due to their easy computation and reduced computation time, the time domain representation of EMG signal has been used extensively for locomotion classification (Miller et.al. 2013; Huang H et.al. 2009). However, limited signal representation in the time domain demands high number of features (Huang H.

Figure 2. A subject stepping down in stair terrain wearing EMG and accelerometer sensor on foot and ankle

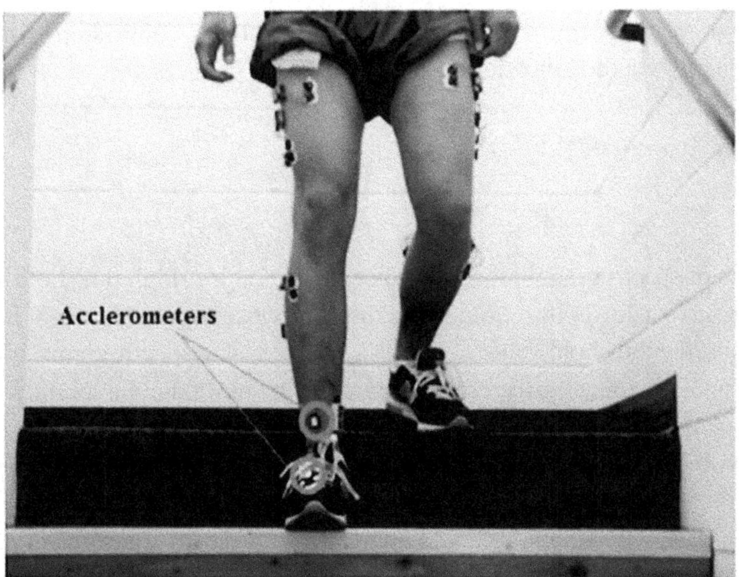

et.al. 2011), leading to high dimensionality for good classification accuracy close to 95%. Moreover, the significantly enhanced classification accuracy of activity identification by introducing frequency domain features (S J Preece et.al. 2009) is appealing for exploration of the simultaneous time-frequency representation of EMG signals in locomotion and transition classification. Such a time-frequency representation can be served by two means:

1. Spectrogram, and
2. Wavelet transform.

Though the wavelet transform offers multi resolution analysis in time and frequency domains compared to fixed resolution in spectrogram, wavelet transform provides redundant information in terms of a large number of wavelet coefficients, thus overburdening the classifier, and wavelet transform is suited to specific applications (Fernandes FCA et.al. 2001; Valens CA 1999). Spectrogram representation of EMG was first presented to analyze fast movement and constant contraction of human hand muscles (Hannaford B and Lehman S, 1986), however little is known about its utility in classifying locomotion modes or transitions using lower extremity EMG. A spectrogram, fixed resolution time-frequency representation, of the data segment uses periodogram approach to calculate the spectral density as following:

where N is the total number of data points in the data segment, ω is the frequency and m is the length of the window. The spectrogram is then calculated, using Matlab 2015, as the magnitude square of each periodogram as follows:

$$Spectrogram\left\{x\left(n\right)\right\}\left(m,\omega\right)=\left|P_x\left(m,\omega\right)\right|^2 \tag{2}$$

The periodogram gives a good estimate of spectral density of non-stationary signals like EMG, calculating the Fourier Transform of auto-correlation to give a better estimate of spectral density. Spectrogram of a 256ms EMG with 64 ms window and 50 percent overlap is shown in Figure 3. A detailed description of periodogram can be found in (Cooper GR and McGillem CD 1999).

Such a periodogram is transformed to threshold based binary conversion (TBBC) by utilizing a threshold (0.5) in energy via the following equation:

$$\begin{aligned} F_{i,j} &= 1, if(|\,F_{i,j}\,|)^2 \geq 0.5 * \max((|\,F_{i,j}\,|)^2)\forall i,j \\ &= 0, otherwise \end{aligned} \tag{3}$$

where F is the value of spectrogram in the bin indices, by i and j. A high threshold value of 1 may lose critical information while a lower threshold value may introduce noisy, redundant information. For this method development, the threshold value of 0.5 was selected. The spectrograms, after TBBC, from all training trials were pooled to develop the 2D histogram. Prior knowledge was extracted from the previous gait cycle. This prior knowledge was integrated into the system as follows: If the previous class is walk then there is no possibility that next class can be stair ascent. The only possibility for next class is either walk or the transition from walk to stair ascent. Hence, for a given EMG data set with prior knowledge of locomotion as walk, the classification should not return stair ascent. Thus, the prior knowledge is able to restrict the possible intended locomotion state, effectively reducing computation time and increasing

Figure 3. Spectrogram of a 256ms EMG signal with 64 ms window and 50 percent overlap

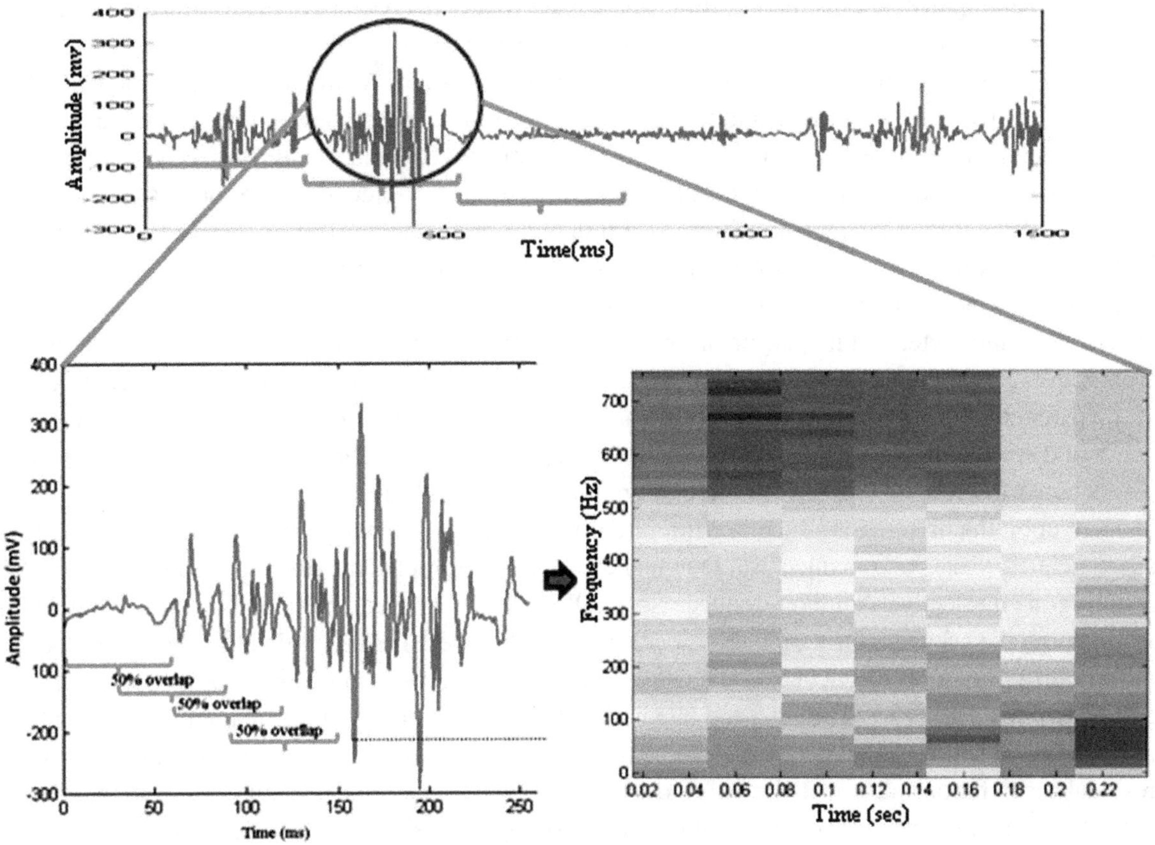

classification accuracy. By training a few if-else rules using developed 2D histogram of seven lower extremities EMG, bandwidth between 3-500 Hz, namely – Tibialis Anterior (TA), Medial Gastrocnemius (MG), Rectus Femoris (RF), Vastus Lateralis (VL), Biceps Femoris (BF), Gluteus Maximus (GMax) and Gluteus Medius (GMed), of thirteen healthy subjects an overall classification error of less than 20% for over ground walking (W), stair ascent (SA) and the transition from over ground walking to stair transition (W-SA) was achieved, using leave-one-subject-out-cross validation. This error was further reduced to less than 11% by utilizing knowledge of previous gait cycle i.e. prior knowledge. More details of classification method and neural input can be found in (Deepak Joshi et. al. 2015). Spectrogram involves frequency transformation and hence requires obvious computational time resources. It was observed that with the computational resources of Intel Core i7 CPU @ 3.40 GHz and 8 GB RAM it took 53.5 ms and 2.5 ms for calculation of spectrogram information and classification decision, respectively. The fast classification is due to if-else rules which are computationally easy to calculate.

WAVELET APPLICATION OF ACCELEROMETRY DATA

Once the classification for locomotion is performed it is desirable to provide appropriate damping for swing and stance phase separately for the respective locomotion. Hence it becomes critical to correctly identify gait events like toe off to separate the swing and stance phase in real time. This becomes critical when the amputee is transitioning from one terrain to another. Ground reaction forces (GRF) and kinematic data from motion capture have been the golden standard for toe identification of toe off in over ground walking and treadmill walking (Y H Chang et. al. 2000; A Hreljac and R N Marshall 2000; J K De Witt 2010). Both of these sources are limited to laboratory settings and hence are not suitable for some applications like Functional Electrical Stimulation (FES) and monitoring of activity of daily living (ADL) where ambulatory monitoring systems are required. Moreover, these sources have not been tested in different terrains or in transitions. With the advent of miniaturization sensor technology and high end signal processing like wavelet it is appealing to explore inertial sensors like accelerometers with high end signal processing for identification of toe off in different terrains and the transitions. A tri-axial accelerometer and its placement on dorsum of the foot along with its axis towards the movement are shown in Figure 4. With respect to a global coordinate reference of anterior-posterior (X) and vertical direction (Z), placement of the accelerometer on the foot led to primary measurement directions as Ax and Az (Figure 4), with Ay representing the medial-lateral direction, orthogonal to Ax and Az.

As noted in Figure 4, Az and Ax were not purely aligned with the global vertical and Z, being dependent upon the orientation of the dorsum of the foot. Foot movement during walking is generally in a low frequency range. To reduce data redundancy, we down-sampled the original data by a factor of 5, resulting in an effective sampling frequency of 300Hz. Down sampling reduced the redundancy while maintaining the critical information. The accelerometer data were filtered with a low pass second order Butterworth filter with 10Hz cut off frequency. This cutoff frequency, compared to other options like 20 and 40 Hz, avoided the local minima and maxima in the acceleration data while maintaining meaningful information of source signal to develop the heuristic algorithms. To remove the gravity component, the residual acceleration value in all directions during a period of quiet stance, is removed from the filtered data. Most of the movement of leg during locomotion is in the direction of progression i.e. Anterior Posterior (AP) and vertical. Hence, these two directional data were explored for identification of toe off event. Various signal processing algorithms and classification schemes have been employed for the identification of toe off in a gait cycle. Heuristic approaches have been especially attractive and appealing due to easy computation and ease in real time implementation algorithms (J. M. Jasiewicz et. al. 2006; A. M. Sabatini et.al. 2005). However, due to the advancement in signal processing algorithms and machine learning, researchers have been able to achieve better accuracy in toe off identification (Aung et.al. 2013). Algorithms need to be robust in identifying the toe off event in locomotion as well as in the transition gait cycle. As toe off marks the transition from stance to swing phase, a discontinuity at this

Figure 4. Placement of accelerometer and associated global and local coordinate reference

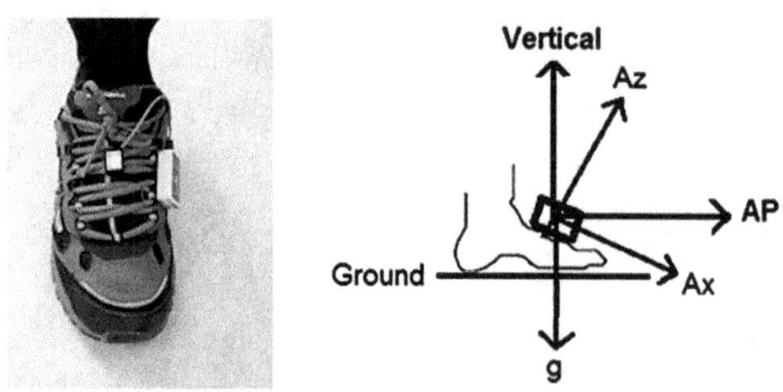

transition in the vertical component of acceleration is expected. Such short period transitions are better highlighted in wavelet analysis due to the high time resolution capability for high frequency in wavelet. Further to reduce the computation time, the transition can be localized in the gait cycle using a heuristic approach before applying the wavelet transform. Figure 5 shows the toe off event localized by points A, B, C, and M. These points can be heuristically identified using the acceleration data in Ax and Az directions. Point A and B were identified utilizing mutual information in the Ax and Ay acceleration data. Specifically, point M is the maximum Ay acceleration peak in a gait cycle, and is the closest unique point in proximity to point A, which is the peak Ax acceleration. Further, point C is the maximum negative Ax peak prior to point A. We segmented Az acceleration of a gait cycle between point A and point B to locally search for the toe off.

Figure 5. The Ax and Ay with foot switch data during ramp walking (ascending, RA). Three separate cycles are shown from one example subject; representing those with minimum, maximum and median stride duration. The Y-axis unit for acceleration and foot switch are ±g and Volt, respectively and are shown with respect to time-normalized gait cycle. The marker C corresponds to the region of Toe-off for all the three stride cycles showing that it lies between point A and B exclusively.

Note: Acceleration in Ay direction is shown with an offset of +2g for visualization purposes.

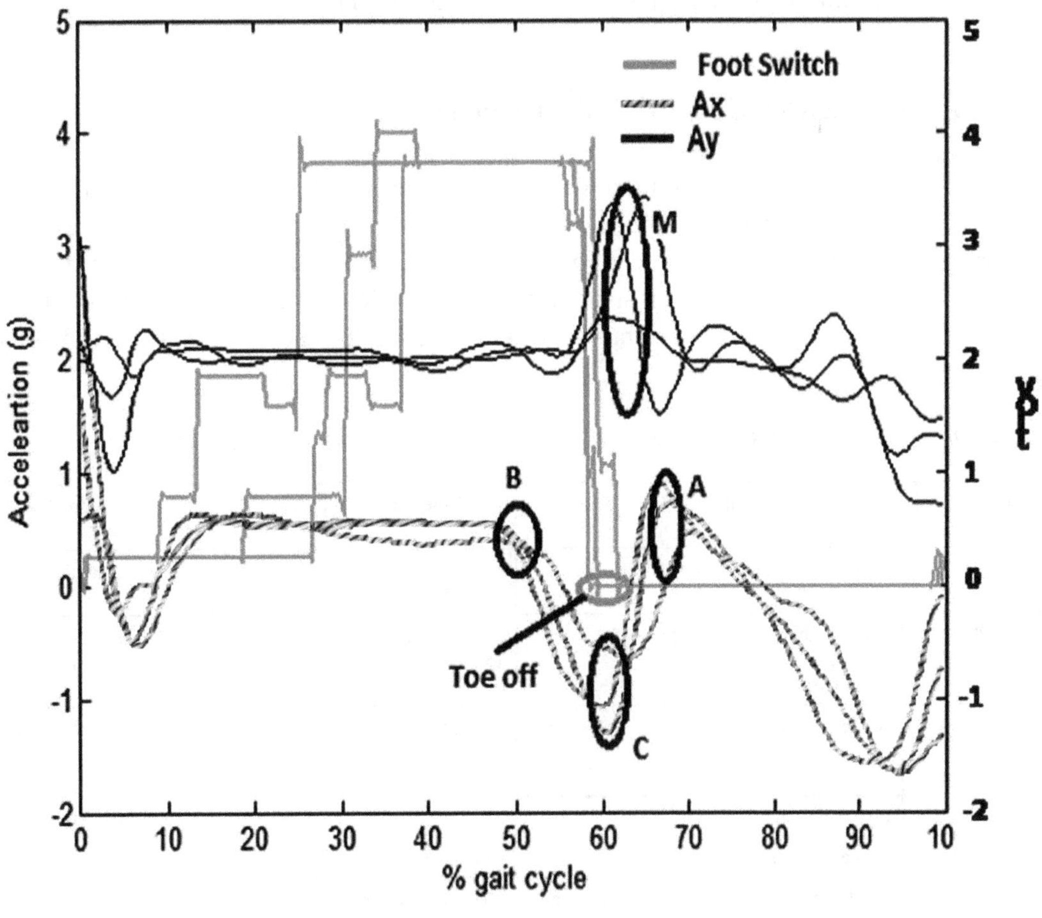

Further, wavelet analysis can highlight the toe off event in the localized segment identified by the heuristic approach. Such an approach has been utilized recently and was demonstrated to be superior to other approaches in the past while detecting the toe off in walk (W), ramp ascent (RA), ramp descent (RD) and both the transitions (W-RA and W-RD) (Deepak Joshi et.al. 2014). Estimation error was first defined as the time difference between the toe off detection by foot switch and toe off detection by the proposed algorithm. Absolute value of this error value was calculated and averaged across the subjects to report mean absolute estimation error. Note: As the effective sampling frequency was 300 Hz, the error of a single sample of time corresponds to 3.3 ms. A comparison of accuracy in correct toe off identification is given in Table 1.

Among the other findings, the average stride durations for steady state locomotion were 1.08 ± 0.078, 1.07 ± 0.10 and 1.06 ± 0.067 seconds for W, RA and RD, respectively and 1.07 ± 0.081 and 1.06 ± 0.076 seconds for the transition W-RA and W-RD respectively. No significant differences were found between any possible pairs of within or between transition and steady state locomotion (paired t-test, $\alpha = 0.05$). Point A, B, C and M were detected with 100 percent accuracy utilizing the Ax and Ay acceleration data; no trial was missed in examining toe off due to misidentification of any instance of point A, B or C. Hence, the Az acceleration was segmented correctly in all the trials across all subjects. The mean absolute estimation error using db2 was 25.6 ± 18.3, 32.5 ± 15.3, 33.2 ± 21.7, 32.5 ± 19.5 and 26.8 ± 16.2ms compared to 17.4 ± 12.5, 13.8 ± 8.5, 22.0 ± 16.4, 20.1 ± 15.5 and 17.1 ± 13.7ms using db1 wavelet, for W, RA, RD, W-RA, and W-RD, respectively. The db1 wavelet performed significantly better than db2 in identifying toe off with high accuracy ($p < 0.01$).

EMG AND ACCELEROMETER COMPARISION

It was concluded in a previous section that the accelerometer and EMG performed with reasonable classification accuracy in different applications for lower limb prosthetics. It will be interesting to see the performance of both sensors in a common application of classification in order to derive a fair comparison of both the sensors. Such an application is to classify the locomotion transition in grouped transition of terrain and direction. For terrain type classification, the data from W-RA and W-RD were

Table 1. Comparison of estimation error (mean ± std) using the reported approaches*

Author	Sensor Placement	Over Ground (ms)	Ramp (ms)	Transition (ms)	Algorithm Type
Jasiewicz et al (2006)	Foot accelerometer	19 ±34	N/A	N/A	Heuristic
Aung et al (2013)	Foot acceleration (simulated + measured)	18.3± 27.0	5.1 ±12.1 (smooth) 15.2± 41.7 (tactile)	N/A	Heuristic + Wavelet + Machine learning
Aung et al (2013)	Ankle accelerometer	19.5± 27.1	32.5± 63.0 (smooth) 21.1± 53.1 (tactile)	N/A	Heuristic + Wavelet + Machine learning
Sabatini et al (2005)	Foot gyroscope	35	35	N/A	Heuristic
Joshi et al (2014)	Foot accelerometer	17.4 ±12.5	13.8 ±8.5	20.1 ±15.5	Heuristic + Wavelet

*The results are shown for db1 wavelet which showed better accuracy than db2 wavelet.

compiled and further class labeled as ramp. Similarly, the data from W-SA and W-SD were compiled and further class labeled as stairs. For direction type classification, data from W-RA and W-SA were compiled and further class labeled as ascent. Lastly, the features from W-RD and W-SD were compiled and further class labeled as descent. In summary, the terrain group represent whether the transition is to stair or to the ramp irrespective of the direction (i.e. up and down). In a similar way the direction group represents whether the transition is to up direction or the down direction. Such a classification scheme is often described as hierarchical classification. Other than classification accuracy, it is important to see the comparison across different events of gait cycle specifically with reference to toe off as the toe off marks the transition from swing to stance phase. The toe off was marked by using foot switch data. Based on the toe off event three windows from a transitional gait cycle were extracted as follows:

1. **Pre Toe Off:** A data segment starting from toe off and extending backward to foot strike of the transitional gait cycle. Window sizes varied from size of 50–350 ms with an increment of 50 ms.
2. **Post Toe Off:** A data segment starting from toe off and extending forward to foot strike on new terrain. Window sizes were similar to pre toe off.
3. **Transitional Window:** A combination of pre and post toe off segments.

EMG and accelerometer sensors were placed exactly as mentioned in previous sections. Data were sampled at 1500 Hz using the Noraxon Telemyo DTS system (Noraxon, Scottsdale, AZ). All post-processing was conducted using custom-written programs in Matlab (Mathworks, Natick, MA). EMG signals were band pass filtered between 20 and 500 Hz using a 4th order digital Butterworth filter. Accelerometer signals were low pass filtered with 10 Hz cut off using a 4th order digital Butterworth filter, in addition to removal of mean before further processing. Figure 6 shows the data from accelerometer and EMG sensor across the gait cycle for mentioned events.

To derive a fair comparison between both sensors it is important to represent the information from both sensors in an equal number of dimensions. Principal component analysis (PCA) is a multivariate technique that transforms the original feature space into a set of new orthogonal variables called principal components such that the variance in new dimensions is maximized. PCA finds these dimensions by directly observing the Eigen vectors of covariance matrix. For the features given in table II for both the sensors, PCA revealed that among top five Eigen vector directions EMG data could capture the 97.45% of variance compared to just 90.36% of variance in accelerometer data (Deepak Joshi et. al. 2015). EMG data were collected from seven channels as mentioned in previous sections; however accelerometer for this study was collected from two tri-axial accelerometers on foot and shank thus constituting six channels as shown in Table 2.

Support vector Machine (SVM) and linear discrimant classifier (LDA) classifiers were used for pattern recognition. LDA is a supervised dimension-reduction technique and well-assessed classification method. The LDA involves finding a linear combination of the independent variables that minimizes the probability of misclassifying the individuals into their respective groups. It projects the dimension into one direction, useful for data classification. The ultimate goal is to find the projection to a line such that the samples from different class are well separated. SVM is a classification method that uses kernel functions to map the original features into high-dimensional feature space for constructing an optimal hyperplane to separate binary classes. A linear kernel was used for the SVM classifier; $k(x_i,x_j) = x_i^T x_j$, where x_i and x_j are the feature vectors of ith and j^{th} classes, respectively, and T denotes transpose. The leave-one-out-cross validation (LOOCV) method was used to test and train the classifiers. Out of total ''n''

Figure 6. EMG and accelerometer data across different events in a gait cycle

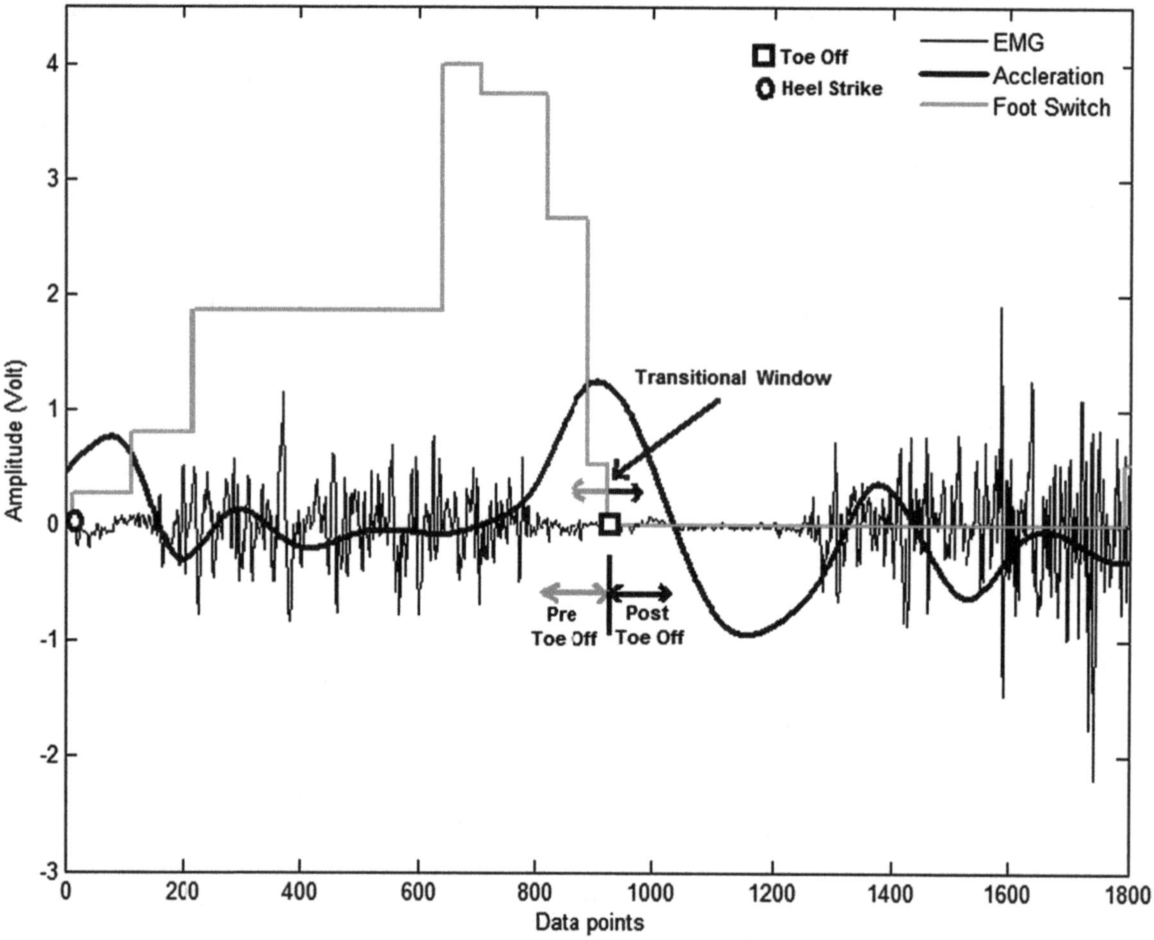

Table 2. Set of features for EMG and accelerometer

EMG (7 Channels)	Accelerometer (6 Channels)
Mean Absolute Value (MAV)	Mean
Number of Zero Crossing (ZC)	Variance
Waveform Length (WL)	Mean Trend
Number of Slope Sign Change (SSC)	Windowed Mean Difference (WMD)
Root Means Square (RMS) value	Variance Trend
Third-order Auto regressive (AR) coefficient	Windowed Variance Difference (WVD)
---	Maximum Difference Acceleration (MDA)
Feature Space = 7 Channels X 8(5+3AR coefficient) features = 56 Dimension	Feature Space = 6 Channels X 7 features = 42 Dimension

trials from all subjects, one trial was used for testing and n-1 trials were used for training the classifier. This procedure was iterated until all the trials had been included in training and testing. Classification accuracy (CA) was then calculated as a percentage; (number of correctly classified trials/total number of trials)*100. Comparison of classification accuracy between terrain and direction type was evaluated statistically, using a paired two-tailed *t* test. For the grouped classification (Terrain vs. Direction), overall the accelerometer performed better than the EMG in the transition gait cycle. However, the performance of both sensors was complementary to each other. In the time windows where accelerometer failed to perform well the EMG could classify the transitions with respectable accuracy. Overall, both the sensors tended toward higher accuracy for terrain type than direction type. Among the three windows the transitional window showed superior performance than the pre-toe off and post-toe off windows. A detailed analysis of the performance of both sensors in different windows of gait cycle can be found in (Deepak Joshi et. al. 2015). In this study, the toe off event during the transitional gait cycle was considered as the gold standard for separation of locomotion modes. It appears to be a good approximation for small distances, where toe off occurs close to the physical transition interface. However, if toe off occurs at a greater distance, this approximation would likely need to be modified. For a short distance, it can be fairly assumed that immediately after toe off the coming locomotion mode is engaged. However, in circumstances where the distance is greater, even after toe off a major part of the gait cycle can still be considered to be within the previous locomotion mode and may violate the assumption. The potential effect of greater distances in transition should be addressed in future studies.

DISCUSSION AND CONCLUSION

The signal processing methods like spectrogram and wavelet have been presented with application to locomotion and transition classification. Frequency domain representation, spectrogram, proved to be successful in classifying the locomotion and the transition. However, it has to be yet tested for an extended number of locomotion and classification. In that case it is advised to explore a greater number of relevant features from the frequency domain representation other than the spectrogram energy only. Accelerometer and EMG data both show reasonable accuracy and complimentary information in a gait cycle. This confirms the result of a recent study (A J Young et. al. 2014) which reported that combining accelerometers and EMG data gives better classification accuracy than using either of them alone while classifying the locomotion, walk, stairs, and ramp from the data of transfemoral amputees. However, the analytical combination was not tested on locomotion transitions.

The wavelet decomposition of just one set of accelerometer data on the foot was able to achieve superior accuracy in toe off identification compared to other algorithms utilizing a machine learning approach. This study allowed us to observe that the combination of signal processing and a heuristic approach is better than a heuristic approach alone at identifying toe off using accelerometry data. This may be due to the fact that heuristic approaches are generally subjective, while signal processing approaches are data driven and hence more adaptive to signal source. The 'gold standard' for toe off detection in this study relied on foot switch data, which itself has some inherent error, due to variations in the size and shape of subjects' feet. This can lead to large variation in estimation error across subjects. It may be necessary to determine any biasing or offset between the estimations derived from foot switch and GRF plates. This offset could be further added or subtracted from the estimation of the proposed algorithm to test it against the GRF true estimation.

It was observed that throughout the transitional gait cycle the high classification performances of EMG and accelerometry were complementary to each other. This difference in window-dependent performance can be explained by the fact that EMG appears prior to the corresponding motion while acceleration is actuated during the motion, demonstrating the well-known electromechanical delay observed in skeletal muscle activation. Seemingly, an optimal combination of both sensor types across the transitional gait cycle can strengthen the revelation of transition patterns. It appears that transitions are better classified as terrain than direction type. A terrain focused approach may thus be ideal for an efficient classification structure. Our findings demonstrate that EMG and accelerometry data sources complement each other across transitional gait cycles. This presents the opportunity for an optimal sensor fusion for robust classification in application. Overall, the findings of this study suggest that a terrain and direction focused classification approach will be useful for inclusion in classification approaches utilized in lower limb amputee samples and possibly in future efforts to enable smooth locomotion transitions using powered prostheses and assistive devices.

LIMITATIONS AND FUTURE DIRECTIONS

Able bodied participants were selected for the studies described in this chapter. With amputation the movement pattern and hence EMG and accelerometer will change as well. In future, it will be crucial to see how these sensors and the classification schemes perform with amputee data. With the complementary nature of both sensors across the gait cycle, it will be worthwhile to explore the fusion of both sensors in order to develop an optimal classification strategy. To recognize the intent of type of transition (direction/terrain) it may be important to include the visual cue as a precursor for the classification. Such a preparatory cue for obstacles and locomotion has been reported previously (R. M. Wilkie et al. 2010; R. M. Wilkie et. al. 2008), however there is a need to effectively integrate such cues into a seamless real-time classification strategy.

ACKNOWLEDGMENT

The studies described in this chapter were carried out under financial support from the U.S. Department of Defense; grant W81XWH-09-2-0144. The authors are grateful to Bryson Nakamura, Eileen Deming, and Daniel Jones for their help in data collection and post processing.

REFERENCES

Aaron, J. Y., Kuiken, T. A., & Hargrove, L. J. (2014). Analysis of using EMG and mechanical sensors to enhance intent recognition in powered lower limb prosthesis. *Journal of Neural Engineering*, *11*, 1–12.

Allen, F. R., Ambikairajah, E., Lovell, N. H., & Celler, B. G. (2006). Classification of a known sequence of motions and postures from accelerometry data using adapted Gaussian mixture models. *Physiological Measurement*, *27*(10), 935–951. doi:10.1088/0967-3334/27/10/001 PMID:16951454

Au, S., Berniker, M., & Herr, H. (2008). Powered ankle-foot prosthesis to assist level-ground and stair-descent gaits. *Neural Networks*, *21*(4), 654–666. doi:10.1016/j.neunet.2008.03.006 PMID:18499394

Aung, M. S., Thies, S. B., Kenney, L. P., Howard, D., Selles, R. W., Findlow, A. H., & Goulermas, J. Y. (2013). Automated detection of instantaneous gait events using time frequency analysis and manifold embedding. *IEEE Transactions on Neural Systems and Rehabilitation Engineering*, *21*(6), 908–916. doi:10.1109/TNSRE.2013.2239313 PMID:23322764

Chang, Y. H., Huang, H. W., Hamerski, C. M., & Kram, R. (2000). The independent effects of gravity and inertia on running mechanics. *The Journal of Experimental Biology*, *203*, 229–238. PMID:10607533

Chowdhury, R. H., Reaz, M. B., Ali, M. A., Bakar, A. A., Chellappan, K., & Chang, T. G. (2013). Surface electromyography signal processing and classification techniques. *Sensors (Basel, Switzerland)*, *13*(9), 12431–12466. doi:10.3390/s130912431 PMID:24048337

Cooper, G. R., & Mc Gillem, C. D. (1999). Probabilistic methods of signal and system analysis (3rd ed.). New York: Oxford University Press.

Culhane, K. M., Lyons, G. M., Hilton, D., Grace, P. A., & Lyons, D. (2004). Long-term mobility monitoring of older adults using accelerometers in a clinical environment. *Clinical Rehabilitation*, *18*(3), 335–343. doi:10.1191/0269215504cr734oa PMID:15137565

De Witt, J. K. (2010). Determination of toe-off event time during treadmill locomotion using kinematic data. *Journal of Biomechanics*, *43*(15), 3067–3069. doi:10.1016/j.jbiomech.2010.07.009 PMID:20801452

Dillingham, T. R., Pezzin, L. E., & MacKenzie, E. J. (2002). Limb amputation and limb deficiency: Epidemiology and recent trends in the United States. *Southern Medical Journal*, *95*, 875–883. PMID:12190225

Doukas, C., & Maglogiannis, I. (2008). *Advanced patient or elder fall detection based on movement and sound data*. Tampere, Finland: IEEE Pervasive Health Conference and Workshops. doi:10.1109/PCTHEALTH.2008.4571042

Drost, G., Stegeman, D. F., van Engelen, B. G. M., & Zwarts, M. J. (2006). Clinical applications of high-density surface EMG: A systematic review. *Journal of Electromyography and Kinesiology*, *16*(6), 586–602. doi:10.1016/j.jelekin.2006.09.005 PMID:17085302

Ermes, M., Parkka, J., Mantyjarvi, J., & Korhonen, I. (2008). Detection of daily activities and sports with wearable sensors in controlled and uncontrolled conditions. *IEEE Transactions on Information Technology in Biomedicine*, *12*(1), 20–26. doi:10.1109/TITB.2007.899496 PMID:18270033

Fernandes, F. C. A., Spaendonck, R. L. V., & Burrus, C. S. (2001). A directional, shift-insensitive, low-redundancy, wavelet transform. In *IEEE Proceedings international conference on image processing*. doi:10.1109/ICIP.2001.959121

Goen & Tiwari, D. C. (2013). Review of Surface Electromyogram Signals: Its Analysis and Applications. *International Journal of Electrical, Computer, Energetic. Electronic and Communication Engineering.*, *7*(11), 11–19.

Graupe, D., Salahi, J., & Kohn, K. H. (1982). Multifunctional prosthesis andorthosis control via microcomputer identification of temporal pattern differences in single-site myo-electric signals. *Journal of Biomedical Engineering*, *4*(1), 17–22. doi:10.1016/0141-5425(82)90021-8 PMID:7078136

Graupe, D., Salahi, J., & Zhang, D. S. (1985). Stochastic analysis of myoelectric temporal signatures for multifunctional single-site activation of prostheses and orthoses. *Journal of Biomedical Engineering*, *7*(1), 18–29. doi:10.1016/0141-5425(85)90004-4 PMID:3982004

Hannaford, B., & Lehman, S. (1986). Short time Fourier analysis of the electromyogram: Fast movements and constant contraction. *IEEE Transactions on Bio-Medical Engineering*, *33*(12), 1173–1181. doi:10.1109/TBME.1986.325697 PMID:3817851

Hreljac, A., & Marshall, R. N. (2000). Algorithms to determine event timing during normal walking using kinematic data. *Journal of Biomechanics*, *33*(6), 783–786. doi:10.1016/S0021-9290(00)00014-2 PMID:10808002

Huang, H., Kuiken, T. A., & Lipschutz, R. D. (2009). A strategy for identifying locomotion mode using surface electromyography. *IEEE Transactions on Bio-Medical Engineering*, *56*(1), 65–73. doi:10.1109/TBME.2008.2003293 PMID:19224720

Huang, H., Zhang, F., Hargrove, L. J., Dou, Z., Rogers, D. R., & Englehart, K. B. (2011). Continuous locomotion-mode identification for prosthetic legs based on neuromuscular-mechanical fusion. *IEEE Transactions on Bio-Medical Engineering*, *58*(10), 2867–2875. doi:10.1109/TBME.2011.2161671 PMID:21768042

Huang, Y., Englehart, K. B., Hudgins, B., & Chan, A. D. (2005). A Gaussian mixture model based classification scheme for myoelectric control of powered upper limb prostheses. *IEEE Transactions on Bio-Medical Engineering*, *52*(11), 1801–1811. doi:10.1109/TBME.2005.856295 PMID:16285383

Jasiewicz, J. M., Allum, J. H., Middleton, J. W., Barriskill, A., Condie, P., Purcell, B., & Li, R. C. T. (2006). Gait event detection using linear accelerometers or angular velocity transducers in able-bodied and spinal-cord injured individuals. *Gait & Posture*, *24*(4), 502–509. doi:10.1016/j.gaitpost.2005.12.017 PMID:16500102

Joshi, Nakamura, & Hahn. (2014). A novel approach for toe off estimation during locomotion and transitions on ramps and level ground. *IEEE Journal of Biomedical and health informatics*. DOI: 10.1109/JBHI.2014.2377749

Joshi, Nakamura, & Hahn. (2015). High energy spectrogram with integrated prior knowledge for EMG-based locomotion classification. *Journal of Medical Engineering and Physics*. DOI: 10.1016/j.medengphy.2015.03.001

Joshi & Hahn. (2015). Terrain and Direction Classification of Locomotion Transitions Using Neuromuscular and Mechanical Input. *Annals of Biomedical Engineering*. doi:10.1007/s10439-015-1407-3

Kobetic, R., To, C., Schnellenberger, J., Audu, M., Bules, T., & Gaudio, R. (2009). Development of hybrid orthosis for standing, walking, and stair climbing after spinal cord injury. *Journal of Rehabilitation Research and Development*, *46*(3), 447–462. doi:10.1682/JRRD.2008.07.0087 PMID:19675995

Maurer, U., Rowe, A., Smailagic, A., & Siewiorek, D. (2006). Location and activity recognition using eWatch: a wearable sensor platform. Lecture Notes in Computer Science, 3864, 86–102.

Miller, J. D., Beazer, M. S., & Hahn, M. E. (2013). Myoelectric walking mode classification for transtibial amputees. *IEEE Transactions on Bio-Medical Engineering*, *60*(10), 2745–2750. doi:10.1109/TBME.2013.2264466 PMID:23708765

Parkka, J., Ermes, M., Korpipaa, P., Mantyjarvi, J., Peltola, J., & Korhonen, I. (2006). Activity classification using realistic data from wearable sensors. *IEEE Transactions on Information Technology in Biomedicine*, *10*(1), 119–128. doi:10.1109/TITB.2005.856863 PMID:16445257

Pober, D. M., Staudenmayer, J., Raphael, C., & Freedson, P. S. (2006). Development of novel techniques to classify physical activity mode using accelerometers. *Medicine and Science in Sports and Exercise*, *38*(9), 1626–1634. doi:10.1249/01.mss.0000227542.43669.45 PMID:16960524

Sabatini, A. M., Martelloni, C., Scapellato, S., & Cavallo, F. (2005). Assessment of walking features from foot inertial sensing. *IEEE Transactions on Bio-Medical Engineering*, *52*(3), 486–494. doi:10.1109/TBME.2004.840727 PMID:15759579

Salarian, A., Russmann, H., Vingerhoets, F. J. G., Burkhard, P. R., & Aminian, K. (2007). Ambulatory monitoring of physical activities in patients with Parkinson's disease. *IEEE Transactions on Bio-Medical Engineering*, *54*(12), 2296–2299. doi:10.1109/TBME.2007.896591 PMID:18075046

Stephen, P. (2009). Activity identification using body-mounted sensors-a review of classification techniques. *Journal of Physiological Measurement*, *30*(4), R1–R33. doi:10.1088/0967-3334/30/4/R01 PMID:19342767

Sup, F., Bohara, A., & Goldfrab, M. (2008). Design and control of a powered transfemoral prosthesis. *The International Journal of Robotics Research*, *27*(2), 263–273. doi:10.1177/0278364907084588 PMID:19898683

Tucker, M. R., Olivier, J., Pagel, A., Bleuler, H., Bouri, M., Lambercy, O., & Gassert, R. et al. (2015). Control strategies for active lower extremity prosthetics and orthotics: A review. *Journal of Neuroengineering and Rehabilitation*, *12*(1), 1–29. doi:10.1186/1743-0003-12-1 PMID:25557982

Valens, C.A., & Valens C. (1999). *Really friendly guide to wavelets*. Academic Press.

Wilkie, R. M., Kountouriotis, G. K., Merat, N., & Wann, J. P. (2010). Using vision to control locomotion: Looking where you want to go. *Experimental Brain Research*, *204*(4), 539–547. doi:10.1007/s00221-010-2321-4 PMID:20556368

Wilkie, R. M., Wann, J. P., & Robert, S. (2008). Active Gaze, Visual Look-Ahead and locomotor control. *Journal of Experimental Psychology. Human Perception and Performance*, *34*(5), 1150–1164. doi:10.1037/0096-1523.34.5.1150 PMID:18823202

Wu, W. H., Bui, A. A., Batalin, M. A., Liu, D., & Kaiser, W. J. (2007). Incremental diagnosis method for intelligent wearablesensor systems. *IEEE Transactions on Information Technology in Biomedicine*, *11*(5), 553–562. doi:10.1109/TITB.2007.897579 PMID:17912972

Zhang, X., Liu, Y., Zhang, F., Ren, J., Sun, Y. L., & Yang, Q. (2012). On design and implementation of neural-machine interface for artificial legs. *IEEE Trans IndInf*, *8*(2), 418–429.

Chapter 10
Single Electronics for Biomedical Applications

Deep Kamal Kaur Randhawa
Guru Nanak Dev University, India

ABSTRACT

The nanoelectronic circuits based on single electronics would revolutionise the new generation electronic bio-medical gadgets. The high speed nanoelectronic devices would make these gadgets faster and more accurate. The nanoelectronic integrated circuits would be a boon for power saving along with advanced portability. As the scaling down of silicon based integrated circuits is limited in nanometer regime alternative materials like organic molecules, polymers, carbon nanotubes and graphene are focal point of research. These materials exhibit various electrical, electronic and mechanical properties, flexibility being one of very significant ones. Flexible nanelectronic integrated circuits would make biomedical applications very patient friendly. The in-vivo examination and diagnosis would be less injurious to the body. Also the flexible nature will increase the maneuverability of the device by the operator. It will improve the targeted diagnosis and targeted drug delivery procedures. This would further facilitate system-on- chip (soc) that will integrate multiple biomedical signal acquisition (ECG, EEG, EP, and respiration-related signals) with on-chip digital signal processing.

INTRODUCTION

Present day medical and healthcare technology is largely supported by electronic circuits. The performance and efficiency of medical diagnostic, computational and procedural machines are dependent upon the performance of integrated circuits. Development of integrated circuits has been instrumental in the development and improvisation of bio-medical equipment. The present generation has observed enormous development in the field of science and technology. Most of the manually handled bio-medical instruments have been replaced by automatic electronic gadgets that are fast, accurate and portable. The semiconductor industry drives the massive software and hardware development sector, with its successive development in speed and miniaturisation.

The rate of advancement of electronics has followed a roadmap commonly referred to as "Moore's Law". The prophecy was formally presented in 1965 by Gordon Moore, Director of Fairchild Semiconductor's Research and Development Laboratories, in the 35th anniversary issue of *Electronics* magazine

DOI: 10.4018/978-1-5225-0660-7.ch010

(Moore, 1965). He forecasted that transistor density on a computer microchip will double, and costs will halve, each twelve months, and this has been (roughly) borne out by empirical observation to the present time. In the 1990s, the Moore's Law was also understood to imply that computing power at fixed cost would continue to double every 18 months. This exponential growth of component density on a chip has now placed current silicon-chip development "bang-up" against the fundamental physical limits of conventional microelectronics. Moore recently admitted that Moore's Law, in its current form, with CMOS silicon, will "run out of gas" in 2017(Jurveston, 2004). Speculation on the continued application of Moore's Law therefore leans towards essential departures from silicon technology to such newer technologies as molecular electronics, quantum computing, spin devices, bio-computing, DNA computers, and other theoretically possible information processing mechanisms (Tuomi, 2002). The electronic devices fabricated using newer technologies supported by quantum computational techniques would provide a fresh lease of life to Moore's law.

The wish to sustain Moore's law is pushing electronics into the realm of nano-scale dimensions. The science and mechanisms of materials and devices at nanometer scale are studied under the umbrella of nanotechnology. It is a technology with an intention of developing tools, machines, and devices of nanometer range, based on scientific principles, governing at this scale. Paradigms for nanotechnology can be schematized in two classes: (i) the "top-down" approach based on obtaining the desired tiny products by sculpting from bulky precursors; (ii) the "bottom-up" approach that is based on the opposite path, i.e. on assembling the nano-products by using nano-sized bricks. Nature provides scientists with such elementary nano-sized building blocks: atoms and molecules. The fascinating spontaneous procedure and covalent interactions supplemented by the property of *self- recognition* and *self-assembly* help in structuring of various kinds of nanomachines that drive the natural mechanisms. Driven by the observation of these imperative principles that nature uses to operate its machines, scientists are planning research towards the fabrication of artificial nanodevices based on the same rules. There is also a huge interest and effort to construct other kinds of nanodevices on the basis of the same rules of supramolecular chemistry, by employing elementary building blocks that are able to recognize each other and form complex arrangements, adapting their structure to the environment and to the partners. In particular, self-assembling nanodevices that express an electrical functionality are pursued in view of the development of molecular electronics (Braun *et al.,* 1998, Keren *et al.,* 2002, Keren *et al.,* 2003).

Granted, they are not yet at the stage where these molecular devices are ready for production and can be incorporated into circuits. In fact, some may never directly see the actual light of commercialisation. They are enabling technologies — technologies on which commercialised versions will be developed. But the need is defined, the trend is clear, and the maturing process of refining and advancing these designs is moving forward. (Smith, 2007)

These continuous reducing sizes have pushed electronics into the domain of mesoscopic physics. Mesoscopic physics is the study of artificially constructed systems which exhibit quantum behavior. Often the systems fabricated in this way are called artificial atoms because the devices that are produced behave in many ways like atoms. Single-electron effects will play an important role in almost any electronic device with dimensions below 30 nm. These effects will form the basis for study of the nanoelectronic devices. The realization and conceptual understanding of the single electron effects and it prominence in electronic devices scaled in nanometer regime has evolved a new exciting field known as Single Electronics.

The nanoelectronic circuits based on single electronics would revolutionise the new generation electronic gadgets. These would be highly beneficial in the bio-medical sciences. The high speed nanoelectronic devices would be faster, more sensitive and accurate. This would further facilitate System-on- Chip (SoC) that will integrate multiple biomedical signal acquisition (ECG, EEG, EP, and respiration-related signals) with on-chip digital signal processing. The embedded flexibility of the SoC facilitates its use in a multitude of applications.

In the present scenario electronic gadgets are essentially most important tools in medical diagnostics and treatment procedures. Biomedical engineers have to develop and use computer tools to collect and analyze data related to medicine and biology. The performance of the modern medical infrastructure is highly sensitive and efficient. This has been possible due to smaller and smaller electronic devices. The nanoelectronic biomedical gadgets will further enhance the portability. Also as these circuits have faster response and shorter time delays, this would mean more sensitive and prompt responses. The small sizes and flexibility would further assist in the development of nanorobots that may in future perform surgery inside the body, and fabrication of tiny devices that could be implanted inside the body for drug delivery and monitoring of various physical parameters. Also use of molecules and biomaterials in nanoelectronics would help in engineering devices or implants that can interact with living tissue. These new devices will have a dramatic impact in the healthcare of people's lives.

The nanoelectronic integrated circuits would be a boon for power saving along with advanced portability. As the scaling down of silicon based integrated circuits is limited in nanometer regime alternative materials like organic molecules, polymers, carbon nanotubes and graphene are focal point of research. These materials exhibit various electrical, electronic and mechanical properties, flexibility being one of very significant ones. Flexible nanelectronic integrated circuits would make biomedical applications very patient friendly. The in-vivo examination and diagnosis would be less injurious to the body. Also the flexible nature will increase the maneuverability of the device by the operator. It will improve the targeted diagnosis and targeted drug delivery procedures.

NANOELECTRONICS

The past half century of microelectronics has been marked by repetitive radical rhetoric promising electronic miniaturization. Nanotechnology was preceded by neologisms such as 'atomic electronics' and 'angstronics' (Gartner and Wolfgang, 1959). Many institutional conditions elicited visions of futuristic panoramas describing newer technologies that would overcome the boundaries imposed by the present technology.

A revolution of kind was witnessed in the middle of 20th century when the transistor was invented. The transistors helped in making the electronic gadgets portable. The state-of-the-art electronic building blocks– vacuum tubes, crystal diodes, and mercury switches – were replaced by transistors. Harold A. Zahl, research director of the Army Signal Corps Engineering Laboratories, noted that the transistor was an 'apparent promise ... to relieve the GI of one of his biggest headaches – carrying weight, with a smaller radio he could carry more food and bullets' (Zahl, 1968). The transistor, it seemed to Zahl, was a perfect solution to many of the engineering problems. As transistors gained widespread use in the mid-1950s, their advantages became sources of serious obstacles. The smaller component size and superior heat characteristics made possible the realization of complex circuitry that previously existed only in the minds of circuit engineers. Everything went on well till the equipment began to fail much more frequently than the tube-based devices. This was due to weak interlinks among the components. The more the number of components…the more the number of connections…and larger are the chances of failure. The US military was among the first groups subjected to the 'tyranny of numbers'. This paved way for printed circuits and automatic assembly techniques for electronic equipment. Eventually, the circuits were assembled on a silicon chip called integrated circuit. Succumbing to the ever-increasing demand of smaller and faster electronic devices, there has been a continuous miniaturization of devices leading to increasing component densities.

In the context of the difficulties regarding the miniaturization of the electronic devices, Arthur von Hippel, a German physicist formulated the basis of bottom-up approach that he referred to as molecular engineering. He suggested fabrication of novel materials by manipulating atoms and molecules for use in molecular engineering applications. The introduction of the concept of molecular engineering by Hippel led to the idea of molecular electronics. The collaboration between Westinghouse Company and the US Air Force at the end of 1950's resulted in the beginning of a program to implement Hippel's ideas. The Air Force organized a conference on "Molecular Electronics" and this was probably the first time term 'Molecular Electronics' was used though it had little to do with the vision of using individual molecules as electronic elements.

Von Hippel's vision was to design the desired material characteristics from the bottom-up. He argued:

Instead of taking prefabricated materials and trying to devise engineering applications consistent with their macroscopic properties, one builds materials from their atoms and molecules for the purpose at hand…He can play chess with elementary particles according to prescribed rules until new engineering solutions become apparent. (Hippel and Arthur, 1956)

In 1958, the US Air Force and Westinghouse adopted the term 'Molecular Electronics' to describe their fundamental joint research program, which aimed to leapfrog beyond both the conventional approach to circuit integration proposed by RCA and the US Army Signal Corps and the growing efforts to build monolithic integrated circuits at Fairchild Semiconductor and Texas Instruments. This program failed and the term 'Molecular Electronics' lost its spark by mid-sixties. The term again surfaced in 1970s thanks to a small group of chemists led by Forrest L. Carter at the Naval Research Laboratory (NRL) but with a disjunctive change. 'Presumptive anomaly' is the term that historian of technology Edward Constant, coined to explain this kind of disjunctive leap in the technological trajectory, even when existing technology shows satisfactory performance. As opposed to functional anomaly, presumptive anomaly occurs, in Constant's words, when scientists or engineers begin to *perceive* that 'under some future conditions the conventional system will fail (or function badly) or that a radically different paradigm will do a much better job' (Constant, 1973)

Molecular electronics, as we understand today, was conceptualized in late 1960's and early 1970's. Experimental investigations regarding the charge transport through the molecules started during that period. In the early 1970s, one piece of this effort was Bruce Scott's group at IBM's Yorktown Heights lab that was trying to develop new lithographic resists used in patterning of silicon. Resists are lacquer-like organic chemicals that, like photographic film, change their chemical character when exposed to light, x-rays, electron beams or other lithographic beam when they are exposed to the image of a pattern of transistors, an acid can then etch away the areas that have been exposed to the beam, leaving behind a solid negative of the transistor pattern. Further, etches can then be used to transfer that pattern directly into the silicon. The idea of molecular electronics was actively pursued by Ari Aviram. He worked on the theory of electron transfer through single organic molecules in association with Mark Ratner. When a voltage is placed across the diode such that electrons run from the electron-rich region to the electron-poor one, a substantial current is created, when the voltage is reversed, electrons pass poorly through the electron-poor region and little current is created. The theoretical issue now was whether a single organic molecule could be designed that would have a similar current-versus-voltage graph to that of a semiconductor diode. In 1974, they published the famous paper on "Molecular Rectifiers" (Aviram and Ratner, 1974) proposing that modified molecules can be used as traditional diodes. This was probably the first proposal for molecular electronic device and still forms the core of molecular electron devices. This research did spark considerable discussion within IBM. For Ratner, Scott, and Aviram's other colleagues, the paper was a theoretical curiosity which could not be tested experimentally, much less scaled up to a product. Aviram's captivating visualization had its moment at IBM, when it was taken seriously by Scott, Philip Seiden (director of Physical Sciences at IBM) and the Yorktown semiconductor establishment, some of whom (for example Sokrates Pantelides) eventually defected from semiconductors to molecular electronics in the late 1990s. It even found its way into the mainstream media (*Time,*1974). The 'Molecular Rectifiers'- paper that is considered as the founding statement of modern molecular electronics, virtually sank without a trace until Aviram returned to the topic in 1988. Yet in that time, largely independent of Aviram and Ratner, a molecular electronics community – dispersed across regions and organizations and disciplines – came into being for the first time.

Other scientists also started working on the concept of molecular electronics. Forrest Carter, a chemist was influenced by the famous lecture "Room at the bottom" by Richard Feynman. This was much before other nanotechnologists could really appreciate the flavor of Feynman's speech. Aviram and Ratner's 1974 paper was important in spurring Carter as he was one of the few to cite it before 1988, and he included both men in his early community-building. Carter's program developed in parallel and was initially much more successful than Aviram's. He introduced concepts of molecular computing and cellular automata, by using single molecules as electronic components or to store bits of information. Carter was able to ignite interest in the field of molecular electronics by organizing various conferences. The major names in the field like Metzger and Mark Reed participated in these events.

Ari Aviram had re-entered the field, publishing new work on the theory and design of molecular logic (Aviram, 1988) and putting together a team to study the electrical characteristics of single molecules with a scanning tunneling microscope (Aviram *et al.*, 1988). Several experimental technologies initially peripheral to molecular electronics (especially the scanning tunneling microscope(STM)) had, by the late 1980s, matured to where they could make certain aspects of molecular electronics realizable. Mark Ratner, for one, imputes his re-entring to the field to his realization that STM offered access to molecules that was unthinkable in 1974.

In the late eighties and early nineties, atomic-sized contacts were obtained and this was highly beneficial for the nanoscience community. These could be used to provide contacts with individual molecules, which was not possible using the lithographic techniques. In 1997, Mark Reed and James Tour reported first transport experiment in single molecules junctions. More experimentation was carried out in nineties and it was observed that molecules can indeed mimic the behavior of electronic devices. Reed's group showed that junctions based certain organic molecules can exhibit rectifying behavior or a typical negative differential resistance. Single molecules were also shown to act as single electron transistors and they exhibited the phenomenon of Coulomb blockade (Reed *et al.* 1997). The various reports and publications indicate that molecular electronics is here to stay and will lead to new and unexpected applications.

SINGLE ELECTRONICS

Single electronics is the technique based on controlling motion of even a single electron. Millikan displayed the manipulation of single electrons in the start of 20th century. Control of singular electron is possible if a very small conducting particle is placed accurately between external terminals. As this was not feasible till late 1980's to have such an arrangement so single electronics could not be implemented in solid-state circuits. But with the present state of art techniques it is possible to obtain these arrangements. Single-electronics is a promising new technology as single-electron devices retain their scalability even on an atomic scale and, moreover, they can control the motion of even a single electron. Therefore, if the single-electron devices are used as ultra large scale integrated circuits (ULSI) elements, the ULSI will have the features of extremely high integration and extremely low power consumption. Scalability in reference to electron devices and circuits means that the performance of electronic devices increases with a decrease of the device dimensions. Power consumption is roughly proportional to the electron number transferred from voltage source to the ground in logic operations. Therefore, the utilization of single-electron devices in integrated circuits is expected to reduce the power consumption of the integrated circuits.

The concept of single electronics is based on the single electron charging and discharging of a conductor called an island. The magnitude of charge of an electron (e=1.6 X 10^{-19} Coulomb) is very small on human scale. But as the field E due to the charge is inversely proportionate to the size of island and it becomes appreciably strong for a nanoscaled island. Hence the theory of single-electron phenomena shows that a more adequate measure of the strength of single electron effects is not the electric field, but the *charging energy.* The charging energy is given by term $E_c = e^2/C$, where C is the capacitance of the island. When the island size becomes comparable with the de-Broglie wavelength of the electrons inside the island, their energy quantization becomes substantial (Kastner, 1993),(Meirav. and Foxman, 1995), (Kouwenhoven *et al.,* 1997), (Ingold and Nazarov,1992). The thermal fluctuations suppress the single electron effects unless charging energy is larger than the thermal energy at the operating temperature.

Single Electron Box

Single electron box is a quantum dot placed between two electrodes. One of the two electrodes is connected to the quantum dot through a tunneling junction while the other electrode is capacitively coupled to the quantum dot as shown in Figure 1.

The charge is transferred from the electrode to the quantum dot through the tunnel junction. The single electron box is based on the principle of conduction of electrons through the island, which is based

Figure 1. Single electron box

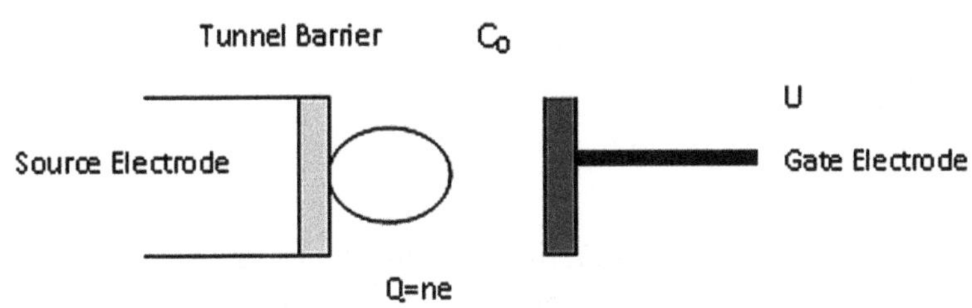

upon charging and discharging of the island by addition and removal of electrons. An electron can hop on to the island from the electrode if its energy level is greater than the single electron charging energy that is given by the relation $E_c = e^2/2C$; where C is the total capacitance of the island. Smaller the size of island, lesser the value of C and higher the value of charging energy. Also for very small sizes the charging energy is much larger than the thermal energy (k_BT). The charging effect that limits the flow of electrons is called coulomb blockade. The charging process can be assisted by application of gate voltage.

The free energy of the system is expressed by the relation:

$$W = \frac{Q^2}{2C_\Sigma} + \frac{C_0}{C_\Sigma} QU + constt \tag{1}$$

where

$Q = -ne$,
n = number of electrons,
e = electronic charge,
C_0 = Island-gate capacitance,
C_Σ = Total island capacitance including C_0,
U = Gate Voltage.

The expression given by Equation (1) is written as:

$$W = \frac{(ne - Q_e)^2}{2C_\Sigma} + constt \tag{2}$$

where $Q_e = UC_0$ is called the external charge.

It is observed from Equation (1) that island charge is discrete while Q_e is continuous in nature. It is also observed Q is a step-like function of Q_e. For a change of external charge ΔQ_e equivalent to 'e', the gate potential should change by an amount $\Delta U = e/C_0$. As 'U', the gate potential is increased, more and more electrons are attracted towards the island. The discreteness of electron transfer through the barriers makes this rise in charge profile resemble a staircase step-like. As the second electrode is not directly connected to the island, there is absence of flow of current through the single electron box. To facilitate flow of current through the device it is restructured by splitting the tunnel junction and applying dc voltage between two parts of external electrode. The restructured arrangement is called Single Electron Transistor.

The electrostatic energy of the system is given by:

$$W = \frac{(ne - Q_e)^2}{2C_\Sigma} - \frac{eV[n_1C_2 + n_2C_1]}{C_\Sigma} + constt \tag{3}$$

where n_1 & n_2 are number of electrons passing through tunnel barriers 1 and 2 and number of electrons on the island $n = n_1 - n_2$ and C_Σ is sum of C_g, C_1 and C_2 along with the stray capacitance of the island. As the size of the island is small the charging energy E_C has a large value. For small temperature $k_BT<<E_C$, so the tunneling rate is low. Cotunneling provides a weak current proportionate to $\frac{R_Q^2}{R_1R_2}$, where R_1 and R_2 are the tunnel barrier resistance. As long as $R_{1,2}> R_Q$ the current is very small at low voltages. For single electron device conceptualization the single island, double tunnel junction is referred to as source electrode-island-drain electrode assembly. The tunnel junctions have capacitances C1 and C2 and resistances R1 and R2 and the total island capacitance is C=C1+C2. Suppression of current for low voltages is called "Coulomb Blockade". At a certain threshold voltage V_t, the coulomb blockade is overcome and current flows through the device. The threshold voltage is a function of gate voltage. Application of appropriate gate voltage equivalent to injection of charge $Q_e = C_0$ U onto the island changes the balance of charges at tunnel barrier capacitance which determine the Coulomb Blockade threshold. Dependence of Threshold voltage V_t on Gate voltage U is piecewise linear and periodic in nature.

Application of voltage across source and drain creates a potential difference between the electrodes. The electrons cannot tunnel from electrode to island till the potential difference is larger than the charging energy. This is called formation of coulomb blockade that leads to zero current through the assembly. The zero current region in the current-voltage characteristics is called coulomb gap that exists for applied voltages $|V_{ds}|< |V_c|$, the coulomb blockade voltage. For values of V_{ds} larger than V_c, electrons are able to tunnel from high energy terminal to island and then onwards to the low energy terminal. This constitutes flow of current through the assembly with repetitive transfer of electron from terminal to island to terminal.

Given the fact that nanoparticles or molecules are much smaller than the mean free path of electrons in typical metals (~ few nanometers at room temperature), bulk resistivity (due to the interactions of electrons with lattice vibrations and impurities of the system) is not a valid concept. This implies that the resistance of a system in which a molecule or monolayer of molecules is attached to the electrodes, does not originate from the inelastic scattering of the electrons at the Fermi energy with the phonons of the molecule. Usually, the molecule is considered as a potential barrier through which electrons tunnel and, to first order, basic theory neglects inelastic scattering in the molecule altogether. Charging effects (Coulomb blockade regime) are taken into consideration depending on the strength of the coupling between the metal-molecule interfaces. The inelastic contributions to current are expected to play a minor role in the low bias regime in simple tunneling junctions.

Electron transport through single molecules placed between two metal electrodes is expected to be very different from transport in bulk structures. This is mainly due to the inherent small size of the molecules. For very small islands, the quantum splitting between electron energy levels may become larger than Ec and k_BT. The generalization of the orthodox theory to this case has been carried out by Averin and Korotkov (Averin and Korotkov,1990) who considered a situation where tunneling is possible between islands with discrete levels.

The electron transport studies in molecular-based structures are described in terms of Molecular Orbitals (MOs). Molecular orbitals are energy levels which are the outcome of electrostatic interaction of atomic orbitals of atoms constituting the molecule. The electrons with unique quantum numbers reside in these MOs. The highest energy level which has electrons is called the Highest Occupied Molecular Orbital (HOMO) and the lowest energy level of the empty MOs is called Lowest Unoccupied Molecular Orbital (LUMO). The Highest Occupied Molecular Orbital (HOMO) is the outermost filled orbital of the molecule. It can be similarised to the valence shell. Surrounding the molecules are probabilistic empty energy levels in which electrons can be added from outside or might jump from HOMO due to energy absorption. The empty orbital with lowest energy level (LUMO) is like the conduction shell. As the size of molecules is very small the charging energy for electrons is very large. Hence there is an appreciable energy difference between corresponding levels leading to discrete energy levels of the molecular orbitals. The gap between HOMO and LUMO called HOMO-LUMO Gap (HLG) of a molecule can be similarised to as the energy band gap (E_g) of bulk materials. The electrons will be able to pass through the molecule if they have energy equal to any of molecular orbital energy level provided that it is coupled to electron reservoirs. The metal contacts act as source and drain whose electrochemical potential determines the equilibrium energy level of the molecule which forms the basis of the flow of electrons.

Coulomb Blockade

In a molecule distribution of electrons in molecules is done one by one, it means the energy gap between energy levels represents charging energy. In neutral form the electrons with highest energy level reside in the outermost MO that is called HOMO. To add another electron the charging energy should be larger than the HOMO-LUMO gap. This means that the phenomenon of coulomb blockade can be explained in terms of energy levels. To study coulomb blockade we concentrate on the quantum dot regime where Energy gap between two levels is larger than the thermal energy (k_BT).

Energy levels come in pairs, one up-spin and one down-spin, which are degenerate (i.e. they have the same energy). Even the smallest device has two levels rather than one and its maximum conductance will be twice the conductance quantum $G_0 \equiv q^2/h$. The expressions for the number of electrons and the current should all be multiplied by two. To explain the concept we consider a channel with two spin-degenerate levels containing one electron when neutral ($N_0 = 1$). The broadened DOS given by,

$$D_\varepsilon(E) = 2 \text{ (for spin)} \times [\gamma/2\pi/ (E - \varepsilon)^2 + (\gamma/2)^2] \quad (4)$$

where the total broadening is the sum of those due to each of the two contacts individually: $\gamma = \gamma_1 + \gamma2$. Since the available states are only half filled for a neutral channel, the electrochemical potential will lie exactly in the middle of the broadened DOS, so that we would expect a lot of current to flow when a bias is applied to split the electrochemical potentials in the source and drain as shown in Figure 2.

Figure 2. A channel with two spin-degenerate levels containing one electron

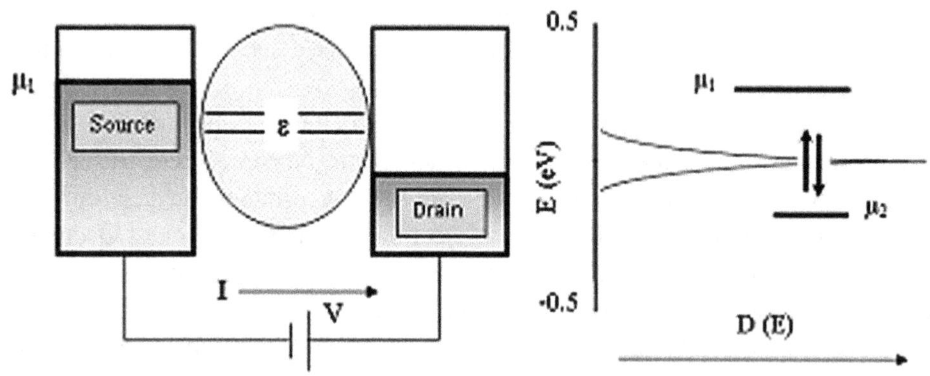

However, under certain conditions the DOS looks like one of the two possibilities shown in Figure 2. The up-spin and the down-spin density of states splits into two parts separated by the single-electron charging energy

$$U_0 \equiv q^2/C_E \tag{5}$$

It is seen that there are hardly any states between μ_1 and μ_2, so very little current flows when we apply a small bias. This is called "Coulomb blockade effect" and has been experimentally observed for systems where the charging energy U_0 exceeds the broadening γ. We need to worry about this effect only if U_0 exceeds both k_BT and $\gamma = \gamma_1 + \gamma_2$.

It is hard to understand why the two peaks should separate based on the simple SCF picture. Two peaks with the same energy ("degenerate") should always remain degenerate as long as they feel the same self-consistent potential U. The point is that no electron feels any potential due to itself. Suppose the up-spin level gets filled first, causing the down-spin level to float up by U_0. But the up-spin level does not float up because it does not feel any self-interaction, leading to the picture shown on the left in Figure 3. Of course, it is just as likely that the down-spin will fill up first leading to the picture on the right. In either case the DOS near μ is suppressed relative to the SCF picture. The magnitude of U_0 depends upon the extent of the electronic wave-function. If an electron is smeared over the surface of a sphere of radius R, the potential of the sphere will be $q/4\pi\varepsilon_r\varepsilon_0R$, so that the energy required to put another electron on the sphere will be $q^2/4\pi\varepsilon_r\varepsilon_0R \approx U_0$. The levels with well-delocalized wave-functions (i.e. large R) have a very small U_0 and the SCF method provides an acceptable description even at the lowest temperatures of interest. But if R is small, then the charging energy U_0 can exceed k_BT and one could be in a regime dominated by single-electron charging effects (Datta, 2005).

Figure 3. Under certain conditions, the up-spin and down-spin density of states splits into two parts separated by the single-electron charging energy, U_0, instead of one single degenerate peak.

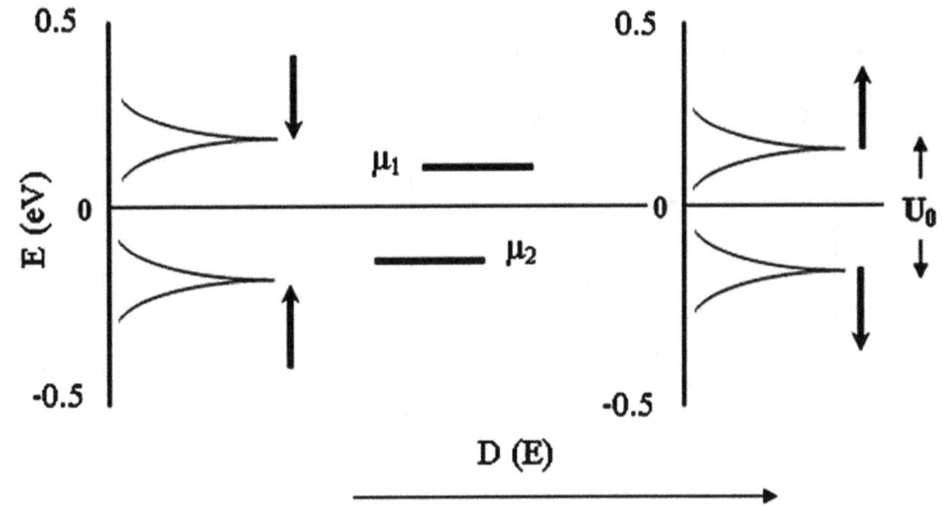

Tunneling

Quantum mechanical transport phenomenon due to wave character becomes relevant when the devices are scaled to nanometer range. Tunneling of electrons through the potential barriers is one of the most exciting quantum-chemical phenomenon. Tunneling is equally important in single electron effects as tunnel junctions are an integral part of single electronics. To understand the concept of tunneling we consider a potential energy barrier as shown in Figure 4. An electron is incident from the left side of the barrier which models a typical metal-insulator-metal junction or an electron bound to an atom or a molecule.

There will be two cases while studying this system when energy of the electron is lesser than the barrier ($E_p < V_0$) and when it is larger than the barrier ($E_p > V_0$). According to classical physics the electron would move past the barrier if $E > V_0$, i.e. the transmission coefficient in this case would be unity while its reflection coefficient would be zero. Opposite will be true for the condition $E < V_0$. It is observed that the classical limiting cases are for $E << V_0$ and $E >> V_0$. In general there is some non-zero probability that the electron will be transmitted through the barrier [Hanson (2008)]. If the electron is transmitted through the barrier in the case $E < V_0$, the electron is said to tunnel through the barrier.

APPLICATIONS

Development of newer techniques to detect biomolecules and cell functions is the dynamic driving force to the advance of biology and medicine. The biological procedures are interrelated by the dynamic actions of molecular machines that are often organized in nanoscale domains. Therefore, there is a dire need to develop biosensors that will offer high sensitivity to detect trace quantity of target molecules or microscopic biological signals, and high spatial and temporal resolution to resolve the delicate biological activities. The promising nanoelectronic biosensors provide amazing possibilities to achieve such targets that are unattainable by the conventional bioanalytical methods. Various materials can be employed for nanoelectronic biosensing, such as, silicon nanowires (SiNWs) (Chen, Li and Chen, 2011), single-walled carbon nanotubes (SWCNTs) (Allen, Kichambare and Star, 2007) and graphene and its derivatives (Liu, Dong and Chen, 2012). Nanoelectronic sensors provide a flexible platform for a large spectrum of bio-

Figure 4. Particle with energy E_p incident on potential barrier

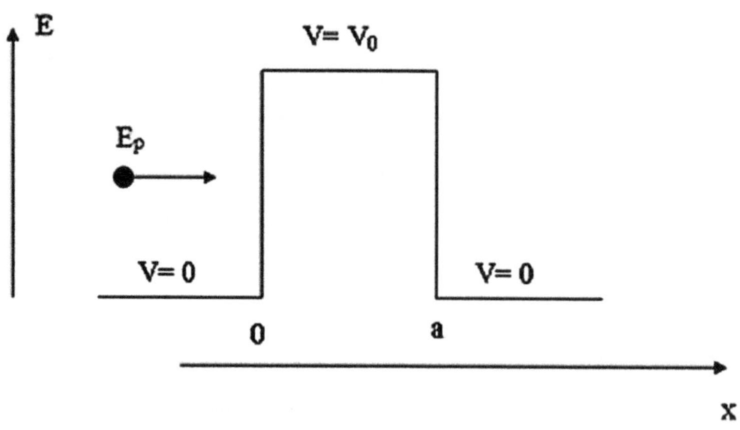

sensing targets and purposes virtue the availability of different sensing materials. This enables various sensing mechanisms and device configurations, and diverse chemistry for biofunctionalization. Depending upon the unique advantages and limitations of a material the choice of nanomaterial should be made based on balanced consideration on specific requirements such as performance, detection mechanisms to be utilized, ease of fabrication and recording, cost, and so on. Efforts are also being done to interface nanoelectronic devices with live cells for detection of dynamic cellular activities, such as, secretion of signaling molecules and generation of bioelectrical signals (Huang, Cai and Chen, 2011)

An array of nanowire transistors can be used for spatially resolved detection, stimulation or inhibition of nerve impulses (electrical spike or action potential produced by ion channel activities in a neuron) and their propagation along individual neurites (slender projection from the cell body of a neuron) (Patolsky et al, 2006). In contrast to the invasive intracellular recording by patch-clamp technique, this nanowire approach provides noninvasive extracellular measurement; as compared to the extracellular recording by metal microelectrode, the nanowire approach offers unraveled spatial resolution. The same group also made a nano-transistor device at the tip of a bent silicon nanowire, and used it, as a novel alternative to patch-clamp yet with minimum invasiveness, to intracellularly record action potentials (Tian et al, 2010). Nanoelectronic sensors can be used to probe at single cell or sub cellular level (even nano-domains). With an array of nanoelectronic sensors, signal distribution and propagation in cell networks could be resolved, e.g., in a brain slice or heart tissue. It is being predicted that nanoelectronics-cell interface would be instrumental or revolutionary to the study of cell functions as well as to the discovery of drugs targeting on these functions (Pui et al, 2010).

Bioinformatics involves developing and using computer tools to collect and analyze data related to medicine and biology. Work in bioinformatics could involve using sophisticated techniques to manage and search databases of gene sequences that contain many millions of entries. Nanoelectromechanical systems (NEMS) are the integration of mechanical elements, sensors, actuators, and electronics on a silicon chip. BioNEMS are the development and application of NEMS in medicine and biology. BioNEMS work include the development of nanorobots that may one day perform surgical procedures inside the living body, and also embed nanoelectronic devices inside the body for delivery of drugs as per the body's demand. As silicon will not be able to handle the shrinking of devices so other alternative materials including biomaterials are being studied for use in electronic devices in nanometer regime. Biomaterials are substances that are engineered for use in devices or implants that must interact with living tissue. The development of coatings that fight infection common in artificial joint implants, materials that can aid in controlled drug delivery, and "scaffolds" that support tissue and organ reconstruction are materials of interest. Newer devices with the latest technologies in term of materials and devices can make a dramatic difference in people's lives. Biomechanics is another aspect of biomedical field that can benefit from nanoelectronics. Biomechanics includes the study of motion, material deformation, and fluid flow. For example, studies of the fluid dynamics involved in blood circulation have contributed to the development of artificial hearts, while an understanding of joint mechanics has contributed to the design of prosthetic limbs. Biosignal Processing deals with extracting useful information from biological signals for diagnostics and therapeutics purposes. This could be studying cardiac signals to determine cardiac health of a patient, developing speech recognition systems that can cope with background noise, or detecting features of brain signals that can be used to control a computer. Radiology is a very important part of medical diagnostics. It refers to the use of radioactive substances such as X-rays, magnetic fields as in magnetic resonance imaging, and ultrasound to create images of the body, its organs and structures. These images are used in the diagnosis and treatment of disease, as well as to assist the doctors in image-guided surgery. X-rays, ultrasound, magnetic resonance imaging (MRI), and computerized tomography (CT) are prominent imaging methods that are used to let us observe the insides of the human body. Work in this area includes developing economical image acquisition systems, image processing algorithms, image/video compression algorithms and standards, and applying advances in multimedia computing systems in a biomedical context. Information Technology in biomedicine covers a varied range of applications and technologies, including the use of virtual reality in medical applications (e.g. diagnostic procedures), the relevance of wireless and mobile technologies in health care settings, artificial intelligence to support diagnostics, and addressing security issues related to making health care information available on the World Wide Web. Instrumentation, Sensors, and Measurement involves the hardware and software design of devices and systems used to measure biological signals. This ranges from developing sensing devices that can capture a biological signal of interest, to applying methods of amplifying and filtering the signal so that it can be further studied, to dealing with sources of interference that could corrupt a signal, to building a complete instrumentation system such as an x-ray machine or a heart monitoring system. whereas microtechology involves development and use of devices on the scale of a micrometer (one thousandth of a millimeter, or about 1/50 of the diameter of a human hair), nanotechnology involves devices on the order of a nanometer (about 1/50 000 of the diameter of a human hair, or ten times the diameter of a hydrogen atom). This field is dedicated to the development of microscopic force sensors that can identify changing tissue properties in a way to help surgeons remove the unhealthy section of the tissue, and nanometer length cantilever beams that bend with cardiac protein levels in ways that can help doctors in the early and rapid diagnosis of heart attacks. As the development of microelectronics in the 1980s has led development of new tools for biomedical instrumentation, the era of nanoelectronics, will in the same way permit further miniaturization towards integrated medical systems, providing proficient methodologies for pathological forecasting. As micro devices have brought a drastic improvement in surgery and medical treatments that have revolutionised clinical procedures in recent times. With the advent of biomolecular science and newer manufacturing techniques due to continuous reduction of devices from micro to nanoelectronics sophisticated applications are being developed for biomedical applications. Nanotechnology prototypes for molecular machines are focus of research in diverse ways, and some interesting devices for propulsion and sensing have been proposed. More complex molecular machines and nanorobots that are embedded with nanoscopic features represent a new class of tools for medical procedures. The revolutionary nanodevices will also assist in dealing with issues related to the replacement or restoration of lost sensory and motor abilities (for example, retinal implants to partially restore sight or electrical stimulation of paralyzed muscles to assist a person in standing). The analysis of the complexities of neural systems in nature, the development of neurorobots (robot arms that are controlled by signals from the motor cortex in the brain) and neuro-electronics (e.g. developing brain-implantable nano-electronics with high computing power) are futuristic proposals for biomedical applications that can be accomplished by lesser invasive nanoelectronic devices and gadgets. Many recently enhanced medical diagnostic techniques and therapeutic innovations have been a consequence of physiological systems modeling. The models of physiological processes (e.g. the control of limb movements, the biochemistry of metabolism) are developed to gain a better understanding of the function of living organisms. Designing augmentative and alternative communication systems for people who cannot communicate in traditional ways is an electronic boon for people with disabilities. Making computers more accessible for people with disabilities, developing new materials and designs for wheelchairs, and making them more interactive have been remarkable achievements. Robotics in surgery includes the use of robotic and image processing systems to interactively assist a medical team both in planning and executing a surgery. These newer nanoelectronics based techniques can minimize the side effects of surgery by providing smaller incisions, lesser trauma, and more precision, while also decreasing the costs. Telemedicine, sometimes refered to as "telehealth" or "e-health," involves the transfer of electronic medical data from one location to another for the evaluation, diagnosis, and treatment of patients in isolated locations. This usually involves the use of network of medical devices, advanced telecommunications technology, video-conferencing systems, and networked computing. Telemedicine has been a boon for remotely located populations in the various parts of the world.

CONCLUSION

The chapter has been focused on the significance of nanoelectronics in biomedical applications. The various avenues of biomedical applications are directly or indirectly dependent upon electronic circuitry. The better the electronics more is the reliability of the electronic applications. Reducing device sizes and higher component densities are making electronic circuits and computational systems more efficient. Revolutionary development has been made in interfacing nanoelectronics with biomolecules, cells, and tissues/organs. No doubt that the convergence of nanoelectronics and biological systems will exhibit profound impacts on fundamental biological studies, diagnosis, drug delivery techniques, and development of human-machine interface. Also the flexible nature of nanoelectronic circuits will help in comfortable in-vivo diagnostics and treatment. Currently nanoelectronic biomedical applications are a scientist's forte. To transform the scientific paradigm into practical and widely accessible techniques, incredible interdisciplinary efforts are required. There is need to understand the concepts of quantum physics, single electronics and nanoelectronic devices.

REFERENCES

Allen, B. L., Kichambare, P. D., & Star, A. (2007). Carbon nanotube field-effect-transistor-based biosensors. *Advanced Materials*, *19*(11), 1439–1451. doi:10.1002/adma.200602043

Averin, D. V., & Korotkov, A. N. (1990). Correlated single-electron tunneling via mesoscopic metal particles: Effects of energy quantization. *Journal of Low Temperature Physics*, *80*(3-4), 173–185. doi:10.1007/BF00683484

Aviram, A. (1988). Molecules for Memory, Logic and Amplification. *Journal of the American Chemical Society*, *110*(17), 5687–5692. doi:10.1021/ja00225a017

Aviram, A., Joachim, C., & Pomerantz, M. (1988). Evidence of Switching and Rectification by a Single Molecule Effected with a ScanningTunneling Microscope. *Chemical Physics Letters*, *146*(6), 490–495. doi:10.1016/0009-2614(88)87486-4

Aviram, A., & Ratner, M. A. (1974). Molecular rectifiers. *Chemical Physics Letters*, *29*(2), 277–283. doi:10.1016/0009-2614(74)85031-1

Braun, E., Eichen, Y., Sivan, U., & Ben-Yoseph, G. (1998). DNA-templated assembly and electrode attachment of a conducting silver wire. *Nature*, *391*(6669), 775–778. doi:10.1038/35826 PMID:9486645

Chen, K.-I., Li, B.-R., & Chen, Y.-T. (2011). Silicon nanowire field-effect transistor-based biosensors for biomedical diagnosis and cellular recording investigation. *Nano Today*, *6*(2), 131–154. doi:10.1016/j.nantod.2011.02.001

Constant, E. W. (1973). A Model forTechnological Change Applied to the Turbojet Revolution. *Technology and Culture*, *14*(4), 553–572. doi:10.2307/3102443

Datta, S. (2005). *Atom to transistor*. New York: Cambridge University Press. doi:10.1017/CBO9781139164313

Gartner, W.W. (1959, December). Integrated Circuitry, Micro-miniaturization and Molecular Electronics. *Semiconductor Products*, 41–46.

Hanson, G. W. (2008). *Fundamentals of Nanoelectronics*. Pearson Education.

Hippel, V., & Arthur, R. (1956). Molecular Engineering. *Science*, *123*(3191), 315–317. doi:10.1126/science.123.3191.315 PMID:17774519

Huang, Y., Cai, D., & Chen, P. (2011). Micro and Nanotechnologies for Study of Cell Secretion. *Analytical Chemistry*, *83*(12), 4393–4406. doi:10.1021/ac200358b PMID:21417447

Ingold, G. L., & Nazarov, Yu. V. (1992). Charge tunneling rates in ultrasmall junctions. In H. Grabert & M. H. Devoret (Eds.), *Single Charge Tunneling* (pp. 21–107). New York: Plenum. doi:10.1007/978-1-4757-2166-9_2

Jurvetson, S. T. (2004). Transcending Moore's Law with Molecular Electronics and Nanotechnology. *Nanotechnology Law and Business*, *1*, 70–90.

Kastner, M. A. (1993). Artificial Atoms. *Physics Today*, *46*(1), 24–31. doi:10.1063/1.881393

Keren, K. et al.. (2002). Sequence-Specific Molecular Lithography on Single DNA Molecules. *Science*, *297*(5578), 72–75. doi:10.1126/science.1071247 PMID:12098693

Keren, K. et al.. (2003). DNA-templated carbon nanotube field-effect transistor. *Science* 302: 1380-1382.
Moore, G.E. (1965). Cramming more Components onto Integrated Circuits. *Electronics*, *38*, 114–117.

Kouwenhoven, L. P. (1997). Electron transport in quantum dots. In B. L. Sohn et al. (Eds.), *Mesoscopic Electron Transfer* (pp. 105–215). Dordrecht: Kluwer, Dordrecht. doi:10.1007/978-94-015-8839-3_4

Liu, Y., Dong, X., & Chen, P. (2012). Biological and chemical sensors based on graphene materials. *Chemical Society Reviews*, *41*(6), 2283–2307. doi:10.1039/C1CS15270J PMID:22143223

Meirav, U., & Foxman, E. B. (1995). Single-electron phenomena in semiconductors. *Semiconductor Science and Technology*, *10*, 255–284.

Patolsky, F., Timko, B. P., Yu, G., Fang, Y., & Greytak, A. B. et al.. (2006). Detection, stimulation, and inhibition of neuronal signals with high-density nanowire transistor arrays. *Science*, *313*(5790), 1100–1104. doi:10.1126/science.1128640 PMID:16931757

Pui, T. S., Sudibya, H. G., Luan, X., Zhang, Q., Ye, F., Huang, Y., & Chen, P. (2010). Non-invasive detection of cellular bioelectricity based on carbon nanotube devices for high-throughput drug screening. *Advanced Materials*, *22*(29), 3199–3203. doi:10.1002/adma.201000548 PMID:20533507

Reed, M. A. (1997). Conductance of a Molecular Junction. *Science*, *278*(5336), 252–254. doi:10.1126/science.278.5336.252

Smith, E. M. (2007). Nano panelist sees molecular devices as next step toward smaller, cheaper, faster devices (James J. Marek, Jr.). *ASME NEWS.* Retrieved from http://www.asmenews.org/archives/backissues/aug01/features/nanopan.html

Tian, B., Cohen-karni, T., Qing, Q., Duan, X., Xie, P., & Lieber, C. M. (2010). Three-dimensional, flexible nanoscale field-effect transistors as localized bioprobes. *Science*, *329*(5993), 830–834. doi:10.1126/science.1192033 PMID:20705858

Time. (1974). Mini-mini Components: Turning Individual Molecules into Electronic Components. *Time Magazine, 103*, 97.

Tuomi, I. (2002). The Lives and Death of Moore's Law. *First Monday*, *7*(11). doi:10.5210/fm.v7i11.1000

Zahl, H. A. (1968). *Electrons Away, or Tales of a Government Scientist*. New York: Vintage.

Chapter 11
Analysis of HRV during the Menstrual Cycle and Postmenopause

Kirti Rawal
Dr. B. R. Ambedkar National Institute of Technology, India

Barjinder Singh Saini
Dr. B. R. Ambedkar National Institute of Technology, India

Indu Saini
Dr. B. R. Ambedkar National Institute of Technology, India

ABSTRACT

Every woman experiences an extensive fluctuation in HRV during her menstrual cycle and even after menopause. A woman who lives long enough will experience menopause as a normal physiologic event. The study of the influence of premenopausal and postmenopausal symptoms on HRV has not been adequate. During this period, health management is an important factor to be considered as it affects the entire quality of women life. Many women having diverse physical, behavioural as well as psychological symptoms at the time of menopause and even after the menopause. Thus, HRV analysis is an appropriate tool to examine the physiological effects of the menstrual cycle in young healthy women and the postmenopause in old women. This chapter intends to study the influence of the menstrual cycle, and postmenopause on autonomic modulation of heart with a perspective of signal processing approach.

INTRODUCTION

The measure of fluctuation in the time interval between heart beats is termed as Heart Rate Variability (HRV). In other words, the regularity of heart beats is monitored by HRV: smaller regularity implies higher HRV and vice versa. Regularity of heart beats is measured from the time elapsed between the consecutive heart beats, *i.e.,* RR intervals in millisecond (ms). The HRV signal is obtained from the Electrocardiogram (ECG) signal by taking time interval between consecutive R peaks of the ECG signal.

DOI: 10.4018/978-1-5225-0660-7.ch011

HRV analysis provides valuable information regarding the functions of the heart and autonomic control through sympathetic and parasympathetic regulation. Higher HRV indicates healthy Autonomic Nervous System (ANS) while lower HRV is associated with poor health and stress. Studying HRV variations gives valuable information regarding stress level, pain, other emotional disturbances, *etc* of women throughout the menstrual cycle (Sato and Miyake, 2004) and after the menopause (Fu et al., 2008; Neves et al., 2007; Ribeiro et al., 2001). The influence and impact of biomedical signals on modern society is tremendous, and signal processing is now a critical component in science and technology. Recording and analyzing HRV signals is continued for several decades but still continue to excite physicians and engineers. Presently variety of tools available for HRV measurement (Acharya et al., 2006; Camm et al., 1996) and assessment but existing techniques are not considered to be accurate analysis method (Mansier et al., 1996; Litvack et al., 1995; Masek et al., 2009). So, decoding HRV variations using signal processing techniques during the menstrual cycle proves to be crucial in determining the health conditions of women and also necessary to decide course of action for treatment of diseases related regularity and irregularity of cycles. In order to gain a deeper insight into the functioning of heart, various physiological maneuvers such as physical activity or postural variation have been used. There is also a strong impact of physical activity on the HRV during the menstrual cycle and the postmenopause. This chapter intends to study the influence of the menstrual cycle, and post menopause on autonomic modulation of heart with a perspective of signal processing approach. For this purpose, it is necessary to evaluate the existing signal processing methods for quantifying the HRV variations during the menstrual cycle (premenopause) and after the menopause (postmenopause) in the lying postures.

The first phase of this chapter is dedicated to application of linear HRV analysis methods for detecting the HRV variations during the menstrual cycle phases in the lying postures. In time domain methods such as (nn50) number of pairs of adjacent NN intervals differing by more than 50ms), and (TINN) Triangular Interpolation of NN intervals are analyzed and implemented on preprocessed menstrual cycle HRV dataset of 74 young women in the menstrual, follicular and luteal phases. nn50 and TINN are used to examine the effects of the menstrual, follicular and luteal phases of the menstrual cycle.

In the second phase of this chapter, the linear time domain methods such as nn50, and TINN are applied on HRV dataset comprising 20 postmenopausal women in the lying postures. Further, a comparative study was made between 74 premenopausal women in the follicular phase of the menstrual cycle and 20 postmenopausal women.

BACKGROUND

Various studies have investigated the effects of menstrual cycle on HRV using linear methods of HRV. Mckinley et al. (2009), Sato et al. (1995), Saeki et al. (1997), Guasti et al. (1999), Yildirir et al. (2002) and Ghildiyal et al. (2011) reported that sympathetic activities were lower in the follicular phase in comparison with the luteal phase. The increase in LF/HF ratio in the luteal phase as compared to the follicular phase was also reported by Sheema et al. (2014). Baker et al. (2008) analyzed that parasympathetic activity was decreased in the late luteal phase of women with premenstrual symptoms as compared to the follicular phase. Ageing effects on HRV in the menstrual cycle was also demonstrated by Bindiya et al. (2011). Some studies such as Nakagawa et al. (2006) and Vishrutha et al. (2012) reported that time domain methods were not able to differentiate the HRV variations between different phases of the menstrual cycle.

Chung and Yang (2011) demonstrated that HRV is decreased in the follicular phase as compared to the luteal phase during sleeping periods of shift work nurses by using frequency domain methods. But, Princi et al. (2005) reported that sympathetic activities were predominant in the follicular phase in comparison to the luteal phase of the menstrual cycle whereas some studies such as Leicht et al. (2003) and Kavitha et al. (2012) found no significant difference of HRV in the menstrual phase with respect to the luteal and follicular phase. Moodithaya and Sandhya (2009) found lower HRV with increase in the LF/HF ratio in the postmenopausal women. Further decreased RR interval and standard deviation in the postmenopausal women is reported by Brockbank et al. (2000) as compared with premenopausal women. Huatamaki et al. (2012), Lee et al. (2011), and Tuomikoski et al. (2011) evaluated the effect of hot flushes in the cardiac functioning of postmenopausal women. Following are the conclusions from the literature survey:

1. There is no concrete study that focuses on the HRV variations in all three phases of menstrual cycle in lying and standing postures.
2. To the best of author's, there is no substantial work that delves down to the details of postmenopausal phase in the lying and standing postures.
3. Most linear methods of HRV analysis fail to detect the HRV variations correctly in different phases of the menstrual cycle.
4. Also, there are limited research published that reveals the HRV variations between follicular phase of the menstrual cycle and postmenopausal phase in the lying and standing postures.

MAIN FOCUS OF THE CHAPTER

Due to these inconclusive results presented by various authors in the literature, linear HRV analysis methods such as nn50 and TINN are evaluated in this chapter for investigating the HRV variations in between the menstrual and follicular phase, follicular and luteal phase, luteal and menstrual phase of the menstrual cycle and in between follicular phase and postmenopausal women.

Linear HRV Analysis Methods

The autonomic balance between the Sympathetic Nervous System (SNS) and Parasympathetic Nervous System (PNS) plays an important role in regulating the heart rate. Increased heart rate is associated with the decreased HRV and vice versa (Camm et al., 1996). The interaction between the sympathetic and parasympathetic branches of ANS originates the HRV signal. Therefore, the variability of the heart rate plays an important role in the regulation of cardiac functioning during normal and pathological conditions. The cardiac autonomic status of women in menstrual, follicular and luteal phases of the menstrual cycle and in postmenopausal stage is presented in this chapter by means of linear methods of HRV analysis. The linear methods are further divided into two types: time domain and frequency domain. Various time-domain measures are used to assess effectual cardiac functioning (Camm et al., 1996). Statistical time domain measures include SDNN (Standard Deviation of NN intervals), SDANN (Standard Deviation of Averages of NN intervals), RMSSD (Root Mean Square value of Successive Differences between adjacent NN intervals), SDNNi (mean of Standard Deviation of all NN intervals), SDSD (Standard Deviation of Differences between Adjacent NN intervals), nn50 (number of pairs of adjacent NN intervals differing by more than 50ms), and pnn50 (percentage of adjacent NN intervals differing by more than 50ms). Geometrical measures include HRV triangular index, TINN (Triangular Interpolation of NN interval histogram), Differential Index and Logarithmic index. All the time domain measures will convey the information about the overall variability in time series but not able to capture the periodic fluctuations of the heart rate (Camm et al., 1996). Frequency domain analysis is the spectral analysis method which decomposes the total variation of data series into its frequency components which can be uttered in the form of a spectral density function that depicts spectral power as a function of frequency. For a given frequency band, spectral power can be quantified by deriving the area beneath the spectral density function within specified frequency range. The mainly common technique for spectral analysis of HRV is the Fast Fourier Transform (FFT) technique. Analysis of FFT analysis assumes that the HRV time series contains only deterministic components and the spectrum computed with the FFT is derived from all data, based on peaks in the spectral distribution (Guasti et al., 1999). The main spectral components which are notable in a spectrum calculated are very low frequency (VLF), low frequency (LF), and high frequency (HF) components.

Time Domain Methods

Time domain methods are the simplest methods used for analysis of HRV. Heart rate at any point in time intervals between consecutive normal complexes is determined using time domain methods. Various time-domain measures are used to assess the effectual cardiac functioning (Camm et al., 1996). The selected time domain methods studied in this chapter were nn50, and TINN (Masek, 1996).

1. **nn50:** nn50 is number of pairs of adjoining NN intervals differing by larger than 50ms in the entire recording. Mathematically it is defined by using (1) (Masek, 1996).

$$nn50 = \sum_{i=1}^{N} \left\{ \left| RR_{i+1} - RR_{i} \right| > 50ms \right\} \tag{1}$$

   where N is the total number of RR intervals in a particular selected segment (Masek, 1996).

2. **Triangular Interpolation of NN Interval (TINN):** TINN is the baseline width of RR interval histogram which is calculated through triangular interpolation. It also expresses overall HRV calculated over 24 hours (Camm et al., 1996; Masek, 1996).

DATA DESCRIPTION AND EXPERIMENTAL PROTOCOLS

In order to accomplish this objective, the Electrocardiogram (ECG) signals of 74 young women during the menstrual cycle and 20 old women in postmenopause were recorded using lead II in the lying position each for 15 minutes in Biomedical Signal Processing and Telemedicine laboratory settings using BIOPAC®MP 150 system. All the signals were recorded at sampling frequency of 500Hz. All the ECG recordings were taken at 8:00AM - 11:00 AM in the morning and at 3:00PM - 6:00PM in the evening. During this study all data were recorded in quiet laboratory settings having maintained temperature levels.

For each ECG recording, three Ag-AgCl electrodes were placed as follows: one electrode is placed on the right arm, one on the left leg, and last is ground which is placed on the right leg. After 10 minutes rest, ECG of healthy young women and old women were recorded for 15 minutes in the lying posture. The RR-intervals were then obtained using software Acknowledge 4.2. In order to remove artifacts in the data, all subjects were instructed to avoid moving of hands, legs and body, talking coughing and sleeping during recording. Also subjects were instructed not to take food, tea or coffee from last two hours prior to recording. The informed written consent was taken from all the subjects.

- **Selection of Subjects:** The subjects in this research work were divided into two groups: (i) Group1 (Premenopausal women/ having menstrual cycle) and (ii) Group2 (Postmenopausal women/ cease of the menstrual cycle).

Group 1: In group1, the subjects selected were 74 healthy young women having regular menstrual cycle of approximately 28 to 32 days in the age group of 18 to 25 yrs. All subjects in this group were confirmed to have regular sleep – wake up schedules, having good health and no heart disease. Also all subjects were confirmed that they were not taken any chronic medication including hormonal contraceptives, and also abstained from smoking, alcoholism and caffeine containing beverages for the previous six months.

The subjects in group1were further divided into three groups: Group 1A, Group1B and Group 1C. Based on the groups, every woman was prescribed to come three times in the laboratory for ECG recording in each phase of the menstrual cycle: once during the menstrual phase (days 1-2 after menses onset), once during the follicular phase (6-10 days) and once during the luteal phase (24-28 days or 28-32 days). The groups were following:

Group 1A: The subjects in this group were prescribed to come in the laboratory for ECG recording during the menstrual phase (days 1-2 after menses onset).

Group 1B: In this group, ECG recordings were carried out in the laboratory for the subjects in the period of follicular phase, *i.e.,* in between 6-10 days of the menstrual cycle.

Group 1C: The subjects in this group were prescribed to come in the laboratory for ECG recording during the luteal phase, *i.e.,* 24-28 days or 28-32 days depending upon the total length of the menstrual cycle.

Group 2: The subjects selected in Group2 were 20 healthy old women in the age group of 48 to 65 yrs having absence of the menstrual cycle for the last 12 months, i.e., postmenopausal state. In this group, every woman was prescribed to come once in the laboratory for ECG recording in the lying and standing postures.

RESULTS

The primary objective of this chapter is as follows:

1. To detect the HRV variations between the menstrual (Group 1A) and follicular phase (Group 1B) in the lying posture.

2. To detect the HRV variations between the follicular (Group 1B) and luteal phase (Group 1C) in the lying postures.
3. To detect the HRV variations between the luteal (Group 1C) and menstrual phase (Group 1A) in the lying posture.
4. To detect the HRV variations between the follicular phase (Group 1B) and postmenopausal phase (Group-2) in the lying posture.

Detecting HRV variations between various phases mentioned above will reveal the autonomic activity of heart during the premenopausal and postmenopausal women. In order to achieve this objective, linear HRV analysis methods including time domain are applied on HRV signals of (i) 74 young healthy women during three phases of the menstrual cycle (Group 1) and (ii) 20 postmenopausal women (Group 2). HRV analysis methods are used to approximate the HRV signals of phases of women so that HRV variations between various phases can be detected accurately. The inaccurate detection of HRV variations within menstrual cycle phases and after the menopause, leads to the inaccurate information regarding health of women during the menstrual cycle like stress. Stress estimation during the menstrual cycle and in postmenopause influences the balance of autonomic nervous system. Investigating HRV variations within the menstrual, luteal and follicular phase using HRV analysis methods is a great challenge for researchers. Analysis of HRV gives important information about the working of the heart and autonomic control through sympathetic and parasympathetic regulations. The effect of HRV variations between three phases of the menstrual cycle and between follicular and postmenopausal phases of women is evaluated using various HRV analysis methods in order to find the autonomic activity of heart.

The mean values are used to find the HRV variations between three phases of the menstrual cycle and between follicular and postmenopausal phases of women in the lying and standing postures. Results are presented in the form of comparing mean values as shown in Table 1.

Application of Linear Methods on HRV Signals of Luteal, Menstrual, and Follicular Phases of the Menstrual Cycle

- **Time Domain Methods:** For finding the effect of luteal, menstrual and follicular phases of the menstrual cycle on HRV variations of premenopausal women, mean values of all linear HRV analysis methods are calculated. Following protocol is followed to find the mean values.

Consider the first linear method in consideration *i.e.,* nn50. Linear method such as nn50 is applied on all 74 premenopausal subjects in the lying and standing postures in order to find out the linear parameter *i.e.,* nn50. Since premenopausal women consists of three phases (Menstrual, follicular and luteal). Thus,

Table 1. HRV variations between phases of the menstrual cycle using time domain methods in the lying posture

S. No.	Time Domain Methods	Phases of Menstrual Cycle (Lying Posture)					
		Menstrual and Follicular Phase		Follicular and Luteal Phase		Luteal and Menstrual Phase	
1.	nn50	252.33	253.63	253.63	228.74	228.74	252.33
2.	TINN	202.31	204.74	204.74	189.73	189.73	202.31

there are total 74 HRV signals per phase per posture for premenopausal subjects. There is one nn50 value pertains to each HRV signal. Mean of 74 nn50 values of each phase in premenopausal subjects in the lying and standing postures are calculated separately. In other words, there is one mean value of nn50 for each phase in the lying posture and one mean value of SDNN in the standing posture. Similarly, the mean values of the linear parameter, i.e., TINN pertain to each linear method for each phase in the lying and posture are calculated.

Table 1 provides the analysis of time domain methods, i.e., nn50 and TINN of HRV of 74 subjects in menstrual (Group 1A), follicular (Group 1B), and luteal phases (Group 1C) of the menstrual cycle in the lying posture.

From Table 1, following observations are made:

- Result shows that mean values of HRV parameters such as nn50, and TINN were lower in the menstrual phase as compared to the follicular phase in the lying postures. Lower mean values of nn50, and TINN parameters of HRV indicates decreased HRV that implies the sympathetic activities are higher in the menstrual phase as compared to the follicular phase of women.
- Further, the HRV parameters, *i.e.,* nn50, and TINN are having lower mean values in the luteal phase as compared to the follicular as well as in the menstrual phase. Lower mean values in the luteal phase imply lower HRV and higher sympathetic activity as compared to the follicular and menstrual phases.

Application of Linear Methods on HRV Signals of Follicular Phases of the Menstrual Cycle and Postmenopausal Women

Similarly, mean values of HRV analysis methods of 20 postmenopausal subjects are calculated. The mean value of 20 postmenopausal is compared with the mean of follicular phase of 20 premenopausal women.

- **Time Domain Methods:** Table 2 provides the analysis of HRV in the lying and standing postures respectively of Group 1C (follicular phase of the menstrual cycle) and Group B (postmenopausal) subjects.

It was also found that mean values of HRV parameters such as nn50, and TINN were lower in the postmenopausal subjects as compared to the subjects in the follicular phase (premenopausal) in the lying postures as shown in Table 2. Lower mean values of the linear parameters of HRV indicate decreased HRV which implies that sympathetic activities are higher in the postmenopausal women as compared to premenopausal women in the follicular phase.

Table 2. HRV variations between follicular phases of the menstrual cycle and postmenopausal women using time domain methods in the lying posture

S. No.	Time Domain Methods	Follicular and Postmenopausal Phases (Lying Posture)	
		Follicular Phases of the Menstrual Cycle	Postmenopausal Phase
1.	nn50	253.63	35.84
2.	TINN	204.74	100.09

Performance Comparison

The mean value is not considered as the reliable method of evaluating methods in detecting HRV variations. Thus, the performance parameter, *i.e.,* accuracy is used for evaluating HRV variations between phases in different postures. The comparative analysis of the time domain HRV parameters, i.e., nn50 and TINN in detecting HRV variations is performed on (i) menstrual cycle dataset of 74 women and (ii) 20 postmenopausal women dataset acquired using BIOPAC®MP150. The accuracy of the algorithm is calculated based upon the ability of detecting the desired relationship of HRV variations (i) between the phases of the menstrual cycle in Group1A, Group1B and Group1C. The accuracy of detecting HRV variations between two phases is defined using (2)

$$Accuracy = \frac{Number\ of\ subjects\ having\ desired\ relation\ of\ HRV\ variations\ between\ phases}{Total\ number\ of\ subjects} \tag{2}$$

The desired relationship of HRV variations using various linear parameters are shown in each case as mentioned in Table 3 and Table 4. The method is considered as better or more accurate that can be able to establish the desired relationship of HRV variations between phases in more number of subjects. The method having high accuracy is considered as better method of detecting HRV variations.

In order to find the accuracy of detecting correct HRV variations between each phase of the menstrual cycle, accuracy of each HRV analysis method is calculated. Figure 1 to Figure 3 showed the comparative analysis of detecting HRV variations in the menstrual, follicular and luteal phases of the menstrual cycle in the lying posture.

Figure 1 demonstrated that nn50 is more accurate in detecting the HRV variations in the menstrual and follicular phase as compared to TINN which corresponds to the desired relationship mentioned in Table 3. It is desirable that HRV in menstrual phase is lower as compared to follicular phase.

Similarly, in Figure 3 it is clearly demonstrated that nn50 gives higher accuracy in detecting HRV variations between menstrual and luteal phases in the lying postures. It is shown in Figure 1 and Figure

Table 3. Interpretation of HRV variations between phases of the menstrual cycle using time domain methods

S. No.	Linear Methods (Time Domain)	Parameters	Correct Relationship of Phases of Menstrual Cycle
1.	Number of pairs of adjacent NN intervals differing by more than 50ms (nn50)	nn50	$nn50_m < nn50_f$ $nn50_f > nn50_l$ $nn50_l < nn50_m$
2.	Triangular Interpolation of NN interval	TINN	$TINN_m < TINN_f$ $TINN_f > TINN_l$ $TINN_l < TINN_m$

Table 4. Interpretation of HRV variations between postmenopausal women and follicular phase of the menstrual cycle using time domain methods

S. No.	Linear Methods (Time Domain)	Parameters	Correct Relationship of Phases of Menstrual Cycle
1.	Number of pairs of adjacent NN intervals differing by more than 50ms (nn50)	nn50	$nn50_p < nn50_f$
2.	Triangular Interpolation of NN interval	TINN	$TINN_p < TINN_f$

Figure 1. Comparative analysis of accuracy of detecting HRV variations between menstrual and follicular phases of the menstrual cycle using nn50 and TINN in the lying posture

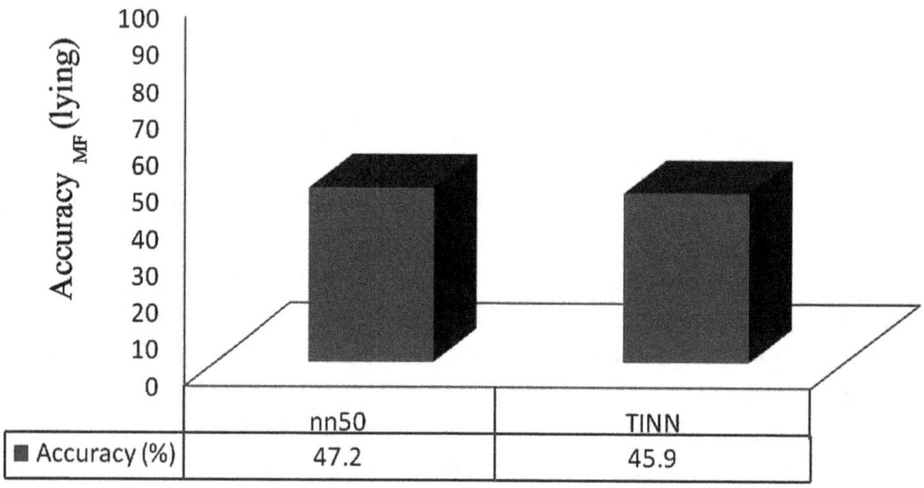

Figure 2. Comparative analysis of accuracy of detecting HRV variations between follicular and luteal phases of the menstrual cycle using nn50 and TINN in the lying posture

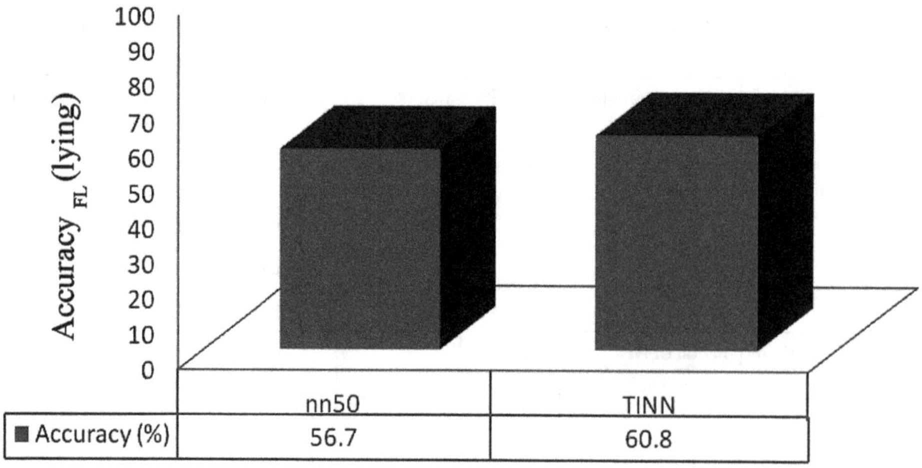

Figure 3. Comparative analysis of accuracy of detecting HRV variations between luteal and menstrual phases of the menstrual cycle using nn50 and TINN in the lying posture

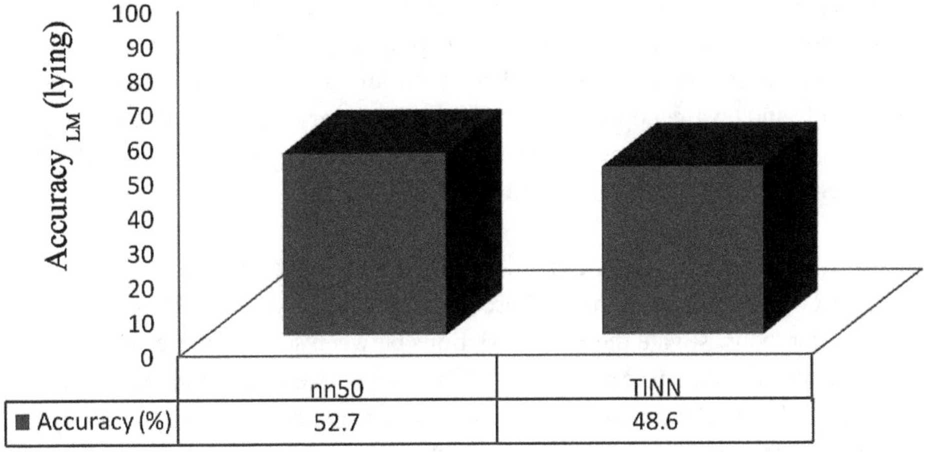

3 the nn50 is more accurate in detecting the desired relationship between the menstrual and follicular phases as well as between the luteal and menstrual phases in the lying postures. But in Figure 2 accuracy of detecting HRV variations between the follicular and luteal phases is higher in TINN as compared to nn50 based HRV analysis method.

In Figure 4, accuracy between postmenopausal women and the follicular phase in the lying posture are calculated by using various time domain methods such as nn50, and TINN based on the Table 4. From Figure 4, it is amply clear that nn50 is having higher accuracy in detecting HRV variations in the postmenopausal and the follicular phase of women as compared to TINN in the lying posture.

Thus, is concluded that the accuracy of detecting HRV variations between phases of the menstrual cycle and also between the follicular and postmenopausal phases is not high in case of linear time domain methods such as nn50 and TINN.

Figure 4. Comparative analysis of accuracy of detecting HRV variations between follicular phase of the menstrual cycle and postmenopausal stage using nn50 and TINN in the lying posture

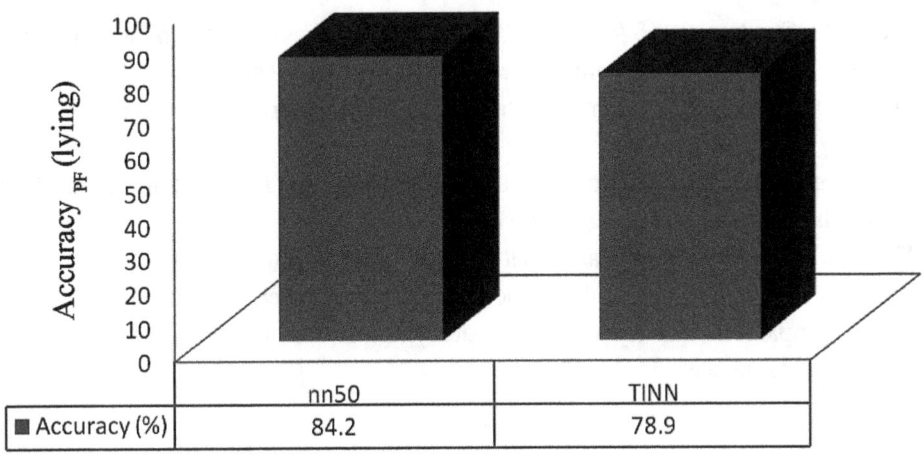

FUTURE RESEARCH DIRECTIONS

There are various applications in which HRV measures are increasingly being employed. The measures of HRV not only provide the fundamental link between the psychological processes and physiological functions as well as basic investigations of cardiac autonomic state. Although the widespread applications (menstrual cycle and postmenopause) of these measures serves as an indication of potential merit, but still there are some issues that are necessary to be resolved, as this would involve the standardization of HRV methods. Some of the issues addressed are following:

1. In this work, the menstrual cycle is divided into three phases such as luteal, menstrual and follicular phases, so, HRV is examined in these phases only. Further, ovulation phase will be desired to be included in order to investigate the HRV variations between several phases of the menstrual cycle.
2. In this work, conventional linear methods of HRV analysis were investigated for finding the correct HRV variations during the menstrual cycle and postmenopause. Based on the limitations of the conventional linear methods, some novel algorithms are required to be proposed.

CONCLUSION

HRV is a noninvasive approach which is used to provide information about the autonomic neural regulation of heart and the circulatory system. HRV signal is a nonstationary signal and in order to accurately measure the variations in the HRV signal, the techniques adopted for its analysis are appropriately selected. In this chapter, an attempt has been made to re-evaluate all the linear HRV analysis methods for detecting HRV variations between the:

1. Menstrual and follicular phase,
2. Follicular and luteal phase,
3. Luteal and menstrual phase of the menstrual cycle, and
4. Between the follicular and postmenopausal phase in the lying and standing postures.

The linear HRV analysis methods such as nn50 and TINN was tested on the

1. Self-recorded ECG data set of 74 young women in three phases of the menstrual cycle, and
2. Self-recorded ECG data set of 20 old women in postmenopausal phase in the lying posture acquired using the BIOPAC®MP150 system. On the basis of work carried, the following conclusions are drawn:
    a. The results proved that the time domain methods are able to differentiate the HRV variations within three phases of the menstrual cycle.
    b. The results clearly demonstrated that HRV is lower in luteal phase as compared to the menstrual and follicular phases of the menstrual cycle. Lower HRV in the luteal phase implies higher sympathetic activity and lower parasympathetic activity as compared to the follicular and menstrual phases.

c. It is demonstrated from the results that HRV is higher in the follicular phase as compared to menstrual and luteal phases of the menstrual cycle which again implies lower sympathetic activity in the follicular phases as compared to other phases of the menstrual cycle.
d. Lastly, sympathetic activities are higher and parasympathetic activities are lower in the postmenopausal women as compared to premenopausal women because of having lower HRV in the postmenopausal women.
e. The accuracy of detecting HRV variations between phases of the menstrual cycle and also between the follicular and postmenopausal phases is not high in case of linear methods. Further consideration is required to find methods that can be able to detect HRV variations accurately.

REFERENCES

Acharya, U., Joseph, K., Kannathal, N., Lim, C., & Suri, J. (2006). Heart rate variability: A review. *Medical & Biological Engineering & Computing*, *44*(12), 1031–1051. doi:10.1007/s11517-006-0119-0 PMID:17111118

Baker, F., Colrain, I., & Trinder, J. (2008). Reduced Parasympathetic activity during sleep in the symptomatic phase of severe premenstrual syndrome. *Journal of Psychosomatic Research*, *65*(1), 13–22. doi:10.1016/j.jpsychores.2008.04.008 PMID:18582607

Bindiya, R., Kishan, K., Damodara, K., Ramaswamy, C., & Bhat, M. (2011). Association between the different phases of menstrual cycle and time domain analysis of Heart Rate Variability in young adult and older adult in Indian Women's. *Research Journal of Pharmaceutical, Biological and Chemical Sciences*, *2*(1), 297–303.

Brockbank, C. L., Chatterjee, F., Bruce, S. A., & Woledge, R. C. (2000). Heart rate and its variability change after the menopause. *Experimental Physiology*, *85*(3), 327–330. doi:10.1111/j.1469-445X.2000.01902.x PMID:10825420

Camm, A. J., Malik, M., Bigger, J. T., Gunter, B., Cerutti, S., & Choen, R. (1996). Task force of the European society of cardiology and the North American society of pacing and electrophysiology Heart rate variability - standards of measurement. Physiological interpretation and clinical use. *Circulation*, *93*(5), 1043–1065. doi:10.1161/01.CIR.93.5.1043 PMID:8598068

Chung, M., & Yang, C. (2011). Heart Rate Variability across the Menstrual Cycle in Shift Work Nurses. *Journal of Experimental and Clinical Medicine*, *3*(3), 121–125. doi:10.1016/j.jecm.2011.04.001

Fu, C., Yang, C., Lin, C., & Kuo, T. (2008). Alteration of cardiovascular autonomic functions by vegetarian diets in postmenopausal women is related to LDL cholesterol levels. *The Chinese Journal of Physiology*, *51*, 100–105. PMID:18666713

Ghildiyal, A., Iqbal, B., Singh, S., Verma, D., & Singh, S. (2011). Changes in sympathovagal balance during mensturalcycle. *Current Neurobiology*, *2*(1), 49–52.

Guasti, L., Grimoldi, P., Mainardi, L., Petrozzino, M., Piantanida, E., Garganico, D., & Venco, A. et al. (1999). Autonomic function and baroreflex sensitivity during a normal ovulatory cycle in humans. *Acta Cardiologica*, *54*(4), 209–213. PMID:10511897

Hautamaki, H., Haapalahti, P., Piirila, P., Tuomikoski, P., Sovijarvi, A., Ylikorkalaa, O., & Mikkolaa, T. S. (2012). Effect of hot flushes on cardiovascular autonomic responsiveness: A randomized controlled trial on hormone therapy. *Maturitas*, *72*(3), 243–248. doi:10.1016/j.maturitas.2012.04.001 PMID:22537767

Kavitha, C., Jamuna, B., & Vijayakumar, G. (2012). Cardiac chronotropism and sympathovagal balance in young women of reproductive age. *International Journal of Biological & Medical Research*, *3*(4), 2313–2318.

Lee, J. O., Kang, S. G., Kim, S. H., Park, S. J., & Song, S. W. (2011). The Relationship between Menopausal Symptoms and Heart Rate Variability in Middle Aged Women. *Korean Journal of Family Medicine*, *32*(5), 299–305. doi:10.4082/kjfm.2011.32.5.299 PMID:22745867

Leicht, A., Hirning, D., & Allen, G. (2003). Heart rate variability and endogenous sex hormones during the menstrual cycle in young women. *Experimental Physiology*, *88*(3), 441–446. doi:10.1113/eph8802535 PMID:12719769

Litvack, D. A., Oberlander, T. F., Carney, L. H., & Saul, J. P. (1995). Time and frequency domain methods for heart rate variability analysis: A methodological comparison. *Psychophysiology*, *32*(5), 492–504. doi:10.1111/j.1469-8986.1995.tb02101.x PMID:7568644

Mansier, P., Clairambault, J., Charlotte, N., Medigue, C., Vermeiren, C., LePape, G., & Swynghedauw, B. et al. (1996). Linear and non-linear analyses of heart rate variability: A minireview. *Cardiovascular Research*, *31*(3), 371–379. doi:10.1016/0008-6363(96)00009-0 PMID:8681324

Masek, O. (2009). *Heart Rate Variability Analysis*. (Diploma Thesis). Czech Technical University in Prague, Prague, Czech Republic.

Mckinley, P., King, A., Shapiro, P., Slavov, I., Fang, Y., Chen, I., & Sloan, R. et al. (2009). The impact of menstrual cycle phase on cardiac autonomic regulation. *Psychophysiology*, *46*(4), 904–911. doi:10.1111/j.1469-8986.2009.00811.x PMID:19386049

Moodithaya, S., & Sandhya, T. (2009). Comparison of Cardiac Autonomic Activity between Pre and Post Menopausal Women using Heart Rate Variability. *Indian Journal of Physiology and Pharmacology*, *53*, 227–234. PMID:20329369

Nakagawa, M., Ooie, T., Takahashi, N., Taniguchi, Y., Anan, F., Yonemochi, H., & Saikawa, T. (2006). Influence of menstrual cycle on QT interval dynamics. *Pacing and Clinical Electrophysiology*, *29*(6), 607–613. doi:10.1111/j.1540-8159.2006.00407.x PMID:16784426

Neves, V. F., Silva de Sa, M. F., Gallo, L. J. Jr, Catai, A. M., Martins, L. E., Crescencio, J. C., & Silva, E. et al. (2007). Autonomic modulation of heart rate of young and postmenopausal women undergoing estrogen therapy. *Brazilian Journal of Medical and Biological Research*, *40*(4), 491–499. doi:10.1590/S0100-879X2007000400007 PMID:17401492

Princi, T., Parco, S., Accardo, A., Radillo, O., Seta, F., & Guaschino, S. (2005). Parametric evaluation of heart rate variability during the menstrual cycle in young women. *Biomedical Sciences Instrumentation, 41*, 340–345. PMID:15850129

Ribeiro, T. F., Azevendo, G. D., Crescencio, J. C., Maraes, V. R., Papa, V., Catai, A. M., & Siliva, E. et al. (2001). Heart rate variability under resting conditions in post menopausal and young women. *Brazilian Journal of Medical and Biological Research, 34*(7), 871–877. doi:10.1590/S0100-879X2001000700006 PMID:11449305

Saeki, Y., Atogami, F., Takahashi, K., & Yoshizawa, T. (1997). Reflex control of autonomic function induced by posture change during the menstrual cycle. *Journal of the Autonomic Nervous System, 66*(1-2), 69–74. doi:10.1016/S0165-1838(97)00067-2 PMID:9334995

Sato, N., & Miyake, S. (2004). Cardiovascular reactivity to mental stress: Relationship with menstrual cycle and gender. *Journal of Physiological Anthropology and Applied Human Science, 23*(6), 215–223. doi:10.2114/jpa.23.215 PMID:15599065

Sato, N., Miyake, S., Akatsu, J., & Kumashiro, M. (1995). Power spectral analysis of heart rate variability in healthy young women during the normal menstrual cycle. *Psychosomatic Medicine, 57*(4), 331–335. doi:10.1097/00006842-199507000-00004 PMID:7480562

Sheema, U. K., Sarwari, K. N., & Malipatil, B. S. (2014). Influence of different phases of the menstrual cycle on heart rate variability. *International Journal of Basic and Applied Medical Sciences, 4*(3), 168-172.

Tuomikoski, P., Ylikorkala, O., & Mikkola, T. S. (2011). Menopausal hot flushes and vascular health. *Annals of Medicine, 43*(4), 283–291. doi:10.3109/07853890.2010.546364 PMID:21254907

Vishrutha, K., Harini, N., Ganaraja, B., Pavanchand, A., & Susheela, V. (2012). A study of cardiac autonomic control and pulmonary functions in different phases of menstrual cycle. *International Journal of Applied Biology and Pharmaceutical Technology, 3*(3), 306–311.

Yildirir, A., Kabakci, G., Akgul, E., Tokgozoglu, L., & Oto, A. (2002). Effects of menstrual cycle on cardiac autonomic innervation as assessed by heart rate variability. *Annals of Noninvasive Electrocardiology, 7*(1), 60–63. doi:10.1111/j.1542-474X.2001.tb00140.x PMID:11844293

Chapter 12
A Comparative Study on Diabetic Retinopathy Detection Using Texture-Based Feature Extraction Techniques

Azam Asilian Bidgoli
University of Kashan, Iran

Hossein Ebrahimpour-Komleh
University of Kashan, Iran

Seyed Jalaleddin Mousavirad
University of Kashan, Iran

ABSTRACT

Diabetic retinopathy is proved to be one of the most important eye disorders in recent decades that late diagnosis of it may cause low vision or even blindness. Specialist are able to detect retinopathy in retinal images using machine learning as a decision support system which helps accelerate and facilitate the diagnosis. The automated diabetic retinopathy is a difficult computer vision problem –with the goal of detecting features of retinopathy. The present chapter is written with the purpose of analyzing and comparing different feature extraction methods to evaluate the best algorithm for detection retinopathy with least error. Extracted features using these methods are used to classify images into normal and altered groups.

INTRODUCTION

In recent years, machine learning and data mining techniques have been considered as good tools for automated medical diagnosis systems (Kononenko, 2001; Kononenko, Bratko, & Kukar, 1997). Bearing in mind that medical diagnosis is a difficult and visual task, it is often carried out by an expert who commonly takes decisions by evaluating the current test results of a patient or comparing the patient

DOI: 10.4018/978-1-5225-0660-7.ch012

with other patients of the same condition by referring to the previous decisions (Polat & Güneş, 2006). Therefore, medical diagnosis is considered as an important but complicated process that requires to be executed accurately and effectively. Machine learning can help experts automate diagnosis and accordingly, reduce the possibility of error in experts dramatically. And, as a result, providing them with more detailed medical data inspected in a shorter time.

Detection of different disease using machine learning methods has been considered in various research works. Such attempts include diagnosis of hepatitis (Bascil & Oztekin, 2012), using neural network, Breast Cancer least square support vector machine (Polat & Güneş, 2007), and heart disease using artificial immune recognition system (Polat, Güneş, & Tosun, 2006).

Nowadays, diabetic retinopathy is the leading cause of blindness in adults all around the world. Most people with diabetes will develop some form of eye disease (retinopathy) causing reduced vision or blindness. Consistently high levels of blood glucose, together with high blood pressure and high cholesterol, are the main causes of retinopathy which can be managed through regular eye checks and keeping glucose and lipid levels at or close to normal ("International federation diabetes," 2014). Therefore, the Importance of early diagnosis of diabetes based on analysis of retinal images is increasing as this disease is affecting more people every day (Klein, Meuer, Moss, & Klein, 1995). As aforementioned, diabetic retinopathy (DR) has a fundamental role in visual impairment, and automated detection of diabetic retinopathy can reduce its lesion.

Regarding the importance of diagnosing the disease, a great deal of attempt has been made to utilize different methods of machine learning to diagnose diabetic retinopathy from retinal images. The process of detection of disease in images using these methods has two steps roughly. First, it should extract some features from images to describe the nature of image. The second step is the classification of these features using a classifier. There are a variety of methods to perform these two steps. Some researchers focus on improving the diagnosis using defining better features, while others outperform different classification methods. (Di Wu, et al, 2006) use Gabor filters to trace and patch the blood vessels together (Wu, Zhang, Liu, & Bauman, 2006). Pinz et al,(Pinz, Bernögger, Datlinger, & Kruger, 1998) use gradient based techniques and hough transforms (Illingworth & Kittler, 1988) to map and localize blood vessels. (Silberman et al, 2010) utilize SIFT feature extractor to describe the images. The second step support machine classifier(SVM) (Conforti & Guido, 2010) is considered to classify the features(Silberman, Ahrlich, Fergus, & Subramanian, 2010). Neovascularization features extracted from retinal images are among other features in this area. (Vatanparast & Harati, 2012) has classified these features using SVM.

Di Wu et al use gabor filters to trace and patch the blood vessels together (Wu et al., 2006). (Pinz et al., 1998) use gradient based techniques and Hough transforms (Illingworth & Kittler, 1988) to map and localize blood vessels. Silberman et al utilize SIFT feature extractor to describe the image. then support machine classifier(SVM)(Conforti & Guido, 2010) is considered to classify the features(Silberman et al., 2010). Neovascularization features extracted from retinal images are other features in this area. (Vatanparast & Harati, 2012) has classified these features using SVM.

In another work, the optic disc is detected by means of morphological filtering techniques and the watershed transformation (Walter, Klein, Massin, & Erginay, 2002). Also (Hoover & Goldbaum, 2003) used fuzzy convergence to determine the origination of the blood vessel network. Some work is performed on vessel segmentation (Niemeijer, Staal, van Ginneken, Loog, & Abramoff, 2004). Retinal vessel segmentation is important for the detection of numerous eye diseases and plays an important role in automatic retinal disease screening systems. (Niemeijer et al., 2004) compared the performance of retinal vessel segmentation methods. But in all of these researches less attention has paid to use textural features of an image.

As (Tang, 1998) asserts, Texture is the term used to characterize the surface of a given object or region and it is one of the main features utilized in image processing and pattern recognition (Tang, 1998). There are different methods to extract such features from images. These methods are based on statistical features of histogram (Gonzales, Woods, & Eddins, 2004), grey level co-occurrence matrix (GLCM) (Haralick, 1979), grey level run length matrix (GLRLM) (Tang, 1998), wavelet transformation (Vetterli & Herley, 1992), gabor filters (Marčelja, 1980), local binary pattern (LBP) (Ojala, Pietikäinen, & Mäenpää, 2002). Numerous features are extracted from each of these contents. Some of these methods generate features that are not appropriate for classifying images and don't contain useful information; therefore, feature selection methods can be applied to reduce the amount of data in classification phase. Selected features are utilized using a classifier algorithm to classify data into exact group. This chapter compares four mentioned methods to extract texture features, and then the SVM classifier classifies these features based on a class label that is defined in considered dataset. The present experiment which is done on a dataset includes 1200 images. The property of dataset has been explained in experiment section.

TEXTURE BASED FEATURE EXTRACTION

In the present section, several feature extraction methods named, statistical features of histogram, grey-level run lengths, gray-level co-occurrence matrix, local binary pattern, wavelet transform features and gabor are considered. Following that, further details of these algorithms are explained.

Statistical Features of Histogram

Histogram is a graph showing the number of pixels in an image at each different intensity value found in that image. Features based upon statistical information from the histogram of an image can be used as a method to describe its texture. Six statistical features are extracted from histogram. First, the histogram of pixel intensity values is computed and then is normalized to (p(i)). After that, based on these vectors (p(i)) and the probability of intensity value occurrence, six features are extracted. The definition of features are shown in Table 1. The definition of extracted features based on statistical information of histogram where different variables are as below:

μ_n : The nth moments.
Z_i: Random variable related to intensity values.
$P(z_i)$: The histogram of the pixel intensity values.
L: The maximum value of intensity level.
σ^2 : Variance

In addition to these 6features, 25 other features based on frequency of pixel intensity value can be computed. Therefore, the range of intensity (0-255) is divided to 25 intervals. Then the number of pixels in the image that are in every interval defined as a feature, meaning that 25 features are extracted from image.

Table 1. The definition of extracted features based on statistical information of histogram

Feature	Computation	Description
Mean	$m = \sum_{i=0}^{L-1} z_i p(z_i)$	The mean of texture intensity. The variance is a measure of the histogram width, that is, a measure of how much the gray levels differ from the mean.
Variance	$\sqrt{\mu_2(2)}$	The variance of texture intensity.
Smoothness	$1 - \frac{1}{(1+\sigma^2)}$	The value of this feature for smooth area in image is close to zero.
3rd Moment	$\sum_{i=0}^{L-1} (z_i - m)^3 p(z_i)$	This feature shows the skewness of the histogram. Skewness is a measure of the degree of histogram asymmetry around the mean Symmetric histogram causes zero value.
Uniformity	$\sum_{i=0}^{L-1} P^2(Z_i)$	The maximum value of feature is obtained when the intensity value of pixels are same.
Entropy	$-\sum_{i=0}^{L-1} p(z_i)\log_2 p(z_i)$	Entropy is a measure of histogram uniformity. The closer to the uniform distribution (P(I) constant), the higher the entropy.

Gray-Level Run Lengths

As mentioned earlier, an element in Gray-Level Run Lengths (GLRL) matrix, QRL, presents the number of consecutive pixels having the same gray-level value. In this content, the number of these pixels represents the length of the run. GLRL features include textural information related to the number of times each gray-level appears in different frequencies. For example in the GLRL matrix (2,3) the elements give the number of times gray-level 2 appears in the image with run length of 3.

In GLRL matrix, the number of rows indicates possible gray levels in the image (N_g) and the number of columns is equal to the largest possible run length in the image (N_r). A GLRL matrix can be defined in four different directions; horizontal, diagonal, vertical, and anti-diagonal (0o,45o,90o, 135o) as shown in Figure 1. For direction 0, each element specifies the number of times a gray level appears in the image by itself, or in pairs, just in direction 0.

For the following image

$$I = \begin{bmatrix} 0 & 0 & 1 & 0 \\ 2 & 1 & 0 & 0 \\ 3 & 2 & 3 & 3 \\ 3 & 2 & 2 & 2 \end{bmatrix}$$

Figure 1. Four different directions for defining GLRL. m and n show the top and left directions of an image respectively.

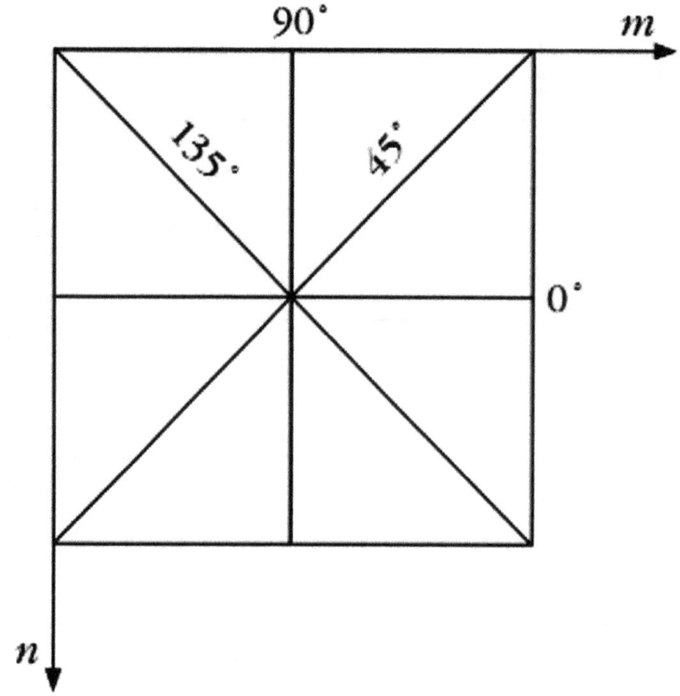

The resulting GLRL matrices for the four principal directions are:

$$Q_{RL}\left(0^{\circ}\right)=\begin{bmatrix}1&2&0&0\\2&0&0&0\\2&0&1&0\\2&1&0&0\end{bmatrix}$$

$$Q_{RL}\left(45^{\circ}\right)=\begin{bmatrix}3&1&0&0\\0&1&0&0\\5&0&0&0\\4&0&0&0\end{bmatrix}$$

$$Q_{RL}\left(90^{\circ}\right)=\begin{bmatrix}3&1&0&0\\2&0&0&0\\3&1&0&0\\2&1&0&0\end{bmatrix}$$

$$Q_{RL}\left(135^{\circ}\right)=\begin{bmatrix}5 & 0 & 0 & 0\\ 2 & 0 & 0 & 0\\ 2 & 0 & 1 & 0\\ 4 & 0 & 0 & 0\end{bmatrix}$$

The first element of the first row of Q_{RL} is the number of times gray-level "0" appears by itself (0 for our example) with direction 45, the second element is the number of times it appears in pairs (2 in the example), and so on. The second row provides the same information for gray-level "1" and so on. Therefore, in matrix (2, 2), for instance, the element indicates the number of times that gray-level "1" appears in pairs.

Based on the preceding dentition of the run length matrix, (Tang, 1998) has defined the following features(Tang, 1998). In all equations N_g and N_r indicate possible gray levels in the image and the largest possible run length in the image respectively, while r(i, j) is the element of GLRL matrix.

1. **Short Run Emphasis (SRE):** $SRE=\dfrac{\sum_{i=1}^{N_g}\sum_{j=1}^{N_r}\dfrac{r\left(i,j\right)}{j^2}}{\sum_{i=1}^{N_g}\sum_{j=1}^{N_r}r\left(i,j\right)}$

2. **Long Run Emphasis (LRE):** $LRE=\dfrac{\sum_{i=1}^{N_g}\sum_{j=1}^{N_r}j^2r\left(i,j\right)}{\sum_{i=1}^{N_g}\sum_{j=1}^{N_r}r\left(i,j\right)}$

3. **Gray Level Non Uniformity (GLNU):** $GLNU=\dfrac{\sum_{i=1}^{N_g}\left(\sum_{j=1}^{N_r}r\left(i,j\right)\right)^2}{\sum_{i=1}^{N_g}\sum_{j=1}^{N_r}r\left(i,j\right)}$

4. **Run Length Non Uniformity (RLNU):** $RLNU=\dfrac{\sum_{i=1}^{N_r}\left(\sum_{j=1}^{N_g}r\left(i,j\right)\right)^2}{\sum_{i=1}^{N_g}\sum_{j=1}^{N_r}r\left(i,j\right)}$

5. **Run Percentage (RP):** $RP=\dfrac{\sum_{i=1}^{N_g}\sum_{j=1}^{N_r}r\left(i,j\right)}{n_p}$

6. **Low Gray Level Run Emphasis (LGRE):** $LGRE=\dfrac{\sum_{i=1}^{N_g}\sum_{j=1}^{N_r}\dfrac{r\left(i,j\right)}{i^2}}{\sum_{i=1}^{N_g}\sum_{j=1}^{N_r}r\left(i,j\right)}$

7. **High Gray Level Run Emphasis (HGRE):** $HGRE=\dfrac{\sum_{i=1}^{N_g}\sum_{j=1}^{N_r}r\left(i,j\right).i^2}{\sum_{i=1}^{N_g}\sum_{j=1}^{N_r}r\left(i,j\right)}$

8. **Short Run Low Gray Level Emphasis (SRLGE):** $SRLGE = \frac{\sum_{i=1}^{N_g}\sum_{j=1}^{N_r}\frac{r(i,j)}{i^2 \cdot j^2}}{\sum_{i=1}^{N_g}\sum_{j=1}^{N_r} r(i,j)}$

9. **Short Run High Gray Level Emphasis (SRHGE):** $SRHGE = \frac{\sum_{i=1}^{N_g}\sum_{j=1}^{N_r}\frac{r(i,j)\cdot i^2}{j^2}}{\sum_{i=1}^{N_g}\sum_{j=1}^{N_r} r(i,j)}.$

10. **Long Run Low Gray Level Emphasis (LRLGE):** $LRLGE = \frac{\sum_{i=1}^{N_g}\sum_{j=1}^{N_r} r(i,j)\cdot i^2 \cdot j^2}{\sum_{i=1}^{N_g}\sum_{j=1}^{N_r} r(i,j)}$

11. **Long Run High Gray Level Emphasis (LRHGE):** $LRHGE = \frac{\sum_{i=1}^{N_g}\sum_{j=1}^{N_r}\frac{r(i,j)\cdot j^2}{i^2}}{\sum_{i=1}^{N_g}\sum_{j=1}^{N_r} r(i,j)}$

Each of features gives different information correspondent to the texture of an image. The value obtained using features is different regarding the smoothness or coarseness of texture. For instance, RP takes low values for smooth images or we expect SRE to be large for coarser and LRE to be large for smoother images.

Gray-Level Co-Occurrence Matrix

Grey-level co-occurrence matrix (GLCM) presents the relative positions among pixels. Let d be the relative distance measured in pixel numbers (d =1 for neighboring pixels, etc.), and N_g is the possible gray levels in the image as described in the previous section. The Co-occurrence matrix Q is a $N_g \times N_g$ matrix, that elements $Q_{CO}(i,j)$ shows the number of pixels at distance d with gray-level values i and j, respectively. This matrix can be constructed in four different directions (0o,45o,90o, 135o) as defined previously. Therefore, each matrix is defined for a special direction (Φ) and distance (d). For the following image

$$I = \begin{bmatrix} 0 & 0 & 1 & 0 \\ 2 & 1 & 0 & 0 \\ 3 & 2 & 3 & 3 \\ 3 & 2 & 2 & 2 \end{bmatrix}$$

The resulting co-occurrence matrices for the four principal directions are as follows:

$$Q_{CO}\left(0^{\circ}, d=1\right) = \begin{bmatrix} 4 & 4 & 0 & 0 \\ 4 & 0 & 2 & 0 \\ 0 & 2 & 4 & 4 \\ 0 & 0 & 4 & 2 \end{bmatrix}$$

$$Q_{CO}\left(90^{\circ}, d=1\right)=\begin{bmatrix} 0 & 2 & 0 & 2 \\ 2 & 0 & 0 & 2 \\ 0 & 0 & 4 & 4 \\ 2 & 2 & 4 & 0 \end{bmatrix}$$

$$Q_{CO}\left(135^{\circ}, d=1\right)=\begin{bmatrix} 2 & 4 & 2 & 4 \\ 4 & 0 & 2 & 0 \\ 0 & 2 & 2 & 6 \\ 4 & 0 & 6 & 2 \end{bmatrix}$$

The first element of the first row of above $Q_{CO}\left(0^{\circ}, d=1\right)$ is the number of times the consecutive pixels (d=1, Φ=0) have the gray value 0. Searching the pixels is performed in the positive and negative directions for each gray level value. So value 4 in the above example, results from searching in the positive and negative directions. From the dentition of the co-occurrence matrix, it is apparent that it is a symmetric one that can be used to reduce subsequent computations.

Based on the preceding definition of co-occurrence matrix, some features can be defined (Haralick, Shanmugam, & Dinstein, 1973). These features give information about the texture of image such as coarseness, smoothness, and so on. 10 features extracted from GLCM are presented below. In all equations, N_g indicates possible gray levels in the image. K is the number of rows in the matrix. p_{ij} refers to the probability of occurrence of element i,j that is calculated as below:

$p_{ij}=\frac{1}{R}q_{ij}$, *R* is the total number of possible pixel pairs and q_{ij} is the element of GLCM matrix.

Extracted features from GLCM matrix.

1. **Max Probability:** $\max(p_{ij})$
2. **Correlation:** $\sum_{i=1}^{k}\sum_{j=1}^{k}(i-j)^2 p_{ij}$
3. **Contrast:** $\sum_{i=1}^{k}\sum_{j=1}^{k}(i-j)^2 p_{ij}$
4. **Uniformity:** $\sum_{i=1}^{k}\sum_{j=1}^{k}p_{ij}^{\ 2}$
5. **Entropy:** $-\sum_{i=1}^{k}\sum_{j=1}^{k}p_{ij}\log_2 p_{ij}$
6. **Homogeneity:** $\sum_{i=1}^{k}\sum_{j=1}^{k}\frac{p_{ij}}{1+|i-j|}$

7. **Dissimilarity:** $\sum_{i=0}^{k}\sum_{j=0}^{k} p_{ij} \mid i - j \mid$

8. **Horizontal Average:** $\mu_i \sum_{i=0}^{k}\sum_{j=0}^{k} i(p_{ij})$

9. **Vertical Average:** $\mu_j \sum_{i=0}^{k}\sum_{j=0}^{k} j(p_{ij})$

10. **Cluster Shade:** $CS = \sum_{i=0}^{k}\sum_{j=0}^{k} ((i - \mu_i) + (j - \mu j))^3 p_{ij}$

11. **Cluster Prominence:** $CP = \sum_{i=0}^{k}\sum_{j=0}^{k} ((i - \mu_i) + (j - \mu j))^4 p_{ij}$

Local Binary Pattern

Local binary pattern (LBP) is a powerful texture based feature extraction method from images that works in a pixel block of them. This block is considered around each pixel of image to extract a feature for corresponding pixel. The size of block in basic LBP is 3×3, but the generic formulation of the operator puts no limitations to the size of the neighborhood. The operator performs the process of thresholding, during which the pixels in the block with the center pixel value is considered as the threshold, and every pixel in the neighborhood with gray value greater than center pixel value is labeled by "1" and otherwise "0". This gives an 8-digit binary number (which is usually converted to decimal for convenience).

The LBP operator performs as in the equation below:

$$LBP_{P,R} = \sum_{i=0}^{P-1} s\left(g_i - g_c\right) 2^i \; S\left(x\right) = \begin{cases} 1 \; x \geq 0 \\ 0 \; x < 0 \end{cases}$$

where P is the number of pixels in the neighborhood. g_i and g_c are the gray value of these pixels and center pixel respectively. These two steps are presented in Figure 2.

A total of $2^8 = 256$ different labels can be obtained depending on the relative gray values of the center and the pixels in the neighborhood. According to the example in figure .if the left top corner be the start

Figure 2. The steps of LBP features formation

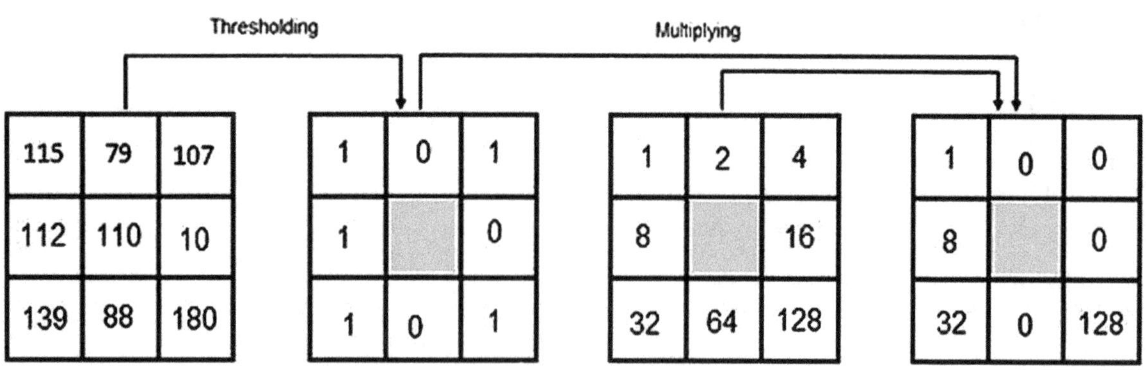

place for constructing binary code with clockwise direction, it will ends up with a binary number, like 10101011. This is 10101110 for start point at top-right. To deal with the difference between patterns, a method is considering largest value of 8 different patterns in clockwise direction. This method also generates rotation invariant features. The corresponding decimal value of the generated binary number is then used for labeling the given pixel. The obtained patterns from any of blocks are used as a feature vector for each image and can describe the texture of the images.

The method is shown in Figure 3. In this example the value 234 is the final pattern.

Features Based on Wavelet

Wavelets are based on small waves of varying frequency and limited duration. Conventional Fourier Transforms is a method for analyzing the signal which is based on sinusoids functions. It separates the Sinusoidal and Cosine components. It provides only the notes or frequency information, temporal information is lost in transformation process. Unlike the Fourier transform, wavelet transform represents a compressed transformation based on different resolutions and scales. The result of every scale and resolution is called wavelet coefficient. In other word wavelet transformation separates the signal to wavelet components in different scales and resolutions as it is presented in Figure 4.

Figure 3. An example of constructing LBP features

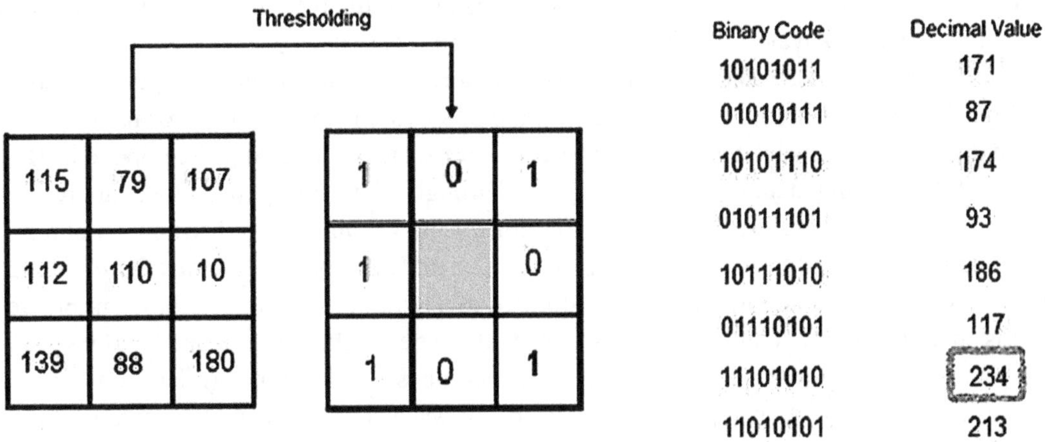

Figure 4. The concept of wavelet transformation
Source: Misiti, Misiti, Oppenheim, & Poggi, 1997.

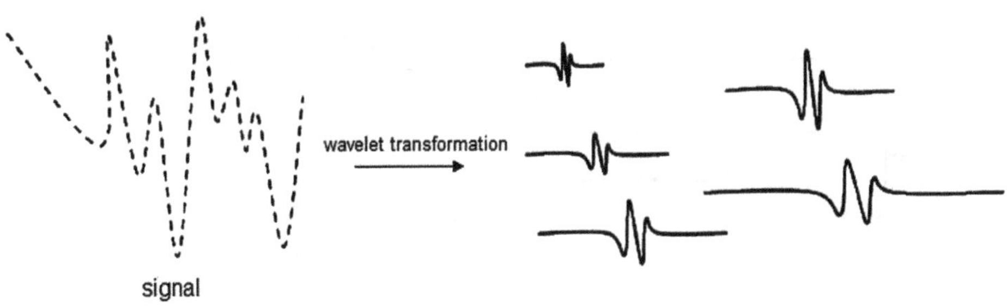

In Continuous wavelet analyzing, the corresponded signal is multiplied to a wavelet function which is Equivalent to window function. The Continuous wavelet is defined as bellow:

$$CWT_x^{\psi}(\tau,s)=\Psi_x^{\psi}(\tau,s)=\frac{1}{\sqrt{|s|}}\int_{-\infty}^{+\infty}x(t)\psi^{*}\left(\frac{t-\tau}{s}\right)dt$$

τ and s are the transition and scaling parameters respectively. Transition parameter controls the amount of movement of window region. Scaling parameter is reversely related to frequency. ψ is the window function called mother wavelet. The most famous mother wavelets are Haar(Haar, 1910), Daubechies(Daubechies, 1992), Meyer(Meyer, 1995). Each wavelet is defined based on some parameters such as, support width, symmetry and the number of vanishing moments. Support width determines the speed of approaching to zero domain in spectral dimension. As a result, large temporal supports for lower frequencies, while maintaining short temporal widths for higher frequencies. The symmetry of wavelet represents the symmetry of signal.

The most digital images don't represent a sinusoidal pattern so it is preferred to analyze the image using a multi resolution wavelet that provides different transformed non sinusoidal pattern (mother wavelet). For calculating wavelet from a discrete signal, it is necessary to apply a low pass filter and high pass filter to signal separately. Through such a pair of filters the signal is decomposed into low- and high-frequency components. In the next step, the obtained low frequency is filtered again using a low pass filter and high pass filter. Through repetition of this procedure, the number of repeating shows the decomposition level of wavelet. This is represented in Figure 5.

For two dimensional cases the transformation is performed as one dimensional; the horizontal and vertical transformation. The figure shows the diagram of a two dimensional transformation.

In two dimensional wavelet, the image with x and y dimension is divided to 4 components (LL، LH، HL and HH). Each component has x/2 and y/2 size. Through the next step, this procedure repeats, and the resulting components are LL^1، LH^1، HL^1 و $HH^1$with x/4 and y/4 dimension. The number of repetitions in time is named decomposition level. Finally, the component LL^n is obtained with $x/2^n$, $y/2^n$ dimension.

So in wavelet transformation, image is transformed to a pyramid structure as shown in Figure 6.

As it is specified, the first and second letters show the type of filter in horizontal and vertical direction, respectively, while the third one represents the decomposition level of wavelet decomposition.

For wavelet analyzing of an image, the coefficients of wavelet are computed. Decomposition is calculated in 5 levels using Daubechies4 wavelet 4 features are extracted from each level including mean,

Figure 5. One dimensional wavelet transformation
Source: Mallat, 1999.

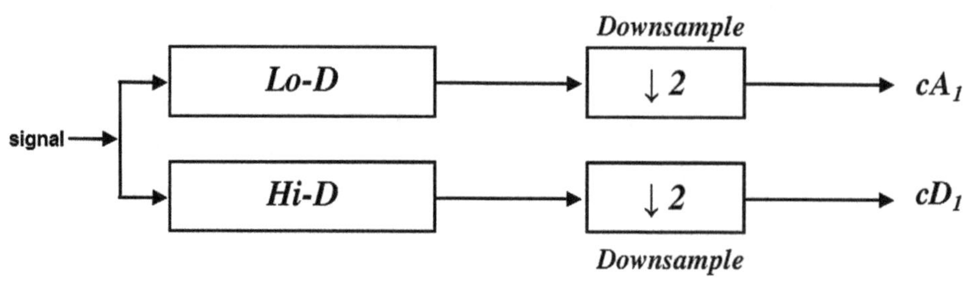

Figure 6. Two dimensional wavelet transformation
Source: Mallat, 1999.

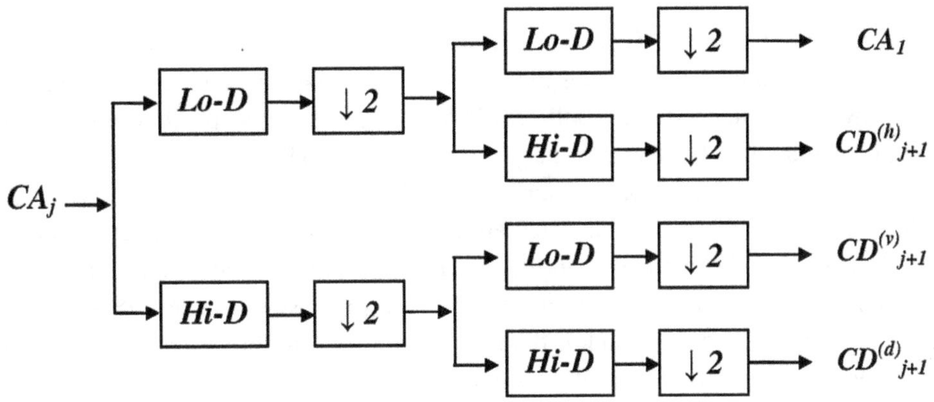

variance, energy and entropy. Consequently, a total of 80 features can be achieved for an image (20 levels *4 features). The 33 features of better results are as below:

- Entropy of horizontal component from levels number 1,2,3.
- Entropy of vertical component from levels number 1,3.
- Entropy of diagonal component from levels number 1,2,3,4.
- Energy of horizontal component from levels number 1,2,3.
- Energy of vertical component from levels number 1,3.
- Energy of diagonal component from levels number 1,2,3,4.
- Variance of horizontal component from level number 2.
- Variance of vertical component from level number 3.
- Variance of diagonal component from level number 2,3,4,5.

Gabor Filter

Gabor feature is obtained based on convolving an image I (x,y) with a 2-D Gabor function g (x,y). The two-dimensional gabor filter is given as the product of a Gaussian low-pass filter with an exponential that is:

$$\frac{1}{2\pi\sigma_x\sigma_y}\exp\left[-\frac{1}{2}\left(\frac{\bar{x}^2}{\sigma_x^{\ 2}}+\frac{\bar{y}^2}{\sigma_y^{\ 2}}\right)\right]\exp[2\pi w\bar{x}]$$

where:

$$\bar{x} = x\cos\theta + y\sin\theta$$

$$\bar{y} = -x\sin\theta + y\sin\theta$$

The parameters σ_x and σ_y are the spatial scaling, which controls the width of the filter, and *w* defines the frequency bandwidths of the filter. The orientation angle θ is usually chosen to be equal to the direction of the filter.

By varying the free parameters θ,σ, and *w* arbitrary orientation and bandwidth characteristics are obtained. Gabor filter banks for analyzing the image in a number of bands, in the context of texture classification, have been successfully employed. If one single value is specified, one convolution per orientation will be computed. If a list of values is given (e.g. 0 and 90 as default), multiple convolutions per orientation will be computed, one for each value in the phase offset list. Filters which are centered at different frequencies and have different orientations are used to cover the frequency range of interest, using various frequency and orientation bandwidths. Images are then filtered through this set of filters, and the features are generated from the resulting output samples. New samples include a matrix *f*×*d* (*f*: the number of different frequencies' and *d:* the number of different directions of filter). Each element of matrix indicates the response at special direction and frequency.

Four different features are extracted from every direction and frequency. These features include the energy, entropy, mean, variance of filtered image.

EXPERIMENTS

In this section, the results of different feature extraction methods on a standard dataset are evaluated. The general steps of experiments are shown in **Error! Reference source not found.**. As it is seen, this chapter focuses on the first step. Evaluation of different feature extraction methods is the main issue in this chapter. The feature reduction step is not important in this scope. The last step is classification that trains a model on training data and then evaluates it by test data. There are different classifiers to build this model. In this chapter, support vector machine (SVM) is utilized. This method is explained in the next section. All methods are implemented in MATLAB R2014a software (Figure 7).

In this chapter, the performance of different feature extraction methods is evaluated based on accuracy, AUC, and confusion matrix criteria.

The definition of accuracy criteria is as bellows:

$$\text{Accuracy} = \frac{\text{TP} + \text{TN}}{\text{P} + \text{N}}$$

Figure 7. A general configuration for medical diagnosis using data mining techniques

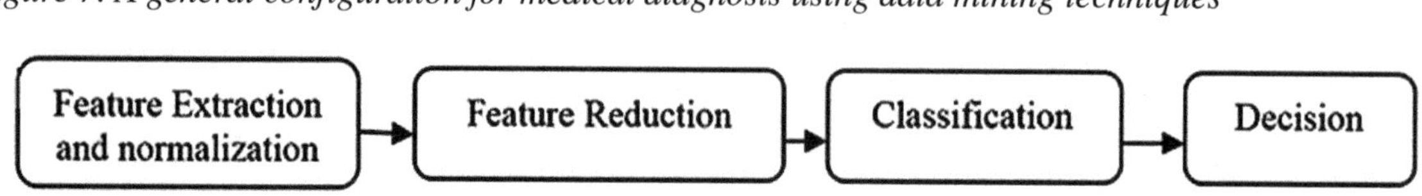

- **True Positives (TP):** These refer to the positive tuples that were correctly labeled by the classier.
- **True Negatives (TN):** These are the negative tuples that were correctly labeled by the classier.
- **False Positives (FP):** These are the negative tuples that were incorrectly labeled as positive.
- **False Negatives (FN):** These are the positive tuples that were mislabeled as negative.

Accuracy is the recognition rate of a method. The accuracy measure works better when the data classes are fairly evenly distributed. Therefore, it is not enough for evaluating a method in unbalanced dataset. In this case, other measures, such as AUC, are better suited. AUC means area under the Receiver Operating Characteristic (ROC) curve. ROC curve is created by plotting the true positive rate (precision) against the false positive rate (recall). It presents the tradeoff between the true positive rate and the false positive rate. The maximum value of AUC is 1.

The confusion matrix is another measure. This measure is a table that each element of it indicates one of the above terms (TP, TN, FP and FN).

For a better generalization of classification, the cross validation method is utilized. For this study 10-fold cross validation is applied. In this method, model assessment is done for 10 times using test set. For this goal the whole dataset is divided into 10 subsets randomly. Each time one part of the data is determined as test set and the remaining parts form training data. The errors of each model at every iteration are accumulated to provide the mean absolute test set error.

All of experiments are performed in different states. All methods of feature extraction have been evaluated using different parameters that should be selected in running the algorithm. Thus, effect of parameters on the performances is shown in the next sections.

Other experiments are related to the evaluation of methods with different number of images. The number of training samples is 140 images (70 images for normal class and 70 images for abnormal class). The number of test images is selected on 10-fold validation. This experiment is performed on two groups of data: training set and test set. The reports of experiments are based on the mean, max, min and standard deviation of accuracy of performance on test data for 10 folds of cross validation. Besides that, for every method, all of train data is utilized to calculate the efficiency of algorithm. Other experiments are performed on 100 selected images. Since some images have noise and bad quality, such as poor lighting conditions. As a result, removing such images will improve the accuracy of diagnosis.

Support Vector Machine

Support vector machine (SVM) is a method for linear and nonlinear classification(Mousavirad & Ebrahimpour-Komleh, 2014). It transforms the original training data into a higher dimension. Within this new dimension, it searches for the linear optimal hyperplane. Suppose that the data set is a linearly separable two class problem. There are an infinite number of hyperplane for separating of data. Figure 8 illustrates a linearly separable two class problem with three hyperplane.

Figure 9 shows two possible hyperplane and their associated margin. Both hyperplane able to classify the data correctly, but hyperplane with the large margin to be more accurate at classifying new instance than the hyperplane with the small margin. SVM searches maximum marginal hyperplane as best hyperplane.

Figure 8. An example of linearly separable two class problem with three hyperplane

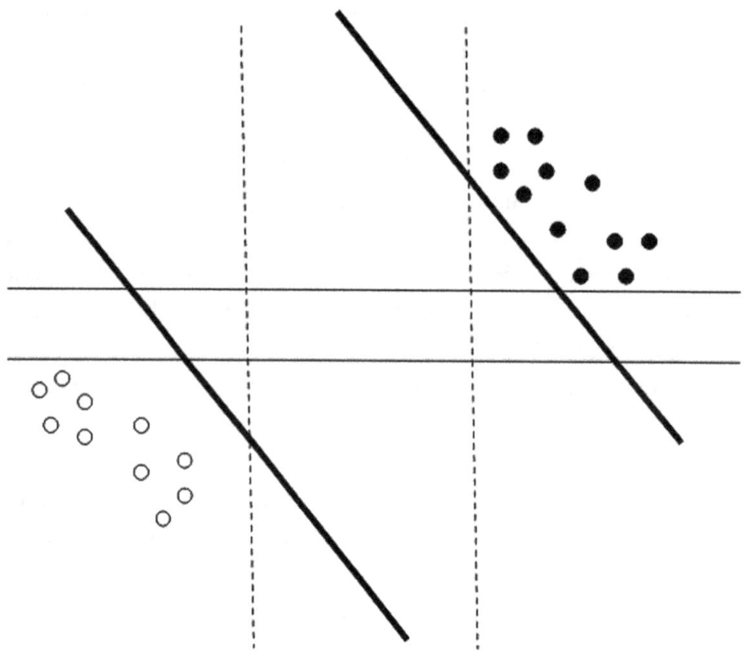

Figure 9. Two hyperplane and their associated margin. Hyperplane with large margin has greater generalization than small margin so is appropriate classification hyperplane

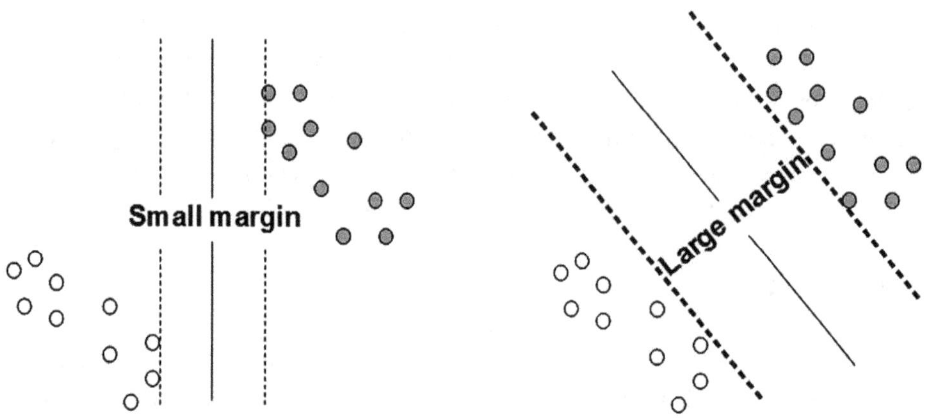

Let us consider a binary classification problem:

$$\{x_i, y_i\},\ i = 1,2,\ldots,L,\ y_i = \{-1,+1\}$$

where x_i are the feature vectors of training set and y_i are the corresponding labels. The goal is to design a hyperplane that classifies correctly all the training vectors. This separating hyperplane can be written as

$$\bar{w}.\bar{x} + b = 0$$

where $\bar{w}$ is a n dimensional weight vector and b is bias. For each training example (x_i, y_i)

$$\bar{w}.\bar{x} + b \leq 0 \quad \text{if } y_i = -1$$
$$\bar{w}.\bar{x} + b \geq 0 \quad \text{if } y_i = +1$$

Combining the above two inequality, we get

$$y_i(\bar{w}.\bar{x} + b) \geq 1 \quad \forall i$$

Support vectors are the closet training data to separating hyperplane. For each support vector, the above inequality is an equality. In Figure 10, the support vectors are shown encircled with a thicker border.

The distance between x_s and the hyperplane is $\frac{1}{\| w \|}$ where $\| w \|$ is the Euclidean norm of w, that is $\sqrt{w_1^2 + w_2^2 + \ldots + w_n^2}$. Therefore, the maximum margin is $\frac{2}{\| w \|}$. The task can be summarized as:

$$\text{minimize} \quad g(w) = \frac{1}{2} \| w \|^2$$
$$\text{subject to } y_i(\bar{w}.\bar{x} + b) \geq 1$$

Figure 10. Support vectors

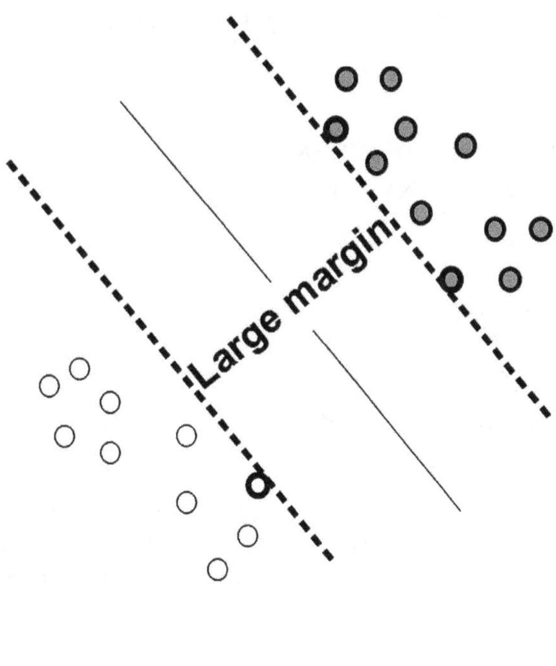

This is a nonlinear optimization task subject to a set of linear inequality constraints. This task can be solve using Karush-Kuhn-Tucker (KKT) conditions. Details can be found in the additional reading list at the end of this chapter.

In order to extend the linear SVMs with nonlinear cases, an extended SVM algorithm is introduced as follows. There are two main steps, first, the original feature vector transforms into a higher dimension space using a non-linear mapping. In the next step, a linear separating hyperplane in the new space is searched.

The computation cost in the training algorithm is very heavy and costly. To overcome this problem, a kernel function, $K(X_i, X_j)$, to the original input vector is applied. That is

$$K(X_i, X_j) = \phi(X_i).\phi(X_j)$$

In other words, $K(X_i, X_j)$ is replaced with $\phi(X_i).\phi(X_j)$ in the training algorithm. In this chapter the kernel function of svm is linear kernel, meaning dot product.

Dataset

The Messidor database ("Messidor project," 2004) has been established to facilitate studies on computer-assisted diagnoses of diabetic retinopathy. Messidor is a research program funded by the French Ministry of Research and Defense within a 2004 TECHNO-VISION program. The 1200 eye fundus color numerical images of the posterior pole for the Messidor database were acquired by 3 ophthalmologic departments using a color video 3CCD camera on a Topcon TRC NW6 non-mydriatic retinograph with a 45 degree field of view. The images were captured using 8 bits per color plane at 1440*960, 2240*1488 or 2304*1536 pixels.

800 images were acquired with pupil dilation (one drop of Tropic amide at 0.5%) and 400 without dilation.

The 1200 images are packaged in 3 sets, one per ophthalmologic department. Each set is divided into 4 zipped sub sets containing each 100 images in TIFF format and an excel file with medical diagnoses for each image. Retinopathy grade has been provided by the medical experts for each image.

- 0 (Normal): (μA = 0) AND (H = 0)
- 1: (0 < μA <= 5) AND (H = 0)
- 2: ((5 < μA < 15) OR (0 < H < 5)) AND (NV = 0)
- 3: (μA >= 15) OR (H >=5) OR (NV = 1)

That:

μA is the number of micro aneurysms.
H is the number of hemorrhages.
NV = 1 indicates neovascularization.
NV = 0 indicates no neovascularization.

In experiments, all images with grade between 1 and 3 is labeled as abnormal. Some sample images with normal and abnormal states are presented in Figure 11 and Figure 12 respectively. The quality of some images is low. Therefore these images can reduce the performance of extracting features and diagnosis.

Figure 11. Some samples of normal eyes

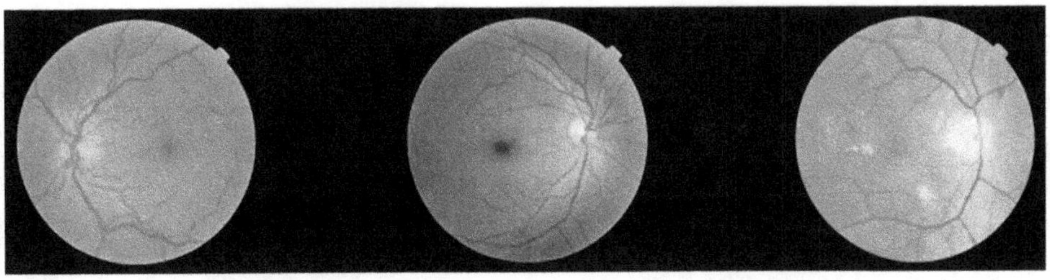

Figure 12. Some samples of altered eyesExperiments on Statistical Feature of Histogram

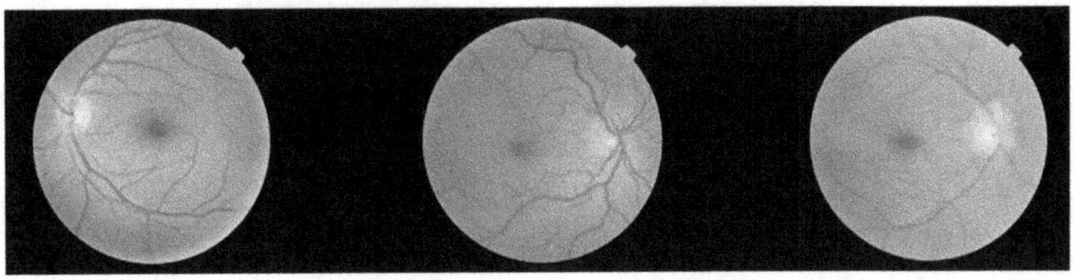

Features extracted from histogram are utilized to classify eye images. The size of vector of these features for every image is 31 including 6 statistical feature that are mean, variance, smoothness, 3rd moment, uniformity and entropy, in addition to 25 features from frequency of gray level values. The feature vectors as inputs are learned using SVM. This method doesn't have any parameter to adjust. Table 2 represents the result of classification for eye images using these features. After selecting images without noise, the accuracy of classification is improved. The results are shown in Table 3. Also the ROC curve of classification in two cases (random images and selected images) are presented in Figure 13 and Figure 14 respectively. The AUC criteria can be obtained from these curves. The value of this important criteria is presented in Table 2 and Table 3.

Table 2. The accuracy of method using Statistical Feature of Histogram

Method	Classification Accuracy					
	Training Set	Test Set				
	Accuracy	Mean	Std. Dev.	Max	Min	AUC
Statistical feature of histogram	79.10	60.5	10.14	83.13	53.44	0.72

Table 3. The accuracy of method using Statistical Feature of Histogram on selected images

Method	Classification Accuracy					
	Training Set	Test Set				
	Accuracy	Mean	Std. Dev.	Max	Min	AUC
Statistical feature of histogram with selected images	93.13	77.45	9.23	80.41	59.30	0.82

Figure 13. The roc curve for classification using Histogram features

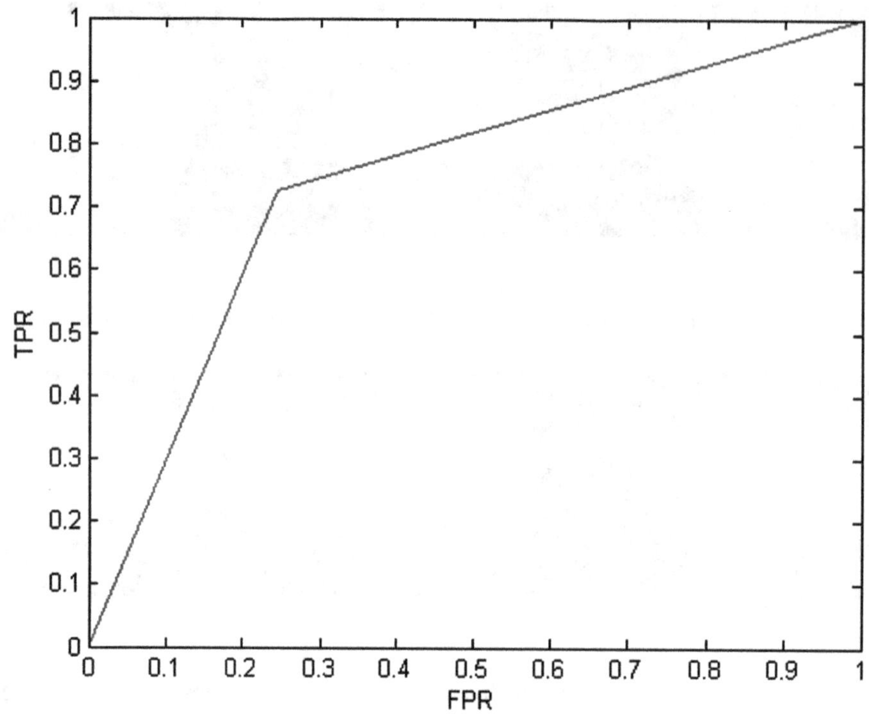

Figure 14. The roc curve for classification using Statistical Feature of Histogram for selected images

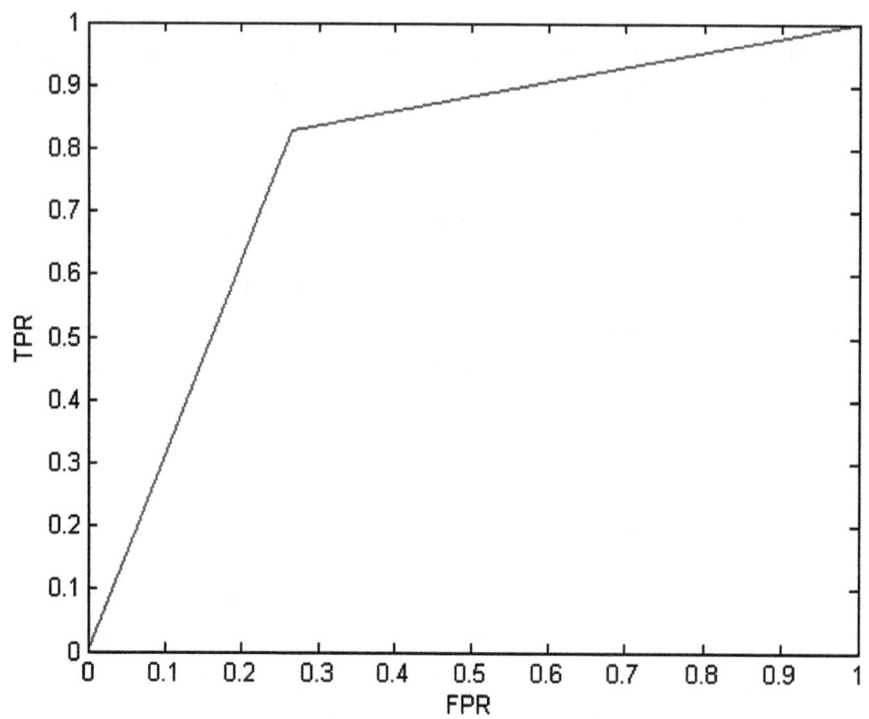

Experiments on Local Binary Pattern

In this Section, the experiment is performed using LBP features extracted from images. The cross validation with k=10 is utilized for the experiments. The performance results of classification using local binary pattern are presented in Table 4. The accuracy of method using LBP features The ROC curve for this case is presented in Figure 15. An important parameter in this method is the size of neighborhood. In the sense that the experiments are evaluated with different size of neighborhood. The worst performance is the result of increasing number of pixels used in extracting features. On the other hand, the best result is obtained when the size of neighborhood is 8 (basic LBP). It is obvious that large size of pixels causes high dimensional feature vectors. Thus more computation is required in this situation. For example, in selection of 8 neighbors, the dimension of feature vectors becomes 256, while the choice of 16 pixels results in 65536 features. Table 5 presents the results of LBP on 100 selected images of dataset. According to the table the improvement of results in this case is visible. The ROC curve of performance for 100 selected images are shown in Figure 16.

Table 4. The accuracy of method using LBP features

Method	Classification Accuracy					
	Training Set	Test Set				
	Accuracy	Mean	Std. Dev.	Max	Min	AUC
LBP	81.06	72.5	7.5	85.71	65.06	0.90

Figure 15. The roc curve for classification using LBP features

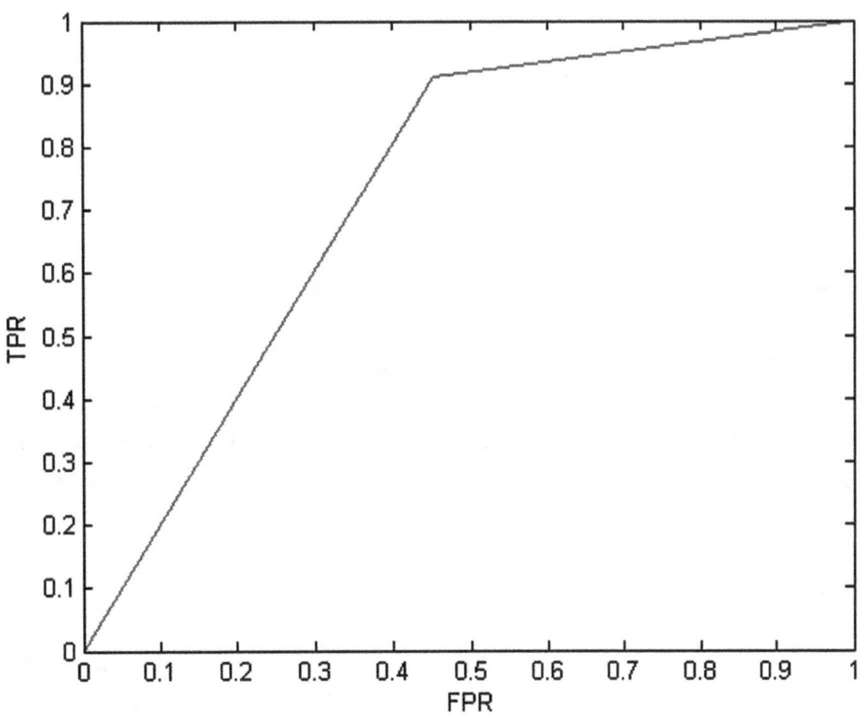

Table 5. The accuracy of method using LBP features on selected images

Method	Classification Accuracy					
	Training Set	Test Set				
	Accuracy	Mean	Std. Dev.	Max	Min	AUC
LBP with selected images	99.01	95.05	3.23	100	90.00	0.98

Figure 16. The roc curve for classification using LBP features for selected images

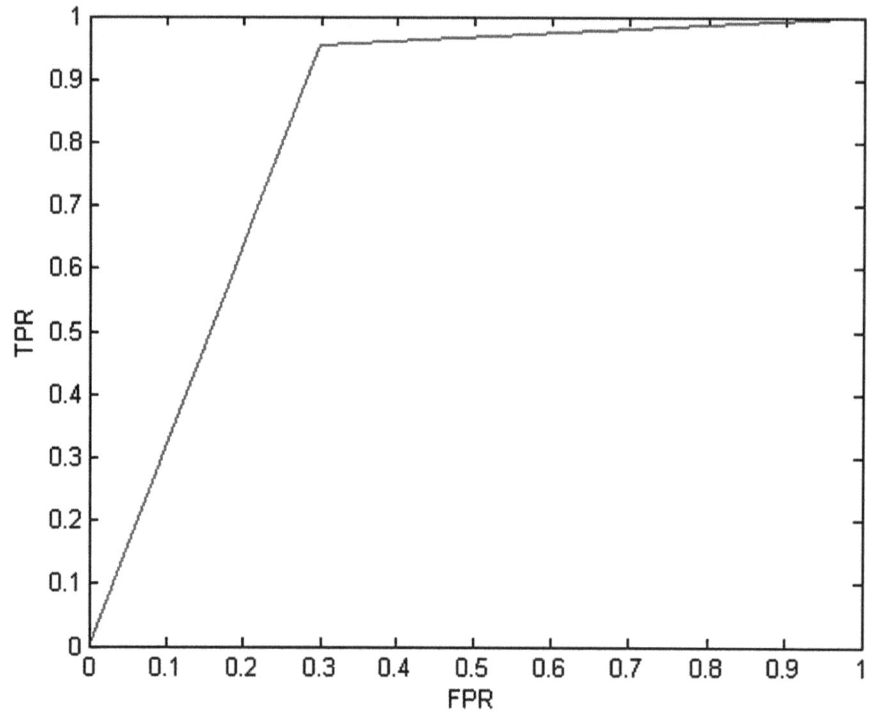

Experiments on Gray-Level Run Lengths

Table 6 shows the results of diagnosis performance using gray-level run length feature extraction method. The size of feature vectors in this case is 44(Eleven features in every directions (0o,45o,90o, 135o)). The definition of extracted features is presented in previous section. Because of low dimensional feature vectors in this method, the computation is lesser. But the performance of the method decreases. Also, the result of evaluation method on selected images is shown in Table 7. As seen in the table, the performance is improved significantly because of removing some images with bad quality. Figure 17 and Figure 18 show the ROC curve of these classification.

Experiment on Gray-Level Co-Occurrence Matrix

In this section the result of classification of data using gray-level co-occurrence features have been evaluated. Table 8 shows the accuracy of experiments on 130 images of two classes. The result of these features is weaker than two previous methods. The ROC plot of these results is shown in Figure 19.

Table 6. The accuracy of method using GLRL features

Method	Classification Accuracy					
	Training Set	Test Set				
	Accuracy	Mean	Std. Dev.	Max	Min	AUC
GLRL	98.45	63.78	8.43	75.65	53.22	0.78

Table 7. The accuracy of method using GLRL features on selected images

Method	Classification Accuracy					
	Training Set	Test Set				
	Accuracy	Mean	Std. Dev.	Max	Min	AUC
GLRL with selected images	99.13	80.45	9.78	88.88	69.10	0.89

Figure 17. The roc curve for classification using GLRL features

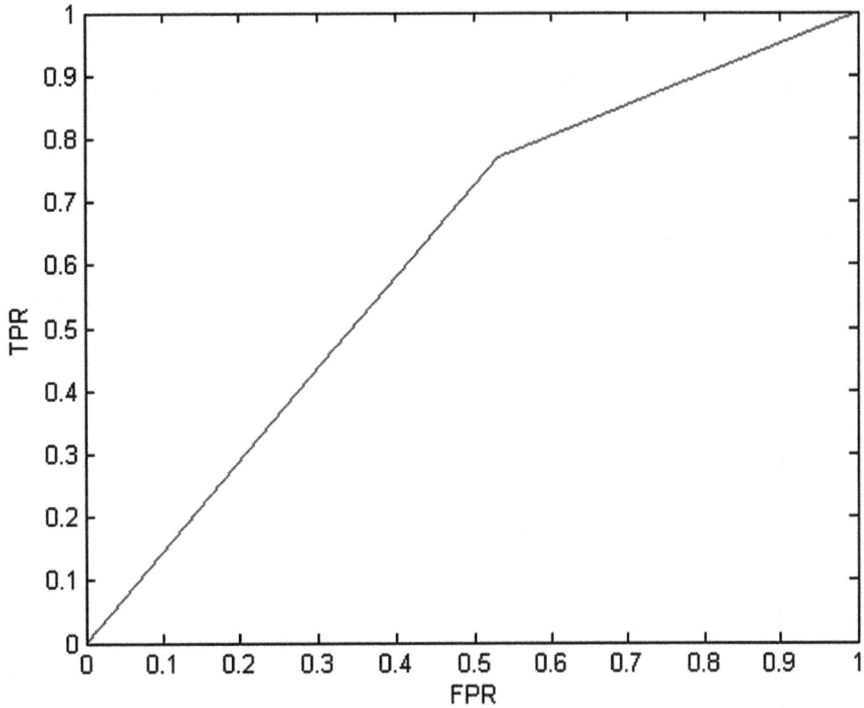

An important parameter in constructing co-occurrence matrix is the relative distance measured in pixel numbers. At the basic GLCM, the distance is set 1. In these experiments, the change of distance doesn't have effect on the performance. Therefore, considering 1 pixel as neighbor results in the best accuracy. Also, the number of features isn't related to the number of bits in binary number, because the number of extracted features is 10 despite of the distance considered for constructing matrix. These features have been calculated in 4 different directions (directions (0o,45o,90o, 135o).

Figure 18. The roc curve for classification using GLRL features for selected images

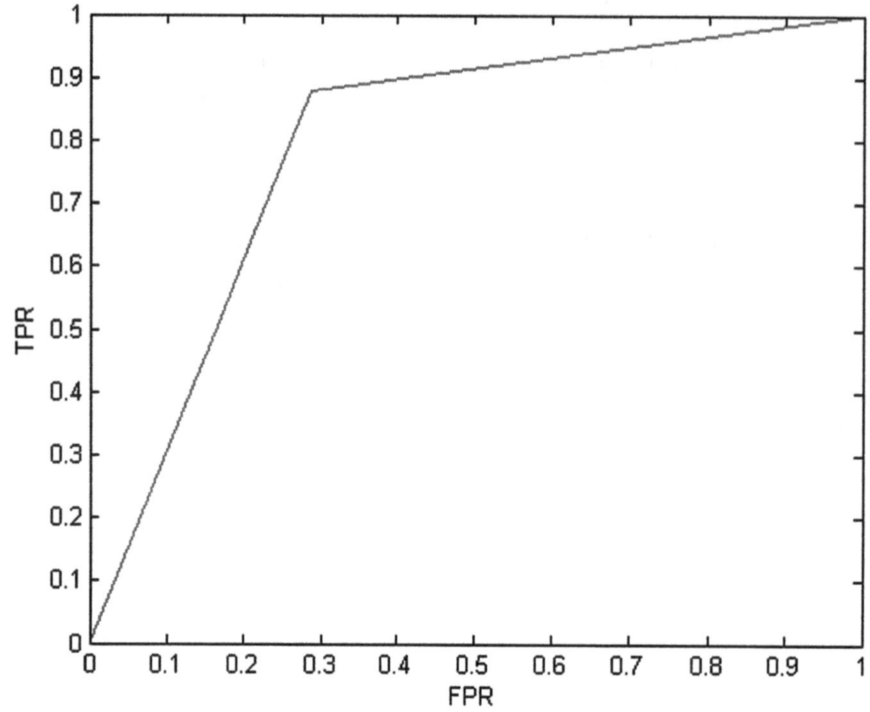

Figure 19. The roc curve for classification using GLCM features

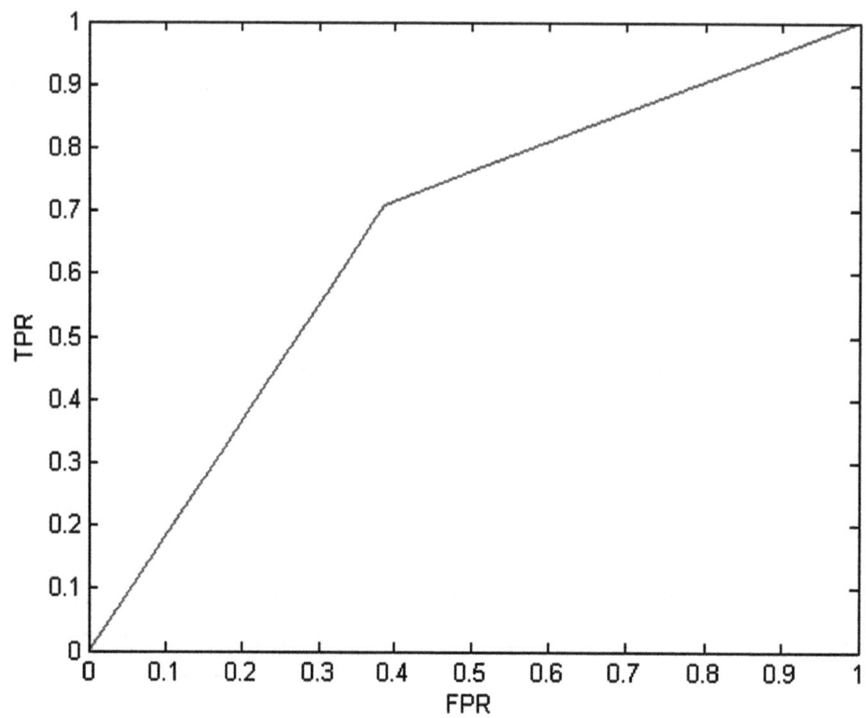

Table 8. The accuracy of method using GLCM features

Method	Classification Accuracy					
	Training Set	Test Set				
	Accuracy	Mean	Std. Dev.	Max	Min	AUC
GLCM	75.45	61.30	12.01	72.12	55.81	0.72

Another experiment for this method is based on 100 selected images. Table 9 exhibits the accuracy of this case. The improving performance is explicit. Some noisy images affect the result of diagnosis. ROC plot of this experiment is also demonstrated in Figure 20.

Table 9. The accuracy of method using GLCM features on selected images

Method	Classification Accuracy					
	Training Set	Test Set				
	Accuracy	Mean	Std. Dev.	Max	Min	AUC
GLCM with selected images	90.51	77.54	9.75	90.12	71.40	0.85

Figure 20. The roc curve for classification using GLCM features for selected images

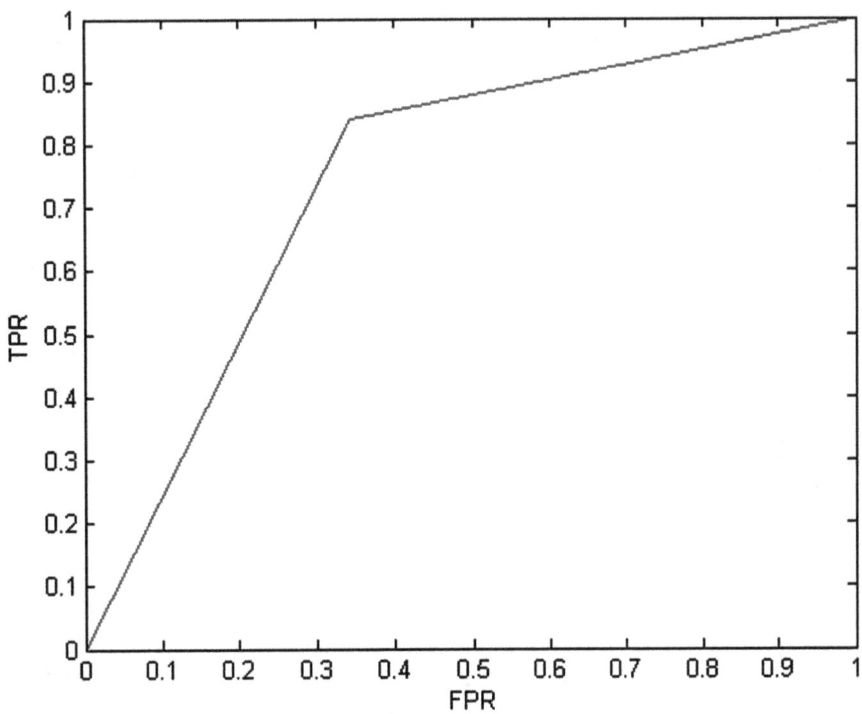

Experiments on Wavelet Features

As explained in previous section, the 4 types of features (mean, variance, entropy and energy) can be extracted from resulting components of wavelet transformation. From each component resulting from wavelet transformation, 4 features are extracted so the size of feature vector in this method is 80. But all of these features are not adequate for classification. An optimization algorithm like Imperialist Competitive Algorithm (ICA)(Atashpaz-Gargari & Lucas, 2007) can be utilized to select the best feature for classification. Table 10 and Table 11show the result of classification using these features from random and selected images. The ROC plot of classification based on these experiment also is presented in Figure 21 and Figure 22.

Experiments on Gabor Filter

The last method for evaluation is gabor filter. The parameter frequency is 8 and the orientation is along 4 basic directions. The accuracy of this method with 10-fold validation is showed in Table 12. This method has weaker results compared to previous feature extraction methods. Using 100 selected images in dataset improves the performance as presented in Table 13. Figure 23 and Figure 24 show the obtained ROC curve of classification results.

Figure 21. The roc curve for classification using wavelet features

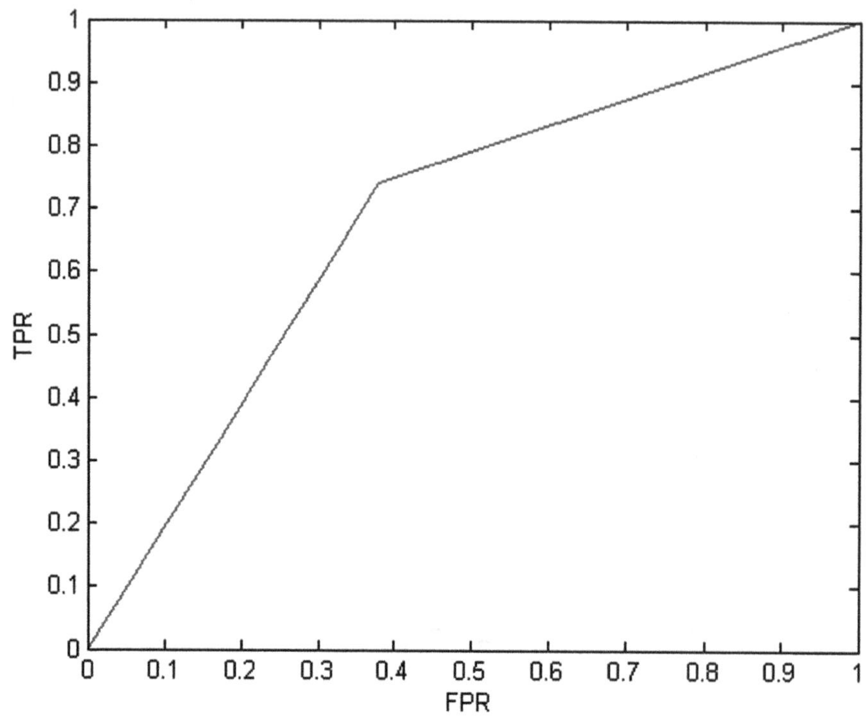

Table 10. The accuracy of method using wavelet features

Method	Classification Accuracy					
	Training Set	Test Set				
	Accuracy	Mean	Std. Dev.	Max	Min	AUC
Wavelet features	91.58	65.12	4.76	69.01	52.20	0.74

Figure 22. The roc curve for classification using wavelet features for selected images

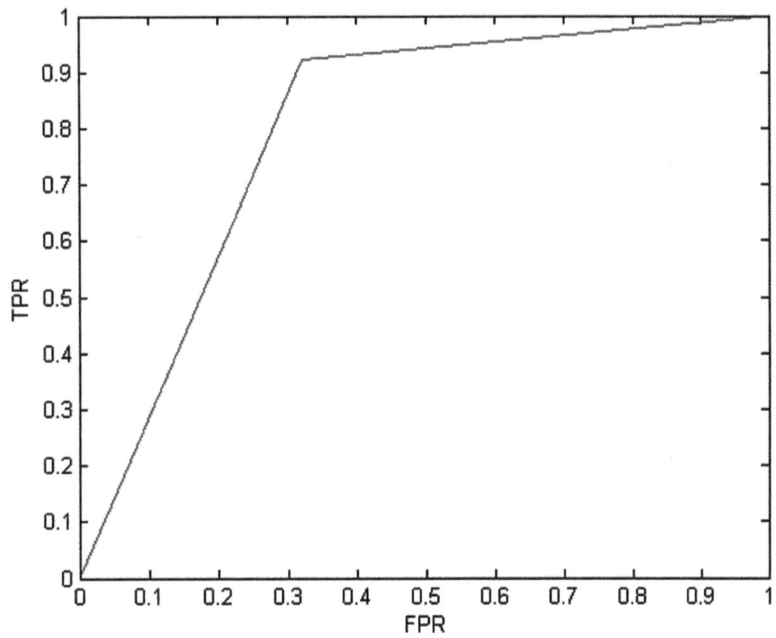

Table 11. The accuracy of method using wavelet features on selected images

Method	Classification Accuracy					
	Training Set	Test Set				
	Accuracy	Mean	Std. Dev.	Max	Min	AUC
Wavelet features with selected images	97.5	80.20	3.45	70. 30	61.00	0.92

Table 12. The accuracy of method using Gabor filer features

Method	Classification Accuracy					
	Training Set	Test Set				
	Accuracy	Mean	Std. Dev.	Max	Min	AUC
Gabor filer	77.58	54.47	3.28	57.43	50.00	0.55

Table 13. The accuracy of method using Gabor filer features on selected images

Method	Classification Accuracy					
	Training Set	Test Set				
	Accuracy	Mean	Std. Dev.	Max	Min	AUC
Gabor filter with selected images	91.11	65.71	3.15	71.00	63.63	0.62

Figure 23. The roc curve for classification using Gabor Filter features

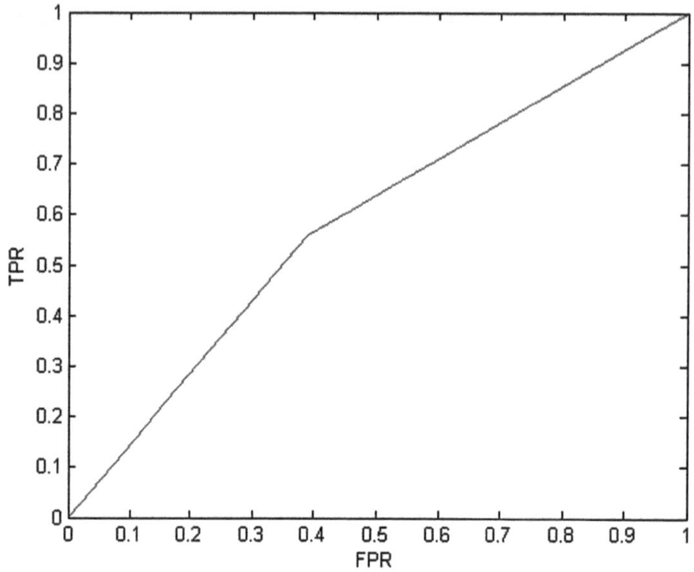

Figure 24. The roc curve for classification using Gabor Filter features for selected images

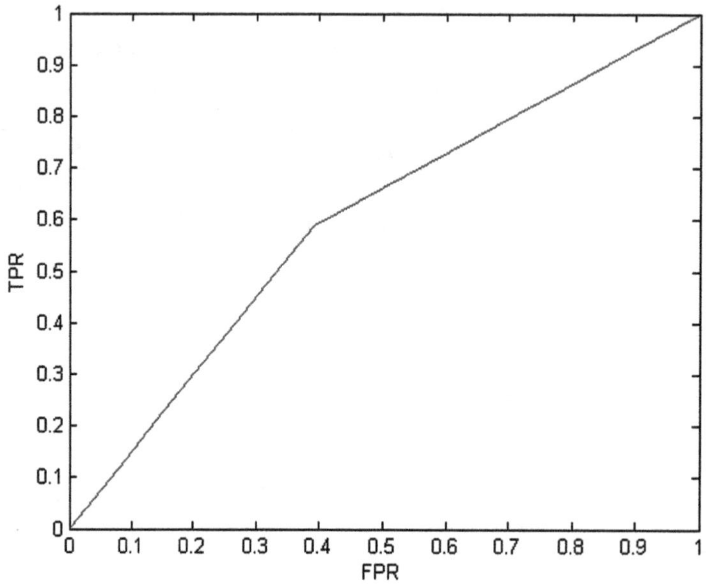

Table 14. The comparison result of different textural feature extraction methods

Method	Accuracy
Statistical feature of histogram	60.5
LBP features	72.5
GLRL features	63.78
GLCM features	61.30
Wavelet features	65.12
Gabor feature	54.47

DISCUSSION

In this section all results from different methods are compared with each other. According to results represented in Table 14 the classification of normal and altered images using features extracted by LBP method has best result. The detection retinopathy can be performed with 72.5 percent accuracy. The other methods outperform LBP method. However some of them such as wavelet features results close to LBP.

CONCLUSION

This chapter presented some predictive techniques for diabetic retinopathy detection. For this purpose, different texture based feature extraction techniques such as statistical features of histogram, grey level co-occurrence matrix, grey level run length matrix, wavelet transform features, gabor filter and local binary pattern has been considered. The results of classification of diabetic retinopathy images is compared. Based on these results, machine learning methods can be utilized to help expert's diagnosis diabetic retinopathy.

REFERENCES

Atashpaz-Gargari, E., & Lucas, C. (2007). *Imperialist competitive algorithm: an algorithm for optimization inspired by imperialistic competition.* Paper presented at the Evolutionary Computation, 2007. CEC 2007. IEEE Congress on. doi:10.1109/CEC.2007.4425083

Bascil, M. S., & Oztekin, H. (2012). A study on hepatitis disease diagnosis using probabilistic neural network. *Journal of Medical Systems*, *36*(3), 1603–1606. doi:10.1007/s10916-010-9621-x PMID:21057884

Conforti, D., & Guido, R. (2010). Kernel based support vector machine via semidefinite programming: Application to medical diagnosis. *Computers & Operations Research*, *37*(8), 1389–1394. doi:10.1016/j.cor.2009.02.018

Daubechies, I. (1992). *Ten lectures on wavelets* (Vol. 61). SIAM. doi:10.1137/1.9781611970104

Gonzales, R. C., Woods, R. E., & Eddins, S. L. (2004). *Digital image processing using MATLAB*. Pearson Prentice Hall.

Haar, A. (1910). On the theory of orthogonal function systems. *Math. Ann, 69*(3), 331–371. doi:10.1007/BF01456326

Haralick, R. M. (1979). Statistical and structural approaches to texture. *Proceedings of the IEEE, 67*(5), 786–804. doi:10.1109/PROC.1979.11328

Haralick, R. M., Shanmugam, K., & Dinstein, I. H. (1973). Textural features for image classification. *Systems, Man and Cybernetics, IEEE Transactions on,* (6), 610-621.

Hoover, A., & Goldbaum, M. (2003). Locating the optic nerve in a retinal image using the fuzzy convergence of the blood vessels. *Medical Imaging. IEEE Transactions on, 22*(8), 951–958.

Illingworth, J., & Kittler, J. (1988). A survey of the Hough transform. *Computer Vision Graphics and Image Processing, 44*(1), 87–116. doi:10.1016/S0734-189X(88)80033-1

International Federation Diabetes. (2014). Retrieved from http://www.idf.org/complications-diabetes

Klein, R., Meuer, S. M., Moss, S. E., & Klein, B. E. (1995). Retinal microaneurysm counts and 10-year progression of diabetic retinopathy. *Archives of Ophthalmology, 113*(11), 1386–1391. doi:10.1001/archopht.1995.01100110046024 PMID:7487599

Kononenko, I. (2001). Machine learning for medical diagnosis: History, state of the art and perspective. *Artificial Intelligence in Medicine, 23*(1), 89–109. doi:10.1016/S0933-3657(01)00077-X PMID:11470218

Kononenko, I., Bratko, I., & Kukar, M. (1997). Application of machine learning to medical diagnosis. *Machine Learning and Data Mining: Methods and Applications, 389*, 408.

Mallat, S. (1999). *A wavelet tour of signal processing*. Academic Press.

Marčelja, S. (1980). Mathematical description of the responses of simple cortical cells*. *JOSA, 70*(11), 1297–1300. doi:10.1364/JOSA.70.001297 PMID:7463179

Messidor Project. (2004). Retrieved from http://messidor.crihan.fr/download-en.php

Meyer, Y. (1995). *Wavelets and operators* (Vol. 1). Cambridge university press.

Misiti, M., Misiti, Y., Oppenheim, G., & Poggi, J.-M. (1997). Wavelet toolbox. Matlab User's Guide, 64.

Mousavirad, S. J., & Ebrahimpour-Komleh, H. (2014). A Comparative Study on Medical Diagnosis Using Predictive Data Mining: A Case Study. *Data Mining and Analysis in the Engineering Field*, 327.

Niemeijer, M., Staal, J., van Ginneken, B., Loog, M., & Abramoff, M. D. (2004). *Comparative study of retinal vessel segmentation methods on a new publicly available database.* Paper presented at the Medical Imaging 2004. doi:10.1117/12.535349

Ojala, T., Pietikäinen, M., & Mäenpää, T. (2002). Multiresolution gray-scale and rotation invariant texture classification with local binary patterns. *Pattern Analysis and Machine Intelligence. IEEE Transactions on, 24*(7), 971–987.

Pinz, A., Bernögger, S., Datlinger, P., & Kruger, A. (1998). Mapping the human retina. *Medical Imaging. IEEE Transactions on, 17*(4), 606–619.

Polat, K., & Güneş, S. (2006). Hepatitis disease diagnosis using a new hybrid system based on feature selection (FS) and artificial immune recognition system with fuzzy resource allocation. *Digital Signal Processing, 16*(6), 889–901. doi:10.1016/j.dsp.2006.07.005

Polat, K., & Güneş, S. (2007). Breast cancer diagnosis using least square support vector machine. *Digital Signal Processing, 17*(4), 694–701. doi:10.1016/j.dsp.2006.10.008

Polat, K., Güneş, S., & Tosun, S. (2006). Diagnosis of heart disease using artificial immune recognition system and fuzzy weighted pre-processing. *Pattern Recognition, 39*(11), 2186–2193. doi:10.1016/j.patcog.2006.05.028

Silberman, N., Ahrlich, K., Fergus, R., & Subramanian, L. (2010). *Case for Automated Detection of Diabetic Retinopathy.* Paper presented at the AAAI Spring Symposium: Artificial Intelligence for Development.

Tang, X. (1998). Texture information in run-length matrices. *Image Processing. IEEE Transactions on, 7*(11), 1602–1609.

Vatanparast, M., & Harati, A. (2012). *A feasibility study on detection of Neovascularization in retinal color images using texture.* Paper presented at the Computer and Knowledge Engineering (ICCKE), 2012 2nd International eConference on. doi:10.1109/ICCKE.2012.6395382

Vetterli, M., & Herley, C. (1992). Wavelets and filter banks: Theory and design. *Signal Processing. IEEE Transactions on, 40*(9), 2207–2232. doi:10.1109/78.157221

Walter, T., Klein, J.-C., Massin, P., & Erginay, A. (2002). A contribution of image processing to the diagnosis of diabetic retinopathy-detection of exudates in color fundus images of the human retina. *Medical Imaging. IEEE Transactions on, 21*(10), 1236–1243.

Wu, D., Zhang, M., Liu, J.-C., & Bauman, W. (2006). On the adaptive detection of blood vessels in retinal images. *Biomedical Engineering. IEEE Transactions on, 53*(2), 341–343.

Chapter 13
Analysis of Electrocardiogram Data Compression Techniques:
A MATLAB-Based Approach

Anukul Pandey
Dr. B. R. Ambedkar National Institute of Technology, India

Butta Singh
Guru Nanak Dev University Regional Campus, India

Barjinder Singh Saini
Dr. B. R. Ambedkar National Institute of Technology, India

Neetu Sood
Dr. B. R. Ambedkar National Institute of Technology, India

ABSTRACT

In this Chapter, a MATLAB-based approach is presented for compression of Electrocardiogram (ECG) data. The methodology employs in three different domains namely direct, transformed and parameter extraction methods. The selected techniques from direct ECG compression methods are TP, AZTEC, Fan, and Cortes. Moreover selected techniques from transformed ECG compression methods are Walsh Transform, DCT, and Wavelet transform. For each of the technique, the basic implementation of the algorithm was explored, and performance measures were calculated. All 48 records of MIT-BIH arrhythmia ECG database were employed for performance evaluation of various implemented techniques. Moreover, based on requirements, any basic techniques can be selected for further innovative processing that may include the lossless encoding.

INTRODUCTION

In current era, patient monitoring systems are gaining importance which results in ever increasing data volume of various biomedical signals such as Electrocardiogram (ECG), Electroencephalogram (EEG) and Electromyogram (EMG). One of the open research problem in biomedical signal processing is the development of efficient data reduction technique (Sabarimalai Sur & Dandapat, 2014). Such techniques rely on maintaining a trade-off between minimization of reconstruction error and maximization of Compression Ratio (CR). ECG monitoring facilitates in providing faster health status of the concerned

DOI: 10.4018/978-1-5225-0660-7.ch013

patient to the health care centre in case of the hostile cardiac behaviour. Cardiac monitoring using ECG signal is the best representative of heart electrical functionality and had proven to be effective in the diagnosis of most of the heart diseases. For continuous monitoring of patient's health status, the ECG signal is recorded for long time durations typically for several hours or few days. The storage of such huge volume of data requires large memory space, for example, a three-channel ECG signal sampled at a frequency of 1 kHz with 11 bits of resolution in three lead system of a particular patient, recorded for 24 h requires 928 MB of memory size per channel without any overhead. Such huge volume of data is also expected to have inter and intra beat correlation or inherent sparsity (Lee, Kim, & Lee, 2011; Ma, Zhang, & Dong, 2015).

So in the present chapter, a brief analysis of algorithms, mathematical background and its simulation implementation using MATLAB, for ECG data compression will be discussed. In order to make the ECG compression technique as a practical tool, this chapter is intended to refer to the MATLAB based routines. Matlab code (.m) of the most common ECG compression methods and algorithms are demonstrated in this chapter.

The performance evaluation of any ECG data compression techniques can be broadly assessed through following six parameters namely 1) Compression Ratio (CR), 2) Percent Root Mean Square Difference (PRD), 3) Percent Root Mean Square Difference Normalized (PRDN), 4) Root Mean Square (RMS) error, 5) Signal to Noise Ratio (SNR), 6) Quality Score (QS). These six qualitative performance evaluation parameters mentioned above are extensively used in literature for accessing the efficiency of any of the compression techniques.

The compression measure CR is equally applicable to both domains where there is difference or same sample resolution in compressed data. The degree of distortion measure in reconstructed ECG signal is primarily computed with respect to the original data, based on the visual as well the qualitative evaluation. The six qualitative performance evaluation parameters mentioned above are extensively used in literature for the comparison purpose (Batista, Melcher, & Carvalho, 2001; Blanco-Velasco et al., 2005; Lee et al., 2011).

The comparison of existing ECG compression methods using the above mentioned performance measures can be carried out, by performing experimentations over most cited Massachusetts Institute of Technology - Beth Israel Hospital (MIT-BIH) database.

Any digital data source has inherent redundancy, if the generated symbols are not equi-probable. The fundamental goal of any data compression approach is efficient data transmission or storage while preserving the significant diagnostic features. The process of data compression seeks to reduce the number of bits of information required to store or transmit digitized ECG signals without a significant reduction in the signal quality (ECG features). Data reduction of ECG signal is achieved by discarding digitized samples that are not vital for rhythm interpretation. For such data reduction, compression techniques are designed, which are classified as lossless or lossy techniques.

The lossless data compression guarantees the integrity of reconstructed data at a compromised CR, typically CR level of 2 to 1 with exact replication of original ECG while the lossy data compression achieves a high compression ratio with varying level of reconstruction error.

For ECG data compression, mostly the lossy type has been applied due to its capability of a high data compression ratio. The efficiency of any compression algorithm can only be evaluated after reconstructing the original signal through the process of decompression. The PRD is used as a similarity measure for the reconstructed and original ECG. The ECG data compression methods can also be broadly divided into three categories namely direct method, transformed method and parameter extraction method.

The direct data compression method analyzes and reduces data points in the time domain. Various direct data ECG compression schemes which includes Turning Point (TP), Amplitude Zone Time Epoch Coding (AZTEC), improved modified AZTEC technique, Co-ordinate Reduction Time Encoding System (CORTES), the delta algorithm and the Fan algorithm. They all have shown their ability for the efficient ECG data reduction.

Typically, AZTEC algorithm has the advantage of high data reduction ratio but suffers from loss of data fidelity due to the presence of discontinuity that occurs in the reconstructed ECG waveform. ASCII based encoding methods are also employed for compression due to its simplicity, which enables them to be used in portable and mobile data ECG data monitoring systems.

The transformed method analyzes energy distribution of the ECG samples by converting the time domain to some other domain, like Fourier transform, Fourier descriptor, Karhunen–Loeve Transform (KLT), the Walsh transform, the Discrete Cosine Transform (DCT) and the wavelet transform etc. This methods falls in category of lossy ECG compression methods as it mostly employs thresholding at some level. The main parameters which needs to be optimized are namely, CR, PRD and threshold value. The transformed based ECG compression method generally consist of following stages, i) pre-processing; for noise removal, ii) transformation; for visualization in other domain, iii) retention of significant coefficients, iv) application of quantization and v) lossless encoding. In the proposed chapter each and every stage was mathematically analyzed and the simulation results has been produced with MATLAB.

The parameter extraction method is based upon dominant feature extraction from the raw signal. The extracted parameter are quantized and then entropy coder is applied for enhancing the compression efficiency. This method includes the processes like vector quantization, peak picking and linear prediction method. There is scope of combining two or more ECG data compression techniques to get better compression efficiency in one or other domain which is an open research problem.

An extensive survey of the various compression methods highlighting their advantages, disadvantages, mathematical analysis and simulation results using MATLAB platform is presented in this chapter proposal thereby facilitating the future research in this direction.

Need of ECG Data Compression

In brief, ECG data compression techniques is the art of signal processing preserving the diagnostic information in a compact form. For any individual under cardiac observation, the ECG data is retrieved continuously online or offline as per prescribed by the cardiac expert. The digitation of ECG data is carried through at the acquisition stage by selecting appropriate sampling frequency and quantization levels. For example as shown in Figure 1, a three-channel ECG signal sampled at a frequency of 1 kHz with 11 bits of resolution in three lead system of a particular patient, recorded for 24 h requires 928 MB of memory size per channel without any overhead. Such huge volume of data is expected to have inter and intra beat correlation or inherent sparsity. For monitoring purpose three lead configuration for ECG acquisition is appropriate. In general for clinical acceptability 12 lead configuration is recommended. This voluminous data can only be handled via appropriate compression technique with varying level of compression ratio and degree of distortion.

Figure 1. ECG data memory size requirement with and without compression technique

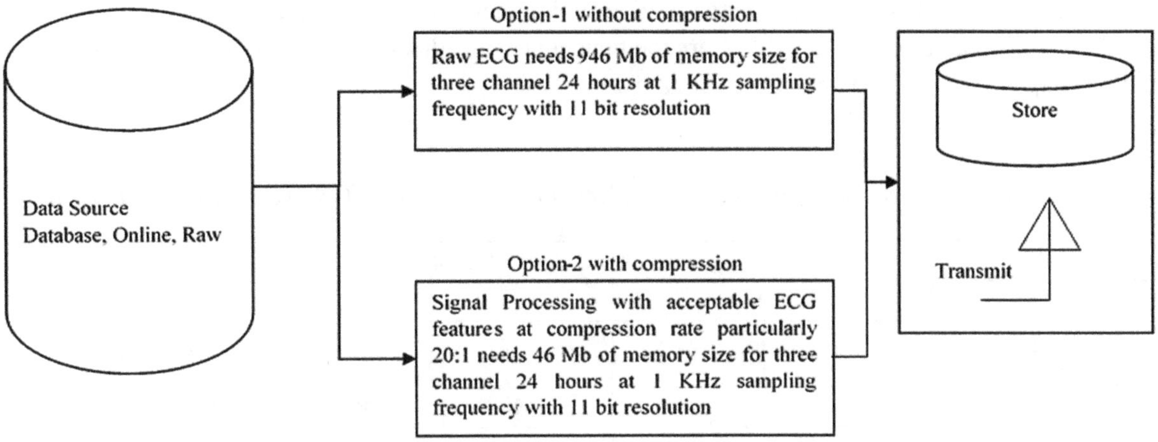

Redundancy in the ECG Data

ECG data compression is possible, because ECG, in general, are highly correlated in inter and intra beat which leads to redundancy. High rate of compression can be achieved through reduction in redundancy and correlation present in ECG data. Redundancy can be inferred as repeated intra beat data in ECG as quasi-stationary sense and higher statistical correlation in inter beat ECG represent plateaus.

DATABASE AND PERFORMANCE MEASURE

In the emerging field of medical engineering, research subjects like cardiac arrhythmia detection (Baibars, Kanjwal, & Marine, 2014), heart rate variability (Singh & Singh, 2012), cardiovascular and pulmonary dynamics (Cheng, 2015), artificial intelligence based medical decision support (Hebert, Korabek, & Scott, 2006)and ECG data compression(Jalaleddine, Hutchens, Strattan, & Coberly, 1990; Ma et al., 2015; Sabarimalai Sur & Dandapat, 2014), etc. are of major interest. The Massachusetts Institute of Technology (MIT) supplies some invaluable resources for such research projects. These resources include databases containing recorded physiological signals and software for analyzing, viewing and creating such recordings. In the present study, ECG samples from Arrhythmia Database (Goldberger et al., 2000) (http://ecg.mit.edu) have been taken for investigation of the efficiency of the various methods. The Database contains 48 half-hour excerpts of two-channel ambulatory ECG recordings, obtained from 47 subjects studied by the BIH Arrhythmia Laboratory. The 11-bit resolutions over 10 mV range with a sampling frequency of 360 Hz per sample channel were recorded. To access the compressor efficiency, first 21,600 samples (10 min duration) were used and evaluated with following six data objective compression performance measure metric (Batista et al., 2001; Blanco-Velasco et al., 2005; Lee et al., 2011).

The .mat file can be extracted from (http://www.physionet.org/cgi-bin/atm/ATM) by selecting appropriate database which is MIT-BIH Arrhythmia Database (mitdb). The record number and appropriate time duration can be selected for export signal as .mat file from toolbox provided by website. For typical record 100, 117 and 119 the extracted transposed sample values for different leads are given in Table 1. The total 6, 50,000 ECG samples per lead is presented per record for 30 minutes of duration at 360 Hz sampling frequency. This total number of samples can be calculated approximately as 360×60×30.09 (sampling frequency× second to minute unit conversion factor × time in minutes).

The sample values stated in Table 1 are the benchmark for illustrating different preceding examples in this chapter. The performance measures are

Table 1. Extracted discrete sample values for selected records from MIT-BIH Arrhythmia Database

	Record					
	100		117		119	
Sample Number	MLII	V5	MLII	V2	MLII	V1
1	995	1011	839	930	825	930
2	995	1011	839	930	825	930
3	995	1011	839	930	825	930
4	995	1011	839	930	825	930
5	995	1011	839	930	825	930
6	995	1011	839	930	825	930
7	995	1011	839	930	825	930
8	995	1011	840	930	821	930
9	1000	1008	840	930	827	933
10	997	1008	836	927	827	934
11	995	1007	836	926	830	935
12	994	1007	833	922	829	942
13	992	1009	830	921	830	939
14	993	1010	830	921	826	941
15	992	1010	828	921	824	940
16	989	1011	828	923	820	939
17	988	1013	831	924	819	935
18	987	1014	834	923	818	934
19	990	1014	836	928	815	933
20	993	1016	842	929	819	935
-	-	-	-	-	-	-
100	957	989	833	910	945	943
101	958	985	835	917	940	941
102	957	987	836	913	935	942
-	-	-	-	-	-	-
498	960	985	839	903	1236	735
499	961	987	840	906	1276	690
500	963	990	840	903	1312	650
-	-	-	-	-	-	-
650000	768	1024	1024	1024	1280	768

Compression Ratio (CR)

The CR provides information about the degree by which the compression algorithm removes the redundant data. Higher the *CR* less number of bits required to store or transmits the data that can be defined as

$$CR = \frac{B_0}{B_c} \tag{1}$$

where, B_0 is the total number of bits required to represent original data and B_c total number of bits required to represent compressed data along with the side information needed for retrieval of original data.

Percentage Root Mean Square Difference (PRD)

It is a measure of acceptable fidelity and degree of distortion introduced during compression and decompression algorithm. Usually, the clinical acceptability of reconstructed signal after decompression is determined through visual inspection. The numerical evaluation of the level of distortion in reconstructed signal in comparison to original signal can be carried out via PRD measure, defined as

$$PRD(\%) = 100 \times \sqrt{\frac{\sum_{n=1}^{N} (X_s(n) - X_r(n))^2}{\sum_{n=1}^{N} (X_s(n))^2}} \tag{2}$$

where, X_r is reconstructed signal with respect to original signal X_s.

Percentage Root Mean Square Difference, Normalized (PRDN)

It is a normalized version of PRD, is PRDN, which does not depend on the mean signal value $\overline{X}$. For any signal, the information lies in its variance. The mean value of the data does not actively contribute to the reconstructed signal fidelity issue. PRDN provides better error estimation in reconstructed signal than PRD.

$$PRDN(\%) = 100 \times \sqrt{\frac{\sum_{n=1}^{N} (X_s(n) - X_r(n))^2}{\sum_{n=1}^{N} (X_s(n) - \overline{X})^2}} \tag{3}$$

Percentage Root Mean Square Difference, Normalized with Respect to Database (PRD_1024)

As for storage purpose, MIT-BIH database adds a 1024 in the original signal. So in order to evaluate the fidelity of reconstructed signal 1024 must be subtracted from the original signal.

$$PRD\_1024 = 100 \times \sqrt{\frac{\sum_{n=1}^{N}(X_s(n) - X_r(n))^2}{\sum_{n=1}^{N}(X_s(n) - 1024)^2}} \tag{4}$$

Root Mean Square Error (RMS)

It provides a measure of error in a reconstructed signal with respect to original signal having signal length N.

$$RMS = \sqrt{\frac{\sum_{n=1}^{N}(X_s(n) - X_r(n))^2}{(N-1)}} \tag{5}$$

Signal to Noise Ratio (SNR)

SNR, measure of degree of noise energy introduced by compression algorithm in decibel (dB) scale.

$$SNR = 10 \times \log\left(\frac{\sum_{n=1}^{N}(X_s(n) - \overline{X})^2}{\sum_{n=1}^{N}(X_s(n) - X_r(n))^2}\right) \tag{6}$$

Quality Score (QS)

QS is defined as the ratio between the CR and PRD. The QS is a very rational performance indicator when it is difficult to estimate the best compression method while taking into account the reconstruction errors as well. A high score represents a superior compression method.

$$QS = \frac{CR}{PRD} \tag{7}$$

All the seven measures are simultaneously used in literature for accessing the efficacy of any ECG compression algorithm. The MATLAB script for calculation for above mentioned performance metric are as follows, which will be used in this chapter for all compression techniques.

If gain (200) and base (1024) are removed before ECG signal processing, then before metric computation both gain and base should be incorporated in reconstructed ECG. Thereby making a fair comparison in the same condition with the original ECG.

Performance Metric Computation

```
ecg=ecg*200+1024;
ecg1=ecg1*200+1024;       % reconstructed ECG signal

l=length(ecg1);            % Length of reconstructed ECG signal
err=(ecg1-ecg(1:l)).^2;    % Square error computation between reconstructed ECG
and original ECG
nu=sum(err);               % Summation of square error

de_1024=(1024-ecg(1:l)).^2;    % Denominator for PRD_1024 computation
du=sum(de_1024);               % Summation of Denominator for PRD_1024
PRD_1024=100*sqrt(nu/du);

de=(ecg(1:l)).^2;          % Denominator for PRD computation
du=sum(de);                % Summation of Denominator for PRD

PRD=100*sqrt(nu/du);

de_mean=(ecg(1:l)-mean(ecg)).^2;   % Denominator for PRDN computation
du=sum(de_mean);                   % Summation of Denominator for PRDN
PRDN=100*sqrt(nu/du);

RMS=sqrt(nu/(length(err)-1));     % RMS computation

SNR=10*log10(du/nu);                % SNR computation
bit_resolution_original=11;      % Original sample resolution
bit_resolution_compressed=11;    % Compressed sample resolution
cr=(bit_resolution_original*length(ecg1))/(bit_resolution_
compressed*length(ecg_tp));

QS=cr/PRD;                             % QS computation
```

Published with MATLAB® R2015a

ECG Data Compression Methods

ECG data compression is broadly classified into two types: (i) lossless ECG data compression and (ii) lossy ECG data compression scheme. Lossless ECG data compression is preferred in case of critically ill patient monitoring where each subtle features are needed to be reproduced. Lossy ECG data compression is preferred in case of non-critical patient monitoring conditions and the elderly or regular monitoring purposes. In Lossless ECG compression exact replica of the original signal can be reproduced. But the achieved compression ratio is less than its counterpart i.e. lossy compression scheme. The achieved higher compression ratio in case of lossy ECG compression is at the cost of quality of reconstructed ECG signal. Figure 2, represents the flow chart giving a diversified classification of ECG data compression methods.

Lossless ECG Data Compression Methods

In lossless ECG data compression, the ECG after decompression and compression is identical to original ECG. Every bit of features and other information in reconstructed ECG is preserved. In other words we can state that the reconstructed ECG is exact replica of the original signal. Although this method provides the one of the conflicting requirements of compression, but fails to achieve the higher compression ratio.

Figure 2. Broad classification scheme for ECG data compression methods

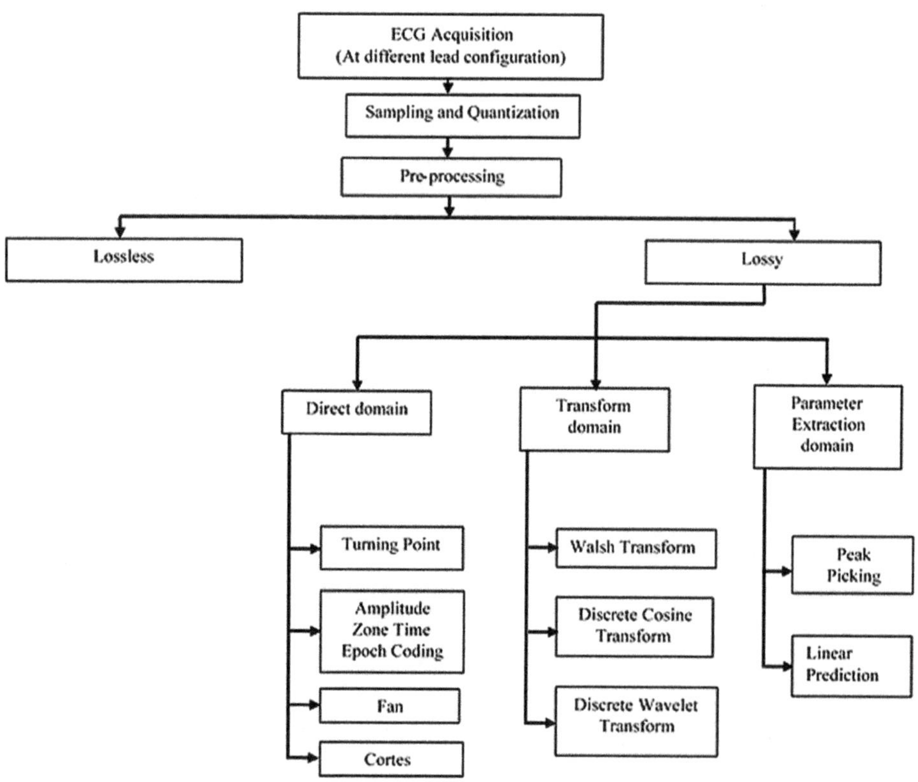

Advantage

- Higher reconstruction signal fidelity.
- Exact replication of original signal is possible.
- Reversible compression.

Disadvantage

- Lower compression ratio.
- Not applicable.

Application

- Critical patient monitoring.

Lossless ECG data compression technique (Horspool & Windels, 1994; Koski, 1997; Sayood, 2010) includes

1. Huffman Encoding
2. LZ Encoding
3. DPCM Encoding

Lossy ECG Data Compression Methods

In lossy compression method reconstructed ECG signal contains degradation with respect to original ECG signal. In this methodology of signal processing perfect reconstruction is sacrificed by the elimination of some amount of redundancies in the original ECG data to in order to achieve a higher compression ratio. Compared to lossless ECG compression method a higher compression ratio can be achieved with varying reconstruction error. For subjective evaluation of the compression scheme these reconstruction errors are not significantly visible. So, lossy ECG data compression methods under certain conditions are regarded as '*visually lossless*'. These certain conditions are preserving the diagnostic features, maintaining the base line. Depending upon the domain of operation on signal the lossy ECG data compression is further subdivided into three groups.

THREE METHODS FOR ECG DATA COMPRESSION

ECG data compression methods can be divided into three different groups namely i) Direct method ii) Transformed domain and iii) Parameter extraction method.

Direct Method

In direct ECG data compression method the digitized ECG samples directly analyzes and compresses the ECG data in the time domain. This section presents a brief overview of the each of basic algorithm along with simulation mechanism especially for ECG data compression. These includes TP, AZTEC, CORTES and Fan algorithm.

Turning Point Method

The basic idea in TP method for ECG data reduction is *to reduce the sampling frequency* of original ECG signal by a factor of two. The maximum possible CR that can be obtained using the TP method is ‘2’ because it preserves one of two samples retaining the slope/turning point information.

The algorithm process three ECG samples at a time. Considering the first sample as reference and then retain one of two remaining samples. The retained sample will become the reference for next two samples. The retention criteria of sample depends upon the magnitude of slope of two samples with respect to reference sample. Whichever sample out of two is having higher magnitude of slope that particular sample is retained other will be dropped for further processing. This process iterates till last sample of the ECG signal is encountered.

In past research (Mueller, 1977) author have concluded that at sampling frequency 200 Hz for ECG data, with 12 bit /sample resolution CR and PRD equal to 2 and 5.3 respectively were achieved. The basic TP procedure for compression is described in Algorithm 1, and reconstruction of ECG data is presented in Algorithm 2.

Algorithm 1. TP method for ECG data compression

```
INPUT:
ecg is the original ECG signal
OUTPUT:
ecg_tp is the compressed ECG signal
Begin
X_ref=ecg(1);
ecg_tp(1)=x_ref;                    // Taking the first as reference point
For  i=2:2:length(ecg)-1
// Increment the loop index by 2 till the length of the ecg signal
Compute the slope of two point with respect to reference sample
 Retain the sample whose slope magnitude is higher with respect to reference sample
 Retained sample become the reference sample for next iteration
 Concatenate the retained sample in ecg_tp
 End
```

Algorithm 2. TP method for reconstruction of ECG data

```
INPUT:
ecg_tp is the compressed ECG signal
OUTPUTS:
ecg1 estimate of original signal
Spline interpolation (which inserts one point in between two consecutive compressed ECG samples)
End
```

Matlab Simulation Program

Contents

- ECG Data Acquisition
- Initialization
- TP Method for ECG Data Compression
- Reconstruction
- End of TP Method for ECG Direct Data Compression Method

```
clc
clear
close all
```

ECG Data Acquisition

```
load('119m.mat');
fs = 360;
time_sec=30*60;                      % Time in number of seconds
ecg=(val(1,1:fs*time_sec)-1024)/200;  % Removing the base(1024) and gain(200)
```

Initialization

Initialization of variable ecg_tp, x_ref and ecg_tp(1)

```
ecg_tp=zeros(1,floor(length(ecg)/2));
x_ref=ecg(1);
ecg_tp(1)=x_ref;
```

TP Method for ECG Data Compression

```
j=2;
for i=2:2:length(ecg)-1
```

```
    % Selecting the pair of samples
    x1=ecg(i);
    x2=ecg(i+1);

    s1=x1-x_ref;
    s2=x2-x_ref;
    if abs(s1)>abs(s2) % Comparing the slope
        x_ref=x1;
    else
        x_ref=x2;
    end
    ecg_tp(j)=x_ref; % Updating the compressed ECG by selecting appropriate
data point
    j=j+1;
end
```

Reconstruction

```
ecg1=spline(1:length(ecg_tp),ecg_tp,1:.5:length(ecg_tp));
```

End of .m Script

An illustration for typical record 119 is given in Figure 3 which shows the original, reconstructed and error signal for 2000 samples. The above mentioned matlab script (.m) files is executed for all 48 records from MIT-BIH database. Table 2 shows the performance measure for typical record 100, 117, and 119 along with the average value for all 48 records. It can be noted that a constant CR equal to 2 and varying values of other performance metrics were obtained using this algorithm. These varying parameter results from the changing complexity in the signal and may violate the nyquist theorem in piece-wise sense.

Advantage

- It retains maximum and minimum points at which the sign of the slope of the signal changes.
- Simple and fast ECG compression algorithm to produce fixed CR of 2:1.
- Iterative application of TP method produces dyadic multiple CR, if there is much higher sampling rate the distortion error may be acceptable.

Limitations

- May violate sampling theorem criteria which results higher degree of distortion in reconstructed signal after repeated application of TP method.
- The retained samples are not equally spaced which may result in localized distortion.

Figure 3. Original, compressed, reconstructed and error ECG signal for TP algorithm for typical record 119

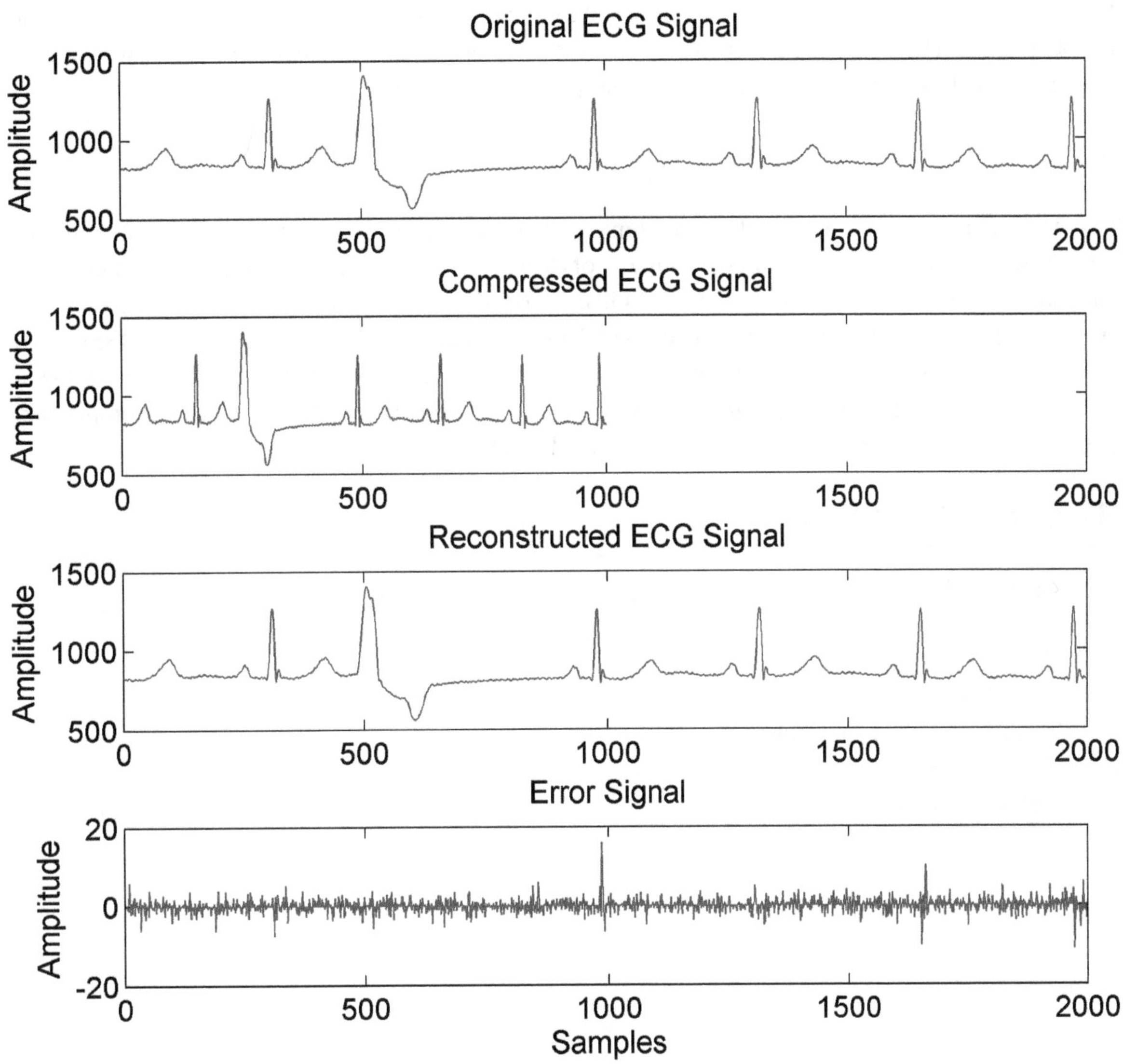

Table 2. Performance measure for selected and averaged value for all 48 records from MIT-BIH database

Record	CR	PRD_1024	PRD	PRDN	RMS	SNR	QS
100	2	1.79	0.13	3.36	1.3	29.47	14.83
117	2	0.77	0.16	2.85	1.36	30.91	12.57
119	2	0.72	0.17	1.37	1.46	37.3	11.74
A*	2±0	1.66±0.75	0.15±0.04	2.28±0.94	1.46±0.35	33.53±3.5	13.81±2.84

A*- for all 48 records average± standard deviation

Summary

TP method retains one of two samples through the maximum slope criteria with respect to reference sample point. The algorithm can provide fixed dyadic CR with varying values of reconstruction error. The reconstruction can be accomplished via interpolation between two consecutive samples.

AZTEC

The AZTEC is original developed for rhythmic analysis in real time monitoring of ECG. The basic AZTEC algorithm was first proposed by authors of (Cox, Nolle, Fozzard, & Oliver, 1968) which further improved modified in (V. Kumar, Saxena, & Giri, 2006). In present chapter we provide step by step illustration of basic AZTEC algorithm with its matlab implementation. The AZTEC algorithm decomposes the signal in terms of plateaus, extremum and slopes. The plateaus and slope detection thresholds are determined empirically. The Algorithm 3 shows the AZTEC algorithm for direct ECG data compression. The combination of plateaus and extremum is called bound.

Matlab Simulation Program

Contents

- Plateau Detection
- Slope Detection
- Reconstruction of ECG signal
- plot
- Performance measure

```
%AZTEC COMPRESSION ON ECG
close all;
clear all;
clc;
load('119m.mat');
ecg=(val(1,1:2077)-1024)/200';
fs = 360;
a=length(ecg);
time = [1: a]/fs;
ln=0;i=1;j=1;tau=0;
vmin=ecg(1);vmax=ecg(1);
vmin1=vmin; vmax1=vmax;
tau_count=1;
```

Algorithm 3. AZTEC algorithm for direct ECG data compression

1: **INPUT:**

2: *ecg* is the original ECG signal

3: **OUTPUT:**

4: *AZTEC* is the compressed ECG data

5: **Begin**

Plateau detection

6: Compare the ECG signal sample with previous extrema point and experimentally determined threshold amplitude.

7: Count the detected consecutive sample which satisfies the above condition

8: Replace the samples with average value of extrema and name it as Line (L)

Slope detection

9: Application of experimentally determined threshold for estimating length of plateau

10: Check for the criteria of the extrema point using the following condition

$$\{(V(L_{i+1}) - V(L_i))(V(L_i) - V(L_{i-1}))\} < 0$$

11: The combined extrema with plateau is called as bound. Except bound left over sample points will fall into the category of slope.

12: The concept of the time list of slope was devised by (Cox et al., 1968) and is given as

$$\tau(S) = \sum_{i=1}^{m-1} \tau(L_i)$$

13: The amplitude of slope is determined by

$$V(S) = V(L_m) - V(L_0)$$

where L_m and L_0 are previous bounds prior to slope.

14: In order to distinguish the slope and bound, we assign -ve sign to slope time list.

15: The complete AZTEC can be determined as an ordered pair of time lists and amplitude list.

16: **End**

Plateau Detection

```
for i=2:a

    if ecg(i)>vmax              % maximum and minimum value updatation
        vmax1=ecg(i);
    elseif ecg(i)<vmin
        vmin1=ecg(i);
    end
    %     avg_L=(vmax+vmin)/2;
    if vmax1-vmin1<=.1            % Check for experimentally determined thresh-
old
        tau_count=tau_count+1;
        avg=(vmax+vmin)/2;
        tau(j)=tau_count;              % duration of line information
        ecg_avg(j)=(vmax+vmin)/2;      % value of the line information
    else
        j=j+1;
        tau_count=1;
        tau(j)=1;
        ecg_avg(j)=ecg(i);

        vmin=ecg(i);vmax=ecg(i);
        vmin1=vmin; vmax1=vmax;
    end
end
loc=find(tau==0);
tau(loc)=1;
```

Slope Detection

A set of AZTEC lines is said to be a “slope” if no line Li is a bound and Lo and Lm are bounds. The slope S is completely specified by its value, v(S)=v(Lm)-v(Lo)

```
j=1;
ecg_all=[];
tau_all=[];
tau_all(j)=tau(j);
ecg_all(j)=ecg_avg(j);
oho=0;
for i=1:length(tau)-1
    if tau(i)<6         % confirmation of not being plaetu
```

```
        if  (ecg_avg(i+1)-ecg_avg(i))*(ecg_avg(i)-ecg_avg(i-1))<0% condition
for extrema detection

            if sum(oho)~=0
                tau_all(j)=sum(oho);
                j=j+1;
                oho=0;
            end
            tau_all(j)=tau(i);
            ecg_all(j)=ecg_avg(i);
            j=j+1;

        else
            % now slope operation
            oho=-(abs(oho)+ tau(i)); % keep eye on adding
        end
    else
        % plaetu
        if sum(oho)~=0
            tau_all(j)=sum(oho);
            j=j+1;
            oho=0;
        end
        tau_all(j)=tau(i);
        ecg_all(j)=ecg_avg(i);
        j=j+1;
    end
end

tau_all=tau_all'; % time list
tau=tau';
ecg_all=ecg_all';
% search for position of slopes
ind=find(tau_all<0);
ecg_all(ind)=ecg_all(ind+1)-ecg_all(ind-1);   % amplitude list

AZTEC(1:2:2*length(tau_all))=tau_all;
AZTEC(2:2:2*length(ecg_all))=ecg_all;
```

Reconstruction of ECG Signal

```
% reverse of slope
AZTEC;
tau_all1=AZTEC(1:2:length(AZTEC)); % should be same as tau_all
ecg_all1=AZTEC(2:2:length(AZTEC));
loc=find(tau_all1<0);
x=ecg_all1;
% inverse of slope
out=x(1:loc(1)-1);
tau1=tau_all1(1:loc(1)-1);
for i=1:length(loc)  % where to insert the slope information
    avg=x(loc(i))/(abs(tau_all1(loc(i)))+1);
    b=x(loc(i)-1)+avg:avg:x(loc(i)+1)-avg;
    % numbers to be inserted

    if loc(i)==loc(end)
        out=[out b x(loc(i)+1:loc(end)) x(end)];
        tau1=[tau1 ones(1,abs(abs(tau_all1(loc(i))))) tau_all1(end)];
    else
        out=[out b x(loc(i)+1:loc(i+1)-1)];
      tau1=[tau1 ones(1,abs(abs(tau_all1(loc(i))))) tau_
all1(loc(i)+1:loc(i+1)-1)];
    end
end
ecg1=[];
for i=1:length(out)
    ecg1=[ecg1 rectpulse(out(i),tau1(i))']; % few ending samples might be
missing
end
```

End of .m Script

Figure 4, the original, reconstructed and error signal is depicted for 2000 samples. The above mentioned matlab script (.m) file is executed for all 48 records from MIT-BIH database and results are presented in Table 3. It shows the performance measure for typical record 100, 117, and 119 and the average value for all 48 records.

Advantage

- Higher compression ratio typically in order of 10.
- Applicable for automatic analysis such as QRS detection, having higher slope regions.

Figure 4. Original, compressed, reconstructed and error ECG signal for AZTEC algorithm for typical record 119

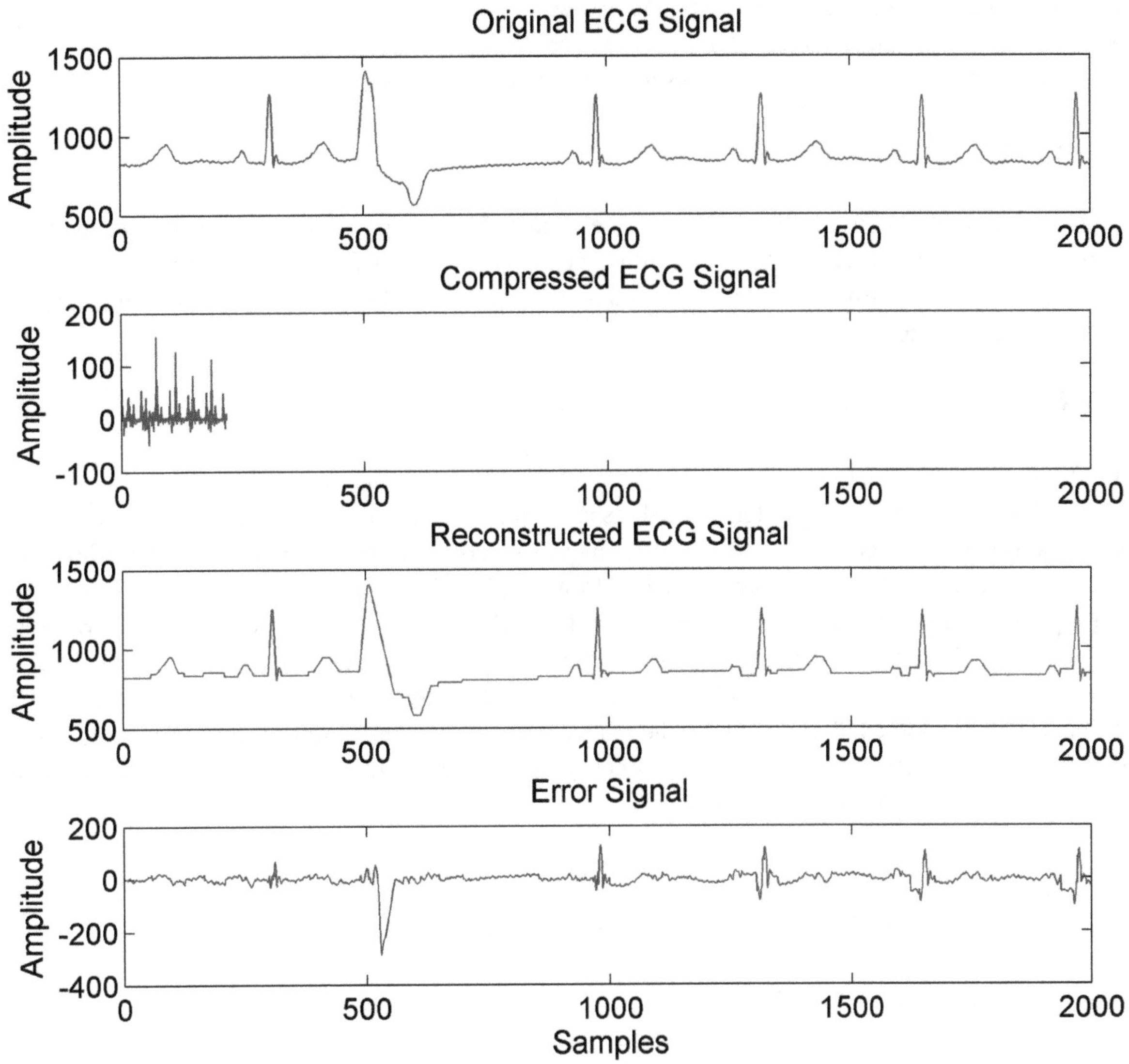

Table 3. Performance measure for AZTEC on selected and averaged value for all 48 records from MIT-BIH database

Record	CR	PRD_1024	PRD	PRDN	RMS	SNR	QS
100	17.06	0	11.8	25.43	0.04	11.89	1.45
117	10.77	0	5.39	19.60	0.05	14.16	2
119	7.64	0.01	14.18	22.73	0.14	11.14	0.54
A*	10.65±3.66	0.01±0.01	20.02±19.38	28.31±20.77	0.09±0.09	12.19±4.10	0.83±0.73

A*- for all 48 records average± standard deviation

Limitations

- The quality of reconstructed signal is very low.
- The reconstructed signal is not acceptable to cardiologist.
- Needs random post processing to resemble the reconstructed signal to original signal.

Summary

The location of important diagnostic features are retained by location of bounds which basically determine the shape of ECG. The AZTEC algorithm keep only extrema (maxima and minima), plateau, and slope. During the reconstruction process plateau and slope are distinguished by introducing a flag of negative sign in time list.

CORTES

The CORTES algorithm (Abenstein & Tompkins, 1982) is the combination of TP and AZTEC method. Depending on the empirically determined threshold value, the length of the lines detected in AZTEC plateaus were retained otherwise the TP data point was saved. If length of the line is less than threshold than in that place of slope operation, TP method was employed. As TP method is efficient in high frequency region and same degree of distortion were added in both high and low frequency regions. Whereas distortion by TP method is tolerated in high frequency region compared to low frequency method. In low frequency region AZTEC algorithm provide low distortion by different length of plateau detection. The interpretation of length of the line is the related with the frequency of the signal, higher the length of the line lower the frequency leads smaller change in the signal and vice-versa. The brief procedure for *CORTES* is described in Algorithm 4.

Algorithm 4. CORTES algorithm for ECG data compression

```
INPUT:
ecg is the original ECG signal
OUTPUT:
CORTES is the compressed ECG data
Begin
Detect plateau as in AZTEC ECG data compression Algorithm 3.
Apply empirically determined threshold (TH) on the length of plateau (L)
    If L < TH
        TP method (Algorithm 1)
     Else
         End
  End
```

Advantage

- Better than AZTEC and TP alone.

Limitations

- The quality of reconstructed signal is still low because of unavoidable distortion.

Summary

Cortes method is hybrid combination of TP and AZTEC method designed to preserve ECG features. The QRS feature of ECG is better preserved compared to AZTEC and isoelectric lines are compressed efficiently in comparison to TP method.

Fan

Fan algorithm for ECG data compression is based on finding the region bounded through the empirically determined threshold. The Fan algorithm draws lines between pairs of starting and ending points so that all intermediate samples are within some specified error tolerance, ε. The step-by-step basic Fan algorithm was illustrated by authors of (Jalaleddine et al., 1990; Tompkins, 1993). The brief procedure is presented in Algorithm 5. The visual representation for record number 119 in depicted in Figure 5. In Table 4 performance measure for Fan algorithm on selected and averaged value for all 48 records from MIT-BIH database is represented.

Matlab Simulation Program

Contents

- Initilization
- Fan algorithm for ECG data compression
- Reconstruction of ECG signal

```
clc;
clear all;
close all;
% Acquisition of ECG
load('100m.mat');
fs = 360;                                 % Sampling Rate
time_sec=6*30;                            % time in number of seconds
ecg=(val(1,1:fs*time_sec))/200;   % Selecting lead II and removing the
base(1024) and gain(200)
```

Figure 5. Original, compressed, reconstructed and error ECG signal for Fan algorithm for typical record 119

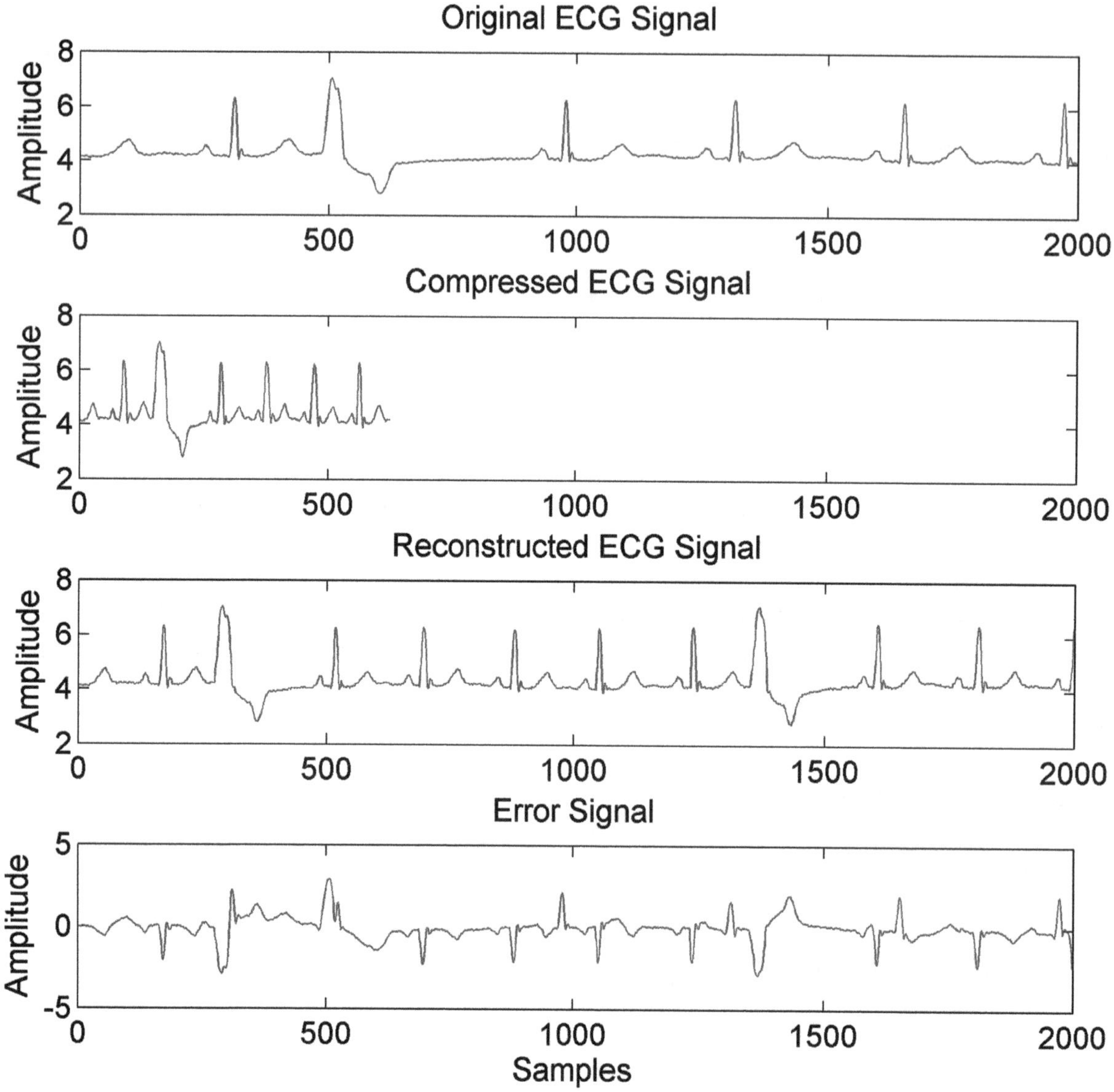

Table 4. Performance measure for Fan algorithm on selected and averaged value for all 48 records from MIT-BIH database

Record	CR	PRD_1024	PRD	PRDN	RMS	SNR	QS
100	2.23	0.03	6.63	180.87	0.32	-5.15	0.34
117	1.96	0.06	13.07	243.79	0.56	-7.74	0.15
119	1.96	0.08	20.01	164.58	0.86	-4.33	0.1
A*	1.9±0.11	0.06±±0.02	12.67±4.04	187.18±47.26	0.6±0.18	-5.22±1.88	0.17±0.05

A*- for all 48 records average± standard deviation

Algorithm 5. Fan algorithm for ECG data compression

1: **INPUT:**

2: *ecg* is the original ECG signal

3: ε error tolerance

4: **OUTPUT:**

5: *Fan* is the compressed ECG data

6: **Begin**

7: X_0=*ecg(1)*; Non-redundant permanent sample point or originating point

8: X_1=*ecg(1)*; Taking second sample and drawing two lines (U_1, L_1)

U_1- passes through sample point (X_0, $X_1+ \varepsilon$)

L_1- passes through sample point (X_0, $X_1- \varepsilon$)

9: If the 3rd sample X_2 falls within the area bounded by two slopes, generate two new slopes (U_2, L_2) that passes through sample point (X_0, $X_2+ \varepsilon$) and (X_0, $X_2- \varepsilon$)

10: Compare the two pair of slopes and retain the most convergent pair. Which imply lower magnitude of U and higher of magnitude of L is retained.

11: Assign $X_1= X_2$ and read the next sample into $X_{2.}$ X_2 always the most recent sample point and X_1 holds the sample immediately preceding to $X_{2.}$

12: Repeat the process by comparing X_2 to values of most convergent slopes.

13: If the sample point falls outside the area, save the line length '*len*' & final amplitude X_1, which then becomes the new originating point X_0 and repeat the process.

14: **End**

Initialization

```
j=1;i=1;k=1;
X0=ecg(i);                          %originating point
fan_compressed(j)=X0;               %save first permanent point
len=1;                              %initialize line length
Epsilon=.01;                          %error tolerance limit
l=length(ecg)-2;                    % length of ECG
T=1;
X1=ecg(i+1);                  % Considering point 2
```

Fan Algorithm for ECG Data Compression

```
  XU1=X1+Epsilon;    XL1=X1-Epsilon;  % upper and lower bound of X1
 while (i<l-3)
     X2=ecg(i+2);           % get next sample point
%      XU1=X1+Epsilon;    XL1=X1-Epsilon;  % upper and lower bound of X1

     XU2 = (XU1 - X0)/T + XU1; % upper bound of X2
     XL2 = (XL1 - X0)/T + XL1; % lower bound of X2
     if (X2>=XL2 && X2<=XU2)   % within bound\

         % obtain the most restrictive bound
         if XU2 < X2 + Epsilon
             XU2=XU2;
         else
             XU2= X2 + Epsilon;
         end

         if XL2 > X2 - Epsilon
            XL2= XL2;
         else
             XL2=X2 - Epsilon;
         end

        len=len+1;
        X1 = X2 ; % X1 hold sample preceding X2
     else        % X2 out of bound, save line
       j=j+1; fan_compressed(j)=X1;  % save final amplitude
       k=k+1; fan_len(k)=len;        %  save line length

      % reset all variables
       X0=X1;
       X1=X2;
       len=1;
       T = 1 ;
XU1 = X1 + Epsilon ;
XL1 = X1 - Epsilon ;

     end
   i=i+len;

 end
```

Reconstruction of ECG Signal

```
z=1; %Sample number for reconstructed ECG
n=2; %To access the array storing lengths

for m=1:length(fan_compressed)-2
    len=fan_len(m+1);
    ecg1(z)=fan_compressed(m);
    for i=1:len
       ecg1(z+i)=ecg1(z); % reconstructed ECG
    end
   z=z+len;
end
```

Published with MATLAB® R2015a

Advantage

- Better than AZTEC and TP alone.
- Simple and faster implementation.
- Higher fidelity of reconstructed signal.

Limitations

- The quality of reconstructed signal is still low because of unavoidable distortion.

Summary

The fan algorithm incorporates the actual sample points which are bounded in the slopes. The three algorithms based on Scan-along polygonal approximation (SAPA) technique closely resemble to Fan algorithm.SAPA-2 proved best result among them. SAPA-2 calculates three slopes between origination sample and actual future sample point. The minor difference between SAPA-2 and Fan is the third slope calculation which is center slope criterion in place of actual sample value criteria.

Transformed Domain

The original ECG samples are subjected to a (linear) transformation in the new domain. The energy compaction property can be further utilized for compression. The basic property of energy compaction is "higher number of samples are clustered in certain region. In current scenario the certain region is near to the origin". The data compression is achieved in any of domains are only through two ways 1) Thresholding and 2) Quantization.

1. **Thresholding:** There are different approaches for thresholding. When thresholding is applied in transformed domain only significant coefficient whose absolute value is above the threshold is retained. The selection of threshold may be user defined or via optimization algorithm.
2. **Quantization:** The thresholded significant coefficient is represented at lower bit rate through quantization scheme.

Walsh Transform

The Walsh transform amuses the ECG data compression application because it decomposes a signal into a set of orthogonal basis, rectangular waveforms of states are solely either +1 or -1. No multiplier is required and provides only real values as output. It is a asymmetrical and orthogonal transformation.

$$WAL(8) = \begin{pmatrix} 1 & 1 & 1 & 1 & 1 & 1 & 1 & 1 \\ 1 & 1 & 1 & 1 & -1 & -1 & -1 & -1 \\ 1 & 1 & -1 & -1 & -1 & -1 & 1 & 1 \\ 1 & 1 & -1 & -1 & 1 & 1 & -1 & -1 \\ 1 & -1 & -1 & 1 & 1 & -1 & -1 & 1 \\ 1 & -1 & -1 & 1 & -1 & 1 & 1 & -1 \\ 1 & -1 & 1 & -1 & -1 & 1 & -1 & 1 \\ 1 & -1 & 1 & -1 & 1 & -1 & 1 & -1 \end{pmatrix}$$

The Walsh transform pair with forward and inverse for a signal x(n) of having length N are given by following

$$y_n = \frac{1}{N}\sum_{i=0}^{N-1} x_i WAL(n,i), n = 1,2\ldots\ldots\ldots\ldots, N-1 \tag{8}$$

$$x_i = \sum_{n=0}^{N-1} y_n WAL(n,i), n = 1,2\ldots\ldots\ldots\ldots, N-1 \tag{9}$$

As Walsh transform is symmetric and orthogonal the only difference between forward and its inverse is a multiplication of '1/N' the normalization factor.

The basic application of Walsh Transform in ECG data compression is previously demonstrated by authors of (Kulkarni, Kumar, & Verma, 1997) and its Matlab implementation is also available and explained in its application program. (http://in.mathworks.com/help/signal/examples/discrete-walsh-hadamard-transform.html). The visual representation for record number 119 in depicted in Figure 6. Table 5 and Table 6 represents the performance measure for Walsh transform on selected and averaged value for all 48 records from MIT-BIH database at Th=1 and 0.5 respectively.

Figure 6. Original, compressed, reconstructed and error ECG signal for Walsh transform

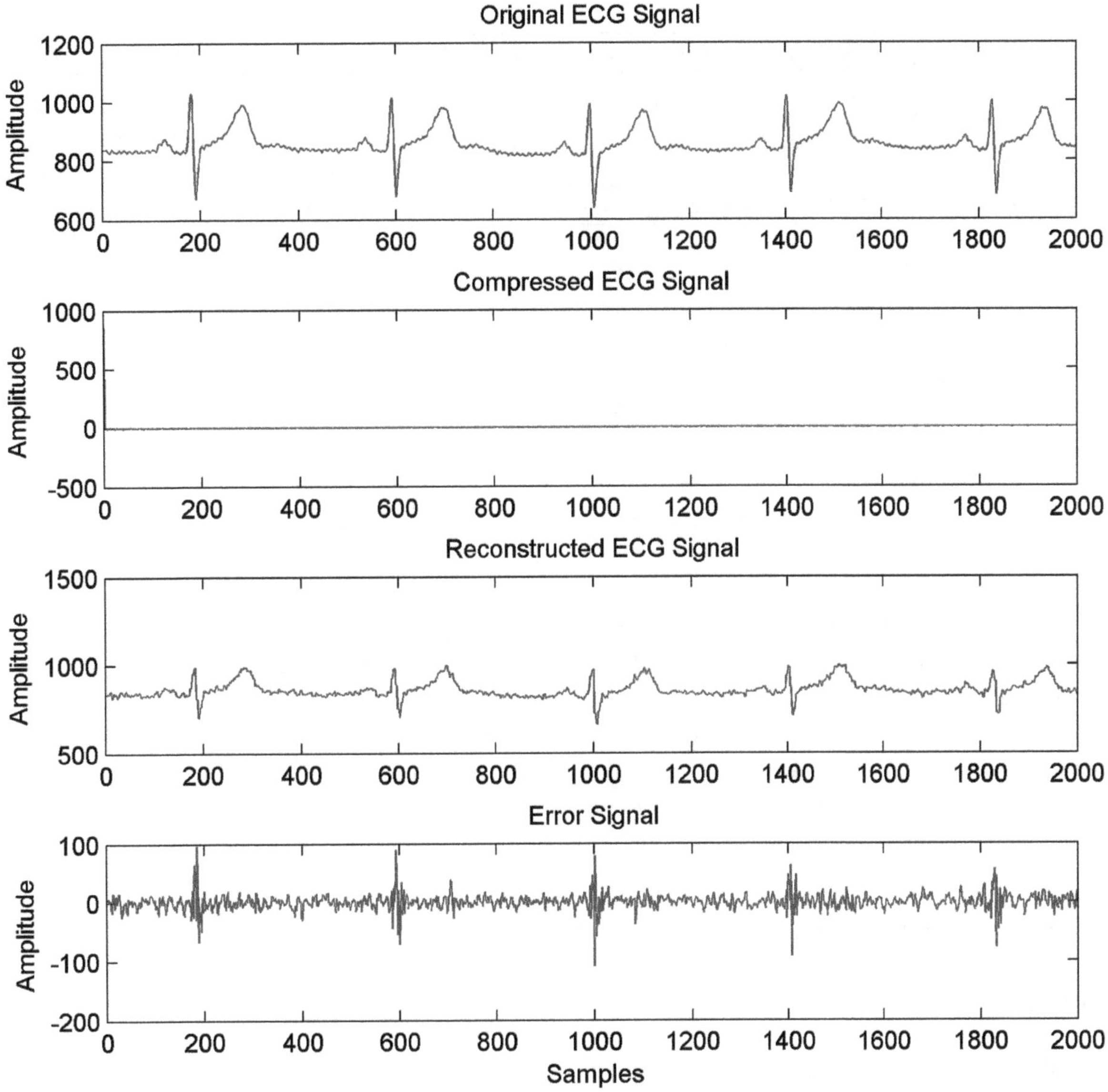

Table 5. Performance measure for Walsh transform on selected and averaged value for all 48 records from MIT-BIH database at Th=1

Record	CR	PRD_1024	PRD	PRDN	RMS	SNR	QS
100	28.44	30.71	2.31	65.56	22.15	3.67	12.34
117	21.79	11.87	2.3	42.93	19.88	7.34	9.47
119	9.79	12.38	2.72	24.62	23.52	12.17	3.6
A*	20.99±18.81	24.64±9.67	2.24±0.36	36.78±13.37	21.33±3.03	9.25±3.16	10.75±12.46

A*- for all 48 records average± standard deviation

Table 6. Performance measure for Walsh transformation selected and averaged value for all 48 records from MIT-BIH database at Th=0.5

Record	CR	PRD_1024	PRD	PRDN	RMS	SNR	QS
100	8.94	18.59	1.4	39.7	13.41	8.02	6.41
117	9.3	7.07	1.37	25.57	11.84	11.85	6.79
119	5.39	7.46	1.64	14.83	14.17	16.57	3.29
A*	8.67±4.82	15.2±6.29	1.37±0.18	22.75±9.13	13.01±1.47	13.52±3.37	6.84±4.88

Algorithm 6.

```
INPUT:
ecg is the original ECG signal
Define  Th (Threshold)
OUTPUT:
Walsh  transformed coefficient for representation of compressed ECG data
Begin
Take forward Walsh transform by using fwht command
Replace the Walsh coefficient with 0 whosoever is less than the empirically determined threshold
Reconstruct the original signal by using the inverse Walsh transform equation via iwht command in Matlab.
Compute the performance measure
End
```

Matlab Simulation Program

Contents


```
clc
clear all
close all
```

Initialization

```
fs=360;                   % sampling frequency
sec=120;                  % time duration of consideration
```

```
t=0:1/fs:sec-1/fs;       % relating time duration and sampling frequency with
number of samples
```

Acquisition of ECG Signal

```
load('117m.mat');  % load ecg data from database

ecg=val(1,1:fs*sec);  % fs*(number of seconds)                  % selecting
appropriate lead i.e. 1st row for lead II
mean_ecg=mean(ecg);
zxecg=ecg-mean(ecg);  % mean removal
```

DCT Transform and Thresholding

```
th=20*2;               % Emperically determined threshold
block_size=64*5;        % block size represents in how much size the DCT is
calculated over th signal

for i=1:length(zxecg)/block_size     % Block wise DCT coefficient computation
   dctzx((i*block_size)-(block_size-1):(i*block_size))=dct(zxecg((i*block_
size)-(block_size-1):i*block_size));
end

% Thresholding

ind_th=find(abs(dctzx)<th); % it calculates number of samples in Discrete Co-
sine Transformed version less the th threshold;
dctzx_th=dctzx;
dctzx_th(ind_th)=0;          % compressed DCT coefficients which is ready for
quantization and grouping
```

Reconstruction

```
for i=1:length(ecg)/block_size      % Inverse DCT computation
    inv_dctzx_th((i*block_size)-(block_size-1):(i*block_size))=idct(dctzx_
th((i*block_size)-(block_size-1):i*block_size));
end

est_ecg_th=mean_ecg+inv_dctzx_th; % Reconstructed ECG
```

Published with MATLAB® R2015a

Advantage

- Orthogonal transformation.
- Used power spectrum analysis, useful for characterizing non-linear signals & solving non-linear differential equations etc.

Limitations

- Computationally expensive with respect to wavelet transform.

Discrete Cosine Transform

The DCT is applied to ECG data compression field for improvement in the compression efficiency(Batista et al., 2001; Bendifallah, Benzid, & Boulemden, 2011). Researchers (Lee et al., 2011) have applied, the length of DCT block size should be same as the length of RR interval of ECG to capture the inter beat correlation. The basic formula for DCT is given below for computation of coefficients

$$y(k) = w(k)\sum_{n=1}^{L} X_s(n)\cos\left(\frac{\pi}{2L}(2n-1)(k-1)\right),\ k = 1,2,\ldots,L$$
$$w(k) = \begin{cases} \dfrac{1}{\sqrt{L}}, & k = 1 \\ \sqrt{\dfrac{2}{L}}, & 2 \le k \le L \end{cases} \tag{10}$$

where, $w(k)$ is scale factor

- After thresholding the significant DCT coefficient can be further quantized and grouped based on desired requirement.

The Algorithm 7 and its Matlab simulation code is basic implementation of DCT. After empirical estimation, a value equal to 40 was used for thresholding the raw DCT coefficients. Table 7 provide the

Table 7. Performance measure for CORTES on selected and averaged value for all 48 records from MIT-BIH database

Record	CR	PRD_1024	PRD	PRDN	RMS	SNR	QS
100	7.66	11.07	0.86	23.3	8.21	12.65	8.95
117	10.12	3.66	0.72	13.53	6.21	17.38	14.05
119	7.24	3.37	0.81	6.63	6.89	23.57	8.97
A*	9.30±3.19	8.90±4.61	0.78±0.11	12.82±6.53	7.43±1.14	18.74±3.76	12.31±4.95

A*- for all 48 records average± standard deviation

Figure 7. Original, compressed, reconstructed and error ECG signal for DCT

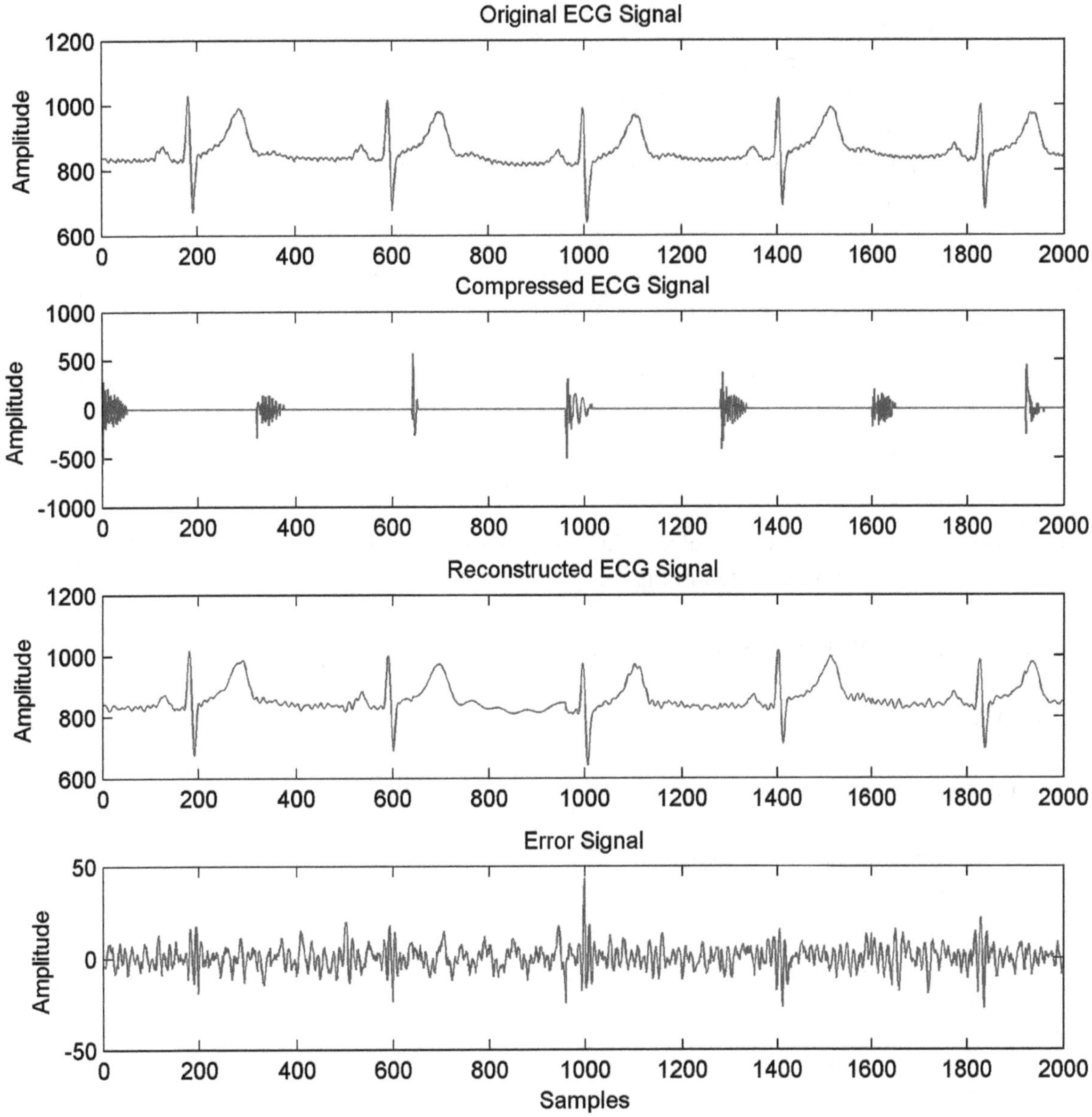

Algorithm 7. DCT coefficients computation for ECG data compression

```
INPUT:
ecg is the original ECG signal
Define block size and empirical threshold
OUTPUT:
dctzx_th is the DCT coefficients after thresholding
Begin
Remove average value in the ecg data points
Apply block wise DCT iteratively until last block
Finding the index in the DCT domain for coefficients to be greater than threshold
Retain the indexed DCT coefficient and replace the remaining sample with zeros.
End
```

values of performance measures for selected and average values of all records. The visual representation for record number is 119 in depicted in Figure 7.

Matlab Simulation Program

Contents

- Initialization
- Acquisition of ECG Signal
- DCT Transform and thresholding
- Reconstructtion

```
clc
clear all
close all
```

Initialization

```
fs=360;                 % sampling frequency
sec=120;                % time duration of consideration
t=0:1/fs:sec-1/fs;      % relating time duration and sampling frequency with
number of samples
```

Acquisition of ECG Signal

```
load('117m.mat');  % load ecg data from database
ecg=val(1,1:fs*sec);  % fs*(number of seconds)                  % selecting
```

```
appropriate lead i.e. 1st row for lead II
mean_ecg=mean(ecg);
zxecg=ecg-mean(ecg);  % mean removal
```

DCT Transform and Thresholding

```
th=20*2;              % Empirically determined threshold
block_size=64*5;       % block size represents in how much size the DCT is
calculated over th signal

for i=1:length(zxecg)/block_size    % Block wise DCT coefficient computation
   dctzx((i*block_size)-(block_size-1):(i*block_size))=dct(zxecg((i*block_
size)-(block_size-1):i*block_size));
end

% Thresholding

ind_th=find(abs(dctzx)<th); % it calculates number of samples in Discrete Co-
sine Transformed version less the th threshold;
dctzx_th=dctzx;
dctzx_th(ind_th)=0;          % compressed DCT coefficients which is ready for
quantization and grouping
```

Reconstruction

```
for i=1:length(ecg)/block_size      % Inverse DCT computation
    inv_dctzx_th((i*block_size)-(block_size-1):(i*block_size))=idct(dctzx_
th((i*block_size)-(block_size-1):i*block_size));
end

est_ecg_th=mean_ecg+inv_dctzx_th; % Reconstructed ECG
```

Published with MATLAB® R2015a

Advantage

- The DCT is falling in the category of orthogonal transform.
- The DCT coefficient generally consists of large amount of near zero values which is main cause of compression.

Limitations

- While DCT operate on real valued input and typically real valued output. Thus there is a need of quantization step in block to achieve compression in same data format.
- Error propagation within the block size arises due to quantization and rounding during reconstruction process.

Discrete Wavelet Transform

The Wavelet Transform is an effective and efficient tool for time-frequency localization. This time-frequency localization is also called as multi-resolution analysis (MRA) representation. The MRA is the basic fundamental approach of the wavelet transform that employed in wide variety of signal processing applications. The localized MRA approach has risen the processing capabilities in stationary and non-stationary domain. Further, it can be successfully applied to the signal feature detection, denoising, and compression. Several reference material for wavelet analysis are available (Daubechies, 1992; Stéphane Mallat, 2009). Wavelet transform is defined in both continuous as well in discrete domain.

The continuous wavelet transform (CWT) is one method of investigating the MRA of data whose frequency content varies with time. CWT maps *x(t)* which is a one dimensional signal to two-dimensional plane formulated by scale and translation defined as.

$$W(s,\tau) = \int x(t)\psi^{*}_{s,\tau}(t)dt \tag{11}$$

where *s* is scale and τ is measure of translation and $\psi^{*}_{s,\tau}(t)$ is the conjugate of mother wavelet formed by orthonormal basis functions. The CWT is computed for the particular scale (variable) by correlating the signal *x(t)* with translated mother wavelet $\psi^{*}_{s,\tau}(t)$. Higher the scale higher the frequency resolution or coarse frequency components and vice-versa. Its reverse is true for time resolution. The *x(t)* can be reconstructed back via inverse wavelet transform (Daubechies, 1992).

The explicit generation of mother wavelet from single wavelet $\psi(t)$ is defined through scaling and translation

$$\psi_{s,\tau}(t) = \frac{1}{\sqrt{s}}\psi\left(\frac{t-\tau}{s}\right) \tag{12}$$

The CWT applied on sampled data, with the smooth shifting process over the length of sampled data points, whereas the scaling is defined from the minimum (original signal scale) to a maximum as determined by the user, thus resulting in coarser resolutions in time and frequency domain. This improved resolution demands higher computational time and memory requirement for estimating the wavelet coefficients. The inherent redundancy and difficultly in analytical description of mother wavelet limits the usability of CWT in current scenario. Thus fast algorithm for wavelet coefficient computation is needed. To overcome above mentioned problem Discrete Wavelet Transform (DWT) has been profound. The DWT scales and translates only on discrete steps. In other words DWT is not time or frequency discrete rather than only translation and the scale step are discrete. Definitely it made a trade of between resolution and above mentioned problem but this compromise is widely acceptable.

The intuitively implementation for wavelet transform as the digital filter bank using Eq. 8 and 9 results in DWT defined as follows

$$DWT(m,k) = \frac{1}{\sqrt{s_0^m}} \sum_k x(k)\psi(s_0^{-m}n - k) \tag{13}$$

As mother wavelet takes various forms depending upon applications, a brief review of their utility for ECG signal processing is available in (Addison, 2005). Most wavelets can be formulated by estimating digital filter coefficients with its impulse response i.e. $\psi(s_0^{-m}n - k)$. The various diagrammatic illustration of forward and inverse DWT as filter banks is available in literature(Al-Shrouf, Abo-Zahhad, & Ahmed, 2003; Hilton, 1997; R. Kumar, Kumar, & Kumar, 2012) which all have the same meaning. The meaning is simple, which deals with the scaling function of the DWT represented as a tree of low and high pass filter bank, within each level only decimated (factor=2) low-pass signal will be transformed further. The subsequent larger scale decomposition results in lower resolution because of the lesser number of samples are available for analysis along with discarded high-frequency components analysis. A dyadic data size is a necessity of filter bank illustration for DWT. which means for *N* decomposition scale the data length must be 2^N. A wide range of literature for ECG data compression using wavelet transform is available with quantization and coding applied after decomposition (Al-Shrouf et al., 2003; Blanco-Velasco, Cruz-Roldán, Godino-Llorente, & Barner, 2007; Djohan, Nguyen, & Tompkins, 1995; Hilton, 1997; Isa, Noviyanto, Jatmiko, & Arymurthy, 2012; Wang & Meng, 2008).

In this Chapter, for ECG signal compression and reconstruction three procedure were adopted. Firstly *N*, level decomposition for given mother wavelet ('haar', 'db2', 'db10', & 'sym8') for input ECG signal was computed. Secondly, thresholding the detail coefficients at empirically or visually determined threshold value and lastly for reconstruction inverse wavelet transform is applied with the help of approximate and modified detail coefficient (exact low pass component and zeros replaced non- significant thresholded detail coefficient with same size) from all levels. The chapter focus is to implement DWT based ECG data compression so we left the quantization and coding part and demonstrated the wavelet based decomposition of ECG signal with its simulation program. The processing of ECG on DWT was operated for dyadic grid and *N=3* was selected for obtaining fixed *CR* by hard thresholding the detail coefficient. Table 8 represents the performance measure for DWT on selected and averaged value for all 48 records from MIT-BIH database over 'haar', 'db2', 'db10', & 'sym8' mother wavelet.

Matlab Simulation Program

Contents

- Initialization
- Decomposition/ Compression part
- Synthesis/Reconstruction Part

Table 8. Performance measure for DWT on selected and averaged value for all 48 records from MIT-BIH database over 'haar', 'db2', 'db10', & 'sym8' mother wavelet

Haar							
Record	CR	PRD_1024	PRD	PRDN	RMS	SNR	QS
100	8	37.11	2.79	78.82	26.77	2.07	2.87
117	8	13.7	2.66	49.53	22.95	6.1	3.01
119	8	23.78	5.22	47.18	45.16	6.53	1.53
A*	8±0	36.74±13.11	3.67±1.56	53.4±13.17	34.77±14.02	5.74±2.32	2.69±1.41
db2							
100	8	35.15	2.64	74.64	25.35	2.54	3.03
117	8	12.62	2.45	45.63	21.14	6.81	3.27
119	8	21.09	4.63	41.85	40.05	7.57	1.73
A*	8±0	32.86±12.97	3.26±1.48	47.96±14.47	30.86±13.13	6.82±2.87	3.04±1.55
db10							
100	8	35.8	2.69	76.04	25.83	2.38	2.98
117	8	12.47	2.42	45.11	20.9	6.92	3.31
119	8	19.87	4.36	39.44	37.75	8.08	1.83
A*	8±0	30.72±13.29	3.03±1.43	45.09±15.86	28.65±12.79	7.55±3.48	3.34±1.8
sym8							
100	8	35.29	2.65	74.98	25.45	2.5	3.02
117	8	12.78	2.48	46.26	21.42	6.7	3.23
119	8	19.49	4.28	38.7	37.02	8.25	1.87
A*	8±0	30.87±13.61	3.04±1.45	45.27±16.24	28.74±12.99	7.55±3.58	3.37±1.92

A*- for all 48 records average± standard deviation

Algorithm 8.

```
INPUT:
ecg is the original ECG signal
OUTPUT:
Wavelet transformed coefficient for representation of compressed ECG data
Begin
Take forward wavelet transform by using dwt command
Replace the wavelet coefficient with 0 whosoever is being the part of high frequency content or details component
Reconstruct the original signal by using the inverse wavelet transform equation via idwt command in Matlab.
Compute the performance measure
End
```

```
clc
clear
close all
```

Initialization

```
fs=360;                    % sampling frequency
sec=60;                   % time duration of consideration
t=0:1/fs:sec-1/fs;         % relating time duration and sampling frequency with
number of samples
load('117m.mat');  % load ecg data from database
ecg=val(1,1:fs*sec);  % fs*(number of seconds)                    % selecting
appropriate lead i.e. 1st row for lead II
ecg_=(ecg(1:2^13)-1024)/200;
```

Decomposition/ Compression Part

```
mother_wave='sym8'; % Select any Mother Wavelet 'haar','db2', 'db10', or 'sym8'

[cA1 cD1]=dwt(ecg_,mother_wave);
[cA2 cD2]=dwt(cA1,mother_wave);
[cA3 cD3]=dwt(cA2,mother_wave);
[cA4 cD4]=dwt(cA3,mother_wave);
```

Synthesis/Reconstruction Part

```
X3 = idwt(cA4,zeros(1,length(cA4)),mother_wave);
X2 = idwt(X3,zeros(1,length(X3)),mother_wave);
X1 = idwt(X2,zeros(1,length(X2)),mother_wave);
X= idwt(X1,zeros(1,length(X1)),mother_wave);
ecg1=X; % Reconstructed ECG
```

Advantage

- Ability to handle non-stationary data.
- Good localization both in time and frequency domain.
- Better ECG performance measure.
- Ability of automatic removal of outliers.

Limitations

- Functional form representation of many wavelets is difficult.
- The DWT is shift sensitive because input-signal shifts generate unpredictable changes in DWT coefficients.
- The DWT suffers from poor directionality because DWT coefficients reveal only three spatial orientations.
- The DWT analysis lacks the phase information that accurately describes non-stationary signal behavior.

Summary

The formalism of the one-dimensional discrete wavelet transform (DWT) based on different mother wavelet is outlined for ECG data decomposition.

Parameter Extraction Method

The parameter extraction method uses pre-processing tool to obtain a set of set-points or features (typical cycles, extreme locations, etc.) that applied to model the original signal. These features are further quantized using the scalar or the vector quantizer and then some lossless coder is utilized to increase the compression efficiency. Reconstruction of original data is carried out by adopting suitable interpolation scheme. The parameter extraction technique is based on the assumption that the ECG signal is formulated through replication of the number of beats at the frequent rate. Review of some ECG data compression method can be readily found in reference (Jalaleddine et al., 1990; Sabarimalai Sur & Dandapat, 2014). Parameter extraction ECG compression methods mainly classified into prediction models(Al-Shrouf et al., 2003; Arnavut, 2007; Cohen & Zigel, 1998; Nave & Cohen, 1993; Ramakrishnan, 1997). Others are also significant for ECG compression includes scalar/ vector quantization (Cohen & Zigel, 1998; Huang, Wang, & Chen, 2013; Shaou-Gang & Yen, 2001) and template matching method (Paggetti et al., 1994).

In Linear prediction model method the instantaneous sample ($\hat{x}$ (n)) is forecasted by (a) weighted combination past (p) samples.

$$\hat{x}(n) = -a(2)x(n-1) - a(3)x(n-2) - \ldots - a(p+1)x(n-p) \tag{14}$$

Then, the error among the forecasted and original samples is sent or stored in place of the original samples. The error is quantized using any efficient quantizer (scalar/vector) which is further encoded with lossless encoding. In this process major compression is achieved in two stages first in by reducing the dynamic range and secondly in process of quantization.

The vector quantization is mainly based on the code book creation and transmitting the only codebook number instead of the wide range of samples which are assigned to that particular codebook number. Codebook may be the signal dependent or universal which is available to both of encoder and decoder.

The template matching based parameter extraction method for ECG compression is similar to vector quantization. The template matching for ECG data compression include steps of the beat segmentation, normalization, matching and subtraction with the coding of the residual signal.

The MATLAB code can be made by implementing the any of individual diverse methodology available in the literature.

CONCLUSION

In this chapter, the implementation of different selected techniques for ECG data compression in MATLAB was presented. The implemented ECG compression algorithm may vary with the exact algorithm for particular technique available in the literature due to the focus of this chapter is on the basic methodology of technique rather than pre-or-post algorithm involved with methods. The selected techniques from direct ECG compression methods are TP, AZTEC, Fan, and Cortes. Moreover selected techniques from transformed ECG compression methods are Walsh Transform, DCT, and Wavelet transform. The performance measure for implemented algorithm is also represented. This study seems to be of selection for the appropriate algorithm as needed.

REFERENCES

Abenstein, J. P., & Tompkins, W. J. (1982). A new data-reduction algorithm for real-time ECG analysis. *IEEE Transactions on Bio-Medical Engineering*, *29*(1), 43–48. doi:10.1109/TBME.1982.324962 PMID:7076268

Addison, P. S. (2005). Wavelet transforms and the ECG: A review. *Physiological Measurement*, *26*(5), 155–199. doi:10.1088/0967-3334/26/5/R01 PMID:16088052

Al-Shrouf, A., Abo-Zahhad, M., & Ahmed, S. M. (2003). A novel compression algorithm for electrocardiogram signals based on the linear prediction of the wavelet coefficients. *Digital Signal Processing*, *13*(4), 604–622. doi:10.1016/S1051-2004(02)00031-3

Arnavut, Z. (2007). ECG signal compression based on Burrows-Wheeler transformation and inversion ranks of linear prediction. *IEEE Transactions on Bio-Medical Engineering*, *54*(3), 410–418. doi:10.1109/TBME.2006.888820 PMID:17355052

Baibars, M., Kanjwal, K., & Marine, J. E. (2014). AF Detected on Implanted Cardiac Implantable Electronic Devices: Is There a Threshold for Thromboembolic Risk? *Current Treatment Options in Cardiovascular Medicine*, *16*(3), 289. doi:10.1007/s11936-013-0289-7 PMID:24500679

Batista, L. V., Melcher, E. U. K., & Carvalho, L. C. (2001). Compression of ECG signals by optimized quantization of discrete cosine transform coefficients. *Medical Engineering & Physics*, *23*(2), 127–134. doi:10.1016/S1350-4533(01)00030-3 PMID:11413065

Bendifallah, A., Benzid, R., & Boulemden, M. (2011). Improved ECG compression method using discrete cosine transform. *Electronics Letters*, *47*(2), 87. doi:10.1049/el.2010.3191

Blanco-Velasco, M., Cruz-Roldán, F., Godino-Llorente, J. I., & Barner, K. E. (2007). Wavelet packets feasibility study for the design of an ECG compressor. *IEEE Transactions on Bio-Medical Engineering*, *54*(4), 766–769. doi:10.1109/TBME.2006.889176 PMID:17405386

Blanco-Velasco, M., Cruz-Roldán, F., Godino-Llorente, J. I., Blanco-Velasco, J., Armiens-Aparicio, C., & López-Ferreras, F. (2005). On the use of PRD and CR parameters for ECG compression. *Medical Engineering & Physics*, *27*(9), 798–802. doi:10.1016/j.medengphy.2005.02.007 PMID:15869896

Cheng, A. C. (2015). *Real-Time Cardiovascular Diseases Detection on a Smartphone*. Academic Press.

Cohen, A., & Zigel, Y. (1998). Compression of multichannel ECG through multichannel long-term prediction. *IEEE Engineering in Medicine and Biology Magazine: The Quarterly Magazine of the Engineering in Medicine & Biology Society*, *17*(1), 109–115. Retrieved from http://www.ncbi.nlm.nih.gov/pubmed/9460626

Cox, J. R., Nolle, F. M., Fozzard, H. A., & Oliver, G. C. (1968). AZTEC, a preprocessing program for real-time ECG rhythm analysis. *IEEE Transactions on Bio-Medical Engineering*, *15*(April), 128–129. doi:10.1109/TBME.1968.4502549 PMID:5648088

Daubechies, I. (1992). Ten Lectures on Wavelets. *IEEE Symposium on Computer Based Medical Systems* (Vol. 61).

Djohan, A., Nguyen, T. Q., & Tompkins, W. J. (1995). ECG compression using discrete symmetric wavelet transform. In *IEEE International Conference on Engineering in Medicine and Biology Society* (pp. 167–168). Montreal, Canada: IEEE. doi:10.1109/IEMBS.1995.575053

Goldberger, A. L., Amaral, L. A., Glass, L., Hausdorff, J. M., Ivanov, P. C., Mark, R. G., & Stanley, H. E. et al. (2000). PhysioBank, PhysioToolkit, and PhysioNet: Components of a new research resource for complex physiologic signals. *Circulation*, *101*(23), e215–e220. doi:10.1161/01.CIR.101.23.e215 PMID:10851218

Hebert, M., Korabek, B., & Scott, R. E. (2006). Moving research into practice: A decision framework for integrating home telehealth into chronic illness care. *International Journal of Medical Informatics*, *75*(12), 786–794. doi:10.1016/j.ijmedinf.2006.05.041 PMID:16872892

Hilton, M. L. (1997). Wavelet and wavelet packet compression of electrocardiograms. *IEEE Transactions on Bio-Medical Engineering*, *44*(5), 394–402. doi:10.1109/10.568915 PMID:9125824

Horspool, R. N., & Windels, W. J. (1994). An LZ approach to ECG compression. In *Computer-Based Medical Systems, 1994.,Proceedings 1994 IEEE Seventh Symposium on* (pp. 71–76). http://doi.org/doi:<ALIGNMENT.qj></ALIGNMENT>10.1109/CBMS.1994.315990

Huang, B., Wang, Y., & Chen, J. (2013). ECG compression using the context modeling arithmetic coding with dynamic learning vector–scalar quantization. *Biomedical Signal Processing and Control*, *8*(1), 59–65. doi:10.1016/j.bspc.2012.04.003

Isa, S. M., Noviyanto, A., Jatmiko, W., & Arymurthy, A. M. (2012). The Effect of Electrocardiogram Signal Compression Using Beat Reordering and SPIHT on Automatic Sleep Stage Classification. *Procedia Engineering*, *41*, 888–896. http://doi.org/<ALIGNMENT.qj></ALIGNMENT>10.1016/j.proeng.2012.07.259

Jalaleddine, S. M., Hutchens, C. G., Strattan, R. D., & Coberly, W. A. (1990). ECG data compression techniques-a unified approach. *IEEE Transactions on Bio-Medical Engineering*, *37*(4), 329–343. doi:10.1109/10.52340 PMID:2186997

Koski, A. (1997). Lossless ECG encoding. *Computer Methods and Programs in Biomedicine*, *52*(1), 23–33. doi:10.1016/S0169-2607(96)01779-8 PMID:9034667

Kulkarni, P. K., Kumar, V., & Verma, H. K. (1997). ECG data compression using fast Walsh transform and its clinical acceptability. *International Journal of Systems Science*, *28*(8), 831–836. doi:10.1080/00207729708929443

Kumar, R., Kumar, A., & Kumar, R. (2012). Electrocardiogram Signal Compression Using Beta Wavelets. *Journal of Mathematical Modelling and Algorithms*, *11*(3), 235–248. doi:10.1007/s10852-012-9181-9

Kumar, V., Saxena, S. C., & Giri, V. K. (2006). Direct data compression of ECG signal for telemedicine. *International Journal of Systems Science*, *37*(1), 45–63. doi:10.1080/00319100500412337

Lee, S., Kim, J., & Lee, M. (2011). A real-time ECG data compression and transmission algorithm for an e-health device. *IEEE Transactions on Bio-Medical Engineering*, *58*(9), 2448–2455. doi:10.1109/TBME.2011.2156794 PMID:21606020

Ma, J., Zhang, T., & Dong, M. (2015). A Novel ECG data compression method using adaptive fourier decomposition with security guarantee in e-Health applications. *IEEE Journal of Biomedical and Health Informatics*, *19*(3), 986–994. PMID:25222961

Mallat, S. (2009). A wavelet tour of signal processing (S. Mallat, Ed.). Academic Press.

Mueller, W. C. (1977). Arrhythmia detection program for an ambulatory ECG monitor. *Biomedical Sciences Instrumentation*, *14*(1), 81–85. PMID:687739

Nave, G., & Cohen, A. (1993). ECG compression using long-term prediction. *IEEE Transactions on Bio-Medical Engineering*, *40*(9), 877–885. doi:10.1109/10.245608 PMID:8288278

Paggetti, C., Lusini, M., Varanini, M., Taddei, A., Marchesi, C., & Sistemi, D. (1994). *A Multichannel Template Based Data Compression Algorithm*. Academic Press.

Ramakrishnan, A. G., & Saha, S. (1997). ECG Coding by Wavelet-Based Linear Prediction. *IEEE Transactions on Bio-Medical Engineering*, *44*(12), 1253–1261. doi:10.1109/10.649997 PMID:9401225

Sabarimalai Sur, M., & Dandapat, S. (2014). Wavelet-based electrocardiogram signal compression methods and their performances: A prospective review. *Biomedical Signal Processing and Control*, *14*(1), 73–107. Retrieved from http://linkinghub.elsevier.com/retrieve/pii/S1746809414000998

Sayood, K. (2010). Introduction to data compression. (K. Sayood, Ed.). Elsevier Inc.

Shaou-Gang, M., & Yen, H.-L. (2001). Multichannel ECG compression using multichannel adaptive vector quantization. *IEEE Transactions on Bio-Medical Engineering*, *48*(10), 1203–1207. doi:10.1109/10.951524 PMID:11585045

Singh, B., & Singh, D. (2012). Effect of threshold value r on multiscale entropy based heart rate variability. *Cardiovascular Engineering and Technology*, *3*(2), 211–216. doi:10.1007/s13239-012-0082-x

Tompkins, W. J. (1993). *Biomedical digital signal processing*. Editorial Prentice Hall.

Wang, X., & Meng, J. (2008). A 2-D ECG compression algorithm based on wavelet transform and vector quantization. *Digital Signal Processing*, *18*(2), 179–188. doi:10.1016/j.dsp.2007.03.003

Chapter 14
Energy Efficient Particle Optimized Compressed ECG Data over Zigbee Environment

Dilip Kumar
SLIET, India

Rajeev Kumar
DAVIET, India

Tony Singla
DAVIET, India

ABSTRACT

Standard Electrocardiogram Tracking instruments are huge to carry away over the remote areas for the surveillance. Holter is the compact instrument meant for collecting ECG of a patient without a pause while the patient is on the go of their daily activities. Holter works on battery for 48 hours without any angle of transmission but when allowed to transmit battery power dies soon, for these purposes some energy saving techniques is required. In this chapter the authors have proposed a Wavelet based Compression Technique, followed by Optimization under Genetic Algorithm and Particle Swarm Optimization. Compressed and Optimized ECG data has been transferred over Zigbee IEEE 802.15.4 with the intention of saving energy implicating it on a hardware chip. Transferred data will be available to the Doctor for on time treatment and further examination and storage. Embedded prior techniques in Holter can enhance its life, with fact of sending crucial data.

INTRODUCTION

Present time reveals the truth that there is a raise in the aging population, busy world and life taking diseases (Maneesha V. Ramesh et al., 2012). Ongoing era demands the early detection and prevention of death threatening diseases [2], out of a huge number here the main focus is on cardiovascular diseases (S. Muthulakshmi and K. Latha, 2012). Cardiovascular diseases take a handsome share in the chart of

DOI: 10.4018/978-1-5225-0660-7.ch014

death threatening diseases. People are too busy in their lives; this thing added a lot in pre death (UK. Jin Yoon et al., 2010). Scenario demands a system that will have a high check over the heart's abnormality, any oddness in daily life demands a Electrocardiogram (ECG) check up (Agus Dwi Swarjaya, 2012). This demands the idea of a technology that is fast, reliable and easy to communicate. In order to satisfy this desire we have to think for a new and efficient wireless technology called Wireless Sensor Network (Ali N. Akansu et al., 2010).Moreover, this has a revolutionary impact over the various research areas, out of a large number of areas our intention is on biomedical area which cover ups a large number of diseases that comes in human lifecycle (R. Gupta and M.mitra, 2012). Electrocardiogram is one of biomedical application which is closely related to WSN (Youssouf Zatout, 2012). Rhythm of heart is a electrical activity which is governed by the traditional ECG machine by placing various electrodes (which work as sensors) that senses the electric change and the same is passed onto the machine through wires which is reportedly drawn on a graph paper in the form of waves with each represented by P,QRS, T and U (S. Karpagachelvi et al., 2010). But our scenario has changed the traditional fact by miniaturizing the size of machine and making the sensing wire free and placing it on proximity of humans by keeping in mind sometime an instant check may not report the abnormalities, so some device need to monitor the patient continuously for a period of time (Benny P.L. Lo et al.). Holter is a monitoring device which actually works in the same way as the normal ECG machines work but on a go. Usually works for 24 or 48 hours after which the stored data will be used by the doctor to report the abnormalities (Shao. Yen Tseng et al., 2009). Where if Holter instead of storing large amount of data keep on sending its acquired data continuously, but this procedure will eat up all the battery cells and Holter machines dies soon before even lasting for 24 hours because during wireless communication most of the energy is wasted. Various authors have tried to overcome this drawback to certain extent they succeeded, out of a number of reach, some have tried to work with the compression method whose job is to cut down the irrelevant data as in the previous work Discrete Cosine transformation is used which creates discrete samples, compresses them and send them wirelessly (Tellez Camiilo et al., 2009). Lack to overcome the battery life of Holter machine as Bluetooth transmission is being used and only the frequency component of ECG is taken into consideration. Our work has overpowered the drawbacks by implementing discrete wavelet transformation (DWT) as a compression method, which discretely compresses the various frequency and time samples over discrete times before compression pre-filtration is done with the help of various filters depending upon the noise ECG data contains (Li Xuemei et al., 2008). Compression only removes the unwanted or less important data from the main data but this is not enough to save energy, this puts up with the idea of optimization (Emran Mohammad Abu Anas et al.,2010).Optimization means how well the compressed data can be further enhanced without changing the meaning of the overall data (Sateh M.S. Jalaleddine et al., 1990). Optimization works on the mirror image samples, whose removal will not lead the data in unwanted state or non-meaningful (Jos Hulzink et al.,2011). Great optimization techniques have been proposed out of large category some of them are listed below-Genetic algorithm, Particle swarm optimization, Ant colony optimization etc (Rozeha A. Roshid et al., 2008).

Genetic algorithm basically gives a simple solution termed as chromosome, where its collection called as population (Hossein Mamaghanian et al., 2011). Each chromosome undergoes a process of fitness evaluation in order to check the suitability of the candidate solution for the problem. Some chromosomes undergo the process of crossover as chromosomes exchange their values or genes, where some undergo mutation where an old value is replaced by new value. Chromosomes that undergo crossover process and mutation process is based upon their crossover rate and mutation rates respectively (Manpreet Kaur et al., 2011). Generation puts a boundary over the evaluation of chromosome that passes through a different above mentioned processes.

Particle swarm optimization gives us a solution as particle; each particle is set to move in a space where it compares its fitness with neighbours (Mehdia Ajana EI Khaddar et al., 2012). Each particle carries two things one is the fitness value and other is its velocity. Fitness factor has two values one the value of particle it has reached so far (pbest) and second is the global value (gbest) that is decided by Particle swarm optimizer and broadcast the value to each particle in the space or population, sometime local value is broadcasted based upon topological location. Every iteration bring up with a updated value that the particle will carry, updated values include the pbest, gbest and velocities of respective particles. Iterations and velocity (Vmax) are predefined parameters.

Compression and optimization have reduced the sample rate in order to match the sample rate media for transmission is selected that is Zigbee Standard is designed and named by IEEE as 802.15.4 which actually works at low cost and low power wireless communication (Guojun Li et al., 2012). Zigbee works on the radio frequency bandwidth of 2.4 GHz / 868MHz/915 MHz. India is specified to use the 2.4 GHz range with 16 channels available with data rate of 250kb/s (P. Manimegalai et al.,2012) .Zigbee is the proprietary standard used in Wireless Communication or more precisely in Wireless Sensor communication. Zigbee operates with low power best paired with Holter machine; this in totality results in saving the battery power and allows battery to stay for few more hours.

PREVIOUS METHODS

Compression and transmission plays a pivotal and subsequent role in the field of health monitoring. Death chart grabs our attention as there is vigorous rise, due to the deadly chronic diseases that are prevailing around the humans. Among the huge number of diseases cardiac diseases are the one that need immediate attention. Cardiac diseases are visualized by the fact of Electrocardiogram (ECG) data which represents the usual heart activity of the humans in a wave cycle representing peaks as P, QRS, T and U. Various devices have been proposed but how efficient these are still a question. Efficiency depends upon the concept of data acquisition and its transmission over terrains of range while dealing with the energy optimization. Energy optimization is considered at both the hardware level and software level, there is great revolution in the field of hardware for saving energy as it gives only 30% of its share in energy saving cycle, while the rest 70% is maintained by the software part which is still in research. So far numerous software techniques have been implemented and their results have shown some satisfaction. Software part is broadly categorized as 1) Compression Techniques, 2) Optimization Techniques and 3) Transmission techniques. Over the years of research a heap of compression techniques have been proposed and modified timely. Compressing the ECG data of the patient's heart, gives us a picture to rectify the symptoms of the particular cardiac disease a patient is going through so that on time help can be availed. In our system a remarkable attention has been paid to work out with the prominent features of ECG. Discrete cosine transformation and LZW hybrid scheme has been proposed by Bo Yu et al. (2010) in their research paper. Drawbacks are as considered hybrid approach only works in the time domain of ECG and consumes more energy with lesser data rate during its transmission as media used is Bluetooth. A low power wearable cardiac device has been proposed by Maneesha V. Ramesh et al. (2012) in their research paper. Drawback different set of modes have been proposed, switching among different modes is time consuming and non-efficient as energy is wasted unnecessarily while transition happens. Our proposed system is far away from the fact of mode changer and attention has been paid to the compression method's reliability and transmission media for communication. An adaptive cosine Fourier Transform approach is proposed by Patompon Chaiyakum and Paramote WardKein (2012) in their paper. Drawback is neglecting the period can put the ECG data in an unrecognizable form as time is one of the prominent factor in ECG. An optimal thresholding algorithm for denoising ECG has been proposed by Sami M. Isa et al. (2011) in their paper. Drawback although thresholding is good concept but when limited to a small section of data samples if samples are in large number it fails deliberately resulting ECG in a fix. In our proposed system has nothing to do with the thresholding concept as Samples are pre de-noised using certain set of filters which makes the compression task quite easy.

A new algorithm has been proposed by Anubhuti Khare et al. (2011) to compress the lossy ECG data in their research paper. Drawback is considering the lossy nature of ECG certain hidden corruptive signals have been neglected, and will be modified or compressed with the technique that has been used. Our proposed system deals with the hidden corruptive signals produced due to the body artifacts, and are removed quietly before compression. Wearable wireless sensor equipment has been designed to compute oxygen saturation and Heart rate and sending it on a wireless media as presented by Cristian Rotaria and Vasile Mante (2012) in their paper. Drawback of proposed system wireless media used is access point to send data over Wi-Fi, it eats up the battery soon with lesser amount of data travelled in totality. Our proposed system has tried to rectify this flaw by using another set of wireless media, which is capable of sending data efficiently with lesser energy consumption and good data rate. New compression technique has been proposed by Mohammad Abo. Zahhad et al. (2012) in which data is considered in 2D format for compression, with attention paid over the single part of ECG. Drawback of the proposed scheme is it only works for images not for digital signals in 1D, secondly it has considered only the QRS factor among the number of factors that represents ECG in more appropriate way and thirdly conversion of 1D data to 2D consumes more energy and space. Mostly the data acquisition equipments are liable to collect data in digital form; this is taken into consideration in our proposed system, working with digital signals is bit easy as compared to analog signals, whose handling is a difficult task. Optimization techniques followed by compression techniques are quite energy saving schemes.

Optimal algorithm has been designed by Grisha Garg et al. (2010) which are based upon the various thresholding concepts added with the DWT compression method shown in their research paper. Drawback in the in this chapter main focus is on the various thresholding techniques instead the kind of DWT scheme is used, thresholding adds a bit difficulty in determining the exact value for each set of thresholding schemes. Our in this chapter has nothing to do with thresholding as sample space is large but instead of thresholding concept optimization techniques have been used to remove redundancy in the samples. Ubiquitous health care monitoring equipment has been designed by Wan. Young et al. (2008) for evaluation of ECG, Accelerometer and SpO_2 presented in their research paper. Major flaw in the proposed system is that acquired data is transmitted directly without any set of compression or optimization technique, this can increment the energy and space usage during transmission. In our proposed system all these flaws have been rectified by proper usage of compression, optimization and transmission techniques. This wholesome reduces a remarkable amount of energy usage that is consumed during transmission of the data after specific steps of denoising, compression and optimization. Health decision support system is designed by Sing. Hui Toh et al. (2009) for monitoring biomedical signals as shown in their research paper. Major flaw in the proposed scheme is type of transmission media used; CDMA consumes more energy when uncompressed data travels from patient's cell phone to server where this is analyzed with the preset of values. Two set of communication medias have been used that will consume more power than single media and this kind of system is feasible in local domain as its global application can lead this into complications. Wearable equipment is designed by Antonio J.Jara et al. (2012) for continuous data transmission via a Bluetooth medium as shown in their respective work. Drawback can be seen in the flow of continuous data over a media that provides lesser data rate, range and consumes more energy, for one time this can be ignored but the continuous flow of data from a wearable device can end up very early as continuous monitoring leads to the more usage of battery and the device can die soon. In our proposed system samples have been evaluated over discrete levels and treated separately over discrete times as this in whole will save the energy consumption and device can work for few more hours. Whereas the transmission media is concerned optimized wireless technology is preferred over Bluetooth for sending and receiving the discrete compressed packets.

Dealing with the redundancy found in the ECG coefficients a new algorithm has been proposed by S. Akhter and M.A. Haque (2010) entitled in their research paper. Disadvantage algorithm works only in time domain but our proposed system has taken this into consideration. ECG is represented in two broader domains as time domain and amplitude domain. ECG data holds the various corruptive signals which hide its functionality, steps to be considered in order to remove those corruptive signals produced by the various movements of the body before the compression. Optimal way of recognizing the various abnormalities in ECG data using Neuro-Fuzzy approach shown by P.D. Khandait et al. (2012) in their research paper. In this paper major drawback is more energy, time and space consuming with less concentration on the artifacts that causes abnormalities every set of abnormality whose negligence cannot be afforded is not recognized by Neuro-Fuzzy technique. In our in this chapter we have statically mentioned the major abnormalities and removed them under a course of steps this saves time, energy and space, precisely design comes up with the data that is important and make it ready for transmission after removing set of abnormality as the received data is an impression for the doctor to find out the oddness so as to reach the patient instantly and timely.

CHAPTER'S HIGHLIGHTS

Electrocardiogram (ECG) data can be compressed by number of techniques but technique mentioned in the base paper is DCT (Discrete Cosine Transform) followed by LZW (Emran Mohammad Abu Anas et al.,2010) and compressed data is sent over the Bluetooth environment, as DCT is restricted to the certain compressed ratio and it blocks some of the important features of the signal and another drawback of the DCT (Anubhuti Khare et al., 2011)is that it represents the signal in the frequency domain but ECG composed of two domains as frequency and time domains. Both domains are equally important to extract the right meaning of the ECG data, for this Discrete wavelet transform (DWT) is used to represents the signal in the frequency and time domain. After compression the second important thing is the transmission of data, whereas in the base paper transmission is done over the Bluetooth media. Medium that has been chosen seems unreliable and more power consumer which results in early dying of the Holter's battery, these drawbacks have been corrected in our chapter with full attention has been paid to the energy utilization. Wavelet transformation compression technique and Zigbee environment overcomes the drawbacks of DCT (Patompon Chaiyakum & Paramote WardKein, 2012) and Bluetooth respectively. Some set of add-on is done in the proposed scheme that is optimization technique, which further reduces the number of samples to be sent over the wireless media.

NEED AND SIGNIFICANCE OF THIS CHAPTER

Need of the in this chapter is illustrated by the Related work as said that ECG data that is evaluated continuously while patient is involved in his daily activities, and secondly its transmission consumes more energy than energy consumed during its compression. Continuous ECG (Uk.Jin Yoon et al., 2010) will be compressed in discrete form under wavelet transformation and transmitted over the Zigbee IEEE802.15.4 protocol and reaches the Doctor or care taker for immediate assistance. Continuous monitoring of data and its transmission without compression can lead the device out of power after few hours but if we correct the transmission by just sending the compressed data over time-domain as a constraint and better protocol for transmission, by this power can be saved and the device can operate for few more hours under set of various environmental conditions. Whereas the significance is concerned it is illustrated by the fact that energy is being saved on account of Compression method and transmission is made better by use of Zigbee IEEE802.15.4 (Wan.Young Chung et al., 2008) protocol as it consumes less power for transmission, easy to operate than Bluetooth (Antonio J. Jara et al., 2012) along with these techniques some optimization techniques have been proposed which further reduces the number of samples to be sent. Results signify the better working of the proposed system under set of parameters as energy. IEEE802.15.4 has a peculiar significance that although its data rate is less than the Bluetooth but consumes less power while transmitting the data as compared to the Bluetooth wireless technology.

EXPERIMENTAL DESIGN

In this paper we have proposed a approach to compress the ECG data after removal of noise from the raw ECG data collected which is obtained from the real time simulator through Virtual Labs (Vlabs) and then passing it through optimizers and then the optimized data is tested over the Zigbee (802.15.4) Environment. Although some performance metrics have been used for evaluation. Once the different ECG data (normal, muscle, respiration and baseline wandering) are obtained from the simulator these undergo a noise removal process respectively at very first step of the proposed signal processing algorithm. Three basic types of noises such as muscle artifact, respiration artifact and baseline wandering will be eliminated which can be probably caused by muscle movement, breathing problem and in contact with high voltage respectively. The first step is to eliminate the baseline drift/wandering (Manpreet Kaur et al., 2011) which is a type of noise got generated during the signal recording process. Baseline drift will be eliminated using a smooth filter.

The next step is to remove the muscle artifact using median Filter. After removing the muscle artifact, the next objective is to remove the spikes or respiration artifact from the ECG data that arises because of any voltage fluctuation using average Filter. Various metrics have been evaluated before and after filtration process using equations 1, 2 and 3.

Then the single-level one-dimensional wavelet decomposition is performed on the ECG signal, which decomposes the signal using discrete wavelet, DWT compression usually compresses the whole received pre-processed signal and transforms it in two components one is approximation coefficient and other is detail coefficient. Coefficients designed above envelopes vital information that is passed on for further processing respectively. Along with Compression some metrics have been evaluated like PSNR (GirishaGarg et al., 2010), MSE (Sani M. Isa et al., 2011) and PRD (Mohammed Abo.Zahhad et al., 2012) by following equations 1,2 and 3.

$$PSNR = 10 * \log_{10}\left(\frac{255 * 255}{MSE}\right) \tag{1}$$

$$MSE = \frac{1}{n} * \left(\sum_{i=0}^{n} (x[i] - x'[i])^2\right) \tag{2}$$

$$PRD = \sqrt{\frac{\sum_{n-0}^{n-1} (x[i] - x'[i])^2}{\sum_{n-0}^{n-1} (x[i])^2} * 100} \tag{3}$$

x[i]- Original ECG data, x'[i]- Transformed ECG data, n- Number of samples.

Above metrics are evaluated at two stages that is at the former stage of compression and secondly at the latter stage of compression. The decomposed signal is passed to the particle swarm optimization and genetic algorithm for the signal optimization process. The ECG signal is optimized using the above two algorithm to get the best ECG signal out of the obtained ECG signal.

The detail of our execution of GA has been described as follow;

Genetic Algorithm Procedure

Input: Compressed ECG data
Output: Optimized ECG data
Step 0: attribute the various variables (population size, crossover rate, mutation rate and utmost number of generations)
Step 1: initialize population randomly as (G(0))
Step 2: calculate present population (find the fitness of chromosomes/genes)
Step 3: while (condition not met) do [step 4-8]
Step 4: select G(u) from G(u+1) [execute selection process]
Step 5 again combine G(t)[do mutation and crossover]
Step 6: caluculate present population (find the fitness of chromosomes/genes).
Step 7: u=u+1
Step 8: go to step 3 repeat the process again

The detail of our execution of PSO has been described as follow;

Particle Swarm Optimization Procedure

Input: Compressed ECG data
Output: Optimized ECG data
Step 1: For each bird/value
Step 2: attribute the values/birds
Step 3: End
Step 4: Do

Step 5: For each bird/value
Step 6: apply fitness check
Step 7: If resulted fitness is enhanced than pBest in history
Step 8: set pBest equal to current value
Step 9: End
Step 10: Choose the pbest among all the birds/values assign it as the gBest for all the birds repeatedly.
Step 11: evaluate bird velocity with equation (a)
Step 12: Update bird position with equation (b)
Step 13: End

$$\mathrm{a[i]} = \mathrm{a[i]} + \mathrm{d}1 * \mathrm{rand}() * (\mathrm{pb[i]} - \mathrm{pre[i]}) + \mathrm{d}2 * \mathrm{rand}() * (\mathrm{gb[i]} - \mathrm{pb[i]}) \tag{4}$$

$$\mathrm{pre[i]} = p\,\mathrm{re[i]} + a\mathrm{[i]} \tag{5}$$

a[i] - particle velocity, pre[i] -current solution that particle holds randomly, pb[i] and gb[i]-local and global best fitness values respectively for each particle

rand ()- random number (0,1), d1, d2 -are learning factors [0 2].

Energy is calculated for both of the optimization processes that is for Genetic algorithm and Particle Swarm Optimization. The one with the lesser energy will be allowed to forward its Optimized compressed ECG data (noise free) for transmission to the medical database server for further analysis by doctor via Zigbee environment experimented on a hardware module. Zigbee consumes lesser power and work without any fatal error. This allows ZigBee networks to form ad-hoc, with no control from the centralized department or high-power transmitter/receiver able to reach all of the devices. Received ECG data is the optimized data along with position where the best sample is residing is used for decompression process. The examined result and all the vital information is later saved to the medical database along with the received ECG signal under the patient ID from where it was received earlier, by this immediate medical assistance is stipulated to the targeted patient and further patient is under regular surveillance (Figure 1).

Figure 1. Flowchart of experimental design

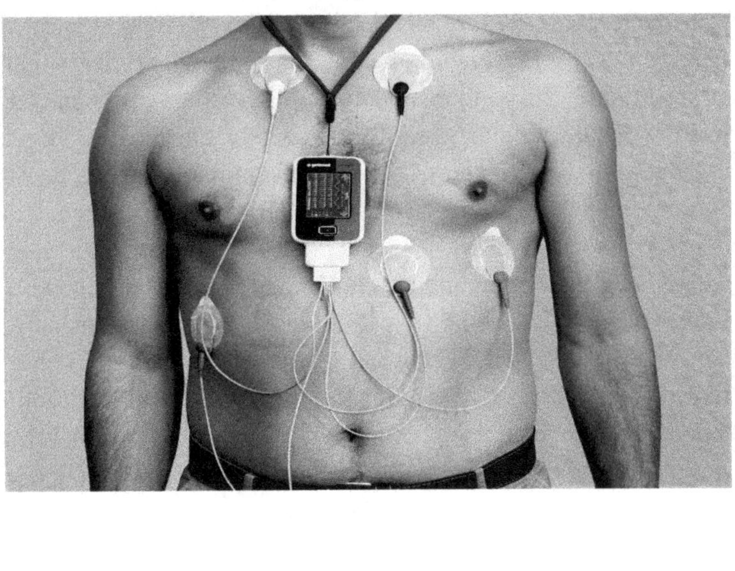

Step 1: Different types of ECG data are collected from the online virtual lab (Vlab) site simulated in real Time

Step 2: Collected ECG data are termed as normal, muscle artifact, baseline wandering and respiration artifact.

Step 3: Extracted data is passed on to different filters for removal of noise based upon the type of collected data filter is used.

Step 4: Muscle artifact data is passed to the median filter for removal of spikes, baseline wandering data is passed to smoothing filter and respiration artifact data is passed to average filter respectively.

Step 5: Performance metrics have been evaluated before and after filtration.

Step 6: Pre-processed data is ready to undergo a wavelet Transformation DWT

Step 7: Performance metrics have been evaluated before and after compression according to equation number 1,2 and 3 respectively.

Step 8: while (iteration terminated)

Do (Step 8)

Step 9: Compressed ECG data passed through optimizers named as Genetic algorithm and Particle swarm optimization.

Step 10: Best optimized ECG data obtained based upon energy consumed by both optimizers, one with less is preferred

Step 11: Optimized compressed ECG data ready for transmission over Zigbee environment.

Step 12: Received ECG data analyzed and stored in medical database for further analysis

Step 13: End.

SIMULATION RESULTS

In this research, a novel heart beat signal propagation and computation model is developed for the patients using body wearable sensors for heart rate monitoring (also known as Holter) connected through Zigbee Environment with the medical database. These kinds of scenarios are usually designed for the special medical environment where patients are monitored on the regular basis to avoid the critical health hazard situations. In this research project, the aim is to improve the ECG signal propagation process by making the whole process energy efficient. The energy consumption can be minimized by optimizing the signal, which will yield out a small-sized equally detailed optimized ECG signals. This optimized ECG signal can be propagated on the ZigBee environment by consuming less energy than the non-optimized signal, for sake of easiness hardware Zigbee module is designed for communication. Also, one more aim of this research is to compute the energy consumption by Genetic Algorithm and Particle Swarm Optimization on the Holter (Body Wearable Heart Rate Recording Wireless Sensor). The signal with the lower energy consumption will be propagated on the ZigBee environment and other complex signal consuming more energy will be discarded.

Various patients have been put on test and evaluation under same set of conditions and various set of performance metrics have been evaluated as- peak signal to noise ratio, mean square error and percentage root mean square difference, all these when taken into consideration have come up with new results that shows remarkable difference among the values before and after filtration and compression respectively based upon different filter size. Tabular representation shown in Table 1 shows that peak signal to noise ratio is more after compression than before compression, whereas mean square error is less after compression than before and same is with the percentage root mean square value which shows a decrement in its value after compression than before compression. Simulated results show that error or corruptive signals have been removed during compression before the signal is ready for transmission.

Table 1 shows the various values of performance metrics before filtration of noisy ECG data with different window sizes (5, 6, 7, 8, 9) respectively. Comparison represents that in case of normal data the value of PSNR is infinite for respective window size, value for MSE is zero and value for PRD is 100 for respective window size, this shows that the normal data is accurate and further comparisons can be drawn from this normal ECG data. Various values of Peak signal to noise ratio, mean square error and percentage root mean square difference for the muscle artifact, respiration artifact and baseline wandering ECG data are listed below with respect to the normal ECG data.

Record shows that values differ from their parent values; apart from their parent values they have values that are different, which gives us a sign that may be some noise is present which needs certain methods for their removal.

The results in the below Table 2 has proved that after filtration of noise from muscle artifact, respiration artifact and baseline wandering ECG data various performance metrics have changed where PSNR has decreased constantly and the same fall is seen in PRD Values and but there is a increase in MSE values with different window sizes respectively which illustrates that there is an noise/error in the signal has with respect to the parent data. Calculated values in Table 2 also represent the values before compression of ECG data (Muscle artifact, respiration artifact and baseline wandering free).

Table 3 shows the values of various performance metrics after the compression process which shows that there is an increase in the PSNR, same increase in seen in PRD values but there is a fall in MSE

Table 1. Recorded performance parameters (statistical errors) before filtration

Window Size	Normal ECG Data			Muscle Artifact			Respiration Artifact			Baseline Wandering		
	PSNR	MSE	PRD	PSNR	MSE	PRD	PSNR	MSE	PRD	PSNR	MSE	PRD
5	Inf	0	100	60.39	0.05	93.13	61.5	0.04	96.6	61.4	0.04	98.3
6	Inf	0	100	60.39	0.05	93.13	61.5	0.04	96.6	61.4	0.04	98.3
7	Inf	0	100	60.39	0.05	93.13	61.5	0.04	96.6	61.4	0.04	98.3
8	Inf	0	100	60.39	0.05	93.13	61.5	0.04	96.6	61.4	0.04	98.3
9	Inf	0	100	60.39	0.05	93.13	61.5	0.04	96.6	61.4	0.04	98.3

Table 2. Recorded performance parameters (statistical errors) after filtration or before compression

Window Size	Muscle Artifact			Respiration Artifact			Baseline Wandering		
	PSNR	MSE	PRD	PSNR	MSE	PRD	PSNR	MSE	PRD
5	69.7	0.006	69.4	66.0	0.016	72.55	83.47	0.0002	95.508
6	67.7	0.011	60.1	65.58	0.017	67.65	83.47	0.0002	95.508
7	66.5	0.014	55.5	65.26	0.019	63.47	74.55	0.0022	87.75
8	65.9	0.013	52.0	65.00	0.02	59.77	74.55	0.0022	87.75
9	65.4	0.018	51.0	64.79	0.021	56.40	70.58	0.0056	80.72

Table 3. Recorded performance parameters (statistical errors) after compression

Window Size	Muscle Artifact			Respiration Artifact			Baseline Wandering		
	PSNR	MSE	PRD	PSNR	MSE	PRD	PSNR	MSE	PRD
5	63.4	0.02	91.92	63.83	0.021	93.87	61.66	0.044	85.38
6	64.69	0.022	93.98	64.31	0.024	94.99	61.66	0.044	85.38
7	65.73	0.01	95.52	64.72	0.02	95.54	62.72	0.03	89.08
8	66.36	0.01	96.44	65.10	0.020	95.95	62.72	0.03	89.08
9	66.74	0.013	96.60	65.48	0.018	96.30	63.77	0.02	92.26

values with different window sizes respectively which shows that error has been removed now the data is error free as shown in tabular form.

In Table 4 particle swarm optimization outperformed Genetic Algorithm. PSO has taken almost less than half energy than GA for the ECG signal optimization. Each patient's ECG data is examined in this project is of the length 40 seconds and has recorded on the 100 samples per second as a sampling rate.

This research project has been developed along with a GUI using the graphical user interface developer called GUIDE in the MATLAB software. The GUI contains various push buttons, text fields and signal plot axis. The buttons are used to process all of the tasks listed in the project one after one in a particular sequence. The processes listed to run on the buttons are main simulation, import signal (normal, muscle artifact, respiration artifact and baseline wandering ECG data), filtration (median, average and smooth filter), DWT filter, optimization (GA & PSO) and Comparison (GA and PSO). The general GUI is shown in the Figure 2.

Figure 2 and 3 shows the imported ECG data from the Virtual Labs. The various noises in the signal are removed is the step after plotting the original signal as shown in Figure 3 and 4.

After the respiration artifact and muscle artifact are being removed a significant change occurs in the signal structure shown in the Figure 5.

Noise produced by the baseline wandering is being removed such that the structure of the signal is changed as shown in Figure 6.

After the process of filtration process each ECG data is passed through compression module which in turn decreases the number of samples to be sent as shown in Figure 7 and 8 respectively.

After the compression process, compressed ECG data still contains certain mirror samples which further are removed with the optimization process under genetic algorithm and particle swarm optimization, individual algorithm is checked for the energy consumed by them during optimization process and one with lesser energy is preferred as shown in Figure 9 and 10 respectively then this data is allowed to be sent over wireless environment.

Table 4. Energy consumption by PSO, Genetic Algorithm and ZigBee -Environment

Sample Types	Energy Computed by GA	Energy Computed by PSO
Normal ECG data	49.03	27.42
Muscle artifact ECG data	50.49	26.98
Respiration artifact ECG data	48.10	37.75
Baseline wandering ECG data	49.04	25.22

Figure 2. GUI interface figure

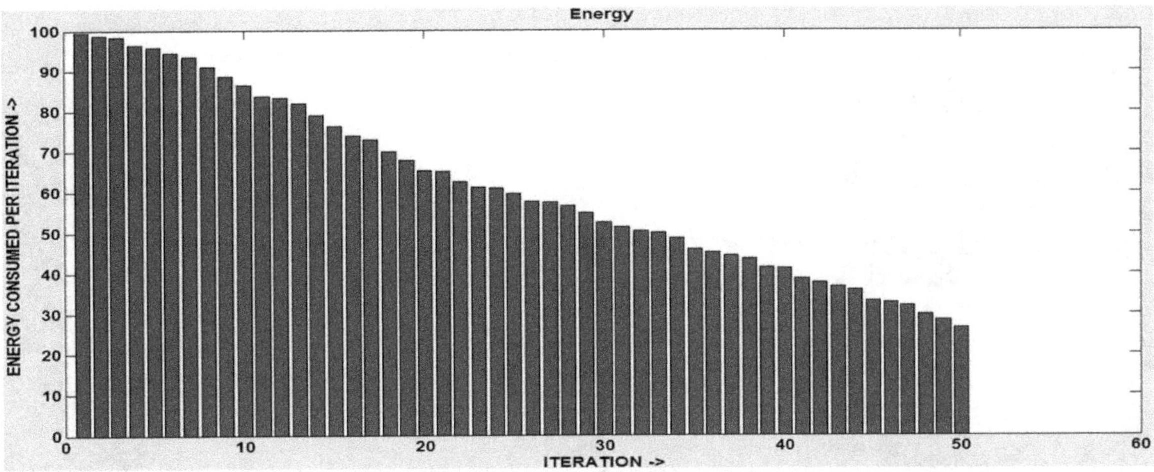

Figure 3. Displaying normal and muscle artifact ECG signal

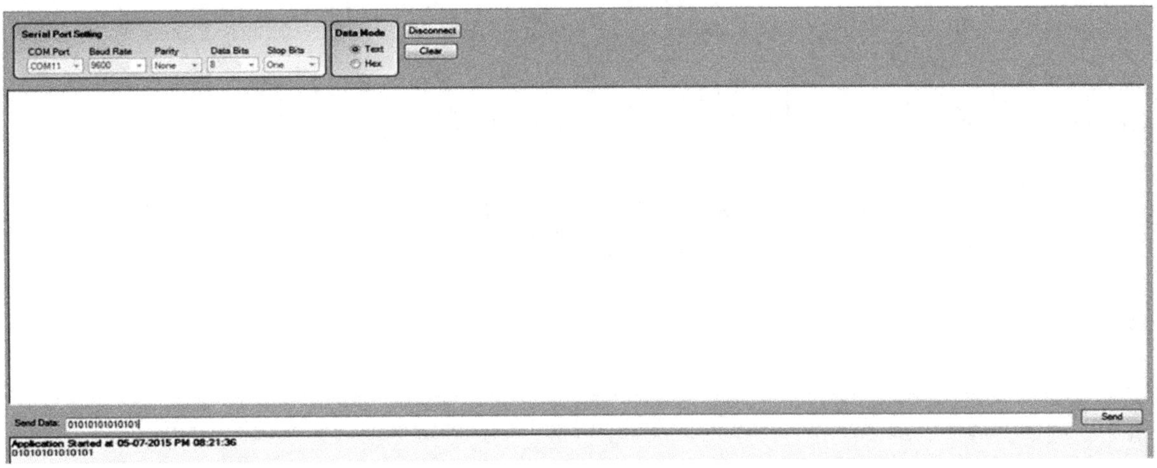

Figure 4. Displaying respiration artifact and baseline wandering in ECG signal

Figure 5. Plot of respiration, muscle artifact ECG data after application of average, median filter respectively

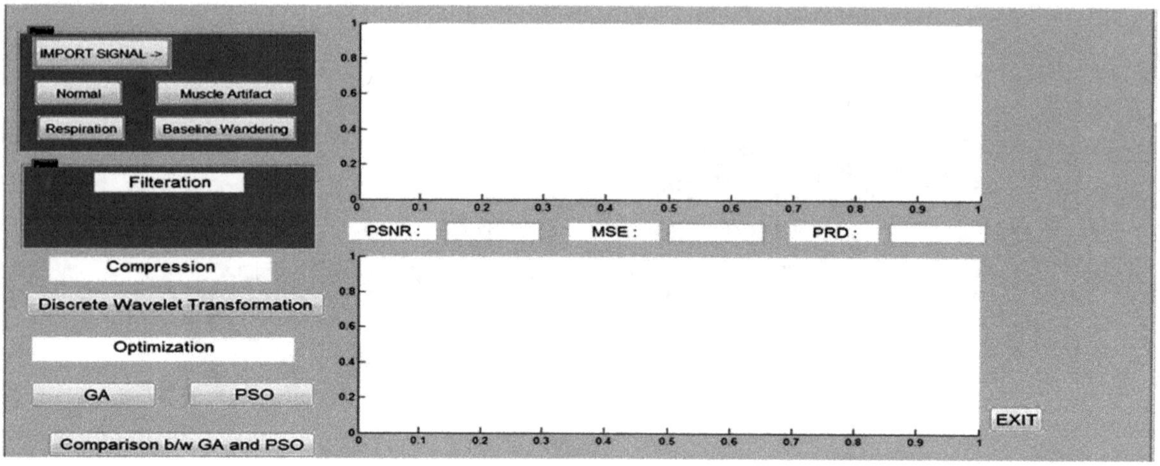

Figure 6. Plot of baseline wandering ECG data after application of smoothing filter

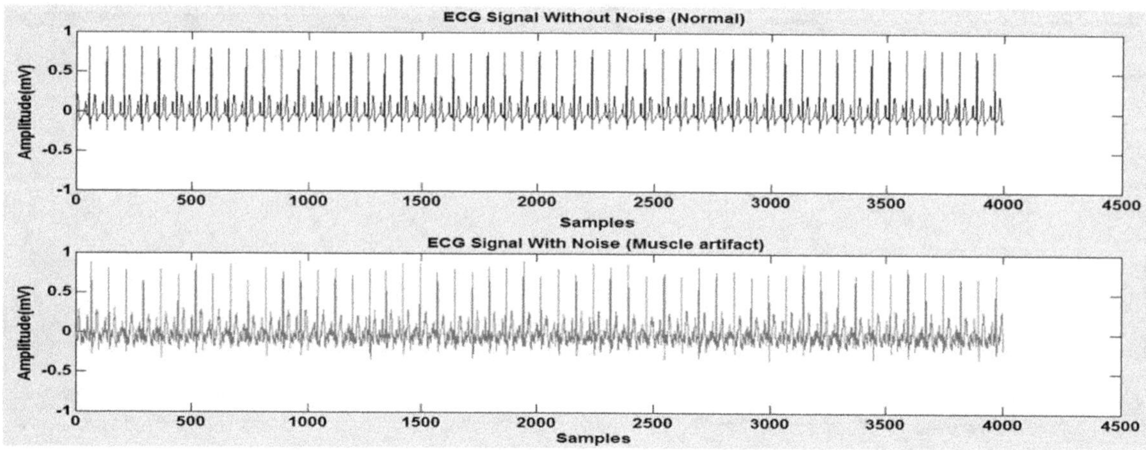

Figure 7. Compression of normal and muscle artifact free ECG data respectively

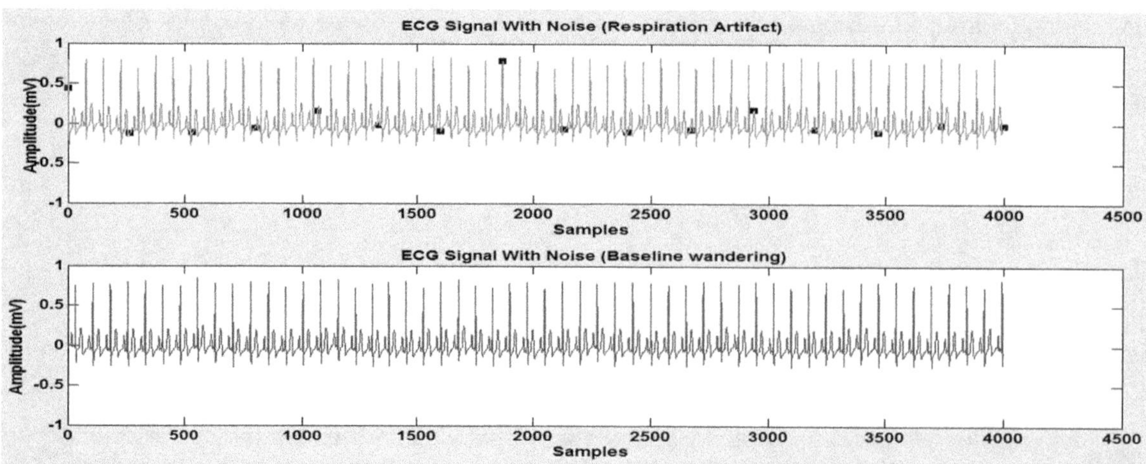

Figure 8. Compression of respiration artifact and baseline wandering free ECG data respectively

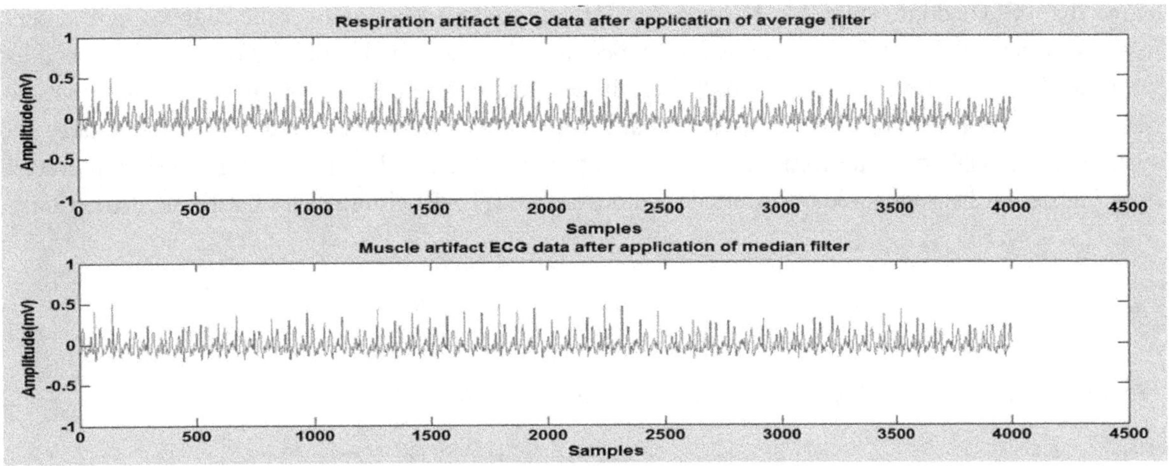

Figure 9. Energy consumption of muscle artifact ECG data under GA

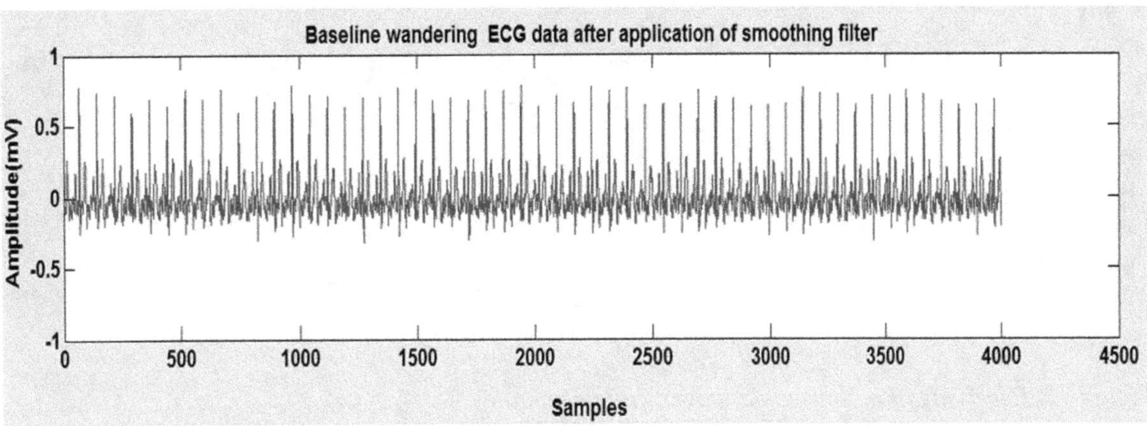

Figure 10. Energy consumption of muscle artifact ECG data under PSO

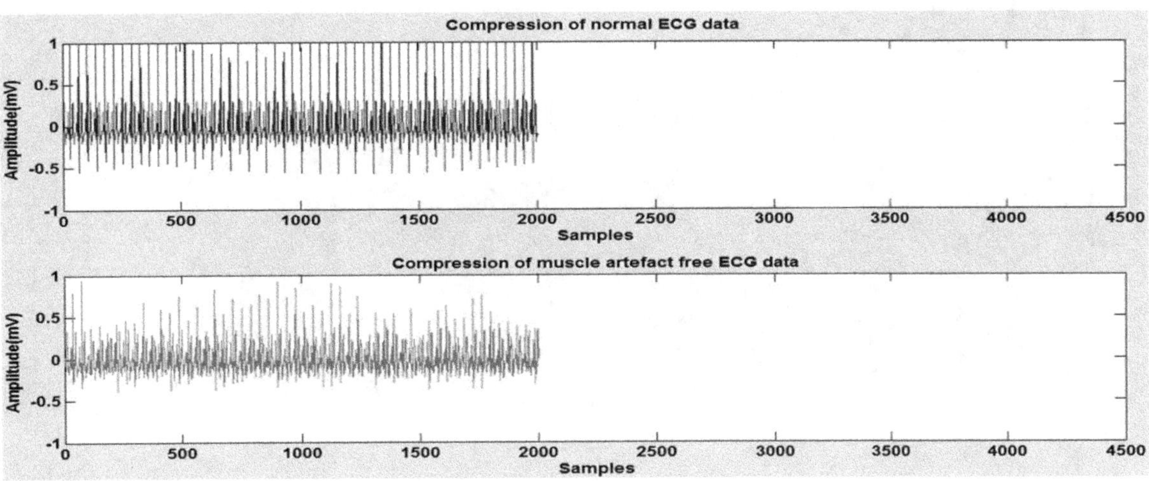

Optimized data received from the algorithm that consumes lesser energy, in our scenario which shows that PSO is dominating GA. Former data is ready for transmission over the Zigbee environment, in order to ease the transmission a hardware Zigbee module is designed which a circuit board embedded with transformer, followed by microcontroller, diodes, resisters, capacitors, Zigbee transmission mote, MAX-232 cable to connect it with the Personal computer, and the whole system takes the battery and system of personal computer for its proper working. Figures 11 and 12 shows the transmission process over Zigbee hardware module transmitted to and from MATLAB with the set of various instructions.

Figure 11. Transmission of optimized data over Zigbee module

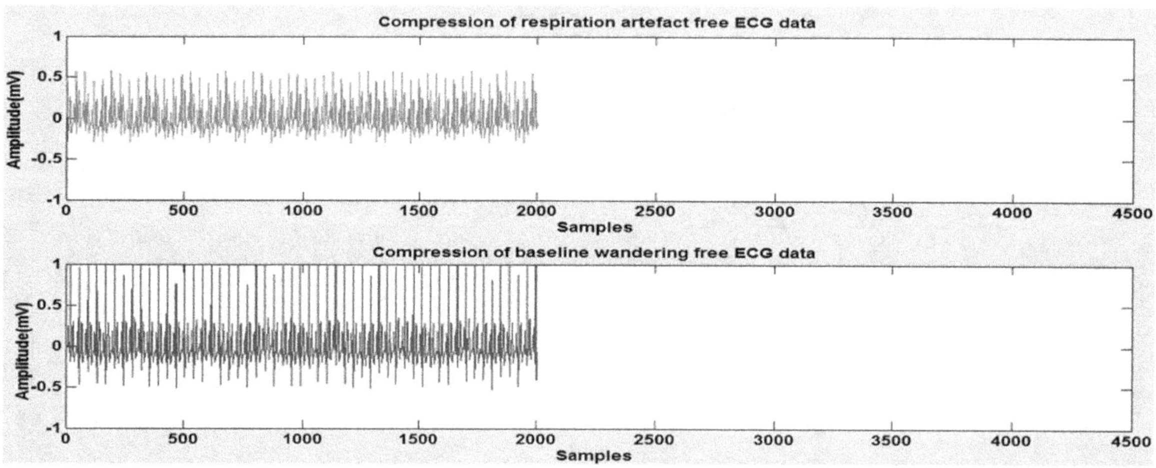

Figure 12. Receiving of optimized data over Zigbee module

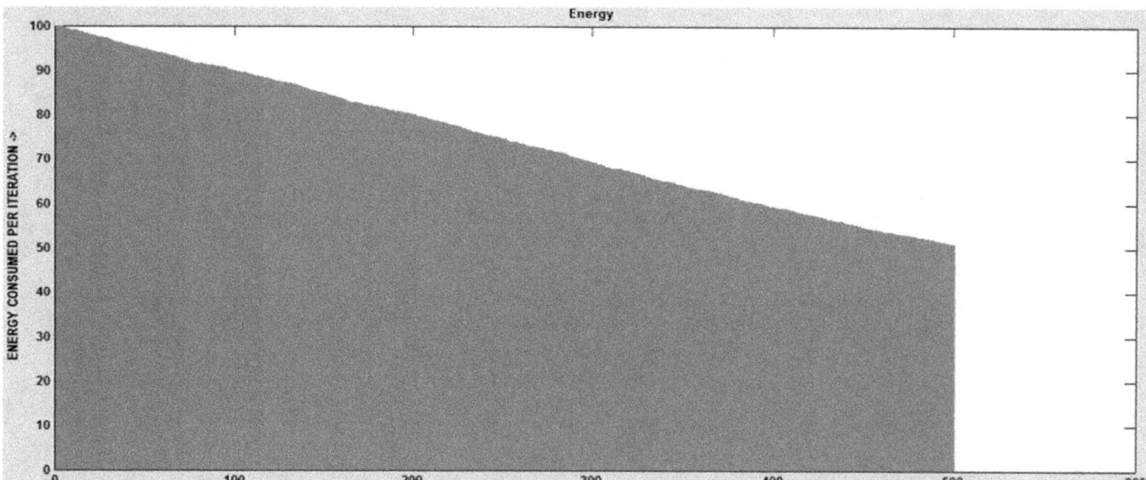

FUTURE RESEARCH DIRECTIONS

There is a future scope that further takes this to another level as the combination of various compression algorithms can be implemented on the various types of ECG data. Pre-filtering of the noisy ECG data can be done by the applications of various hybrid filters further work can be considered based upon the transmission process of wireless communication. Moreover, bandwidth dedication, channel allocation and delay related factors are some of the issues on which the work can be performed, as this will not only enhance the data transmission but will allow the device to send the more accurate data on-demand. In addition to this, certain other artifacts that can be identified with the help of the ECG transmitted will be an icing on the cake. What's more, work can be further carried forward by considering the various uproars near the patient who is under surveillance. Further, this chapter gives someone a platform to deal with the high prioritised discipline that is health, which nowadays demands a lot more attention than any other field of the education, as this field highly represents the way to deal with all the detrimental problems and how to curb with those diseases by initiating certain steps before it is too late for the patient, who actually needs this kind of help for themselves.

CONCLUSION

In this research project, we have proposed an effective ECG signal optimization and propagation framework using particle swarm optimization (PSO), Genetic Algorithm (GA), ZigBee wireless environment, discrete wavelet transform, noise removal filters and signal drift removal filter techniques and technologies. All of the technologies have been combined on one platform to increase the performance of the ECG signal recording using body wearable wireless sensors for ECG monitoring and low energy propagation of the ECG signal by compressing the signal using optimization techniques irrespective of the loss of ECG signal details. When compared with the base paper which includes only DWT compression over different mode consumes more energy when devices switch from one mode to other. In the base paper [1] compressed data was allowed to traverse through Bluetooth technology which is not efficient and consumes lot of energy and data packets are of low rate which is not feasible. Above two problems have been rectified in the proposed chapter with due concentration over the Energy consumption as there is no mode change it operates continuously but sends data discretely based upon the DWT compression technique. Maximum energy is consumed during transmission so Zigbee environment is preferred over Bluetooth to send the data with data rate higher than Bluetooth. Proposed paper do include another set of energy saving technique that is optimization techniques which are missing in the base paper, this overall saves more energy while data that is meant for sending is lesser in amount as unwanted or repeated data will be flushed away by PSO and GA . Out of two one that has consumed significantly lower energy than the other for the process of ECG signal optimization will be traversed over communication channel. Whereas it is also recorded that ZigBee environment has also consumed significantly lower amount of energy than the non optimized ECG signal propagation environment. Transferred data is being stored in a database for further analysis.

REFERENCES

Akansu, A. N., Serdijn, W. A., & Selesnick, I. W. (2010). *Emerging applications of wavelets: A review*. Elsevier.

Akhter, S., & Haque, M. A. (2010, August). Ecg Comptression Using Run Length Encoding. In *18th European Signal Processing Conference EUSIPCO-2010* (pp. 1645-1649).

Camiilo, T., Oscar, R., & Carlos, L. (2009). *Biomedical Signal Monitoring Using Wireless Sensor Networks*. IEEE.

Chaiyakum & Wardkein. (2012, May). A New ECG Compression by Using Adaptive Cosine Fourier Transform. In Electrical Engineering/Electronics, Computer, Telecommunication and Information Technology (ECTI.CON) (pp. 1-4).

Chung, L., & Jung. (2008, August). A Wireless Sensor Network Compatible Wearable U.Healthcare Monitoring System Using Integrated ECG, Accelerometer and SPO2. In *30th Annual International IEEE EMBS conference* (pp. 1529-1532).

Garg, S. Gupta, & Mittal. (2010). Optimal Algorithm for ECG Denoising using Discrete Wavelet Transforms. IEEE.

Gupta, R., & Mitra, M. (2012, December). An ECG compression technique for telecardiology application. In *India Conference* (p. 4). IEEE.

Hossain, Afran, & Sayed. (2010, December). Compression of ECG signals exploiting correlation between ECG cycles. In *6th International Conference on Electrical and Computer Engineering ICECE 2010, Dhaka, Bangladesh* (pp. 622-625).

Hulzink, Konijnenburg, Ashouei, Breeschoten, Berset, Huisken, … Van Ginderdeuren. (2011, December). An Ultra Low Energy Biomedical Signal Processing System Operatng at Near Threshold. *IEEE Transactions on Biomedical Circuits and Systems, 5*(6), 546-554.

Isa, Noviyanto, & Arymurthy. (2011). Optimal Selection of Wavelet Thresholding Algorithm for ECG signal denoinsing. In ICACSIS (pp. 365-370).

Jalaleddine, Hutchens, Strattan, & Coberly. (1990, April). ECG Data Compression Techniques. A Unified Approach. *IEEE Transactions on Bio-Medical Engineering*, *37*(4), 329–343.

Jara. (2012, July). Evaluation of Bluetooth Low Energy capabilities for continuous data transmission from a wearable electrocardiogram. In Innovative Mobile and Internet Services in Ubiquitous Computing (IMIS) (pp. 912-917).

Karpagachelvi, Arthanari, & Sivakumar. (2010, April). ECG Feature Extraction Techniques-A Survey Approach. *International Journal of Computer Science and Information Security*, *8*(1), 76–80.

Kaur, M., Singh, B., Ubhi, & Rani. (2011). Digital Filtration of ECG Signals for Removal of Baseline Drift. In *International Conference on Telecommunication Technology and Applications Proc. of CSIT*. IACSIT Press.

Khaddar. (2012, May). Emerging Wireless Technologies In E-Health. In Multimedia Computing and System (ICMCS), (pp. 440-445).

Khandait, Bawane, Limaye, & Khandait. (2012, April). Efficient ECG Abnormalities Recognition Using Neuro-Fuzzy Approach. International Journal of Advanced Research in Computer Science and Software Engineering, 2, 402-407.

Khare, Saxena, & Nerkar. (2011). ECG Data Compression Using DWT. *International Journal of Engineering and Advanced Technology*, *1*(1), 11–13. doi:10.1109/HealthCom.2012.6379443

Li, J., & Li. (2008, May). Home healthcare platform based on Wireless Sensor Networks. In *5th International Conference on Informational Technology and Application in Biomedicine*, China (pp. 263-266). doi:10.1109/LATINCOM.2009.5305161

Li. (2012, May). Genetic Particle Filtering for Denoising of ECG Corrupted by Muscle Artifacts. In *Natural Computation (ICNC)* (pp. 562-565).

Lo, Thiemjarus, King, & Yang. (n.d.). *Body Sensor Network – A Wireless Sensor Platform For Pervasive Healthcare Monitoring*. Academic Press.

Mamaghanian, Khaled, Atienza, & Vandergheynst. (2011, September). Compressed Sensing for Real Time Energy Efficient ECG Compression on Wireless Body Sensor Nodes. *IEEE Transactions on Biomedical Engineering, 58*(9), 2457-2466.

Maneesha, V., Ramesh, R. G. R., & Abhishek, T. K. (2012). Low Power Intelligent Wearable Cardiac Sensor Using Discrete Wavelet Compression. In *International Conference on Advances in Mobile Network, Communication and its Application* (pp. 107-110). IEEE.

Manimegalai, P. (2012, March). Estimation of Cardiovascular Parameters from ECG and PPG Signals. In *Bioengineering Conference (NEBEC)* (pp. 237-238). doi:10.1109/NEBC.2012.6207051

Muthulakshmi, S., & Latha, K. (2012). Classification of ECG Waveform Using Feature Selection Algorithm. In *International Conference on Advanced Communication Control and Computing Technologies* (pp. 162-165). IEEE.

Rashid, A., & Rahim, S. & Mahalin. (2008, December). Home healthcare via Wireless Biomedical Sensor Network. In *IEEE International Rf And Microwave Conference Proceedings* (pp. 511-514). IEEE.

Rotariu & Manta. (2012). Wireless System for Remote Monitoring of Oxygen Saturation and Heart Rate. In *Proceedings of Federated Conference on Computer Science and Information System* (pp. 193-196). IEEE.

Suarjaya. (2012). A New Algorithm for Data Compression Optimization. *International Journal of Advanced Computer Science and Applications, 3*(8), 14-17. doi:10.1109/ICACCCT.2012.6320762

Toh, Do, Chung, & Lee. (2009). Health Decision Support for Biomedical Signals Monitoring System over a WSN. In *2nd International Symposium on Electronic Commerce and Security* (pp. 605-608). IEEE.

Tseng, Tsai, Lai, & Fang. (2009). *A Wireless Biomedical Sensor Network using IEEE802.15.4*. IEEE.

Yoon, Hwang, Noh, Cheol, & Royoon. (2010, July). Comparison Of Cwt With Dwt For Detecting QRS Complex On Wearable Ecg Recorder. In *IEEE, International Conference on Wavelet Analysis and Pattern Recognition, Qingdao* (pp. 300-303). IEEE.

Yu, Yang, & Chong. (2010). ECG Monitoring over Bluetooth: Data Compression and Transmission. In *Communication Society WCNC Proceedings*. IEEE.

Zahhad, Ahmed, & Zakaria. (2012). Electrocardiogram Signals Compression Technique Based on QRS. Complex Estimation and 2.D DWT. In ICCIT (pp. 554-559).

Zatout, Y. (2012). Using Wireless Technologies for Healthcare Monitoring at Home: a Survey. In 14th International Conference on e.Health Networking, Applications and Services (pp. 383-386). IEEE.

Chapter 15
Optimized Clustering Techniques with Special Focus to Biomedical Datasets

Anusuya S. Venkatesan
Saveetha University, India

ABSTRACT

The clinical data including clinical test results, MRI images and drug responses of patients are documented and analyzed with machine learning and data mining tools. The scale and complexity of these datasets is a big challenge to machine learning and data mining community as the data is of mixed type. The extraction of meaningful or desired information from these datasets provides knowledge in decision making process which in turn helps for the diagnosis and treatment of the diseases. Biomedical datasets are a collection of data with diverse types as it involves images, clinical studies, statistical reports etc. The recent researches have focused on different clustering and classification methods to manage and analyze the biomedical datasets. The objective of this chapter is to cluster or classify the patterns of interest from Brain MRI images, Liver disorder and Breast cancer datasets using efficient clustering methodologies. Among the different algorithms in data mining for clustering, classification, visualization and interpretation, K Means, Fuzzy C Means and Neural Networks(NN) are frequently used for clustering and classification of biomedical datasets. The performance of these methods are greatly influenced by the initialization of K value and its convergence speed. This chapter discusses about FCM and K Means clustering methods and its optimization with meta heuristics such as Particle Swarm Optimization (PSO) and Quantum Particle Swarm Optimization (QPSO). The experimental section of this paper exhibits analysis in terms of Intra cluster distances, elapsed time and Davis Bouldin Index (DBI).

INTRODUCTION

Data mining is an interdisciplinary area involves artificial intelligence, soft computing, database system etc. The tools of data mining infer information from the databases and this information converted to knowledge of patterns and relationships. The relationships among data are referred as Classes, Clusters, Associations and Sequential Patterns. Data clustering have been applied in the area of data mining and machine learning. The specific applications include statistics (McLachlan et al., 1997), bioinformatics

DOI: 10.4018/978-1-5225-0660-7.ch015

(He et al. 2006), machine learning (Ethem Alpaydin., 2004) exploratory data analysis, image segmentation, security, medical image analysis, web handling and mathematical programming (Pyle 1999; Panov et al. 2008). The process of clustering split the data into homogeneous and inhomogeneous classes with respect to similarity between data.

Clusters are formed by finding the distance between data points. The existing tools explore the data and help to visualize it in different models. The cluster representation is one of the widely accepted exploratory models to analyze the data with the different levels of observation. Clustering is applied to biomedical datasets to understand the characteristics of bio information and to find interesting patterns associated to prior information. Most of the bio medical datasets have inherent noise and inconsistency, sometimes mixed with semantic information and experimental results. Hence, generating quality clusters on biomedical datasets is a challenging task. The role of clustering in biomedical datasets is to derive meaningful information which assists pathologists on decision making.

In case of medical image segmentation, the system works by segmenting the whole image into multiple segments and extracts only the specific region for investigation. In image segmentation, the intensities of all pixels within a homogenous cluster are similar but the intensities of inhomogeneous clusters are different from homogeneous one. Medical image analysis is mainly dependent on effective image segmentation to extract suspicious regions from complex medical images (Neeraj et al., 2010).

Clustering is categorized as an optimization problem to satisfy the criteria of minimizing the similarity within a cluster and maximizing the dissimilarity between clusters. Table 1 shows the different distance measures used to find the distance between data points. Some clustering techniques use heuristic algorithms (Bandyopadhyay S, 2002)(Das S et al.,2008)(S. Ouadfel et al.,2010) to obtain centres for clusters. The objectives of using Optimization techniques with clustering techniques are 1) to find global optima 2) to enforce robustness against initialization 3) to improve the partitioning quality 4) to deal with unknown and known number of clusters 5) to speed up convergence etc. Clusters are represented in different forms such as Connectivity models, Centroid models, Distribution models, Density models and Graph-based models.

- **Hierarchical Clustering (Ward et al, 1963):** Is an example for connectivity models which fall into two types, they are Agglomerative and Divisive. Agglomerative is bottom up approach while Divisive is top down approach.
- **Centroid Models:** Clusters are formed based on the centroids found on the original data, the number of centroids is fixed to K, the clusters are formed by assigning the data items to the nearest cluster centroid. Example: K Means (Hartigan et al, 2009).
- **Density Based Models:** Martin Ester et al. (1996) defines clusters as connected dense regions in the data space. Example: Density Based Spatial Clustering of Applications with Noise (DBSCAN) and Ordering Points to Identify the Clustering Structure (OPTICS).
- **Distribution Models (Bishop, 2006):** Clusters are modeled using statistical distributions, such as multivariate normal distributions using Expectation-Maximization algorithm.

In this chapter the term FCM-PSO refers as the procedure of FCM is optimized with PSO while FCM-QPSO refers optimization of FCM using QPSO. K Means-PSO and K Means QPSO refers the optimization of K Means using PSO and QPSO. The main objective of this chapter is to find the clusters or abnormal structures present in the biomedical datasets such as MRI images, Liver disorder and Breast cancer datasets (Table 1).

Table 1. The various distance measures of clustering

Distance Measures	Formula	Comments
Euclidean	$d = \sqrt{\sum_{i=1}^{n}(x_i - y_i)^2}$	Computes the square root of the sum of the squares of the differences between corresponding values.
City block	$d = \sum_{i=1}^{n}\lvert x_i - y_i \rvert$	Computes the sum of the differences of their corresponding components.
Cosine	$d_\alpha(x,y) = \cos(\theta) = \frac{x \cdot y}{\lVert x \rVert \cdot \lVert y \rVert}$	The Cosine Similarity takes into only the angle and discards the magnitude.
Pearson correlation	$r_{xy} = \frac{S_{x,y}}{\sqrt{S_x}\sqrt{S_y}} = \frac{\sum_{i=1}(x_i - \overline{x})(y_i - \overline{y})}{\sqrt{\sum_{i=1}(x_i - \overline{x})^2 \sum_{i=1}(y_i - \overline{y})^2}}.$ $d_R(x,y) = 1 - r_{xy}$	The Pearson Correlation Distance computes the distance of each point from the linear regression line.
Minkowski Distance	$d_M k(x,y) = \left\{ \lvert x_1 - y_1 \rvert^m + \lvert x_2 - y_2 \rvert^m + \ldots + \lvert x_n - y_n \rvert^m \right\}^{\frac{1}{m}} = \left\{ \sum_{i=1}^{n} \lvert x_i - y_i \rvert^m \right\}^{\frac{1}{m}}$	Minkowski Distance is a generalization of Euclidean and Manhattan distance.
Manhattan distance	$d_M(x,y) = \lvert x_1 - y_1 \rvert + \lvert x_2 - y_2 \rvert + \ldots + \lvert x_n - y_n \rvert = \sum_{i=1}^{n} \lvert x_i - y_i \rvert$	Manhattan distance represents distance that is measured along directions that are parallel to the x and y axes.
Chebychev distance	$d_{\max}(x,y) = \max_i \lvert x_i - y_i \rvert$	Chebychev distance simply picks the largest difference between any two corresponding coordinates.

Hybrid clustering algorithms attempt to make use of the merits of various optimization techniques to find global optimal clusters. Table 2 shows the widely used biomedical datasets processed using nature inspired meta heuristics techniques.

BACKGROUND

Related Work of Clustering and Its Optimized Performance

The process of clustering split the data into homogeneous and inhomogeneous classes with respect to similarity between data. Clustering is a process of data mining aids to investigate patterns in financial statement disclosures in detection of fraud (Glen et al.,2014). The partition clustering K Means is used

Table 2. Widely used Bio medical datasets optimized with Nature inspired meta heuristics

Dataset	Creator	Optimization Techniques
Breast cancer [683 x 9], Cl-2	W.H. Wolberg O. Mangasarian	GA (Abraham. A, 2007)(H. He et al.,2012), ACO – (A. Chowdhury et al.,2012) PSO – (L. Chuang, 2011, T. Cura 2012, F. Yang 2009), BFO – (J.R. Olesen,2009)
Thyroid [215 x 5], Cl-3	R. Quinlan	ACO(A. Ghosh, 2008)PSO(T.Cura 2012)
Dermatology [366 x 34], Cl-6	N. Ilter Guvenir	AIS – (S.J. Nanda, 2012), Firefly – (J. Senthilnath, 2011)
Diabetes [768 x 8], Cl-2	V. Sigillito	ACO – (H. Azzag,2003), BFO – (J.R. Olesen,2009), Firefly – [J. Senthilnath,2011),

to cluster the data from retail stores in order to reduce the transportation cost. The factors considered for clustering are stores location, order, goods, transportation vehicles, road and traffic information (MehrdadKargari et al.,2012). Ant based clustering is applied to clustering medical database followed by association rule mining to mine the rules for each group (Kuo R.J et al., 2007). A two level approach comprising Kohonen's Self-Organizing Map and K Means clustering applied to discover hidden structures from the database of accidental occupational accidents occurred in the Italian wood processing industry. The turnover rates of Taiwanese companies were analyzed using Artificial Neural Network (ANN) and Self Organizing Map (SOM) clustering (Chin-Yuan Fan et al., 2012). In case of medical image analysis, the diseases are diagnosed or examined from the images of non-invasive medical imaging modalities such as CT, MRI, PET, X-ray etc. Generally, the classification systems include the processes such as the 1) Extraction of region of interests (ROIs) represent lesion, 2) Feature extraction from ROI and 3) The classification of ROI from extracted features. ROI detection system helps to visualize and interpret the Objects of interest according to the requirement of specific domain. The system works by segmenting the whole image into multiple segments and extracts only the specific region for investigation. Medical image analysis is mainly dependent on effective image segmentation to extract suspicious regions from complex medical images (Neeraj et al., 2010). Clustering is strongly connected to machine learning because a solution to the clustering problem may be used to propagate labels from observed data to unobserved data. Table 3 shows the various biomedical applications of K Means and Fuzzy C Means.

Clustering with PSO-FCM has been proposed by Hsuan-mingFeng et al in 2006. The outliers are easily found and removed by sliding PCA-Fuzzy (Paulo Salgado et al., 2012). A combination of Support Vector Machine (SVM) with PSO and FCM (Kun Chang Lee et al., 2012) overcomes the limitations of basic FCM in terms of the accuracy of classification. The clustering results of Fuzzy C-Means is further improved by Quantum based PSO (Hao Wang et al., 2007). Fuzzy-PSO (HesamIzakian et al., 2011, Cheng Jian Lin et al., 2008) clustering is found to be very efficient in many clustering problems. Particle Swarm Optimization(PSO) has been introduced to find the fuzzy threshold and parameters for fuzzy entropy. The results showed that the search ability of the method is superior to exhaustive search method in segmenting remote sensing images (Linyi et al., 2008). Performance analysis between GA-Fuzzy and PSO-Fuzzy (Amitava, 2012) showed that PSO–Fuzzy outperforms GA-Fuzzy technique even when Signal to Noise Ratio (SNR) is low (Du Feng et al., 2005).

QPSO was proposed to improve the search ability of PSO and is used to find global optimal threshold on images (Tian, 2009). Fuzzy Tsallis Entropy optimization using PSO is proposed (Yinggan, 2008) to improve the performance of Shannon Entropy. An elite learning optimization approach (Leung et al.,

Table 3. Applications of FCM and K Means on Biomedical datasets

FCM in Biomedical Analysis	Author, Year
Mammogram Image Segmentation to detect breast cancer.	Guru Kalyan et al., 2015.
Classification of brain MRI.	N. V. S. Natteshan et al., 2015.
The automated algorithm of tissue-specific analysis to assist functional MRI studies with different modalities of response in different brain regions.	MJ Chiu et al., 2011.
To segment bone from air and soft tissues.	Mohammad HadiAarab et al., 2014.
To find optimum number of clusters for liver CT image segmentation.	Abder-Rahman Ali et al., 2014.
To detect prostate boundary in ultrasound images.	Aboul Ella Hassanien et al., 2010.
Segmentation of tumor from brain MRI images.	M. Shasidha et al., 2011.
K Means in Biomedical Analysis	**Author, Year**
To segment brain tumour.	Deepak, K.S et al., 2013.
To track the tumour objects from brain MRI.	Li-Hong Juang et al., 2010.
Medical image segmentation.	Ng, H.P 2006.
To segment 2D echocardiography images for clinical analysis.	Nandagopalan S et al., 2010.
To extract ventricle and atrium borders for detecting heart abnormalities using automatic segmentation of echocardiographic images of different views.	Nandagopalan, S. et al., 2010 .
To segment white matter and gray matter from brain MRI images.	Kumbhar, A.D.et al., 2011.

2012), Radial Basis Function Neural Network(RBFNN) using Augmented Lagrangian PSO(ALPSO) proposed for classification problem. Velocity vectors of PSO are updated with linearly decreasing inertia weight and the proposed structure optimizes weight matrix and other controlling parameters. A PSO based optimized learning method used to (Vahid et al., 2013) optimize RBF unit centres. Different architectures using PSO such as RBF1, RBF2,RBF3 and RBF4 (George et al., 2013) are discussed and result shows that the number of hidden node increases as the values of fitness function decreases. PSO-RBFNN structure proposed for Electro Cardiogram (ECG) beat classification (Mehmet et al., 2010). A method of FCM optimized using Ant Colony Optimization (ACO) and Genetic Algorithm (GA) proposed to provide optimal RBF centres to increase accuracy rate (Zhide et al., 2009; Zhen et al.,2008). FCM with GA and PSO (Gopal et al., 2010) has been proposed to identify tumors from MRI brain image. Similarly, partitional clustering, K-means followed by Support Vector Image (SVM) proposed to study the statistical features of ROI from the mammogram (Aarthi et al., 2011).

The eminent property of fuzzy clustering allow data points to belong to more than one group, influences gene clustering (Ioannis A et al.,2012) where a semi supervised Fuzzy clustering has been applied to know the functioning and cooperation of genes. Swarm optimization techniques have been developed implemented successfully in many areas such as image segmentation, clustering, pattern identification, classification etc. An improved biogeography based optimization technique using the principle of maximizing fuzzy entropy has been applied on CT images of human head and analyzed that the performance is better than GA,PSO and basic Biogeography-Based Optimization. To identify early diagnosis of brain tumour, FCM clustering has been optimized with GA and PSO (Gopal et al., 2010).

K Means and Fuzzy C-Means (FCM) clustering methods have been adapted in many disciplines to partition the data elements efficiently. The performance of these two clustering methods greatly influenced by the initialization of K value and convergence speed. The recent researches have shown that the hybridization of Particle Swarm Optimization(PSO) and Quantum Particle Swarm Optimization(QPSO) with K Means and Fuzzy C Means produces better optimized clustering results.

OVERVIEW OF OPTIMIZATION

Optimization refers the best selection of an element among available alternatives based on some criteria. There is no universal optimization algorithm. The algorithm chosen must ensure for robustness, efficiency and accuracy. Generally, the optimization methods differentiated in terms of generic/approximate and problem specific/exact. Among them, the nature inspired meta heuristic population based methods provide better solution to solve optimization problems. Meta heurists are usually non deterministic algorithms which are powerful than heuristic search based algorithms. Meta heuristics algorithms perform well in trapping local minima, provides guaranteed solutions and they are more generic while heuristic methods are problem specific. The meta heuristics are classified based on the criteria such as population based or single point search, dynamic or static objective function, single neighbourhood or various neighbourhood structures and memory usage or memory-less methods. Some of the meta heuristic optimization methods with advantageous and weakness are given in the Table 4.

The goal of optimization is to find the values of the variables that minimize or maximize the objective function while satisfying the constraints.

An optimization algorithm is a set of steps executed iteratively till satisfactory or optimal solution is found. The aim of optimization is to minimize the cost function or maximize the efficiency (Panos et al., 2000). Given a function f: $Q \rightarrow R$ from set Q to the R, set of real numbers, the aim is to find an element x0 in R such that $f(x0) \leq f(x), \forall x \in R$ ("Minimization") or such that $f(x0) \geq f(x), \forall x \in R$ ("Maximization"), where f is the objective function/cost function. A feasible solution that optimizes f is called an optimal solution.

Table 4. Strength and weakness of heuristic approaches GA,SA,AIS and ACO

Method	Author, Year	Strength	Weakness
GA	Holland,1975	• Different types of optimization problems can be solved using GA. • Finds global best solution. • Portable with other algorithms.	• Encoding scheme is complex. • Convergence depends on crossover and mutation operations. • Convergence rate is slow. • Provides sub optimal solution.
SA	Kirkpatrick, 1983	• Computation time is low. • Easy. • Implementation • Property of convergence.	• Inner loop iterations. • Initial temperature to be set.
AIS	J.D Farmer,1986	• Self adaptive method. • New search area is explored.	• Provides sub optimal solution. • Number of Property settings.
ACO	M. Dorigo,1992	• Suitable for graph structured problems. • Scalability and robustness is high.	• Implementation is complex. • Parameter initialization based on trial and error. • Support of discrete search space.

Mathematical models are abstract models describe the mathematical relationships among elements in a system. The general form of an optimization model is

min or max $f(x_1,\ldots,x_n)$ (objective function)

subject to $g_i(x_1,\ldots,x_n) \geq 0$ (functional constraints)

$x_1,\ldots,x_n \in S$ (set constraints)

$x_1,\ldots,x_n$ are called decision variables. The goal is to find $x_1,\ldots,x_n$ by satisfying the constraints and to achieve min (max) objective function value.

The conventional optimization techniques have convergence at local optimal point and more parameters are to be set with respective to the technique. Therefore the recent researches make use of swarm based optimization techniques to aid for global convergence with better optimal solution.

OPTIMIZATION TECHNIQUES USING SWARM INTELLIGENCE (SI)

Swarm intelligence (SI) is a self-organized and collective behavioral system. It was firstly introduced in the context of cellular robotic systems by Gerardo Beni and Jing Wang in year of 1989. SI is an intelligent optimization technique, inspired by the collective behaviour of birds, fishes and colonies of insects (Abraham et al., 2006, Engelbrecht et al., 2005) while searching for food. There is no centralized controller but they exhibit complex global behaviour and all individuals follow simple rules to interact with neighbours. The general rules of birds flocking are 1) Collision Avoidance 2) Velocity matching 3) Flock Centring. The optimization potential of collective behaviours of insects has been studied by many researches. An insect may have only a few hundreds of brain cells but the colonies are capable to elaborate communication systems, to develop terrific resistance to the threats, to develop complex social relationships and creation of intelligent skills. The similar behaviours are also observed in birds flocking and fish schooling. SI methods are part of meta heuristic family of algorithms (Talbi E., 2002) have been used in the various areas of research.

SI techniques have been used efficiently in data mining techniques such as classification, clustering, feature selection, pre processing and outlier detection. Swarm intelligence algorithms have proved to be very efficient in solving real world optimization problems and it has been applied in Military Applications, Robotics Navigation and Space Research. SI algorithms include Particle Swarm Optimization, Ant Colony Optimization, Stochastic Diffusion Search, and Bacteria Foraging etc. Figure 1 shows the collective behavior of ants and bees.

Particle Swarm Optimization (PSO)

PSO is a population based stochastic optimization technique developed by Dr. Eberhart and Dr. Kennedy in 1995, inspired by social behaviour of bird flocking or fish schooling and has been rapidly applied to data mining tasks such as classification and clustering to optimize the results. In PSO, particles in the swarm fly around in D dimensional space and interact with each other for optimal solution. Each particle in the population iteratively discovers its own position according to velocity and its previous positions. The individual best positions of particles are stored in order to find global best positions in each iteration. The positions of ith particle in D dimensions is represented with position vector $Xi =(x_{i1},$

Figure 1. Ant colonies and swarm of bees

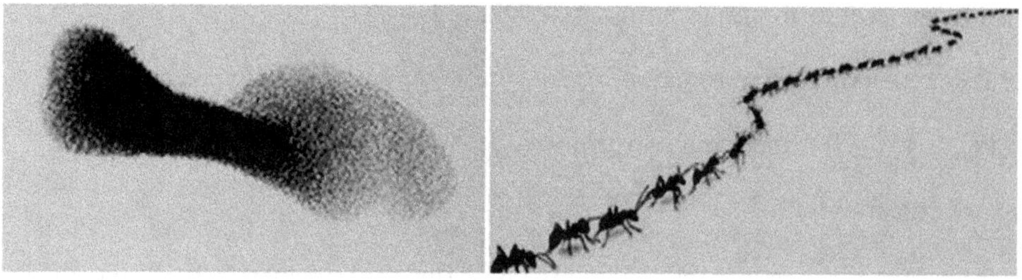

$x_{i2}, x_{i3}, \ldots, x_{in}$) as given in Equation 2 and velocity vector Vi = ($v_{i1}, v_{i2}, v_{i3}.. v_{in}$) given in Equation 1. The optimal solution of the problem is determined according to fitness function.

$$V_i(t+1) = \omega V_i(t) + c_1 rand()(Pbest(t) - X_i(t)) + c_2 rand()(Gbest(t) - X_i(t)) \quad (1)$$

$$X_i(t+1) = X_i(t) + V_i(t+1) \quad (2)$$

Each particle maintains two positions; 1) Personal best position (Pbest) is the best position experienced so far and 2) Global best position (Gbest) is the best position over entire swarm. The Equation1 and Equation 2 are updated iteratively based on Pbest and Gbest values where ω is the inertia weight controls the speed of algorithm. The local and social search of PSO influenced by two positive parameters c_1 and c_2, generally set between the range [0,2]. The steps involved in PSO have been listed below, where Swarm_Size represents the population size of the swarm participating in the search, pbest is the personal best position of individual particles experienced so far and gbest is the global best positions in the swarm.

Procedure of PSO

```
Generate random population of N solutions(particles);
For(i=0;i<Swarm_Size;i++)
Evaluate fitness f(x_i)
Initialize the value of weight factor  ω;
while (termination condition is not true)
{
for(i=0;i<Swarm_Size;i++)
{
if(f(x_i)>pbest_i) pbest_i=x_i;
if(pbest_i>gbest_i) gbest_i=pbest_i;
Update(Position x_i, Velocity v_i);
Evaluate f(x_i);
}
}
```

In PSO, the agents are referred as particles and particles move around the solution space. The movement of particles evaluated using fitness criterion at every timestamp and best move is found. The main difference between PSO and other algorithms is that the number of particles involve in search process is higher in PSO and the error minimization of PSO is higher than GA. The variants of PSO are classified based on fuzziness, accordance, attraction, activity, grouping, mobility, divisibility, interaction, uncertainty, continuity, topology, hierarchy, restriction, cooperation, objective, recursively etc.

Quantum Particle Swarm Optimization (QPSO)

Quantum Particle Swarm Optimization (QPSO) is a variant of PSO and is proposed for better search ability and good convergence speed. The quantum model of PSO referred as Quantum PSO was proposed by Sun et al., in 2004 where the movement of particles are dynamic on the basis of quantum mechanics. According to uncertainty principle of quantum mechanics, the velocity and the positions of particles cannot be determined simultaneously in QPSO. Hence, the probability of finding a particle's position in quantum search space mapped into actual position in the search space by the method collapsing. QPSO has been used in wide range of optimization problems (Leandro dos Santos, C, 2010; Debao et al., 2012; Jun et al., 2012). PSO has the limitation of converging at local optima, to improve the searching ability of PSO, QPSO and Chaos theory based application is introduced in the image matching problem (Maolong, 2008). A variant of QPSO called Multi Elicit QPSO (MEQPSO) on gene expression analysis is tested and superiority of MEQPSO is proved (Jun et al., 2012). Effectiveness of QPSO on time complexity and convergence rate are analysed and improvements in these factors are proposed through algorithms such as QPSO with random mean position (Maolong et al., 2008), QPSO with ranking operator and Multi-Elitist QPSO (Jun et al., 2012).

In the model of QPSO, the particles are moving in quantum space and the state of particle is characterized by wave function $\left|\Psi_{(x,t)}\right|^2$. $\Psi(x,t)$ is the probability density function which denotes the probability of particles appearing in a certain position and particles changes its position according to following iterative equations 3 and 4.

$$x_i(t+1) = P_i + \beta\left|Mbest_i - x_i(t)\right| * \ln(1/u), \text{If k} \geq 0.5 \tag{3}$$

$$x_i(t+1) = P_i - \beta\left|Mbest_i - x_i(t)\right| * \ln(1/u), \text{If k} < 0.5 \tag{4}$$

where β is called Contraction–Expansion coefficient to determine the convergence speed of algorithm. M is the population size, P_i is calculated using Equation 6 and Mbest is the mean of Pbest values calculated using Equation 5

$$\text{Mbest} = (1/\text{M}\sum_{i=1}^{M}\text{P}_{i1}, 1/\text{M}\sum_{i=1}^{M}\text{P}_{i2}, \ldots\ldots, 1/\text{M}\sum_{i=1}^{M}\text{P}_{iD}) \tag{5}$$

$$P_i = \varphi * pBest_i + (1-\varphi) * gBest_i \tag{6}$$

The parameters k, u and φ are random numbers distributed in the range [0,1].

Procedure of QPSO

```
Initialize population size M, the positions of particles X and Dimension D.
Evaluate fitness of all particles
Calculate Pbest(P_id) positions of all particles and find Gbest(P_gd) among par-
ticles.
While(condition)
        Calculate mbest positions according to Equation  5
                for i= 1 to Population Size(M)
                                For j = 1 to dimension D
                        update particles positions as per Equation  3 and
Equation 4
                endfor
endWhile
```

K MEANS OPTIMIZED USING PSO AND QPSO METHODS

The objects or particles are clustered or grouped based on the principle of maximizing the intra class similarity and minimizing the interclass similarity. That is, the clusters of objects are formed so that objects within a cluster have high similarity in comparison to one another, but are very dissimilar to objects in other clusters. K-means is the most commonly used partitional clustering algorithm but the major problem of K-means is the selection of the initial partition and its convergence to local optima. The users usually run the algorithms repeatedly with different values of k and compare the clustering results in order to detect the optimal number of clusters.

K means algorithm operates on a set of d-dimensional vectors, $D = \{\mathbf{x}_i \mid i = 1, \ldots, N\}$,

where $\mathbf{X}_i \in R^d$ denotes the ith data point.

The algorithm is initialized by picking k points in R^d as the initial k cluster representatives or "centroids".

1. Choose K centroids at random.
2. Make initial partition of objects into K clusters by assigning objects to closest centroid.
3. Calculate the centroid (mean) of each of the K clusters.
    a. For object i, Calculate its distance to each of the centroids.
    b. Allocate object i to cluster with closest centroid.
    c. If object was reallocated, recalculate centroids based on new clusters.
4. Repeat Step3 for object i= 1 to N
5. Repeat steps 3 & 4 until no reallocations occur.
6. Assess cluster structure for fit and stability.

The above algorithm is optimized using PSO and QPSO for better clustering results.

Procedure of K Means-PSO

The optimization of K Means using PSO (TaherNiknam et al., 2010) is described in the following steps.

1. In the context of K Means-PSO clustering, before initializing the particles, the data points are randomly assigned to K clusters first.
2. Particle fitness is evaluated using Eq.7

$$F(j) = 1 / N\sum_{1}^{K} \sum x \in K_i \left\| x_j - C_i \right\|^2 \tag{7}$$

F(j) in Equation 7 is the fitness function of the particle j, between a data point $x_{j=1..N}$ and the cluster center C_i where N represents the total number of data points in the clustering process. Minimizing the sum of squared distance from all points to their cluster centres would result in compact clusters.

3. Find the velocity and position of the particles using Equation 1. and Equation 2
4. The new generation is optimized by K Means as given below.
   a. The data set is reassigned to clusters according to nearest rule.
   b. Cluster centroids, fitness value are recalculated and positions are updated.
5. If the position is satisfactory or the maximum iteration is reached then the process is stopped.

Otherwise, return to step 2.

Procedure of K Means – QPSO

In the derived K Means-QPSO, each particle maintains the positions Xi = (C_1, C_2, …, C_i, .., C_k), where Ci represents the ith cluster centroid vector and K is the number of clusters. The particles adjust its centroid vectors based on its own experience and its neighbours.

The proposed hybrid K Means - QPSO clustering consists of following steps

1. Each particle chooses K data vectors from the given dataset as the initial clusters centroid vectors and data points are randomly assigned to K clusters.
2. Calculate the fitness of particles using Equation 7
   a. Update the local and mean best positions as given in Equation 3,4 and 5.
   b. Update the global best positions from Mean best positions.
   c. Set Gbest positions as the cluster centroids.
3. Perform step 2 for maximum number of iterations.

FCM AND ENTROPY BASED CLUSTERING OPTIMIZED USING PSO AND QPSO

Fuzzy C Means clustering (FCM) is an efficient clustering algorithm (Dunn J.C, 1973, Bezdek J.C., 1981) used in the area of pattern recognition widely. In FCM-PSO and FCM-QPSO the partitioning of elements is done by optimizing the objective function of FCM i.e, the sum of square error function between data elements and centre using Euclidean distance. Fuzzy partitioning allows data items belonging to more than one cluster according to their level of membership. FCM clustering provides better results than traditional threshold based hard clustering in boundaries. The membership of such elements would be between 0 and 1 to indicate their partial membership. Researchers (Ghazanfari M.,2007, Kun Chang Lee, 2012) use Particle Swarm Optimization(PSO) and Genetic Algorithm (GA) to optimize the objective function of FCM. Fuzzy C-Means algorithm separates a finite set of n elements X={x_1,x_2... x_n} into cluster collections based on a standard criteria and it gives list of partition matrix $U = u_{ij} \in \left[0,1\right]$ and cluster centers C={c_1...c_c}, for i=1,2..c and j=1,2..n with each element u_{ij} providing the degree to which each element x_i belongs to $c_{j.}$ The objective function is determined by Equation 8

$$\min J_{FCM} = \sum_{i=1}^{c}\sum_{j=1}^{n}\mu_{ij}^{m} d_{ij}^{2} = \sum_{i=1}^{c}\sum_{j=1}^{n}\mu_{ij}^{m} \| x_j - a_i \|^2 \tag{8}$$

where μ represents the degree of membership of cluster data objects, c represents the cluster number, m represents fuzzy index (m>1) that controls fuzziness.

$$a_i^{(t)} = \frac{\sum_{j=1}^{n}\left[\mu_{ij}^{(t-1)}\right]^m x_j}{\sum_{j=1}^{n}\left[\mu_{ij}^{(t-1)}\right]^m}; i = 1,2...c \tag{9}$$

$$\sum_{i=1}^{c}\sum_{j=1}^{n}\mu_{ij}^{m} d_{ij}^{2} = \sum_{i=1}^{c}\sum_{j=1}^{n}\mu_{ij}^{m} \| x_j - a_i \|^2 \tag{10}$$

$$\mu_{ij}^{(k)} = \left[\sum_{1=1}^{c}\left[\frac{\left[(x_j - a_i^{(k)})'(x_j - a_i^{(k)})\right]}{(x_j - a_i^{(k)})'(x_j - a_i^{(k)})}\right]^{1/m}\right]^{-1}$$

The steps of FCM are given below:

1. Initialize fuzzy factor m, clustering number K, and U.
2. Find membership function and cluster centers using Equation 9 and 10.

Repeat step (2), until $\left|J_{FCM}(t) - J_{FCM}(t-1)\right| \le \varepsilon$ where ε is a predefined positive number and t is the maximum number of iterations.

FCM-PSO

FCM - PSO is a hybrid clustering method where fuzzy partitioning method, Fuzzy C Means(FCM) is optimized using Particle Swarm Optimization(PSO). In PSO, particles in the swarm fly around in D dimensional space and interact with each other for optimal solution. Each particle in the population iteratively discovers its own position according to velocity and its previous positions. The individual best positions of particles are stored in order to find global best positions in each iteration. The positions of ith particle in D dimensions is represented with position vector $Xi = (x_{i1}, x_{i2}, x_{i3}, \ldots, x_{in})$ and velocity vector $Vi = (v_{i1}, v_{i2}, v_{i3} .. v_{in})$. The optimal solution of the problem is determined according to fitness function mentioned in Equation 8. Each particle maintains two positions; 1) Personal best position (Pbest) is the best position experienced so far and 2) Global best position (Gbest) is the best position over entire swarm. The Procedure of FCM - PSO is given below;

Procedure of FCM - PSO

```
Begin
Randomly generate the random population of N particles
        For(i=0;i<populationsize;i++)
        Evaluate fitness f(X[i]) as in Equation 8
            End For.
        Initialize the value of weight factor ω, c1 and c2;
        while (termination condition is not true)
        for(i=0;i<populationsize;i++)
                if(f(X[i])>pbest_i) pbest_i=X[i];
                          End If.
                Update gbest;
                Update(Position X[i], Velocity V[i]);
                Evaluate f(X[i]);
                Assign gbest as the cluster centres(Optimized Cluster cen-
ters).
                 End For.
        End While.
                    Partition the dataset with the optimized cluster centers.
End.
```

FCM-QPSO

In FCM-QPSO, the objective function of FCM is optimized with Quantum Particle Swarm Optimization. The procedure for FCM-QPSO is mentioned below.

Procedure of FCM-QPSO

```
1.        Initialize the cluster numbers c, number of iterations T and   swarm
2.        Randomly generate pbest and gbest positions
3.        For t= 1 to T
      a. Find mbest
```

```
b. For each ido
        i.          Partition the dataset into clusters based on the gbest
positions.
        ii.         Update fitness function and particle positions
    End For i;
End For t;
```

ENTROPY BASED CLUSTERING

Maximum entropy principle was introduced in the year 1957 by Jaynes. Entropy is defined as the uncertainty that is expressed quantitatively by the information. The entropy is the measurement of information content within the system. The clustering problem can be formulated with objective function to minimization of uncertainty or maximization of the partition entropy. The concept of maximum entropy preserves the entropy of the input space. The entropy usually is the measure of dissimilarity between objects. The clustering result or the detection of lesion is determined according to the principle of maximizing entropy. Entropy based methods exploits the entropy on the distribution of gray levels, the maximum entropy being an indication of detecting objects of interest in the thresholded image. Threshold T lies in range ($0<T<L-1$, L=0, 1, 2….255) and the image is divided into two classes or two regions C_O and C_B based on T, where C_O is the object region and C_B is the background region. Shannon's entropy (Shannon 1949) is defined as in Equation 11;

$$H = -\sum_{i=0}^{n} p_i \log(p_i) \tag{11}$$

where p_i is the probability of occurrence of gray value i. The theory of maximum entropy is to select i which makes entropy as the maximum one. In order to arrive to the solution, attempted to maximize the entropy to increase information gain. When the sum of two class entropies, the image foreground and the image background reaches its maximum then the image is said to be optimally thresholded and it is defined as in Equation(12);

$$H_F(T) = -\sum_{g=0}^{T-1} \frac{p_g}{P_F} \log \frac{p_g}{P_F} \tag{12}$$

$$T_{opt} = \arg\max[H_f(T) + H_b(T)] \tag{13}$$

and

$$H_B(T) = -\sum_{g=T+1}^{255} \frac{p_g}{P_B} \log \frac{p_g}{P_B} \tag{14}$$

$$\text{Fitness}=H(t) = H_F(t)+H_B(T) \tag{15}$$

To solve the Equation 12 directly without involving optimization technique would cost more. Thus, the computational intelligence technique with maximum entropy proposed to enhance the speed and accuracy.

ME-WQPSO Clustering

The accurate brain image segmentation is very important for correct diagnosis. Most brain images contain noise and inhomogeneity. The segmentation process must be structured properly to process the data of this type. In case of QPSO, the mbest is calculated as the average of personal best positions of particles. The importance is not given to any specific particles. All the particles are treated equally. But in WQPSO, the particles elitism is accounted. The particles best positions are marked according to its fitness. If the fitness is high, the particle is reaching the destination. Particles are ranked according to its fitness ranging from high to low and then each particle is assigned a weight coefficient α_i decreasing from 1.5 to 0.5 with particles rank. Thus the mean best position is updated as

$$mbest = 1/M \sum_{i=1}^{M} a_{i1}P_{i1}, 1/M \sum_{i=1}^{M} a_{i2}P_{i2}, \ldots\ldots, 1/M \sum_{i=1}^{M} a_{iD}P_{iD}) \qquad (16)$$

where *M* is the size of the swarm and a_{iD} (i=1 to M, D=dimension) is the weight coefficient P_{id}(i=1 to M, D=dimension) best positions of particles.

The steps for implementing WQPSOME are presented below;

1. Initialize the population size, the positions X[i], dimensions and set P[i]=X[i];
2. Compute Maximum Entropy as in Equation 15 for the population sizes.
3. Find out threshold=Max(ME).
4. Update pbest positions for the population based on the threshold obtained in step 3.
5. P_g=Max(pbest), accordingly update particles positions.
6. Compute Beta value and mbest as in Equation (16).
7. If gbest(global best position)<X[i] Tseg=1; else Tseg=0;
8. Repeat steps 2 to 7 for Maximum number of iterations.

The global convergence capability of WQPSO and QPSO is different from PSO. In the case of PSO the particles fly within bounded region while in QPSO, the particles fly across n-dimensional search space at each iteration. WQPSO and QPSO are good global convergent algorithms and seem to be a promising optimization problem solvers.

EXPERIMENTAL RESULTS

The data considered for this chapter are Brain MRI, Liver disorder and Breast cancer datasets. The brain MRI images of 50 patients are collected from Scan World diagnostic centre, Chennai for experimental analysis. The data set liver disorder consists of 345 rows and 7 columns. The first five variables depict the blood test parameters sensitive to liver disorders arise from excessive alcohol consumption. The dataset breast cancer consists of 699 rows and 10 columns concerned with the chronological grouping of the clinical data of patients.

Implementation Results of FCM-PSO and FCM-QPSO on Brain MRI Images

Medical image analysis is mainly dependent on effective image segmentation to extract suspicious regions from complex medical images. In this chapter, optimized FCM and KFCM are applied on Brain MRI to detect abnormal structure present in the images shown in Figures 2 and 3. Gaussian noise(5%) is added to the image to find the robustness of algorithms.

The segmented results are shown in Figures 3-9 are the two classes of the image I. The objective values of class 1 using FCM, FCM-PSO and FCM-QPSO are 0.1471, 0.3999 and 0.4000 and class 2 produces 0.4647,0.5000 and 0.5000. In this experiment fuzzy parameter m is set to 2 and other constant values of PSO is set as c1=c2=1.49,w=0.72,swarm size =30 and Maximum Iterations =100. The same number of iterations is followed in all the algorithms and termination parameter is set as ε=0.001. The objective values of class 1 using FCM, FCM-PSO and FCM-QPSO on the image II are 0.1588, 0.3917 and 0.4100 and 0.4412, 0.4987 and 0.5100 for class 2.

Clustering on Liver Disorder and Breast Cancer

K Means-PSO utilizes the globalized searching of PSO and fast convergence of K Means. Figure 10 shows the clustering results of K Means QPSO on Breast cancer for K=5 with the DBI of 0.1331 with less overlapping as compared to FCM-QPSO. Figures 11 and 12 show the objective values for the corresponding iterations obtained on Liver disorder and Breast cancer. Figures 13 and 14 show the clustering results of FCM for three clusters. The DBI achieved for breast cancer is 0.0659 and 0.0026 for Liver disorder with heavy overlapping of clusters. The Figure 15 shows the obtained principal components on Breast

Figure 2. Original MRI image(I)

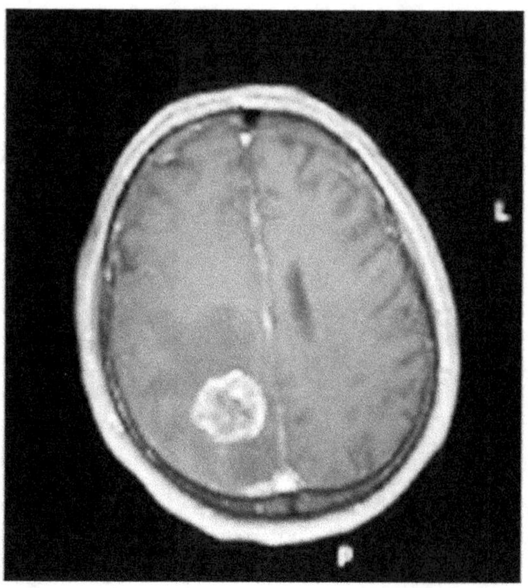

Figure 3. Noisy image (II) of I

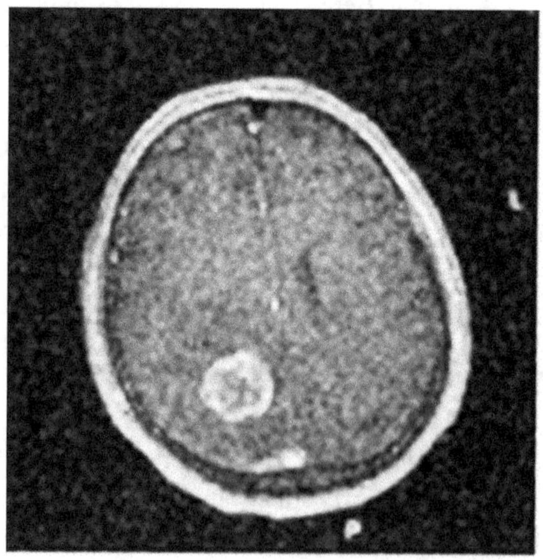

Figure 4. Results of FCM, FCM-PSO and FCM-QPSO on Figure 2

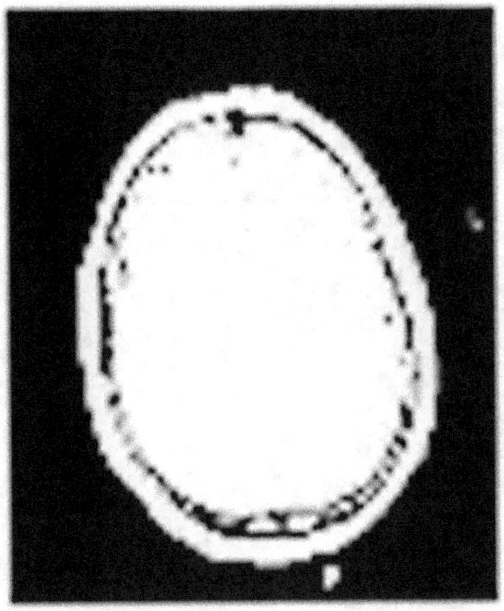

Figure 5. Results of FCM, FCM-PSO and FCM-QPSO on Figure 2

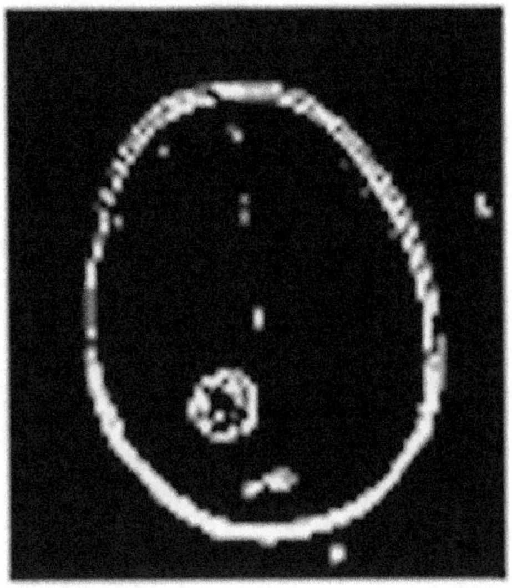

Figure 6. Results of FCM, FCM-PSO and FCM-QPSO on Figure 2

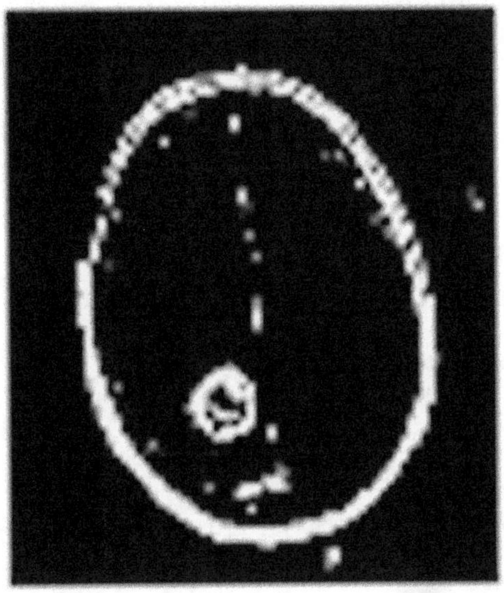

Figure 7. Results of FCM, FCM-PSO and FCM-QPSO on Figure 2

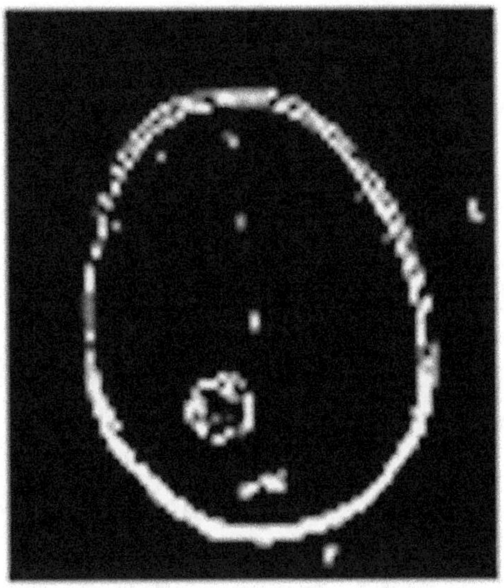

cancer for K=3. The Figure 16 shows the clustering results of PCA – K Means on Breast cancer dataset for K=2. PCA-K Means generates clusters with minimum Sum Square Error (SSE) in less computation time than K Means, K Means-PSO and K Means - QPSO. The experiments show that K Means-QPSO and PCA-K Means are effective methods for partitioning large data sets. K Means based methods and PCA-K Means have less overlapping compared to FCM based Methods. FCM as soft clustering method,

Figure 8. Results of FCM, FCM-PSO and FCM-QPSO on Figure 2

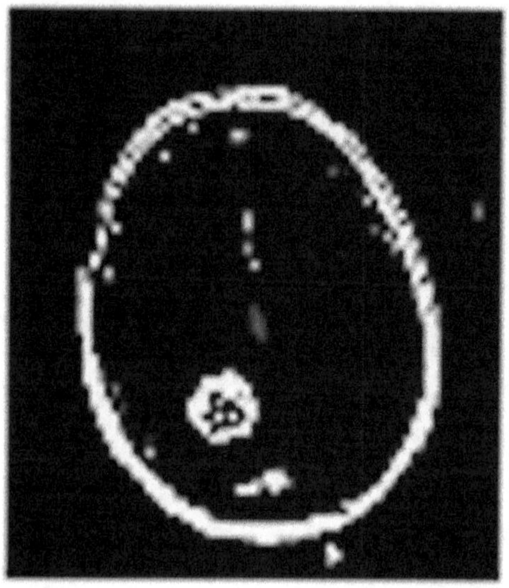

Figure 9. Results of FCM, FCM-PSO and FCM-QPSO on Figure 2

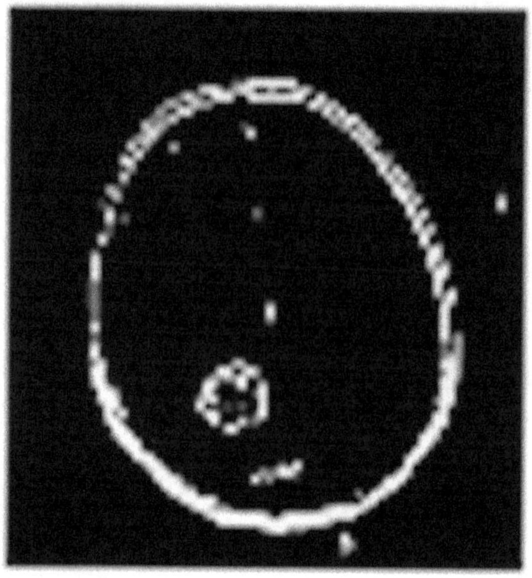

the degree of membership of elements in clusters are considered and the performance of QPSO based clustering is better than other methods with less DBI even on noisy data.

Table 5 shows the evaluation results of existing and proposed FCM algorithms on brain MRI images(I and II) shown in Figures 2 and 3 respectively. DBI of 0.4123 and 0.4136 has been achieved while using FCM-QPSO which is better than other methods.

Figure 10. Clustering results of K means - QPSO for breast cancer data set (K=5)

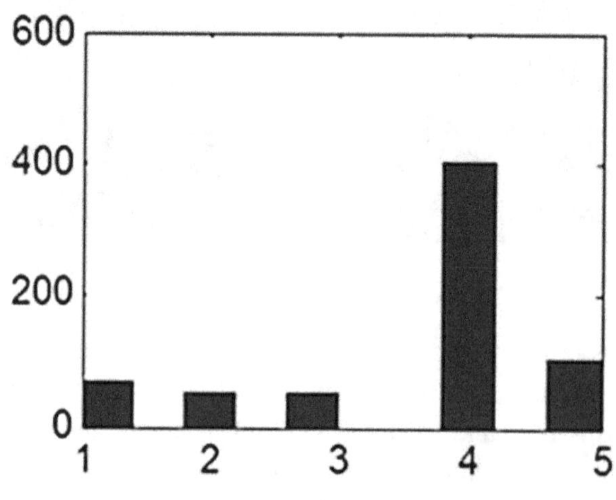

Figure 11. The values of objective function of FCM on Liver disorder dataset

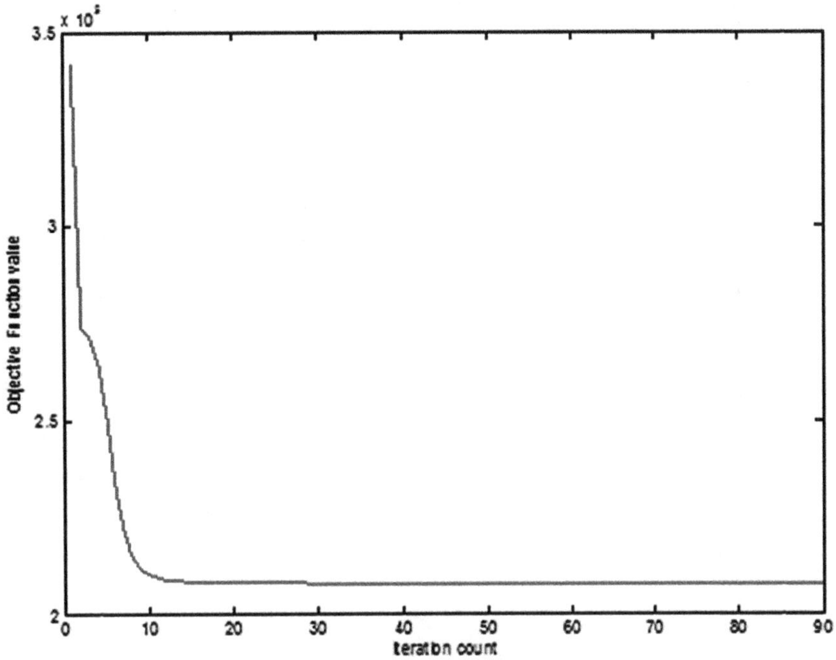

Figure 12. The values of objective function of FCM on Breast Cancer data set

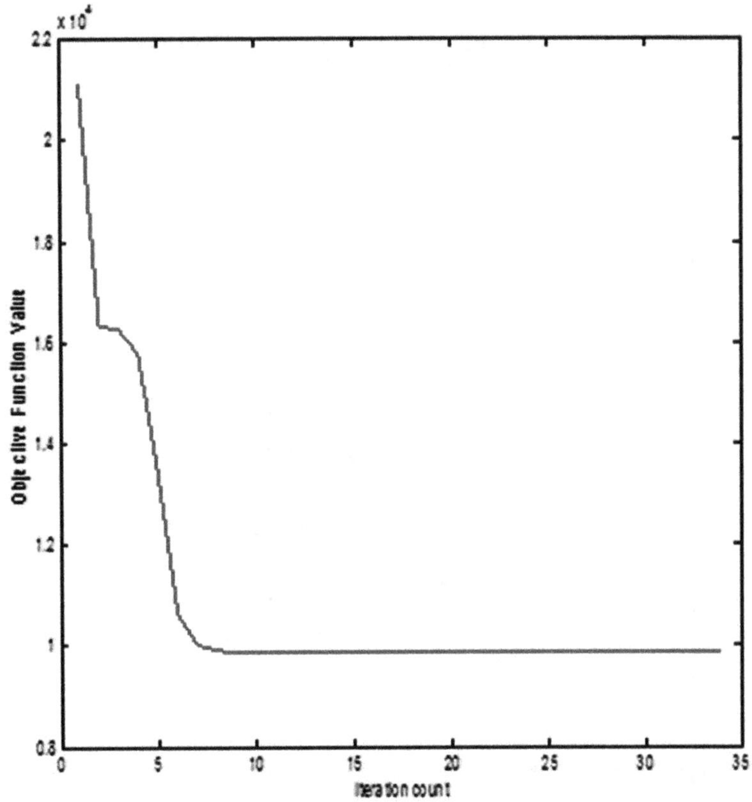

Figure 13. Clustering of Breast cancer dataset using FCM for K=3

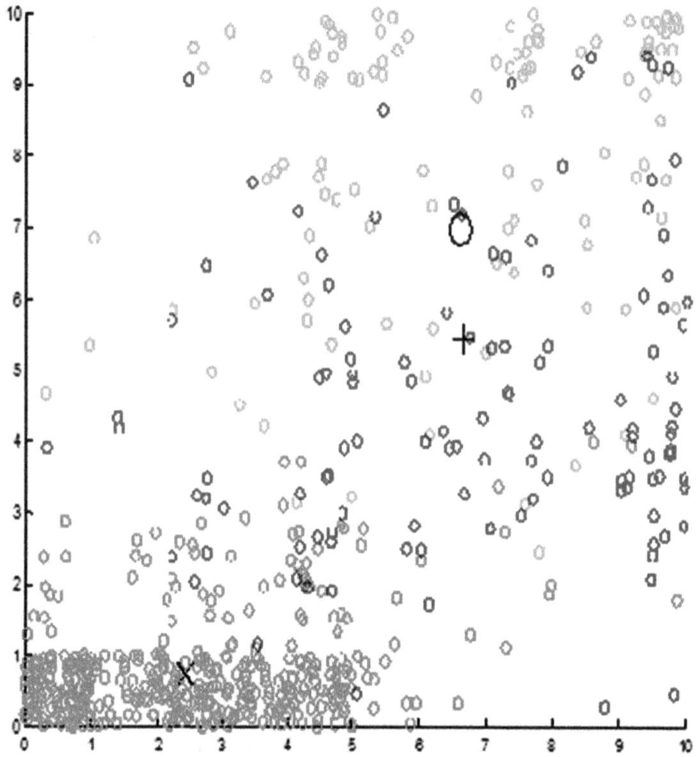

Figure 14. Clustering of Liver disorder using FCM for K=3

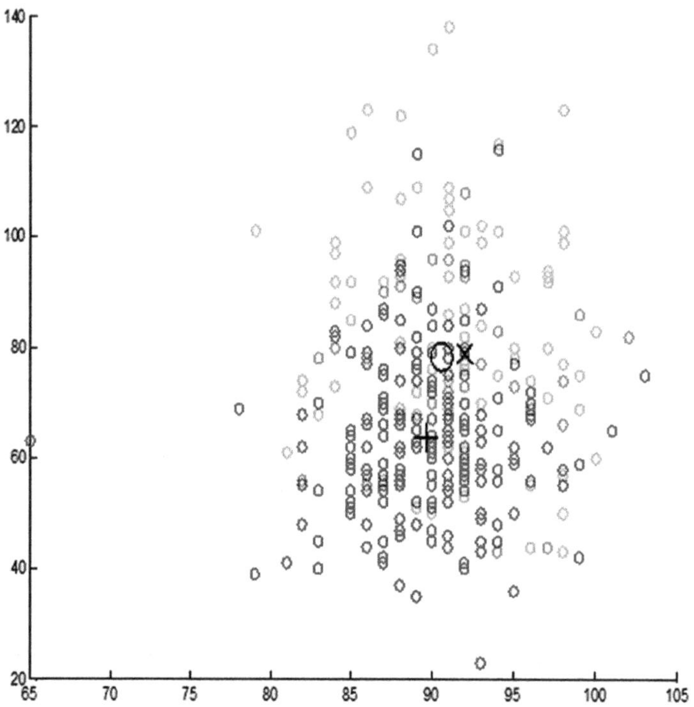

Figure 15. Clustering of Breast cancer using PCA- K Means for K=3

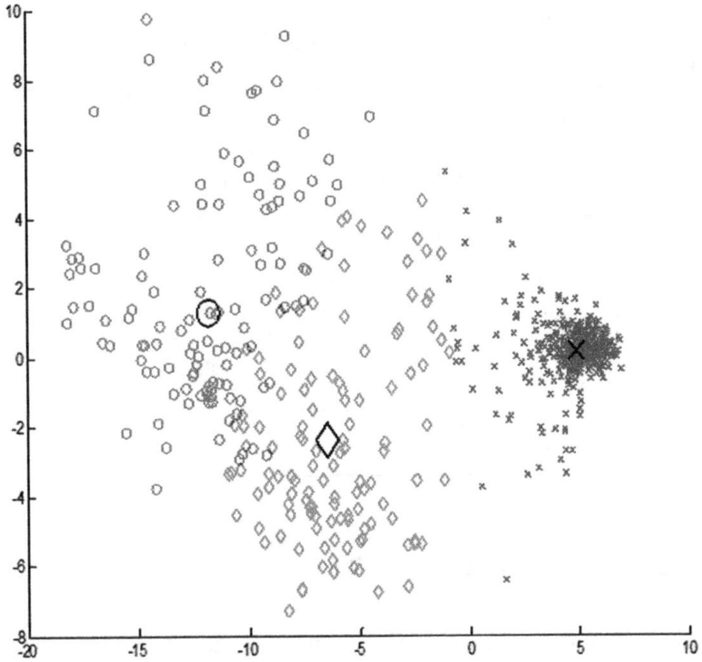

Figure 16. Clustering of Breast cancer using PCA- K Means for K=2

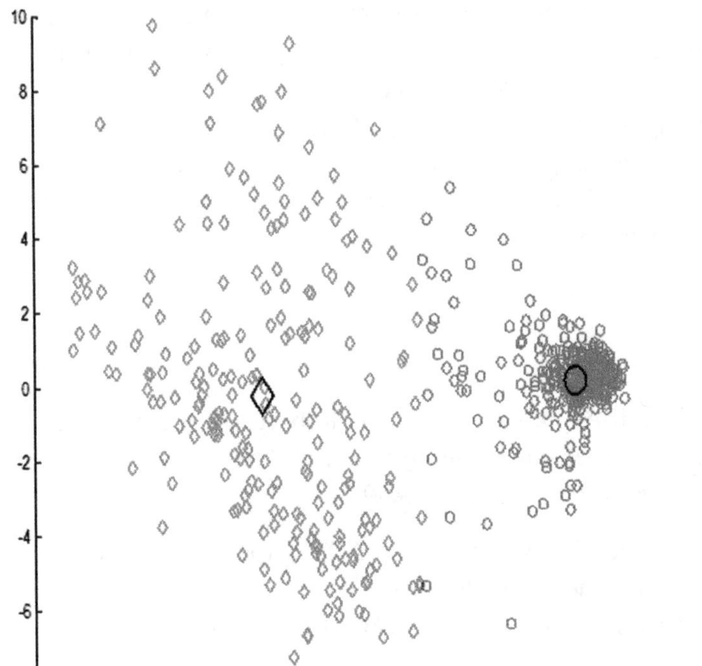

Table 5. Evaluation results of existing and proposed FCM clustering algorithms on Brain MRI images

Method	Image and dataset	Intra Distance (Avg)	Cluster Centres	Number of Classes	Threshold level (Class 1)	Threshold level (Class 2)	Elapsed Time (Secs)	DBI
FCM	Figure 2. 1	0.3020	0.3373, 0.4510	2	0.1471	0.4647	24.6408	0.4156
	Figure 2. 2	0.2990	0.4157 0.7137	2	0.1588	0.4412	26.2200	0.4178
FCM-PSO	Figure 2. 1	0.2933	0.3174 0.4689	2	0.3999	0.5000	26.7892	0.4123
	Figure 2. 2	0.2919	0.4234 0.6790	2	0.3917	0.4987	23.8654	0.4140
FCM-QPSO	Figure 2. 1	0.2921	0.3578 0.4698	2	0.4000	0.5000	22.4567	**0.4123**
	Figure 2. 2	0.2912	0.3988 0.7098	2	0.4100	0.5100	22.691547	**0.4136**

CONCLUSION AND FUTURE RESEARCH

This chapter elaborates different partitional, fuzzy clustering and Maximum Entropy methods and its optimization using PSO, QPSO and WQPSO. A nature inspired meta heuristics swarm intelligence methods particularly PSO and its variants improve the performance of conventional clustering methods in terms of quality of clusters and convergence speed. The experiments on these methods were conducted on Medical images, liver disorder and breast cancer datasets and the analysis reveals that the optimized clustering produces better clustering results than standard clustering in terms of validity measures. The proposed clustering methods are well suited to detect the patterns of interest from diverse data types of biomedical datasets particularly to deal with medical disorders.

There is an increasing trend to improve the performance of clustering methodologies using swarm optimization techniques. The proposed approaches can be extended to multi model brain imaging, CT, mammography and ultrasound images to detect abnormalities. WQPSO based Bayesian networks can be tested on mentioned datasets.

REFERENCES

Aarabi, Kazerooni, Khateri, Ay, & Rad. (2014). A Robust MR-based attenuation map generation in short-TE MR images of the head employing hybrid spatial fuzzy C-means clustering and intensity inhomogeneity correction. *EJNMMI Physics, 1*, A49.

Aarthi, R., Divya, K., Komala, N., & Kavitha, S. (2011). Application of feature extraction and clustering in mammogram classification using Support Vector Machine. *Third International Conference on Advanced Computing (ICoAC)*. doi:10.1109/ICoAC.2011.6165150

Abraham, A., Das, S., & Roy, S. (2007). Swarm intelligence algorithms for data clustering. *Soft Computing for Knowledge Discovery and Data Mining*, 279–313.

Abraham, A., Guo, H., & Liu, H. (2006). Swarm Intelligence: Foundations, perspectives and applications. *Studies in Computational Intelligence*, *6*, 3–25. doi:10.1007/978-3-540-33869-7_1

Ali, A.-R., Couceiro, M., Hassanien, A. E., Tolba, M. F., & Snášel, V. (2014). Fuzzy C-Means based liver CT image segmentation with optimum number of clusters. *Advances in Intelligent Systems and Computing*, *303*, 131–139. doi:10.1007/978-3-319-08156-4_14

Amitava, C., Patrick, S., Amir, N., & Raphael, B. (2012). An improved biogeography based optimization approach for segmentation of human head CT-scan images employing fuzzy entropy. *Engineering Applications of Artificial Intelligence*, *25*(8), 1698–1709. doi:10.1016/j.engappai.2012.02.007

Azzag, H., Monmarche, N., Slimane, M., & Venturini, G. (2003). AntTree: A new model for clustering with artificial ants. In *IEEE Congress on Evolutionary Computation*. doi:10.1109/CEC.2003.1299421

Bandyopadhyay, S., & Maulik, U. (2002). Genetic clustering for automatic evolution of clusters and application to image classification. *Pattern Recognition*, *35*(6), 1197–1208. doi:10.1016/S0031-3203(01)00108-X

Bezdek, J.C. (1981). *Pattern Recognition with Fuzzy Objective Function Algorithms*. Academic Press.

Bishop. (2006). *Pattern Recognition and Machine Learning*. Academic Press.

Chen, D., Wang, J., Zou, F., Hou, W., & Zhao, C. (2012). An Improved group search optimizer with operation of quantum-behaved swarm and its application. *Applied Soft Computing*, *12*(2), 712–725. doi:10.1016/j.asoc.2011.10.021

Chiu, M. J., Lin, C. C., Chuang, K. H., Chen, J. H., & Huang, K. M. (2001). Tissue segmentation-assisted analysis of fMRI for human motor response: An approach combining artificial neural network and fuzzy C-Means. *Journal of Digital Imaging*, *14*(1), 38–47. doi:10.1007/s10278-001-0023-y PMID:11310914

Chowdhury A., & Das, S. (2012). Automatic shape independent clustering inspired by ant dynamics. *Swarm Evol. Comput*, 33–45.

Chuang, L., Hsiao, C., & Yang, C. (2011). Chaotic particle swarm optimization for data clustering. *Expert Systems with Applications*, *38*(12), 14555–14563. doi:10.1016/j.eswa.2011.05.027

Cura, T. (2012). A particle swarm optimization approach to clustering. *Expert Systems with Applications*, *39*(1), 1582–1588. doi:10.1016/j.eswa.2011.07.123

Das, S., Abraham, A., & Konar, A. (2008). Automatic kernel clustering with a multi-elitist particle swarm optimization algorithm. *Pattern Recognition Letters*, *29*(5), 688–699. doi:10.1016/j.patrec.2007.12.002

Deepak, K. S., Gokul, K., Hinduja, R., & Rajkumar, S. (2013). An Efficient approach to predict tumour in 2D Brain image using classification techniques. *International Conference on Information Communication and Embedded Systems (ICICES)*. doi:10.1109/ICICES.2013.6508256

Dorigo, D. (1992). *Optimization, Learning and Natural Algorithms*. (Ph.D. Thesis). Politecnico di Milano, Italy.

Dunn, J. C. (1973). A Fuzzy Relative of the ISODATA Process and its use in detecting compact well-separated clusters. *J. Cybernetics*, *3*(3), 32–57. doi:10.1080/01969727308546046

Engelbrecht, A. P. (2005). *Fundamentals of Computational Swarm Intelligence*. Chichester, UK: Wiley.

Ester, M., Kriegel, H.P., Sander, J., & Xu, X. (1996). A Density-based algorithm for discovering clusters in large spatial databases with noise. *Proc. 2nd Int. Conf. on Knowledge Discovery and Data Mining*.

Ethem, . (2004). *Introduction to Machine Learning*. The MIT Press.

Fan, C.-Y., Fan, P.-S., Chan, T.-Y., & Chang, S.-H. (2012). Using hybrid data mining and machine learning clustering analysis to predict the turnover rate for technology professionals. *Expert Systems with Applications*, *39*(10), 8844–8851. doi:10.1016/j.eswa.2012.02.005

Farmer, J. D. N., Packard, N. H., & Perelson, A. S. (1986). Packard., & A. Perelson.(1986) The Immune system, adaptation and machine learning. *Physica D. Nonlinear Phenomena*, *2*(1-3), 187–204. doi:10.1016/0167-2789(86)90240-X

Feng, D., Wenkang, S., Liangzhou, C., Yong, D., & Zhenfu, Z. (2005). Infrared image segmentation with 2-D maximum entropy method based on particle swarm optimization (PSO). *Pattern Recognition Letters*, *26*(5), 597–603. doi:10.1016/j.patrec.2004.11.002

George, E., & Tsekouras, J. (2013). On Training RBF neural networks using input–output fuzzy clustering and particle swarm optimization. *Fuzzy Sets and Systems*, *221*, 65–89. doi:10.1016/j.fss.2012.10.004

Ghazanfari, M., Alizadeh, S., Fathian, M., & Koulouriotis, D. E. (2007). Comparing simulated annealing and genetic algorithm in learning FCM. *Journal of Applied Mathematics and Computation*, *192*(1), 56–68. doi:10.1016/j.amc.2007.02.144

Ghosh, A., Halder, A., Kothari, M., & Ghosh, S. (2008). Aggregation pheromone density based data clustering. *Journal Information Sciences: an International Journal*, *178*(13), 2816–2831. doi:10.1016/j.ins.2008.02.015

Glen, L. (2014). A Taxonomy to guide research on the application of data mining to fraud detection in financial statement audits. *International Journal of Accounting Information Systems*, *15*(4), 357–380. doi:10.1016/j.accinf.2014.05.006

Gopal, N. N., & Karnan, M. (2010). Diagnose brain tumor through MRI using image processing clustering algorithms such as Fuzzy C Means along with intelligent optimization techniques.*IEEE International Conference on Computational Intelligence and Computing Research (ICCIC)*. doi:10.1109/ICCIC.2010.5705890

Hartigan, E., Axe, M. J., & Snyder-Mackler, L. (2009). Perturbation training prior to ACL reconstruction improves gait asymmetries in non-copers. *Journal of Orthopaedic Research*, *27*(6), 724–729. doi:10.1002/jor.20754 PMID:19023893

Hassanien, A. E., Schaefer, G., & AlQaheri, H. (2010). Prostate boundary detection in ultrasound images based on Type-II fuzzy sets and modified fuzzy C-Means. Soft Computing in Industrial Applications. *Advances in Intelligent and Soft Computing.*, *75*, 187–195. doi:10.1007/978-3-642-11282-9_20

He, P., Shan, L., Lin, N. C., Martin, G. B., Kemmerling, B., Nürnberger, T., & Sheen, J. (2006). Specific bacterial suppressors of MAMP signaling upstream of MAPKKK in Arabidopsis innate immunity. *Cell*, *125*(3), 563–575. doi:10.1016/j.cell.2006.02.047 PMID:16678099

Holland, J. H. (1975). *Adaptation in Natural and Artificial Systems*. University of Michigan Press.

Ioannis, A. (2012). A Semi-supervised fuzzy clustering algorithm applied to gene expression data. *Pattern Recognition*, *45*(1), 637–648. doi:10.1016/j.patcog.2011.05.007

Izakian, H., & Abraham, A. (2011). Fuzzy C-means and fuzzy swarm for fuzzy clustering problem. *Expert Systems with Applications*, *38*(3), 1835–1838. doi:10.1016/j.eswa.2010.07.112

Juang, L.-H., & Wu, M.-N. (2010). MRI brain lesion image detection based on color-converted K-means clustering segmentation. *Measurement*, *43*(7), 941–949. doi:10.1016/j.measurement.2010.03.013

Jun, S., Wei, C., Wei, F., Xiaojun, W., & Wenbo, X. (2012). Gene expression data analysis with the clustering method based on an improved quantum-behaved particle swarm optimization. *Engineering Applications of Artificial Intelligence*, *25*(2), 376–391. doi:10.1016/j.engappai.2011.09.017

Kanungo, & Singh. (2015). Mammogram Image Segmentation using Hybridization of fuzzy clustering and optimization algorithms. *Intelligent Computing. Communication and Devices*, *309*, 403–413.

Kargari, M., & Sepehri, M. M. (2012). Stores clustering using a data mining approach for distributing automotive spare-parts to reduce transportation costs. *Expert Systems with Applications*, *39*(5), 4740–4748. doi:10.1016/j.eswa.2011.09.121

Kennedy, J., & Eberhart, R. C. (1995). Particle Swarm Optimization. *Proceedings of IEEE International conference on Neural Networks*. doi:10.1109/ICNN.1995.488968

Kirkpatrick, S. C. (2010). Optimization by Simulated Annealing. *Science*.

Kumbhar, A. D., & Kulkarni, A. V. (2011). Magnetic Resonant image segmentation using trained K-means clustering. *World Congress on Information and Communication Technologies (WICT)*. doi:10.1109/WICT.2011.6141301

Kuo, R. J., Lin, S. Y., & Shih, C. W. (2007). Mining association rules through integration of clustering analysis and ant colony system for health insurance database in Taiwan. *Expert Systems with Applications*, *33*(3), 794–808. doi:10.1016/j.eswa.2006.08.035

Leandro dos Santos, C. (2010). Gaussian quantum-behaved particle swarm optimization approaches for constrained engineering design problems. *Expert Systems with Applications*, *37*(2), 1676–1683. doi:10.1016/j.eswa.2009.06.044

Lee, K. C., Lee, N., & Lee, H. (2012). Multi-agent knowledge integration mechanism using particle swarm optimization. *Journal of Technological Forecasting and Social Change*, *79*(3), 469–484. doi:10.1016/j.techfore.2011.08.004

Lin, C. J. (2008). An efficient immune-based symbiotic particle swarm optimization learning algorithm for TSK-type neuro-fuzzy networks design. *Journal on Fuzzy Sets and Systems*, *159*(21), 2890–2909. doi:10.1016/j.fss.2008.01.020

Linyi, L., & Deren, L. (2008). Fuzzy entropy image segmentation based on particle swarm optimization. *Progress in Natural Science*, *18*(9), 1167–1171. doi:10.1016/j.pnsc.2008.03.020

Maolong, X., Jun, S., & Wenbo, X. (2008). An Improved quantum-behaved particle swarm optimization algorithm with weighted mean best position. *Applied Mathematics and Computation*, *205*(2), 751–759. doi:10.1016/j.amc.2008.05.135

McLachlan, G., & Krishnan, T. (1997). *The EM Algorithm and Extensions*. John Wiley & Sons.

Nanda, S. J., & Panda, G. (2012). Accurate partitional clustering algorithm based on Immunized PSO. *IEEE International Conference on Advances in Engineering, Science and Management*.

Nandagopalan, S., Adiga, B. S., & Dhanalakshmi, C., & Deepak. (2010). Automatic Segmentation and ventricular border detection of 2D echocardiography images combining K-Means clustering and active contour model. Second International Conference on Computer and Network Technology (ICCNT).

Nandagopalan, S., Dhanalakshmi, C., Adiga, B.S., & Deepak, N. (2010). A Fast K-Means algorithm for the segmentation of echocardiographic images using DBMS-SQL. *The 2ndInternational Conference Computer and Automation Engineering* (ICCAE).

Natteshan, N. V. S., & Angel Arul Jothi, J. (2014). Automatic classification of brain MRI Images using SVM and neural network classifiers. *Advances in Intelligent Systems and Computing*, *311*, 157–166.

Neeraj, S., & Lalit, M. (2010). Automated medical image segmentation techniques. *Journal of Medical Physics*, *35*(1), 3–14. doi:10.4103/0971-6203.58777 PMID:20177565

Ng, H. P., Ong, S. H., Foong, K. W. C., Goh, P. S., & Nowinski, W. L. (2006). Image Segmentation Using K-Means Clustering and Improved Watershed Algorithm.*IEEE Southwest Symposium on Image Analysis and Interpretation*. doi:10.1109/SSIAI.2006.1633722

Olesen, Cordero, & Zeng. (2009). Auto-Clustering using particle swarm optimization and bacterial foraging, in: Agents and Data Mining Interaction. Lecture Notes in Computer Science, 5680, 69–83.

Ouadfel, S., Batouche, M., & Teleb-Ahmed, A. (2010). A modified particle swarm optimization algorithm for automatic image clustering.*Proceedings of the 1st International Symposium on Modeling and Implementing Complex Systems*.

Panos, M., Pardalos, H., Romeijn, & Tuy. (2000). Recent developments and trends in global optimization. *Journal of Computational and Applied Mathematics, 124*(1-2), 209–228.

Panov, P., Dzeroski, S., & Soldatova, L. (2008). OntoDM: An ontology of data mining.*IEEE International Conference on Data Mining Workshops*.

Pyle, D. (1999). *Data Preparation for Data Mining*. Morgan Kaufmann.

Salgado, P., & Igrejas, G. (2012). A PCA-fuzzy clustering algorithm for contours analysis. *Advances in Intelligent and Soft Computing*, *107*, 305–311. doi:10.1007/978-3-642-24001-0_28

Senthilnath, J., Omkar, S. N., & Mani, V. (2011). Clustering using firefly algorithm: Performance study. *Swarm and Evolutionary Computation*, *1*(3), 164–171. doi:10.1016/j.swevo.2011.06.003

Shasidha, M., & Sudheer Raja, V., & Kumar. (2011). MRI Brain image segmentation using modified fuzzy c-means clustering algorithm. *International Conference on Communication Systems and Network Technologies*.

Talbi, E. (2002). A Taxonomy of hybrid metaheuristics. *Journal of Heuristics*, *8*(5), 541–564. doi:10.1023/A:1016540724870

Tan, H. H. Y. (2012). A two-stage genetic algorithm for automatic clustering. *Neurocomputing*, *81*(1), 49–59.

Tian, J., & Zeng, J. (2009). 2D Fuzzy Maximum Entropy Image Threshold Segmentation Method Based on QPSO. *Computer Engineering.*, *35*(3), 230–232.

Vahid, F., & Gholam Ali, M. (2013). An Improvement in RBF learning algorithm based on PSO for real time applications. *Neurocomputing*, *111*, 169–176. doi:10.1016/j.neucom.2012.12.024

Wang, Shiqin, & Xu. (2007). Scalability of hybrid fuzzy C-Means algorithm based on quantum-behaved PSO. *Fourth International Conference on Fuzzy Systems and Knowledge Discovery*.

Ward, J. H. Jr. (1963). Hierarchical grouping to optimize an objective function. *Journal of the American Statistical Association*, *58*(301), 236–244. doi:10.1080/01621459.1963.10500845

Yang, F., Sun, T., & Zhang, C. (2009). An efficient hybrid data clustering method based on K-harmonic means and Particle Swarm Optimization. *Expert Systems with Applications*, *36*(6), 9847–9852. doi:10.1016/j.eswa.2009.02.003

Yinggan, T., Qiuyan, D., Xinping, G., & Fucai, L. (2008). Threshold Selection Based on Fuzzy Tsallis Entropy and Particle Swarm Optimization. *NeuroQuantology*, *6*(4), 412–419. doi:10.14704/nq.2008.6.4.197

Zhide, L., Jiabin, C., & Chunlei. (2009). A New RBF Neural Network with GA-based Fuzzy C-Means Clustering Algorithm for SINS Fault Diagnosis. *Chinese Control and Decision Conference*. doi:10.1109/CCDC.2009.5195114

ADDITIONAL READING

Jinhui, L., & Yiliang, Z. (2013). Multi threshold image segmentation using maximum fuzzy entropy based on a new 2D histogram. *Optik, Elsevier*, *124*(18), 3756–3760.

Jun, S., Bin, F., & Wenbo, X. (2004). Particle swarm optimization with particles having quantum behaviour. *Congress on Evolutionary Computation*, *1*, 325–331.

Jun, S., Xiaojun, W., Vasile, P., Wei, F., Choi-Hong, L., & Wenbo, X. (2012). Convergence analysis and improvements of quantum-behaved particle swarm optimization. *Information Sciences*, *193*(15), 81–103.

KEY TERMS AND DEFINITIONS

Clustering: Clustering is the process of grouping similar data in a cluster and dissimilar data in different clusters.

Computation Time: Computation Time is the execution time of an algorithm and is measured in seconds.

Davis Bouldin Index (DBI): DBI is the cluster validity measure and the value of DBI is less for clusters with low intra cluster distances and high inter cluster distances.

Entropy: Entropy is defined as the uncertainty that is expressed quantitatively by the information.

Fuzzy C Means (FCM): FCM is the partitioning of elements based on fuzzy membership.

Gbest: It is the global best of Swarm.

Intra Cluster: It is the distance between data points within the cluster.

K Means: K Means is the partitional clustering algorithm where K refers the number of clusters.

Medical Image Processing: Medical image processing is one of the techniques to visualize and analysis the diverse types of medical images from user perspective.

Overlapping of Clusters: It refers belongingness of an object in two or more clusters.

Particle Swarm Optimization (PSO): PSO is a population based stochastic optimization technique and it is abbreviated as Particle Swarm Optimization.

Pbest: It is the personal best position of the particles.

Quantum Particle Swarm Optimization (QPSO): QPSO is Quantum PSO where particles movement are dynamic on the basis of quantum mechanics.

Swarm Intelligence (SI): SI is a self organized and collective behavioral system.

Weighed Quantum Particle Swarm Optimization (WQPSO): WQPSO is Weighted QPSO where each particle is assigned with weight according to fitness.

Compilation of References

Aarabi, Kazerooni, Khateri, Ay, & Rad. (2014). A Robust MR-based attenuation map generation in short-TE MR images of the head employing hybrid spatial fuzzy C-means clustering and intensity inhomogeneity correction. *EJNMMI Physics, 1*, A49.

Aaron, J. Y., Kuiken, T. A., & Hargrove, L. J. (2014). Analysis of using EMG and mechanical sensors to enhance intent recognition in powered lower limb prosthesis. *Journal of Neural Engineering, 11*, 1–12.

Aarthi, R., Divya, K., Komala, N., & Kavitha, S. (2011). Application of feature extraction and clustering in mammogram classification using Support Vector Machine. *Third International Conference on Advanced Computing (ICoAC)*. doi:10.1109/ICoAC.2011.6165150

Abenstein, J. P., & Tompkins, W. J. (1982). A new data-reduction algorithm for real-time ECG analysis. *IEEE Transactions on Bio-Medical Engineering*, *29*(1), 43–48. doi:10.1109/TBME.1982.324962 PMID:7076268

Abraham, A., Das, S., & Roy, S. (2007). Swarm intelligence algorithms for data clustering. *Soft Computing for Knowledge Discovery and Data Mining*, 279–313.

Abraham, A., Guo, H., & Liu, H. (2006). Swarm Intelligence: Foundations, perspectives and applications. *Studies in Computational Intelligence*, *6*, 3–25. doi:10.1007/978-3-540-33869-7_1

Abramoff, M. D., Garvin, M. K., & Sonka, M. (2010). Retinal imaging and image analysis. *IEEE. Reviews in Biomedical Engineering*, *3*, 169–208. doi:10.1109/RBME.2010.2084567 PMID:22275207

Acharya, U. R., Sree, S. V., Alvin, A. P. C., & Suri, J. S. (2012). Use of principal component analysis for automatic classification of epileptic EEG activities in wavelet framework. *Expert Systems with Applications*, *39*(10), 9072–9078. doi:10.1016/j.eswa.2012.02.040

Acharya, U., Joseph, K., Kannathal, N., Lim, C., & Suri, J. (2006). Heart rate variability: A review. *Medical & Biological Engineering & Computing*, *44*(12), 1031–1051. doi:10.1007/s11517-006-0119-0 PMID:17111118

Adam, H., Valentina, K., & Michael, G. (2000). Locating Blood Vessels in Retinal Images by Piecewise Threshold Probing of a Matched Filter Response. *IEEE Transactions on Medical Imaging*, *19*(3), 203–210. doi:10.1109/42.845178 PMID:10875704

Addison, P. S. (2005). Wavelet transforms and the ECG: A review. *Physiological Measurement*, *26*(5), R155–R199. doi:10.1088/0967-3334/26/5/R01 PMID:16088052

Adochiei, N., & David, V. (2012). *QRS time detection using Wavelet Multiresolution Analysis for determining HRV in case of ECG signals with high level noise.* Paper presented at the Electrical and Power Engineering (EPE), 2012 International Conference and Exposition on. doi:10.1109/ICEPE.2012.6463866

Agaian, S. S., Panetta, K. A., & Grigoryan, A. M. (2001). Transform based image enhancement algorithms with performance measure. *IEEE Transactions on Image Processing*, *10*(3), 367–382. doi:10.1109/83.908502 PMID:18249627

Agaian, S. S., Panetta, K. A., Nercessian, S. C., & Danahy, E. E. (2010). Boolean derivatives with application to edge detection for imaging systems. *IEEE Transactions on Systems, Man, and Cybernetics. Part B, Cybernetics*, *40*(2), 371–382. doi:10.1109/TSMCB.2009.2024771 PMID:19884097

Aggarwal, V., & Patterh, M. S. (2012). Quality controlled ECG compression using essentially non-oscillatory point-value decomposition (ENOPV) technique. *Digital Signal Processing*, *22*(1), 878–884. doi:10.1016/j.dsp.2012.06.010

Ahlstrom, C., Johansson, A., Uhlin, F., Lnne, T., & Ask, P. (2005). Noninvasive investigation of blood pressure changes using the pulse wave transit time: A novel approach in the monitoring of hemodialysis patients. *Journal of Artificial Organs*, *8*(3), 192–197. PMID:16235036

Ahmad, S., Chen, S., Soueidan, K., Batkin, I., Bolic, M., Dajani, H., & Groza, V. (2012). Electrocardiogram-assisted blood pressure estimation. Biomedical Engineering. *IEEE Transactions on*, *59*(3), 608–618.

Akansu, A. N., Serdijn, W. A., & Selesnick, I. W. (2010). *Emerging applications of wavelets: A review*. Elsevier.

Akay, M. (Ed.). (2006). *Wiley Encyclopedia of Biomedical Engineering*. Wiley-Interscience.

Akhter, S., & Haque, M. A. (2010, August). Ecg Comptression Using Run Length Encoding. In *18th European Signal Processing Conference EUSIPCO-2010* (pp. 1645-1649).

Akram, M. U., Atzaz, A., Aneeque, S. F., & Khan, S. A. (2009). Blood vessel enhancement and segmentation using wavelet transform.*IEEE International Conference on Digital Image Processing*. doi:10.1109/ICDIP.2009.70

Alacam, B., Yazici, B., Intes, X., & Chance, B. (2006). Extended Kalman filtering for the modeling and analysis of ICG pharmacokinetics in cancerous tumors using NIR optical methods. *Biomedical Engineering. IEEE Transactions on*, *53*(10), 1861–1871.

Alagoz, F., Valdez, A. C., Wilkowska, W., Ziefle, M., Dorner, S., & Holzinger, A. (2010). From cloud computing to mobile internet from user focus to culture and hedonism: The crucible of mobile health care and wellness applications. In *5th International Conference on Pervasive Computing and Applications(ICPCA '10)*. IEEEComputerSociety. doi:10.1109/ICPCA.2010.5704072

Alesanco, A., & Garcia, J. (2010). Clinical assessment of wireless ECG transmission in real-time cardiac telemonitoring. *IEEE Transactions on Information Technology in Biomedicine*, *14*(5), 1144–1152. doi:10.1109/TITB.2010.2047650 PMID:20378476

Ali, A.-R., Couceiro, M., Hassanien, A. E., Tolba, M. F., & Snášel, V. (2014). Fuzzy C-Means based liver CT image segmentation with optimum number of clusters. *Advances in Intelligent Systems and Computing*, *303*, 131–139. doi:10.1007/978-3-319-08156-4_14

Aliaam, A. H., Abdel, R. Y., Atef, Z. G., Amr, A. S., & Ghoneim, A. R. (2008). Optic disc detection from normalized digital fundus images by means of vessels direction matched filter. *IEEE Transactions on Medical Imaging*, *27*(1), 11–18. doi:10.1109/TMI.2007.900326 PMID:18270057

Aliberti, S., Tobaldini, E., Nunziata, V., Suigo, G., Giuliani, F., & D'Adda, A. et al.. (2013). Cardiac autonomic alterations impact early and late outcomes in patients with community-acquired pneumonia. *The European Respiratory Journal*, *42*(Suppl 57), 2765.

Allen, B. L., Kichambare, P. D., & Star, A. (2007). Carbon nanotube field-effect-transistor-based biosensors. *Advanced Materials*, *19*(11), 1439–1451. doi:10.1002/adma.200602043

Allen, F. R., Ambikairajah, E., Lovell, N. H., & Celler, B. G. (2006). Classification of a known sequence of motions and postures from accelerometry data using adapted Gaussian mixture models. *Physiological Measurement*, *27*(10), 935–951. doi:10.1088/0967-3334/27/10/001 PMID:16951454

Allen, J. (2007). Photoplethysmography and its application in clinical physiological measurement. *Physiological Measurement*, *28*(3), R1. PMID:17322588

Al-Shrouf, A., Abo-Zahhad, M., & Ahmed, S. M. (2003). A novel compression algorithm for electrocardiogram signals based on the linear prediction of the wavelet coefficients. *Digital Signal Processing*, *13*(4), 604–622. doi:10.1016/S1051-2004(02)00031-3

Ambrosio, R., Guevara, C., Silva, C., Heredia, A., & Moreno, M. (2014). *Electrical characterization of textile electrodes for an ECG acquisition system.* Paper presented at the Electrical Engineering, Computing Science and Automatic Control (CCE), 2014 11th International Conference on. doi:10.1109/ICEEE.2014.6978306

Amitava, C., Patrick, S., Amir, N., & Raphael, B. (2012). An improved biogeography based optimization approach for segmentation of human head CT-scan images employing fuzzy entropy. *Engineering Applications of Artificial Intelligence*, *25*(8), 1698–1709. doi:10.1016/j.engappai.2012.02.007

Anand, S., Shantha Selva Kumari, R., Thivya, T., Jeeva, S. (2013). Sharpening enhancement of ultrasound images using contourlet transform. *Optik-International Journal for Light and Electron Optics, 124,* 4789–4792.

Anand, S., ShanthaSelvaKumari, R., Jeeva, S., & Thivya, T. (2013). Contourlet transform based sharpening enhancement of retinal images and vessel extraction application. *Biomedizinische Technik. Biomedical Engineering*, *58*, 87–96. PMID:23314502

Anand, S., & Gayathri, S. (2015). Mammogram image enhancement by two stage adaptive histogram equalization. *Optik-International Journal of Light and Electron Optics*, *126*(21), 3150–3152. doi:10.1016/j.ijleo.2015.07.069

Anand, S., Kumari, R. S. S., Jeeva, S., & Thivya, T. (2013). Directionlet transform based sharpening and enhancement of mammographic x-ray images. *Biomedical Signal Processing and Control*, *8*(4), 391–399. doi:10.1016/j.bspc.2013.02.001

Anand, S., & Shantha Selva Kumari, R. (2013). Sharpening enhancement of computed tomography (CT) images using hyperbolic secant square filter. *Optik-International Journal for Light and Electron Optics*, *124*(15), 2121–2124. doi:10.1016/j.ijleo.2012.06.026

Arai, Y.-C. P., Ushida, T., Matsubara, T., Shimo, K., Ito, H., & Sato, Y. (2011). The influence of acupressure at extra 1 acupuncture point on the spectral entropy of the EEG and the LF/HF ratio of heart rate variability. *Evidence-Based Complementary and Alternative Medicine*. PMID:18955366

Arandiga, F., Cohen, A., Donat, R., & Matei, B. (2010). Edge detection insensitive to changes of illumination in the image. *Image and Vision Computing*, *28*(4), 553–562. doi:10.1016/j.imavis.2009.09.002

Arka, H.I., & Chellappan, K. (2014). Collaborative compressed I-cloud medical image storage with decompress viewer. In *Proceedings of Medical and Rehabilitation Robotics and Instrumentation* (MRRI '13). doi:10.1016/j.procs.2014.11.041

Arnavut, Z. (2007). ECG signal compression based on Burrows-Wheeler transformation and inversion ranks of linear prediction. *IEEE Transactions on Bio-Medical Engineering*, *54*(3), 410–418. doi:10.1109/TBME.2006.888820 PMID:17355052

Arnott, P., Pfeiffer, G., & Tavel, M. (1984). Spectral analysis of heart sounds: Relationships between some physical characteristics and frequency spectra of first and second heart sounds in normals and hypertensives. *Journal of Biomedical Engineering*, *6*(2), 121–128. PMID:6708485

Arturo, A., Manuel, E. G., & Diego, M. (2010). Detecting the optic disc boundary in digital fundus images using morphological, edge detection and feature extraction techniques. *IEEE Transactions on Medical Imaging*, *29*(11), 1860–186. doi:10.1109/TMI.2010.2053042 PMID:20562037

Arunachalam, K., Jacob, L. V., & Kamalanand, K. (2014). Design and analysis of finite element based sensors for diagnosis of liver disorders using biocompatible metals. *Technology and Health Care: Official Journal of the European Society for Engineering and Medicine*, *22*(6), 867-875.

Atashpaz-Gargari, E., & Lucas, C. (2007). *Imperialist competitive algorithm: an algorithm for optimization inspired by imperialistic competition.* Paper presented at the Evolutionary Computation, 2007. CEC 2007. IEEE Congress on. doi:10.1109/CEC.2007.4425083

Atlaoui, D., Pichot, V., Lacoste, L., Barale, F., Lacour, J., & Chatard, J. (2007). Heart rate variability, training variation and performance in elite swimmers. *International Journal of Sports Medicine*, *28*(5), 394–400. doi:10.1055/s-2006-924490 PMID:17111320

Aubert, A., Ramaekers, D., Cuche, Y., Lysens, R., Ector, H., & Van de Werf, F. (1996). *Effect of long term physical training on heart rate variability*. Academic Press.

Aubert, A., Beckers, F., & Ramaekers, D. (2001). Autonomic Cardiac Control in Athletes and Non-Athletes at Rest. *Progress in Biomedical Research*, *6*, 318–321.

Aung, M. S., Thies, S. B., Kenney, L. P., Howard, D., Selles, R. W., Findlow, A. H., & Goulermas, J. Y. (2013). Automated detection of instantaneous gait events using time frequency analysis and manifold embedding. *IEEE Transactions on Neural Systems and Rehabilitation Engineering*, *21*(6), 908–916. doi:10.1109/TNSRE.2013.2239313 PMID:23322764

Au, S., Berniker, M., & Herr, H. (2008). Powered ankle-foot prosthesis to assist level-ground and stair-descent gaits. *Neural Networks*, *21*(4), 654–666. doi:10.1016/j.neunet.2008.03.006 PMID:18499394

Averin, D. V., & Korotkov, A. N. (1990). Correlated single-electron tunneling via mesoscopic metal particles: Effects of energy quantization. *Journal of Low Temperature Physics*, *80*(3-4), 173–185. doi:10.1007/BF00683484

Aviram, A. (1988). Molecules for Memory, Logic and Amplification. *Journal of the American Chemical Society*, *110*(17), 5687–5692. doi:10.1021/ja00225a017

Aviram, A., Joachim, C., & Pomerantz, M. (1988). Evidence of Switching and Rectification by a Single Molecule Effected with a ScanningTunneling Microscope. *Chemical Physics Letters*, *146*(6), 490–495. doi:10.1016/0009-2614(88)87486-4

Aviram, A., & Ratner, M. A. (1974). Molecular rectifiers. *Chemical Physics Letters*, *29*(2), 277–283. doi:10.1016/0009-2614(74)85031-1

Azar, A., Balas, V., & Olariu, T. (2014). Classification of EEG-Based Brain–Computer Interfaces. In B. Iantovics & R. Kountchev (Eds.), *Advanced Intelligent Computational Technologies and Decision Support Systems* (Vol. 486, pp. 97–106). Springer International Publishing. doi:10.1007/978-3-319-00467-9_9

Azuaje, F., Dubitzky, W., Wu, X., Lopes, P., Black, N., Adamson, K., et al. (1997). *A neural network approach to coronary heart disease risk assessment based on short-term measurement of RR intervals*. Academic Press.

Azzag, H., Monmarche, N., Slimane, M., & Venturini, G. (2003). AntTree: A new model for clustering with artificial ants. In *IEEE Congress on Evolutionary Computation*. doi:10.1109/CEC.2003.1299421

Babashzadeh, A., Huang, J., & Daoud, M. (2013). Exploiting semantics for improving clinical information retrieval. In *Proceedings of the 36th International ACM Conference on Research and Development in Information Retrieval*. Association For Computer Machinery. doi:10.1145/2484028.2484167

Baek, H. J., Kim, K. K., Kim, J. S., Lee, B., & Park, K. S. (2010). Enhancing the estimation of blood pressure using pulse arrival time and two confounding factors. *Physiological Measurement*, *31*(2), 145. PMID:20009186

Baibars, M., Kanjwal, K., & Marine, J. E. (2014). AF Detected on Implanted Cardiac Implantable Electronic Devices: Is There a Threshold for Thromboembolic Risk? *Current Treatment Options in Cardiovascular Medicine*, *16*(3), 289. doi:10.1007/s11936-013-0289-7 PMID:24500679

Baker, F., Colrain, I., & Trinder, J. (2008). Reduced Parasympathetic activity during sleep in the symptomatic phase of severe premenstrual syndrome. *Journal of Psychosomatic Research*, *65*(1), 13–22. doi:10.1016/j.jpsychores.2008.04.008 PMID:18582607

Baker, S. M., Poskar, C. H., Schreiber, F., & Junker, B. H. (2015). A unified framework for estimating parameters of kinetic biological models. *BMC Bioinformatics*, *16*(1), 104. doi:10.1186/s12859-015-0500-9 PMID:25886743

Ball, M. J., Garets, D. E., & Handler, T. J. (2003). Leveraging information technology towards enhancing patient care and a culture of safety in the US. *Methods of Information in Medicine*, *42*(5), 503–508. PMID:14654884

Bandyopadhyay, S., & Maulik, U. (2002). Genetic clustering for automatic evolution of clusters and application to image classification. *Pattern Recognition*, *35*(6), 1197–1208. doi:10.1016/S0031-3203(01)00108-X

Barros, L. C. (2004, June). Fuzzy set-based model to compute the life expectancy of HIV infected populations. In *Fuzzy Information, 2004. Processing NAFIPS'04. IEEE Annual Meeting of the* (Vol. 1, pp. 314-318). IEEE.

Barrow, M. (2011, December 23). Patients get right to see medical records online. *The Times*. Retrieved from http://www.thetimes.co.uk/tto/health/news/article3266823.ece

Bar-Shalom, Y., & Li, X. R. (1998). Estimation and Tracking: Principles, Techniques, and Software. Artech House.

Bartels, A., & Harder, D. (1992). Non-invasive determination of systolic blood pressure by heart sound pattern analysis. *Clinical Physics and Physiological Measurement*, *13*(3), 249–256. PMID:1424474

Bascil, M. S., & Oztekin, H. (2012). A study on hepatitis disease diagnosis using probabilistic neural network. *Journal of Medical Systems*, *36*(3), 1603–1606. doi:10.1007/s10916-010-9621-x PMID:21057884

Baselli, G., Cerutti, S., Interdonato, T., Orizio, C., Perini, R., & Veicsteinas, A. (n.d.). *HRV during exercise in sedentary subjects and athletes*. Academic Press.

Batista, L. V., Melcher, E. U. K., & Carvalho, L. C. (2001). Compression of ECG signals by optimized quantization of discrete cosine transform coefficients. *Medical Engineering & Physics*, *23*(2), 127–134. doi:10.1016/S1350-4533(01)00030-3 PMID:11413065

Batmani, Y., & Khaloozadeh, H. (2013). Optimal chemotherapy in cancer treatment: State dependent Riccati equation control and extended Kalman filter. *Optimal Control Applications and Methods*, *34*(5), 562–577. doi:10.1002/oca.2039

Belciug, S. (2009). Patients length of stay grouping using the hierarchical clustering algorithm. *Annals of the University of Craiova, 36*(2), 79-84.

Bellazzi, R., & Zupan, B. (2008). Predictive data mining in clinical medicine: Current issues and guidelines. *International Journal of Medical Informatics*, *77*(2), 81–97. doi:10.1016/j.ijmedinf.2006.11.006 PMID:17188928

Bendifallah, A., Benzid, R., & Boulemden, M. (2011). Improved ECG compression method using discrete cosine transform. *Electronics Letters*, *47*(2), 87. doi:10.1049/el.2010.3191

Benzid, R., Messaoudi, A., & Boussaad, A. (2008). Constrained ECG compression algorithm using the block-based discrete cosine transform. *Digital Signal Processing*, *18*(1), 56–64. doi:10.1016/j.dsp.2007.08.003

Bersvendsen, J., Orderud, F., Massey, R., Fossa, K., Gerard, O., Urheim, S., & Samset, E. (2016). Automated Segmentation of the Right Ventricle in 3D Echocardiography: A Kalman Filter State Estimation Approach. *IEEE Transactions on Medical Imaging*, *35*(1), 42–51. doi:10.1109/TMI.2015.2453551 PMID:26168434

Bezdek, J.C. (1981). *Pattern Recognition with Fuzzy Objective Function Algorithms*. Academic Press.

Bhutada, G. G., Anand, R. S., & Saxena, S. C. (2011). Edge preserved image enhancement using adaptive fusion of Images Denoised by Wavelet and Curvelet Transform. *Digital Signal Processing*, *21*(1), 118–130. doi:10.1016/j.dsp.2010.09.002

Bickley, L. S. (Ed.). (2009). *Bates' Guide to Physical Examination and History Taking* (11th ed.). Lippincott Williams & Wilkins.

Bilgin, A., Marcellin, M. W., & Altbach, M. I. (2004). Wavelet compression of ECG signals by JPEG2000. *Data Compression Conference, 2004. Proceedings*. http://doi.org/ doi:10.1109/DCC.2004.1281503

Bilgin, A., Marcellin, M. W., & Altbach, M. I. (2003). Compression of electrocardiogram signals using JPEG2000. *IEEE Transactions on Consumer Electronics*, *49*(4), 833–840. doi:10.1109/TCE.2003.1261162

Bindiya, R., Kishan, K., Damodara, K., Ramaswamy, C., & Bhat, M. (2011). Association between the different phases of menstrual cycle and time domain analysis of Heart Rate Variability in young adult and older adult in Indian Women's. *Research Journal of Pharmaceutical, Biological and Chemical Sciences*, *2*(1), 297–303.

Bishop. (2006). *Pattern Recognition and Machine Learning*. Academic Press.

Blanco-Velasco, M., Cruz-Roldán, F., Godino-Llorente, J. I., & Barner, K. E. (2007). Wavelet packets feasibility study for the design of an ECG compressor. *IEEE Transactions on Bio-Medical Engineering*, *54*(4), 766–769. doi:10.1109/TBME.2006.889176 PMID:17405386

Blanco-Velasco, M., Cruz-Roldán, F., Godino-Llorente, J. I., Blanco-Velasco, J., Armiens-Aparicio, C., & López-Ferreras, F. (2005). On the use of PRD and CR parameters for ECG compression. *Medical Engineering & Physics*, *27*(9), 798–802. doi:10.1016/j.medengphy.2005.02.007 PMID:15869896

Bland, J. M., & Altman, D. G. (1986). Statistical methods for assessing agreement between two methods of clinical measurement. *Lancet*, *1*, 307–310. PMID:2868172

Blásquez, J. C. C., Font, G. R., & Ortís, L. C. (2009). Heart-rate variability and precompetitive anxiety in swimmers. *Psicothema*, (4): 531–536. PMID:19861094

Bock, R., Meier, J., Nyul, L. G., & Michelson, G. (2010). Glaucoma risk index: Automated glaucoma detection from color fundus images. *Medical Image Analysis*, *14*(3), 471–481. doi:10.1016/j.media.2009.12.006 PMID:20117959

Booth, J. (1977). A short history of blood pressure measurement. *Proceedings of the Royal Society of Medicine, 70*(11), 793–799.

Borsali, R., & Na, A. (2004). *ECG Compression Using an Ensemble Polynomial Modeling: Comparison With the DCT Based Technique*. Academic Press.

Boutayeb, M., Rafaralahy, H., & Darouach, M. (1997). Convergence analysis of the extended Kalman filter used as an observer for nonlinear deterministic discrete-time systems. *Automatic Control. IEEE Transactions on*, *42*(4), 581–586.

Bozic, S. M. (1979). *Digital and Kalman filtering*. London: Edward Arnold.

Bramwell, J. C., & Hill, A. V. (1922). The velocity of the pulse wave in man. *Proceedings of the Royal Society of London. Series B, Containing Papers of a Biological Character*.

Braun, E., Eichen, Y., Sivan, U., & Ben-Yoseph, G. (1998). DNA-templated assembly and electrode attachment of a conducting silver wire. *Nature*, *391*(6669), 775–778. doi:10.1038/35826 PMID:9486645

Breiman, L. (1984). *Classification and regression trees*. Chapman & Hall/CRC.

Brigham, R. A. D. (2013). *Department of Radiology, Brigham and Women's Hospital*. Harvard Medical School. Retrieved from http://brighamrad.harvard. edu/Cases/bwh/hcache/group0-index.html

Brignell, J. E., & White, N. M. (1996). *Intelligent Sensor Systems: 2nd*. Institute of Physics Publishing.

Brockbank, C. L., Chatterjee, F., Bruce, S. A., & Woledge, R. C. (2000). Heart rate and its variability change after the menopause. *Experimental Physiology*, *85*(3), 327–330. doi:10.1111/j.1469-445X.2000.01902.x PMID:10825420

Brosnan, M., La Gerche, A., Kalman, J., Lo, W., Fallon, K., MacIsaac, A., & Prior, D. L. (2014). Comparison of frequency of significant electrocardiographic abnormalities in endurance versus nonendurance athletes. *The American Journal of Cardiology*, *113*(9), 1567–1573. doi:10.1016/j.amjcard.2014.01.438 PMID:24641963

Brovko, O., Wiberg, D. M., Arena, L., & Bellville, J. W. (1981). The extended Kalman filter as a pulmonary blood flow estimator. *Automatica*, *17*(1), 213–220. doi:10.1016/0005-1098(81)90096-0

Brzezinski, M., Luisetti, T., & London, M. J. (2009). Radial artery cannulation: A comprehensive review of recent anatomic and physiologic investigations. *Anesthesia and Analgesia*, *109*(6), 1763–1781. PMID:19923502

Budinger, T. F. (2003). Biomonitoring with wireless communications. *Annual Review of Biomedical Engineering*, *5*(1), 383–412. PMID:14527317

Buxi, D., Redout, J.-M., & Yuce, M. R. (2015). A survey on signals and systems in ambulatory blood pressure monitoring using pulse transit time. *Physiological Measurement*, *36*(3), R1. PMID:25694235

Camiilo, T., Oscar, R., & Carlos, L. (2009). *Biomedical Signal Monitoring Using Wireless Sensor Networks*. IEEE.

Camm, A. J., Malik, M., Bigger, J. T., Gunter, B., Cerutti, S., & Choen, R. (1996). Task force of the European society of cardiology and the North American society of pacing and electrophysiology Heart rate variability - standards of measurement. Physiological interpretation and clinical use. *Circulation*, *93*(5), 1043–1065. doi:10.1161/01.CIR.93.5.1043 PMID:8598068

Canny, J. (1986). A Computational Approach to Edge Detection. *IEEE Transactions on Pattern Analysis and Machine Intelligence*, *8*(6), 679–698. doi:10.1109/TPAMI.1986.4767851 PMID:21869365

Carlsson, S. (1988). Sketch Based Coding of Gray Level Images. *Signal Processing*, *15*(1), 57–83. doi:10.1016/0165-1684(88)90028-X

Carvalho, P., Paiva, R., Couceiro, R., Henriques, J., Antunes, M., Quintal, I., Muehlsteff, J., & Aubert, X. (2010). Comparison of systolic time interval measurement modalities for portable devices. In *Engineering in Medicine and Biology Society (EMBC), 2010 Annual International Conference of the IEEE.*

Cattivelli, F. S., & Garudadri, H. (2009, June). Noninvasive cuffless estimation of blood pressure from pulse arrival time and heart rate with adaptive calibration. In *Wearable and Implantable Body Sensor Networks, 2009. BSN 2009. Sixth International Workshop on* (pp. 114-119). IEEE. doi:10.1109/BSN.2009.35

Cazelles, B., & Chau, N. (1995). Adaptive dynamic modelling of HIV/AIDS epidemic using extended Kalman filter. *Journal of Biological System*, *3*(03), 759–768. doi:10.1142/S0218339095000691

Centers for Disease Control and Prevention (CDC). (2013). *Today's HIV/AIDS epidemic*. Author.

Ceylan, R., & Özbay, Y. (2007). Comparison of FCM, PCA and WT techniques for classification ECG arrhythmias using artificial neural network. *Expert Systems with Applications*, *33*(2), 286–295. doi:10.1016/j.eswa.2006.05.014

Chaiyakum & Wardkein. (2012, May). A New ECG Compression by Using Adaptive Cosine Fourier Transform. In Electrical Engineering/Electronics, Computer, Telecommunication and Information Technology (ECTI.CON) (pp. 1-4).

Chamberlain, N. R. (2010). *HIV Infections and AIDS*. Available from: http://www.atsu.edu/faculty/chamberlain/Website/lectures/lecture/aids.htm

Chan, K. W., Hung, K., & Zhang, Y. T. (2001). Noninvasive and cuffless measurements of blood pressure for telemedicine. In *Engineering in Medicine and Biology Society, 2001.Proceedings of the 23rd Annual International Conference of the IEEE* (*Vol. 4*, pp. 3592-3593). IEEE. doi:10.1109/IEMBS.2001.1019611

Chan, A. D. C., Englehart, K., Hudgins, B., & Lovely, D. F. (2001). Myo-electric signals to augment speech recognition. *Medical & Biological Engineering & Computing*, *39*(4), 500–504. doi:10.1007/BF02345373 PMID:11523740

Chandrasekaran, V., Dantu, R., Jonnada, S., Thiyagaraja, S., & Subbu, K. (2013). Cuffless differential blood pressure estimation using smart phones. Biomedical Engineering. *IEEE Transactions on*, *60*(4), 1080–1089.

Chang, Y. H., Huang, H. W., Hamerski, C. M., & Kram, R. (2000). The independent effects of gravity and inertia on running mechanics. *The Journal of Experimental Biology*, *203*, 229–238. PMID:10607533

Chase, N. L., Sui, X., & Blair, S. N. (2008). Swimming and all-cause mortality risk compared with running, walking, and sedentary habits in men. *International Journal of Aquatic Research and Education*, *2*(3), 213–223.

Chen, C. M., Hsu, C. Y., Chiu, H. W., & Rau, H. H. (2011). *Prediction of survival in patients with liver cancer using artificial neural networks and classification and regression trees*. Academic Press.

Chen, D., Pibarot, P., Honos, G., & Durand, L.-G. (1996). Estimation of pulmonary artery pressure by spectral analysis of the second heart sound. *The American Journal of Cardiology*, *78*(7), 785–789. PMID:8857483

Chen, D., Wang, J., Zou, F., Hou, W., & Zhao, C. (2012). An Improved group search optimizer with operation of quantum-behaved swarm and its application. *Applied Soft Computing*, *12*(2), 712–725. doi:10.1016/j.asoc.2011.10.021

Cheng, A. C. (2015). *Real-Time Cardiovascular Diseases Detection on a Smartphone*. Academic Press.

Chen, K.-I., Li, B.-R., & Chen, Y.-T. (2011). Silicon nanowire field-effect transistor-based biosensors for biomedical diagnosis and cellular recording investigation. *Nano Today*, *6*(2), 131–154. doi:10.1016/j.nantod.2011.02.001

Chen, W., Kobayashi, T., Ichikawa, S., Takeuchi, Y., & Togawa, T. (2000). Continuous estimation of systolic blood pressure using the pulse arrival time and intermittent calibration. *Medical & Biological Engineering & Computing*, *38*(5), 569–574. PMID:11094816

Chiu, M. J., Lin, C. C., Chuang, K. H., Chen, J. H., & Huang, K. M. (2001). Tissue segmentation-assisted analysis of fMRI for human motor response: An approach combining artificial neural network and fuzzy C-Means. *Journal of Digital Imaging*, *14*(1), 38–47. doi:10.1007/s10278-001-0023-y PMID:11310914

Chou, H.-H., Chen, Y.-J., Shiau, Y.-C., & Kuo, T.-S. (2006). An effective and efficient compression algorithm for ECG signals with irregular periods. *IEEE Transactions on Bio-Medical Engineering*, *53*(6), 1198–1205. doi:10.1109/TBME.2005.863961 PMID:16761849

Chowdhury A., & Das, S. (2012). Automatic shape independent clustering inspired by ant dynamics. *Swarm Evol. Comput*, 33–45.

Chowdhury, R. H., Reaz, M. B., Ali, M. A., Bakar, A. A., Chellappan, K., & Chang, T. G. (2013). Surface electromyography signal processing and classification techniques. *Sensors (Basel, Switzerland)*, *13*(9), 12431–12466. doi:10.3390/s130912431 PMID:24048337

Chua, E.-P., Redmond, S., McDarby, G., & Heneghan, C. (2010). Towards using photoplethysmogram amplitude to measure blood pressure during sleep. *Annals of Biomedical Engineering*, *38*(3), 945–954. PMID:20049639

Chuang, L., Hsiao, C., & Yang, C. (2011). Chaotic particle swarm optimization for data clustering. *Expert Systems with Applications*, *38*(12), 14555–14563. doi:10.1016/j.eswa.2011.05.027

Chu, J. U., Moon, I., & Mun, M. S. (2006). A real-time EMG pattern recognition system based on linear-nonlinear feature projection for a multifunction myoelectric hand. *IEEE Transactions on Bio-Medical Engineering*, *53*(11), 2232–2239. doi:10.1109/TBME.2006.883695 PMID:17073328

Chung, E., Chen, G., Alexander, B., & Cannesson, M. (2013). Non-invasive continuous blood pressure monitoring: A review of current applications. *Frontiers of Medicine*, *7*(1), 91–101. PMID:23345112

Chung, L., & Jung. (2008, August). A Wireless Sensor Network Compatible Wearable U.Healthcare Monitoring System Using Integrated ECG, Accelerometer and SPO2. In *30th Annual International IEEE EMBS conference* (pp. 1529-1532).

Chung, M., & Yang, C. (2011). Heart Rate Variability across the Menstrual Cycle in Shift Work Nurses. *Journal of Experimental and Clinical Medicine*, *3*(3), 121–125. doi:10.1016/j.jecm.2011.04.001

Cisco. (2009). *The Cisco powered network cloud: An exciting managed ser-vices opportunity.* Available at http://www.cisco.com/en/US/solutions/collateral/ns341/ns525/ns537/whitepaper c11-532553.html

Ciupe, M. S., Bivort, B. L., Bortz, D. M., & Nelson, P. W. (2006). Estimating kinetic parameters from HIV primary infection data through the eyes of three different mathematical models. *Mathematical Biosciences*, *200*(1), 1–27. doi:10.1016/j.mbs.2005.12.006 PMID:16469337

Cohen, A., & Zigel, Y. (1998). Compression of multichannel ECG through multichannel long-term prediction. *IEEE Engineering in Medicine and Biology Magazine: The Quarterly Magazine of the Engineering in Medicine & Biology Society*, *17*(1), 109–115. Retrieved from http://www.ncbi.nlm.nih.gov/pubmed/9460626

Cohen, E. A. Jr. (1981). A note on normal functions of normal random variables. *Computers & Mathematics with Applications (Oxford, England)*, *7*(5), 395–400. doi:10.1016/0898-1221(81)90124-3

Cohn, J. N., Finkelstein, S., McVeigh, G., Morga, D., LeMay, L., Robinson, J., & Mock, J. (1995). Noninvasive pulse wave analysis for the early detection of vascular disease. *Hypertension*, *26*(3), 503–508. PMID:7649589

Conforti, D., & Guido, R. (2010). Kernel based support vector machine via semidefinite programming: Application to medical diagnosis. *Computers & Operations Research*, *37*(8), 1389–1394. doi:10.1016/j.cor.2009.02.018

Constant, E. W. (1973). A Model forTechnological Change Applied to the Turbojet Revolution. *Technology and Culture*, *14*(4), 553–572. doi:10.2307/3102443

Cooper, G. R., & Mc Gillem, C. D. (1999). Probabilistic methods of signal and system analysis (3rd ed.). New York: Oxford University Press.

Cortes, C., & Vapnik, V. (1995). Support-vector networks. *Machine Learning*, *20*(3), 273–297. doi:10.1007/BF00994018

Couceiro, R., Carvalho, P., Paiva, R., Henriques, J., Antunes, M., & Quintal, I. andMuehlsteff, J. (2011). Beat-to-beat cardiac output inference using heart sounds. In *Engineering in Medicine and Biology Society,EMBC, 2011 Annual International Conference of the IEEE.*

Cox, J. R., Nolle, F. M., Fozzard, H. A., & Oliver, G. C. (1968). AZTEC, a preprocessing program for real-time ECG rhythm analysis. *IEEE Transactions on Bio-Medical Engineering*, *15*(April), 128–129. doi:10.1109/TBME.1968.4502549 PMID:5648088

Culhane, K. M., Lyons, G. M., Hilton, D., Grace, P. A., & Lyons, D. (2004). Long-term mobility monitoring of older adults using accelerometers in a clinical environment. *Clinical Rehabilitation*, *18*(3), 335–343. doi:10.1191/0269215504cr734oa PMID:15137565

Cura, T. (2012). A particle swarm optimization approach to clustering. *Expert Systems with Applications*, *39*(1), 1582–1588. doi:10.1016/j.eswa.2011.07.123

Da Silva, P. M. P. (2013). *A pervasive system for real-time blood pressure monitoring*. Academic Press.

da Silva, F. L. (2013). EEG and MEG: Relevance to Neuroscience. *Neuron*, *80*(5), 1112–1128. doi:10.1016/j.neuron.2013.10.017 PMID:24314724

Dai, F., Zheng, N., & Xue, J. (2008). Image smoothing and sharpening based on nonlinear diffusion equation. *Signal Processing*, *88*(11), 2850–2855. doi:10.1016/j.sigpro.2008.05.008

Danielsen, M., & Ottesen, J. (2001). Describing the pumping heart as a pressure source. *Journal of Theoretical Biology*, *212*(1), 71–81. PMID:11527446

Das, S., Abraham, A., & Konar, A. (2008). Automatic kernel clustering with a multi-elitist particle swarm optimization algorithm. *Pattern Recognition Letters*, *29*(5), 688–699. doi:10.1016/j.patrec.2007.12.002

Datta, S. (2005). *Atom to transistor*. New York: Cambridge University Press. doi:10.1017/CBO9781139164313

Daubechies, I. (1992). Ten Lectures on Wavelets. *IEEE Symposium on Computer Based Medical Systems* (Vol. 61).

Daubechies, I. (1992). *Ten lectures on wavelets* (Vol. 61). SIAM. doi:10.1137/1.9781611970104

de Abreu, L. C., Roque, A. L., de Castro, B. C., de Souza, A. C. A., Vanderlei, L. C. M., Ferreira, L. L., et al. (2014). *Responses of the geometric indices of heart rate variability to the active orthostatic test in women*. Academic Press.

de Carvalho, T. D., Pastre, C. M., Rossi, R. C., de Abreu, L., Valenti, V., & Vanderlei, L. M. (2011). Geometric index of heart rate variability in chronic obstructive pulmonary disease. *Revista Portuguesa de Pneumologia*, *17*(6), 260–265. doi:10.1016/j.rppnen.2011.10.001 PMID:21920699

De Saint-Exupery, A. (2009). *Internet of Things: Strategic research roadmap*. Retrieved from http://www.sintef.no/upload/IKT/9022/CERP-IoT%20SRA_IoT_v11_pdf.pdf

De Senneville, B. D., Roujol, S., Hey, S., Moonen, C., & Ries, M. (2013). Extended Kalman filtering for continuous volumetric MR-temperature imaging. *Medical Imaging. IEEE Transactions on*, *32*(4), 711–718.

de Souza, F. M. C. (1999). Modeling the dynamics of HIV-1 and CD4 and CD8 lymphocytes. *Engineering in Medicine and Biology Magazine, IEEE*, *18*(1), 21–24. doi:10.1109/51.740960 PMID:9934596

De Witt, J. K. (2010). Determination of toe-off event time during treadmill locomotion using kinematic data. *Journal of Biomechanics*, *43*(15), 3067–3069. doi:10.1016/j.jbiomech.2010.07.009 PMID:20801452

Deb, S., Nanda, C., Goswami, D., Mukhopadhyay, J., & Chakrabarti, S. (2007, November). Cuff-less estimation of blood pressure using pulse transit time and pre-ejection period. In *Convergence Information Technology, 2007. International Conference on* (pp. 941-944). IEEE. doi:10.1109/ICCIT.2007.206

Deepak, K. S., Gokul, K., Hinduja, R., & Rajkumar, S. (2013). An Efficient approach to predict tumour in 2D Brain image using classification techniques. *International Conference on Information Communication and Embedded Systems (ICICES)*. doi:10.1109/ICICES.2013.6508256

DeGiorgio, C. M., Miller, P., Meymandi, S., Chin, A., Epps, J., Gordon, S., & Harper, R. M. et al. (2010). RMSSD, a measure of vagus-mediated heart rate variability, is associated with risk factors for SUDEP: The SUDEP-7 Inventory. *Epilepsy & Behavior, 19*(1), 78–81. doi:10.1016/j.yebeh.2010.06.011 PMID:20667792

Dennis, A., Michaels, A. D., Arand, P., & Ventura, D. (2010). Noninvasive diagnosis of pulmonary hypertension using heart sound analysis. *Computers in Biology and Medicine, 40*(9), 758–764. PMID:20691967

Desolneux, A., Moisan, L., & Morel, J. M. (2001). Edge Detection by Helmholtz Principle. *Journal of Mathematical Imaging and Vision, 14*(3), 271–284. doi:10.1023/A:1011290230196

Dillingham, T. R., Pezzin, L. E., & MacKenzie, E. J. (2002). Limb amputation and limb deficiency: Epidemiology and recent trends in the United States. *Southern Medical Journal, 95*, 875–883. PMID:12190225

Dixit, N. M., & Perelson, A. S. (2004). Complex patterns of viral load decay under antiretroviral therapy: Influence of pharmacokinetics and intracellular delay. *Journal of Theoretical Biology, 226*(1), 95–109. doi:10.1016/j.jtbi.2003.09.002 PMID:14637059

Djohan, A., Nguyen, T. Q. W. J. T., Djohan, A., Nguyen, T. Q., & Tompkins, W. J. (1995). ECG compression using discrete symmetric wavelet transform. In IEEE -EMBC and CMBEC (pp. 167–168). Montreal, Canada: IEEE.

Djohan, A., Nguyen, T. Q., & Tompkins, W. J. (1995). ECG compression using discrete symmetric wavelet transform. In *IEEE International Conference on Engineering in Medicine and Biology Society* (pp. 167–168). Montreal, Canada: IEEE. doi:10.1109/IEMBS.1995.575053

Dorigo, D. (1992). *Optimization, Learning and Natural Algorithms*. (Ph.D. Thesis). Politecnico di Milano, Italy.

Doukas, C., & Maglogiannis, I. (2008). *Advanced patient or elder fall detection based on movement and sound data*. Tampere, Finland: IEEE Pervasive Health Conference and Workshops. doi:10.1109/PCTHEALTH.2008.4571042

DRIVE. (2013). *Digital Retinal Images for Vessel Extraction*. Retrieved from http://www.isi.uu.nl/Research/Databases/DRIVE/

Drost, G., Stegeman, D. F., van Engelen, B. G. M., & Zwarts, M. J. (2006). Clinical applications of high-density surface EMG: A systematic review. *Journal of Electromyography and Kinesiology, 16*(6), 586–602. doi:10.1016/j.jelekin.2006.09.005 PMID:17085302

Drummond, K. E., & Murphy, E. (2011). *Minimally invasive cardiac output monitors*. Continuing Education in Anaesthesia, Critical Care &Pain.

Duarte, R. C. M., Matos, F. M., & Batista, L. V. (2007). Near-lossless compression of ECG signals using perceptual masks in the DCT domain. In *IV Latin American Congress on Biomedical Engineering IFMBE Proceedings 18* (pp. 229–231). IFMBE. doi:10.1007/978-3-540-74471-9_53

Dunn, J. C. (1973). A Fuzzy Relative of the ISODATA Process and its use in detecting compact well-separated clusters. *J. Cybernetics, 3*(3), 32–57. doi:10.1080/01969727308546046

Einbeck, J., Evers, L., & Bailer-Jones, C. (2008). Representing Complex Data Using Localized Principal Components with Application to Astronomical Data. In A. Gorban, B. Kégl, D. Wunsch, & A. Zinovyev (Eds.), *Principal Manifolds for Data Visualization and Dimension Reduction* (Vol. 58, pp. 178–201). Springer Berlin Heidelberg. doi:10.1007/978-3-540-73750-6_7

Elder, J. (1991). Are edges incomplete. *International Journal of Computer Vision, 34*(2/3), 97–122. doi:10.1023/A:1008183703117

Eltoukhy, M. M., Faye, I., & Samir, B. B. (2010). Breast cancer diagnosis in digital mammogram using multiscalecurvelet transforms. *Computerized Medical Imaging and Graphics, 34*(4), 269–276. doi:10.1016/j.compmedimag.2009.11.002 PMID:20004076

Engelbrecht, A. P. (2005). *Fundamentals of Computational Swarm Intelligence*. Chichester, UK: Wiley.

Engelhart, K., Hudgins, B., Parker, P. A., & Stevenson, M. (1999). Classification of the myoelectric signal using time-frequency based representations. *Medical Engineering & Physics, 21*(6-7), 431–438. doi:10.1016/S1350-4533(99)00066-1 PMID:10624739

Erdogmus, H. (2009). Cloud computing: Does nirvana hide behind the nebula? *IEEE Software, 26*(2), 4–6. doi:10.1109/MS.2009.31

Er, M. J., Wu, S., Lu, J., & Toh, H. L. (2002). Face recognition with radial basis function (RBF) neural networks. *Neural Networks. IEEE Transactions on, 13*(3), 697–710. PMID:18244466

Ermes, M., Parkka, J., Mantyjarvi, J., & Korhonen, I. (2008). Detection of daily activities and sports with wearable sensors in controlled and uncontrolled conditions. *IEEE Transactions on Information Technology in Biomedicine, 12*(1), 20–26. doi:10.1109/TITB.2007.899496 PMID:18270033

Ester, M., Kriegel, H.P., Sander, J., & Xu, X. (1996). A Density-based algorithm for discovering clusters in large spatial databases with noise. *Proc. 2nd Int. Conf. on Knowledge Discovery and Data Mining.*

Ethem, . (2004). *Introduction to Machine Learning*. The MIT Press.

Fan, C.-Y., Fan, P.-S., Chan, T.-Y., & Chang, S.-H. (2012). Using hybrid data mining and machine learning clustering analysis to predict the turnover rate for technology professionals. *Expert Systems with Applications, 39*(10), 8844–8851. doi:10.1016/j.eswa.2012.02.005

Farmer, J. D. N., Packard, N. H., & Perelson, A. S. (1986). Packard., & A. Perelson.(1986) The Immune system, adaptation and machine learning. *Physica D. Nonlinear Phenomena, 2*(1-3), 187–204. doi:10.1016/0167-2789(86)90240-X

Feng, D., Wenkang, S., Liangzhou, C., Yong, D., & Zhenfu, Z. (2005). Infrared image segmentation with 2-D maximum entropy method based on particle swarm optimization (PSO). *Pattern Recognition Letters, 26*(5), 597–603. doi:10.1016/j.patrec.2004.11.002

Fernandes, F. C. A., Spaendonck, R. L. V., & Burrus, C. S. (2001). A directional, shift-insensitive, low-redundancy, wavelet transform. In *IEEE Proceedings international conference on image processing*. doi:10.1109/ICIP.2001.959121

Fernandez-Aleman, J. L., & Lozoya, P. A. A. (2013). To evaluate, Security and privacy in electronic health records: A systematic literature review. *Journal of Biomedical Informatics, 46*(3), 541–562. doi:10.1016/j.jbi.2012.12.003 PMID:23305810

Fiala, J., Bingger, P., Foerster, K., Heilmann, C., Beyersdorf, F., Zappe, H., & Seifert, A. (2010, November). Implantable sensor for blood pressure determination via pulse transit time. In Sensors, 2010 IEEE (pp. 1226-1229). IEEE. doi:10.1109/ICSENS.2010.5690619

Filho, E. B. L., Rodrigues, N. M. M., & da Silva, E. A. B. (1923–1926). da, Faria, S´. M. M. de, & Carvalho, M. B. de. (2008). ECG signal compression based on Dc equalization and complexity sorting. *IEEE Transactions on Bio-Medical Engineering, 55*(7).

Filter, R. A., & Xia, X. (2003). Computer based HIV/AIDS parameter estimation for practitioners and patients. In *Proceedings of the First African Control Conference*.

Filter, R. A., Xia, X., & Gray, C. M. (2005). Dynamic HIV/AIDS parameter estimation with application to a vaccine readiness study in Southern Africa. *Biomedical Engineering. IEEE Transactions on*, *52*(5), 784–791.

Finkelstein, J. (2014). *Classification of cycling exercise status using short-term heart rate variability.* Paper presented at the Engineering in Medicine and Biology Society (EMBC), 2014 36th Annual International Conference of the IEEE.

Fira, C. M., & Goras, L. (2008). An ECG signals compression method and its validation using NNs. *IEEE Transactions on Bio-Medical Engineering*, *55*(4), 1319–1326. doi:10.1109/TBME.2008.918465 PMID:18390322

Foo, J. Y. A. (2007). Pulse transit time in paediatric respiratory sleep studies. *Medical Engineering & Physics*, *29*(1), 17–25. PMID:16495120

Foo, J. Y. A., Lim, C. S., & Wang, P. (2006). Evaluation of blood pressure changes using vascular transit time. *Physiological Measurement*, *27*(8), 685. PMID:16772667

Foo, J. Y. A., Lim, C. S., Wilson, S. J., Williams, G. R., Harris, M.-A., & Cooper, D. M. (2007). Pulse transit time ratio as a potential marker for paediatriccrural and brachial blood pressure index. *Physiological Measurement*, *21*, 415–417. PMID:17287846

Foo, J. Y. A., Wilson, S. J., Williams, G. R., Coates, A., Harris, M.-A., & Cooper, D. M. (2005a). Predictive regression equations and clinical uses of peripheral pulse timing characteristics in children. *Physiological Measurement*, *26*(3), 317. PMID:15798305

Foo, J. Y. A., Wilson, S. J., Williams, G. R., Harris, M.-A., & Cooper, D. M. (2005b). Pulse transit time as a derived noninvasive mean to monitor arterial distensibility changes in children. *Journal of Human Hypertension*, *19*, 723–729. PMID:15920454

Foo, J. Y. A., Wilson, S. J., Williams, G. R., Harris, M.-A., & Cooper, D. M. (2005c). Pulse transit time changes observed with different limb positions. *Physiological Measurement*, *26*(6), 1093. PMID:16311456

Foracchia, M., Grisan, E., & Ruggeri, A. (2004). Detection of optic disc in retinal images by means of a geometrical model of vessel structure. *IEEE Transactions on Medical Imaging*, *23*(10), 1189–1195. doi:10.1109/TMI.2004.829331 PMID:15493687

Foracchia, M., Grisan, E., & Ruggeri, A. (2005). Luminosity and contrast normalization in retinal images. *Medical Image Analysis*, *3*(3), 179–190. doi:10.1016/j.media.2004.07.001 PMID:15854840

Forouzanfar, M., Ahmad, S., Batkin, I., Dajani, H., Groza, V., & Bolic, M. (2013). Coefficient-free blood pressure estimation based on pulse transit time; cuff pressure dependence. Biomedical Engineering. *IEEE Transactions on*, *60*(7), 1814–1824.

Fu, C., Yang, C., Lin, C., & Kuo, T. (2008). Alteration of cardiovascular autonomic functions by vegetarian diets in postmenopausal women is related to LDL cholesterol levels. *The Chinese Journal of Physiology*, *51*, 100–105. PMID:18666713

Fukushima, H., Kawanaka, H., Bhuiyan, M., & Oguri, K. (2013). Cuffless blood pressure estimation using only photoplethysmography based on cardiovascular parameters. In *Engineering in Medicine and Biology Society (EMBC), 2013 35th Annual International Conference of the IEEE.*

Fung, P., Dumont, G., Ries, C., Mott, C., & Ansermino, M. (2004). Continuous noninvasive blood pressure measurement by pulse transit time. In *Engineering in Medicine and Biology Society, 2004. IEMBS '04. 26th Annual International Conference of the IEEE.*

Furedy, J. J., Szabo, A., & Pronnet, F. (1996). Effects of psychological and physiological challenges on heart rate, t-wave amplitude, and pulse-transit time. *International Journal of Psychophysiology*, *22*(3), 173–183. PMID:8835625

Garg, S. Gupta, & Mittal. (2010). Optimal Algorithm for ECG Denoising using Discrete Wavelet Transforms. IEEE.

Gartner, W.W. (1959, December). Integrated Circuitry, Micro-miniaturization and Molecular Electronics. *Semiconductor Products*, 41–46.

Gavrovska, A. M., Jevtic, D. R., & Reljin, B. D. (2009). *Selection of wavelet decomposition levels in ECG filtering*. Academic Press.

George, E., & Tsekouras, J. (2013). On Training RBF neural networks using input–output fuzzy clustering and particle swarm optimization. *Fuzzy Sets and Systems*, *221*, 65–89. doi:10.1016/j.fss.2012.10.004

Ge, S. S., Tian, Z., & Lee, T. H. (2005). Nonlinear control of a dynamic model of HIV-1. *Biomedical Engineering. IEEE Transactions on*, *52*(3), 353–361.

Gesche, H., Grosskurth, D., Kchler, G., & Patzak, A. (2012). Continuous blood pressure measurement by using the pulse transit time: Comparison to a cuff-based method. *European Journal of Applied Physiology*, *112*(1), 309–315. PMID:21556814

Ghaffari, A., Homaeinezhad, M., Khazraee, M., & Daevaeiha, M. (2010). Segmentation of Holter ECG Waves Via Analysis of a Discrete Wavelet-Derived Multiple Skewness–Kurtosis Based Metric. *Annals of Biomedical Engineering*, *38*(4), 1497–1510. doi:10.1007/s10439-010-9919-3 PMID:20087769

Ghazanfari, M., Alizadeh, S., Fathian, M., & Koulouriotis, D. E. (2007). Comparing simulated annealing and genetic algorithm in learning FCM. *Journal of Applied Mathematics and Computation*, *192*(1), 56–68. doi:10.1016/j.amc.2007.02.144

Ghildiyal, A., Iqbal, B., Singh, S., Verma, D., & Singh, S. (2011). Changes in sympathovagal balance during menstural cycle. *Current Neurobiology*, *2*(1), 49–52.

Ghorbanian, P., Jalali, A., Ghaffari, A., & Nataraj, C. (2012). An improved procedure for detection of heart arrhythmias with novel pre-processing techniques. *Expert Systems: International Journal of Knowledge Engineering and Neural Networks*, *29*(5), 478–491. doi:10.1111/j.1468-0394.2011.00606.x

Ghosh, D., Midya, B. L., Koley, C., & Purkait, P. (2005). *Wavelet aided SVM analysis of ECG signals for cardiac abnormality detection*. Academic Press.

Ghosh, A., Halder, A., Kothari, M., & Ghosh, S. (2008). Aggregation pheromone density based data clustering. *Journal Information Sciences: an International Journal*, *178*(13), 2816–2831. doi:10.1016/j.ins.2008.02.015

Gilchrist, M. A., Coombs, D., & Perelson, A. S. (2004). Optimizing within-host viral fitness: Infected cell lifespan and virion production rate. *Journal of Theoretical Biology*, *229*(2), 281–288. doi:10.1016/j.jtbi.2004.04.015 PMID:15207481

Giri, D., Acharya, U. R., Martis, R. J., Sree, S. V., Lim, T. C., Ahamed, T., & Suri, J. S. (2013). Automated diagnosis of Coronary Artery Disease affected patients using LDA, PCA, ICA and Discrete Wavelet Transform. *Knowledge-Based Systems*, *37*, 274–282. doi:10.1016/j.knosys.2012.08.011

Glen, L. (2014). A Taxonomy to guide research on the application of data mining to fraud detection in financial statement audits. *International Journal of Accounting Information Systems*, *15*(4), 357–380. doi:10.1016/j.accinf.2014.05.006

Goen & Tiwari, D. C. (2013). Review of Surface Electromyogram Signals: Its Analysis and Applications. *International Journal of Electrical, Computer, Energetic. Electronic and Communication Engineering.*, *7*(11), 11–19.

Goldberger, A. L., Amaral, L. A., Glass, L., Hausdorff, J. M., Ivanov, P. C., Mark, R. G., & Stanley, H. E. et al. (2000). PhysioBank, PhysioToolkit, and PhysioNet: Components of a new research resource for complex physiologic signals. *Circulation, 101*(23), e215–e220. doi:10.1161/01.CIR.101.23.e215 PMID:10851218

Goldstein, P. (2009). *Alternative IT sourcing strategies: from the campus to the cloud.* EDUCAUSE Center for Applied Research. Available at: https://net.educause.edu/ir/library/pdf/EKF/EKF0905.pdf

Goli, S., & Jayanthi, T. (2014, January). Cuff less Non-Invasive Blood Pressure Measurement Using Pulse Transit Time measurement. *International Journal of Recent Development in Engineering and Technology*, 2(1), 2347–6435.

Gonzales, R. C., Woods, R. E., & Eddins, S. L. (2004). *Digital image processing using MATLAB*. Pearson Prentice Hall.

Gonzalez, & Woods. (2009). *Digital Image Processing*. Prentice Hall.

Gopal, N. N., & Karnan, M. (2010). Diagnose brain tumor through MRI using image processing clustering algorithms such as Fuzzy C Means along with intelligent optimization techniques.*IEEE International Conference on Computational Intelligence and Computing Research (ICCIC)*. doi:10.1109/ICCIC.2010.5705890

Graupe, D., Salahi, J., & Kohn, K. H. (1982). Multifunctional prosthesis andorthosis control via microcomputer identification of temporal pattern differences in single-site myo-electric signals. *Journal of Biomedical Engineering, 4*(1), 17–22. doi:10.1016/0141-5425(82)90021-8 PMID:7078136

Graupe, D., Salahi, J., & Zhang, D. S. (1985). Stochastic analysis of myoelectric temporal signatures for multifunctional single-site activation of prostheses and orthoses. *Journal of Biomedical Engineering, 7*(1), 18–29. doi:10.1016/0141-5425(85)90004-4 PMID:3982004

Grisan, E., Giani, A., Ceseracciu, E., & Ruggeri, A. (2006). Model based illumination correction in retinal images.*IEEE Int. Symposium Biomedical Imaging, Nano to Macro*. doi:10.1109/ISBI.2006.1625085

Gu, W., Poon, C., & Zhang, Y. (2008). A novel parameter from ppgdicrotic notch for estimation of systolic blood pressure using pulse transit time. In *Medical Devices and Biosensors, 2008. ISSS-MDBS 2008. 5th International Summer School and Symposium on.*

Guasti, L., Grimoldi, P., Mainardi, L., Petrozzino, M., Piantanida, E., Garganico, D., & Venco, A. et al. (1999). Autonomic function and baroreflex sensitivity during a normal ovulatory cycle in humans. *Acta Cardiologica, 54*(4), 209–213. PMID:10511897

Güler, N. F., & Koçer, S. (2005). Use of support vector machines and neural network in diagnosis of neuromuscular disorders. *Journal of Medical Systems, 29*(3), 271–284. doi:10.1007/s10916-005-5187-4 PMID:16050082

Guo, L., Chen, F., Chen, L., & Tang, X. (2010). The building of cloud computing environment for e-health. In *Proceedings of the International Conference on e-Health Networking, Digital Ecosystems and Technologies* (EDT' 10). Shenzhen, China: IEEE Computer Society. doi:10.1109/EDT.2010.5496512

Gupta, R., & Mitra, M. (2012, December). An ECG compression technique for telecardiology application. In *India Conference* (p. 4). IEEE.

Gupta, R., & Mitra, M. (2014). Wireless electrocardiogram transmission in ISM Band: An approach towards telecardiology. *Journal of Medical Systems, 38*(10), 90. doi:10.1007/s10916-014-0090-5 PMID:25085695

Gupta, S., Gudapati, R., Gaurav, K., & Bhise, M. (2013). Emerging risk factors for cardiovascular diseases: Indian context. *Indian Journal of Endocrinology and Metabolism, 17*(5), 806–814. doi:10.4103/2230-8210.117212 PMID:24083161

Gupta, S., Kaur, L., Chauhan, R. C., & Saxena, S. C. (2007). A versatile technique for visual enhancement of medical ultrasound images. *Digital Signal Processing*, *17*(3), 542–560. doi:10.1016/j.dsp.2006.12.001

Guyton, A., & Hall, J. E. (Eds.). (2006). *Textbook of Medical Physiology* (11th ed.). Elsevier Saunders.

Guzik, P., Piskorski, J., Krauze, T., Girguś, P., Wykrętowicz, A., & Wysocki, H. (2005). Numerical descriptors of Poincaré plots analysis of RR intervals are related to baroreflex sensitivity and hemodynamic parameters in healthy people. *Analysis, 1*(4), 8-9.

Haar, A. (1910). On the theory of orthogonal function systems. *Math. Ann*, *69*(3), 331–371. doi:10.1007/BF01456326

Han, M., Liu, Y. H., Xi, J. H., & Guo, W. (2007). Noise smoothing for nonlinear time series using wavelet soft threshold. *IEEE Signal Processing Letters*, *14*(1), 62–65. doi:10.1109/LSP.2006.881518

Hannaford, B., & Lehman, S. (1986). Short time Fourier analysis of the electromyogram: Fast movements and constant contraction. *IEEE Transactions on Bio-Medical Engineering*, *33*(12), 1173–1181. doi:10.1109/TBME.1986.325697 PMID:3817851

Hanson, G. W. (2008). *Fundamentals of Nanoelectronics*. Pearson Education.

Haralick, R. M., Shanmugam, K., & Dinstein, I. H. (1973). Textural features for image classification. *Systems, Man and Cybernetics, IEEE Transactions on,* (6), 610-621.

Haralick, R. M. (1979). Statistical and structural approaches to texture. *Proceedings of the IEEE*, *67*(5), 786–804. doi:10.1109/PROC.1979.11328

Haraty, R. A., Dimishkieh, M., & Masud, M. (2015). An Enhanced k-Means Clustering Algorithm for Pattern Discovery in Healthcare Data. *International Journal of Distributed Sensor Networks*, *2015*, 1–11. doi:10.1155/2015/615740

Harrington, D., Presuhn, R., & Wijnen, B. (2002). *An Architecture for Describing Simple Network Management Protocol (SNMP) Management Frameworks*. Standard(STD) 62, RFC 3411.

Hartigan, E., Axe, M. J., & Snyder-Mackler, L. (2009). Perturbation training prior to ACL reconstruction improves gait asymmetries in non-copers. *Journal of Orthopaedic Research*, *27*(6), 724–729. doi:10.1002/jor.20754 PMID:19023893

Ha, S., Kim, C., Chi, Y., Akinin, A., Maier, C., Ueno, A., & Cauwenberghs, G. (2014). Integrated circuits and electrode interfaces for noninvasive physiological monitoring. Biomedical Engineering. *IEEE Transactions on*, *61*(5), 1522–1537.

Hassanien, A. E., Schaefer, G., & AlQaheri, H. (2010). Prostate boundary detection in ultrasound images based on Type-II fuzzy sets and modified fuzzy C-Means. Soft Computing in Industrial Applications. *Advances in Intelligent and Soft Computing.*, *75*, 187–195. doi:10.1007/978-3-642-11282-9_20

Hautamaki, H., Haapalahti, P., Piirila, P., Tuomikoski, P., Sovijarvi, A., Ylikorkalaa, O., & Mikkolaa, T. S. (2012). Effect of hot flushes on cardiovascular autonomic responsiveness: A randomized controlled trial on hormone therapy. *Maturitas*, *72*(3), 243–248. doi:10.1016/j.maturitas.2012.04.001 PMID:22537767

He, X., Goubran, R. A., & Liu, X. P. (2013, May). Evaluation of the correlation between blood pressure and pulse transit time. In *Medical Measurements and Applications Proceedings (MeMeA), 2013 IEEE International Symposium on* (pp. 17-20). IEEE. doi:10.1109/MeMeA.2013.6549697

Hebert, M., Korabek, B., & Scott, R. E. (2006). Moving research into practice: A decision framework for integrating home telehealth into chronic illness care. *International Journal of Medical Informatics*, *75*(12), 786–794. doi:10.1016/j.ijmedinf.2006.05.041 PMID:16872892

Hennig, A., & Patzak, A. (2013). Continuous blood pressure measurement using pulse transit time. *Somnologie-Schlafforschung und Schlafmedizin*, *17*(2), 104–110. doi:10.1007/s11818-013-0617-x

Heo, G., Gader, P., & Frigui, H. (2009). RKF-PCA: Robust kernel fuzzy PCA. *Neural Networks*, *22*(5-6), 642–650. doi:10.1016/j.neunet.2009.06.013 PMID:19592217

He, P., Shan, L., Lin, N. C., Martin, G. B., Kemmerling, B., Nürnberger, T., & Sheen, J. (2006). Specific bacterial suppressors of MAMP signaling upstream of MAPKKK in Arabidopsis innate immunity. *Cell*, *125*(3), 563–575. doi:10.1016/j.cell.2006.02.047 PMID:16678099

Hey, S., Gharbi, A., von Haaren, B., Walter, K., Konig, N., & Loffler, S. (2009, February). Continuous noninvasive pulse transit time measurement for psycho-physiological stress monitoring. In *eHealth, Telemedicine, and Social Medicine, 2009. eTELEMED'09. International Conference on* (pp. 113-116). IEEE.

Hilton, M. L. (1997). Wavelet and wavelet packet compression of electrocardiograms. *IEEE Transactions on Bio-Medical Engineering*, *44*(5), 394–402. doi:10.1109/10.568915 PMID:9125824

Hippel, V., & Arthur, R. (1956). Molecular Engineering. *Science*, *123*(3191), 315–317. doi:10.1126/science.123.3191.315 PMID:17774519

Ho, C. H., Brotherton, B. J., Lewis, K. E., & Uzunyan, M. Y. (2014). A High School Wrestler with Severe Bradycardia. *The Journal of Pediatrics*, *165*(1), 202-202. e201.

Ho, C. Y. F., & Ling, B. W. K. (2010). Initiation of HIV therapy. *International Journal of Bifurcation and Chaos in Applied Sciences and Engineering*, *20*(04), 1279–1292. doi:10.1142/S0218127410026484 PMID:20543654

Holland, J. H. (1975). *Adaptation in Natural and Artificial Systems*. University of Michigan Press.

Holtshousen WS, & Smit A. (2007). A cost-efficiency analysis of a mobile dental clinic in the public *services. South African Dental Association*, *62*(8), 336-338.

Hoover, A., & Goldbaum, M. (2003). Locating the optic nerve in a retinal image using the fuzzy convergence of the blood vessels. *Medical Imaging. IEEE Transactions on*, *22*(8), 951–958.

Horspool, R. N., & Windels, W. J. (1994). An LZ approach to ECG compression. In *Computer-Based Medical Systems, 1994.,Proceedings 1994 IEEE Seventh Symposium on* (pp. 71–76). http://doi.org/ doi:<ALIGNMENT.qj></ALIGNMENT>10.1109/CBMS.1994.315990

Hossain, Afran, & Sayed. (2010, December). Compression of ECG signals exploiting correlation between ECG cycles. In *6th International Conference on Electrical and Computer Engineering ICECE 2010, Dhaka, Bangladesh* (pp. 622-625).

Ho, W. H., & Chan, A. L. F. (2010). Hybrid Taguchi-differential evolution algorithm for parameter estimation of differential equation models with application to HIV dynamics. *Mathematical Problems in Engineering*.

Hreljac, A., & Marshall, R. N. (2000). Algorithms to determine event timing during normal walking using kinematic data. *Journal of Biomechanics*, *33*(6), 783–786. doi:10.1016/S0021-9290(00)00014-2 PMID:10808002

Huang, B., Wang, Y., & Chen, J. (2009). 2-D compression of ECG signals using ROI mask and conditional entropy coding. *IEEE Transactions on Bio-Medical Engineering*, *56*(4), 1261–1263. doi:10.1109/TBME.2008.2009643 PMID:19272868

Huang, B., Wang, Y., & Chen, J. (2013). ECG compression using the context modeling arithmetic coding with dynamic learning vector–scalar quantization. *Biomedical Signal Processing and Control*, *8*(1), 59–65. doi:10.1016/j.bspc.2012.04.003

Huang, G. B., Zhou, H. M., Ding, X. J., & Zhang, R. (2012). Extreme Learning Machine for Regression and Multiclass Classification. *IEEE Transactions on Systems, Man, and Cybernetics. Part B, Cybernetics*, *42*(2), 513–529. doi:10.1109/TSMCB.2011.2168604 PMID:21984515

Huang, H., Kuiken, T. A., & Lipschutz, R. D. (2009). A strategy for identifying locomotion mode using surface electromyography. *IEEE Transactions on Bio-Medical Engineering*, *56*(1), 65–73. doi:10.1109/TBME.2008.2003293 PMID:19224720

Huang, H., Zhang, F., Hargrove, L. J., Dou, Z., Rogers, D. R., & Englehart, K. B. (2011). Continuous locomotion-mode identification for prosthetic legs based on neuromuscular-mechanical fusion. *IEEE Transactions on Bio-Medical Engineering*, *58*(10), 2867–2875. doi:10.1109/TBME.2011.2161671 PMID:21768042

Huang, Y., Cai, D., & Chen, P. (2011). Micro and Nanotechnologies for Study of Cell Secretion. *Analytical Chemistry*, *83*(12), 4393–4406. doi:10.1021/ac200358b PMID:21417447

Huang, Y., Englehart, K. B., Hudgins, B., & Chan, A. D. (2005). A Gaussian mixture model based classification scheme for myoelectric control of powered upper limb prostheses. *IEEE Transactions on Bio-Medical Engineering*, *52*(11), 1801–1811. doi:10.1109/TBME.2005.856295 PMID:16285383

Huang, Y., Liu, D., & Wu, H. (2006). Hierarchical Bayesian methods for estimation of parameters in a longitudinal HIV dynamic system. *Biometrics*, *62*(2), 413–423. doi:10.1111/j.1541-0420.2005.00447.x PMID:16918905

Hughes, D., Babbs, C., & Geddes, L., & Bo. (n.d.). Measurements of young's modulus of elasticity of the canine aorta with ultrasound. *Ultrasonic Imaging*, *1*(4):356 – 367. PMID:575833

Hulzink, Konijnenburg, Ashouei, Breeschoten, Berset, Huisken, … Van Ginderdeuren. (2011, December). An Ultra Low Energy Biomedical Signal Processing System Operatng at Near Threshold. *IEEE Transactions on Biomedical Circuits and Systems, 5*(6), 546-554.

Hwang, K. H., Lee, H., & Choi, D. (2012). Medical image retrieval: Past and present. *Journal of Healthcare Informatics Research*, *18*(1), 3–9. doi:10.4258/hir.2012.18.1.3 PMID:22509468

IEEE-SA. (2014). *IEEE standard for wearable cuffless blood pressure measuring devices*. IEEE P1708/D04.

Ilayaraja, M., & Meyyappan, T. (2013). Mining Medical Data to Identify Frequent Diseases using Apriori Algorithm. In *Proceedings of the 2013 International Conference on Pattern Recognition, Informatics and Mobile Engineering* (PRIME'13). doi:10.1109/ICPRIME.2013.6496471

Illingworth, J., & Kittler, J. (1988). A survey of the Hough transform. *Computer Vision Graphics and Image Processing*, *44*(1), 87–116. doi:10.1016/S0734-189X(88)80033-1

Ingold, G. L., & Nazarov, Yu. V. (1992). Charge tunneling rates in ultrasmall junctions. In H. Grabert & M. H. Devoret (Eds.), *Single Charge Tunneling* (pp. 21–107). New York: Plenum. doi:10.1007/978-1-4757-2166-9_2

International Federation Diabetes. (2014). Retrieved from http://www.idf.org/complications-diabetes

Ioannis, A. (2012). A Semi-supervised fuzzy clustering algorithm applied to gene expression data. *Pattern Recognition*, *45*(1), 637–648. doi:10.1016/j.patcog.2011.05.007

Isa, Noviyanto, & Arymurthy. (2011). Optimal Selection of Wavelet Thresholding Algorithm for ECG signal denoinsing. In ICACSIS (pp. 365-370).

Isa, S. M., Noviyanto, A., Jatmiko, W., & Arymurthy, A. M. (2012). The Effect of Electrocardiogram Signal Compression Using Beat Reordering and SPIHT on Automatic Sleep Stage Classification. *Procedia Engineering, 41*, 888–896. http://doi.org/<ALIGNMENT.qj></ALIGNMENT>10.1016/j.proeng.2012.07.259

Iwasa, Y., Michor, F., & Nowak, M. A. (2005). Virus evolution within patients increases pathogenicity. *Journal of Theoretical Biology, 232*(1), 17–26. doi:10.1016/j.jtbi.2004.07.016 PMID:15498589

Izakian, H., & Abraham, A. (2011). Fuzzy C-means and fuzzy swarm for fuzzy clustering problem. *Expert Systems with Applications, 38*(3), 1835–1838. doi:10.1016/j.eswa.2010.07.112

Jain, H.K., Thao, C., & Zhao, H. (2012). Enhancing electronic medical record retrieval through semantic query expansion. *Journal of Information Systems and e-Business Management, 10*(2), 165–181. doi:10.1007/s10257-010-0133-5

Jalaleddine, Hutchens, Strattan, & Coberly. (1990, April). ECG Data Compression Techniques. A Unified Approach. *IEEE Transactions on Bio-Medical Engineering, 37*(4), 329–343.

Jalaleddine, S. M., Hutchens, C. G., Strattan, R. D., & Coberly, W. A. (1990). ECG data compression techniques-a unified approach. *IEEE Transactions on Bio-Medical Engineering, 37*(4), 329–343. doi:10.1109/10.52340 PMID:2186997

Jara. (2012, July). Evaluation of Bluetooth Low Energy capabilities for continuous data transmission from a wearable electrocardiogram. In Innovative Mobile and Internet Services in Ubiquitous Computing (IMIS) (pp. 912-917).

Jasiewicz, J. M., Allum, J. H., Middleton, J. W., Barriskill, A., Condie, P., Purcell, B., & Li, R. C. T. (2006). Gait event detection using linear accelerometers or angular velocity transducers in able-bodied and spinal-cord injured individuals. *Gait & Posture, 24*(4), 502–509. doi:10.1016/j.gaitpost.2005.12.017 PMID:16500102

Jazwinski, A. H. (1970). *Stochastic Processes and Filtering Theory*. Academic Press.

Jian, C., Jie, T. B., Zichun, T., Jian, X., Yakang, D., & Jian, Z. (2008). Retinal vessel enhancement and extraction based on directional field. *Journal of X-Ray Science and Technology, 16*, 189–201.

Jiang, H., Shen, F., Chen, S., Li, K. C., & Jeong, Y. S. (2015). A secure and scalable storage system for aggregate data in IoT. *Journal of Future Generation Computer Systems., 49*, 133–141. doi:10.1016/j.future.2014.11.009

Johnston, P., Imam, Z., Dempsey, G., Anderson, J., & Adgey, A. (1998). The transthoracic impedance cardiogram is a potential haemodynamic sensor for an automated external defibrillator. *European Heart Journal, 19*(12), 1879–1888. PMID:9886732

Joshi & Hahn. (2015). Terrain and Direction Classification of Locomotion Transitions Using Neuromuscular and Mechanical Input. *Annals of Biomedical Engineering*. doi:10.1007/s10439-015-1407-3

Joshi, G. D., & Sivaswamy, J. (2008). Colour Retinal Image Enhancement based on Domain Knowledge. *Sixth Indian Conference on Computer Vision, Graphics and Image Processing*. doi:10.1109/ICVGIP.2008.70

Joshi, Nakamura, & Hahn. (2014). A novel approach for toe off estimation during locomotion and transitions on ramps and level ground. *IEEE Journal of Biomedical and health informatics*. DOI: 10.1109/JBHI.2014.2377749

Joshi, Nakamura, & Hahn. (2015). High energy spectrogram with integrated prior knowledge for EMG-based locomotion classification. *Journal of Medical Engineering and Physics*. DOI: 10.1016/j.medengphy.2015.03.001

ska, J. A., Gouse, H., Paul, R. H., Stein, D. J., & Flisher, A. J. (2010). Does highly active antiretroviral therapy improve ognitive function? A systematic review. *Journal of Neurovirology, 16*(2), 101–114. doi:10.3109/13550281003682513 345318

Juang, L.-H., & Wu, M.-N. (2010). MRI brain lesion image detection based on color-converted K-means clustering segmentation. *Measurement, 43*(7), 941–949. doi:10.1016/j.measurement.2010.03.013

Jun, S., Wei, C., Wei, F., Xiaojun, W., & Wenbo, X. (2012). Gene expression data analysis with the clustering method based on an improved quantum-behaved particle swarm optimization. *Engineering Applications of Artificial Intelligence, 25*(2), 376–391. doi:10.1016/j.engappai.2011.09.017

Jurvetson, S. T. (2004). Transcending Moore's Law with Molecular Electronics and Nanotechnology. *Nanotechnology Law and Business, 1*, 70–90.

Kahn, C. H. Jr, & Thao, C. (2007). GoldMiner: A radiology image search engine. *AJR. American Journal of Roentgenology, 188*(6), 1475–1478. doi:10.2214/AJR.06.1740 PMID:17515364

Kai, E., Rebeiro-Hargrave, A., Inoue, S., Nohara, Y., Maruf, R. I., Nakashima, N., & Ahmed, A. (2014). Empowering the healthcare worker using the Portable Health Clinic. In *28th International Conference on Advanced Information Networking and Applications (AINA'14)*. doi:10.1109/AINA.2014.108

Kamalanand, K., & Jawahar, P. M. (n.d.). Unscented Transformation for Estimating the Lyapunov Exponents of Chaotic Time Series Corrupted by Random Noise. International Journal of Mathematical Sciences, 7(4), 1–6.

Kamalanand, K., & Srinivasan, S. (2011). Modelling and analysis of normal and atherosclerotic blood vessel mechanics using 3D finite element models. *ICTACT Journal on Soft Computing, special issue on Fuzzy in Industrial and Process Automation, 2*(1), 261-264.

Kamalanand, K., & Jawahar, P. M. (2013). Reconstructed bifurcation diagrams of CD4 cells and HIV-1 viral load dynamics under the effect of antiretroviral drugs. *Network Modeling Analysis in Health Informatics and Bioinformatics, 2*(4), 303–305. doi:10.1007/s13721-013-0047-5

Kamalanand, K., & Jawahar, P. M. (2014). Hybrid BFPSO algorithm based estimation of optimal drug dosage for antiretroviral therapy in HIV-1 infected patients. *BMC Infectious Diseases, 14*(Suppl 3), E14. doi:10.1186/1471-2334-14-S3-E14

Kamalanand, K., & Jawahar, P. M. (2015). Prediction of Human Immunodeficiency Virus-1 Viral Load from CD4 Cell Count Using Artificial Neural Networks. *Journal of Medical Imaging and Health Informatics, 5*(3), 641–646. doi:10.1166/jmihi.2015.1430

Kamalanand, K., & Ramakrishnan, S. (2015). Effect of gadolinium concentration on segmentation of vasculature in cardiopulmonary magnetic resonance angiograms. *Journal of Medical Imaging and Health Informatics, 5*(1), 147–151. doi:10.1166/jmihi.2015.1370

Kanungo, & Singh. (2015). Mammogram Image Segmentation using Hybridization of fuzzy clustering and optimization algorithms. *Intelligent Computing. Communication and Devices, 309*, 403–413.

Karen, F. P., Yicong, Z., Agaian, S., & Hongwei, J. (2011). Nonlinear unsharp masking for mammogram enhancement. *IEEE Transactions on Information Technology in Biomedicine, 15*(6), 918–928. doi:10.1109/TITB.2011.2164259 PMID:21843996

Kargari, M., & Sepehri, M. M. (2012). Stores clustering using a data mining approach for distributing automotive spare-parts to reduce transportation costs. *Expert Systems with Applications, 39*(5), 4740–4748. doi:10.1016/j.eswa.2011.09.121

Karlsson, J. S., Roeleveld, K., Gronlund, C., Holtermann, A., & Ostlund, N. (2009). Signal processing of the surface electromyogram to gain insight into neuromuscular physiology. *Philosophical Transactions of the Royal Society a-Mathematical Physical and Engineering Sciences, 367*(1887), 337-356. doi: DOI 10.1098/rsta.2008.0214

Karpagachelvi, Arthanari, & Sivakumar. (2010, April). ECG Feature Extraction Techniques-A Survey Approach. *International Journal of Computer Science and Information Security*, *8*(1), 76–80.

Kastner, M. A. (1993). Artificial Atoms. *Physics Today*, *46*(1), 24–31. doi:10.1063/1.881393

Katona, P. G., McLean, M., Dighton, D. H., & Guz, A. (1982). Sympathetic and parasympathetic cardiac control in athletes and nonathletes at rest. *Journal of Applied Physiology*, *52*(6), 1652–1657. PMID:7107476

Kaufman, L. M. (2009). Data security in the world of cloud computing. *IEEE Security and Privacy*, *7*(4), 61–64. doi:10.1109/MSP.2009.87

Kaur, M., Singh, B., Ubhi, & Rani. (2011). Digital Filtration of ECG Signals for Removal of Baseline Drift. In *International Conference on Telecommunication Technology and Applications Proc. of CSIT.* IACSIT Press.

Kaur, P.D., & Chana, I. (2014). Cloud based intelligent system for delivering health care as a service. *Journal of Computer Methods and Programs in Biomedicine*, *113*(1), 346-359. doi:10.1016/j.cmpb.2013.09.013

Kavitha, C., Jamuna, B., & Vijayakumar, G. (2012). Cardiac chronotropism and sympathovagal balance in young women of reproductive age. *International Journal of Biological & Medical Research*, *3*(4), 2313–2318.

Kemmotsu, O., Ueda, M., Otsuka, H., Yamamura, T., Winter, D., & Eckerle, J. (1991). Arterial tonometry for noninvasive, continuous blood pressure monitoring during anesthesia. *Anesthesiology*, *75*(2), 333–340. PMID:1859020

Kennedy, J., & Eberhart, R. C. (1995). Particle Swarm Optimization. *Proceedings of IEEE International conference on Neural Networks.* doi:10.1109/ICNN.1995.488968

Keren, K. et al.. (2002). Sequence-Specific Molecular Lithography on Single DNA Molecules. *Science*, *297*(5578), 72–75. doi:10.1126/science.1071247 PMID:12098693

Keren, K. et al.. (2003). DNA-templated carbon nanotube field-effect transistor. *Science* 302: 1380-1382. Moore, G.E. (1965). Cramming more Components onto Integrated Circuits. *Electronics*, *38*, 114–117.

Khaddar. (2012, May). Emerging Wireless Technologies In E-Health. In Multimedia Computing and System (ICMCS), (pp. 440-445).

Khandait, Bawane, Limaye, & Khandait. (2012, April). Efficient ECG Abnormalities Recognition Using Neuro-Fuzzy Approach. International Journal of Advanced Research in Computer Science and Software Engineering, 2, 402-407.

Khare, Saxena, & Nerkar. (2011). ECG Data Compression Using DWT. *International Journal of Engineering and Advanced Technology*, *1*(1), 11–13. doi:10.1109/HealthCom.2012.6379443

Khezri, M., & Jahed, M. (2007). Real-time intelligent pattern recognition algorithm for surface EMG signals. *Biomedical Engineering Online*, *6*(1), 45. doi:10.1186/1475-925X-6-45 PMID:18053184

Kiatpanichagij, K., & Afzulpurkar, N. (2009). Use of supervised discretization with PCA in wavelet packet transformation-based surface electromyrogram classification. *Biomedical Signal Processing and Control*, *4*(2), 127–138. doi:10.1016/j.bspc.2009.02.004

Kim, H. C., Kim, K. Y., Park, J. W., & Lee, H. J. (2001). Electrical impedance tomography reconstruction algorithm using extended Kalman filter. In *Industrial Electronics, 2001. Proceedings. ISIE 2001. IEEE International Symposium on* (Vol. 3, pp. 1677-1681). IEEE. doi:10.1109/ISIE.2001.931960

Kim, J. S., Kim, K. K., Baek, H. J., & Park, K. S. (2008). *Comparable parameter related to arterial stiffness in blood pressure estimation method.* Academic Press.

Kim, J. Y., Cho, B. H., Im, S. M., Jeon, M. J., Kim, I. Y., & Kim, S. I. (2005). Comparative study on artificial neural network with multiple regressions for continuous estimation of blood pressure. In *Engineering in Medicine and Biology Society, 2005. IEEE-EMBS 2005. 27th Annual International Conference of the*.

Kim, Y., & Lee, J. (2010, August). Cuffless and non-invasive estimation of a continuous blood pressure based on ptt. In *Information Technology Convergence and Services (ITCS), 2010 2nd International Conference on* (pp. 1-4). IEEE. doi:10.1109/ITCS.2010.5581266

Kim, J. K., Park, J. M., Song, K. S., & Park, H. W. (1997). Adaptive mammographic image enhancement using first derivative and local statistics. *IEEE Transactions on Medical Imaging*, *16*(5), 495–502. doi:10.1109/42.640739 PMID:9368105

Kim, S. Y., Moon, S. K., Jung, D. C., Hwang, S. I., Sung, C. K., Cho, J. Y., & Lee, H. J. et al. (2011). Pre-Operative Prediction of Advanced Prostatic Cancer Using Clinical Decision Support Systems: Accuracy Comparison between Support Vector Machine and Artificial Neural Network. *Korean Journal of Radiology*, *12*(5), 588. doi:10.3348/kjr.2011.12.5.588 PMID:21927560

Kim, Y. H., & Cho, Y. J. (2008). Feature and noise adaptive unsharp masking based on statistical hypotheses test. *IEEE Transactions on Consumer Electronics*, *54*(2), 823–830. doi:10.1109/TCE.2008.4560166

Kirkpatrick, S. C. (2010). Optimization by Simulated Annealing. *Science*.

Kirschner, D. (1996). Using mathematics to understand HIV immune dynamics. *AMS Notices*, *43*(2).

Klas, G., Rodermund, V. F., Shelby, V. Z., Akhouri, S., & Holler, E. J. (2014). *"Lightweight M2M": Enabling Device Management and Applications for the Internet of Things*. Retrieved from http://archive.ericsson.net/service/internet/picov/get?DocNo=1/28701-FGB101973

Kleeman, L. (1996, January). Understanding and applying Kalman filtering. In *Proceedings of the Second Workshop on Perceptive Systems*. Curtin University of Technology.

Klein, R., Meuer, S. M., Moss, S. E., & Klein, B. E. (1995). Retinal microaneurysm counts and 10-year progression of diabetic retinopathy. *Archives of Ophthalmology*, *113*(11), 1386–1391. doi:10.1001/archopht.1995.01100110046024 PMID:7487599

Kobetic, R., To, C., Schnellenberger, J., Audu, M., Bules, T., & Gaudio, R. (2009). Development of hybrid orthosis for standing, walking, and stair climbing after spinal cord injury. *Journal of Rehabilitation Research and Development*, *46*(3), 447–462. doi:10.1682/JRRD.2008.07.0087 PMID:19675995

Kononenko, I. (2001). Machine learning for medical diagnosis: History, state of the art and perspective. *Artificial Intelligence in Medicine*, *23*(1), 89–109. doi:10.1016/S0933-3657(01)00077-X PMID:11470218

Kononenko, I., Bratko, I., & Kukar, M. (1997). Application of machine learning to medical diagnosis. *Machine Learning and Data Mining: Methods and Applications*, *389*, 408.

Konstantinos, K., Vasudev, B., & Giordano, B. (1999). Image sharpening in the JPEG domain. *IEEE Transactions on Image Processing*, *8*(6), 874–878. doi:10.1109/83.766864 PMID:18267500

Korurek, M., & Nizam, A. (2010). Clustering MIT-BIH arrhythmias with Ant Colony Optimization using time domain and PCA compressed wavelet coefficients. *Digital Signal Processing*, *20*(4), 1050–1060. doi:10.1016/j.dsp.2009.10.019

Koski, A. (1997). Lossless ECG encoding. *Computer Methods and Programs in Biomedicine*, *52*(1), 23–33. doi:10.1016/S0169-2607(96)01779-8 PMID:9034667

Koufi, V., Malamateniou, F., & Vassilacopoulos, G. (2010).Ubiquitous access to cloud emergency medical services.*IEEE International Conference on Information Technology and Applications in Biomedicine*. doi:10.1109/ITAB.2010.5687702

Kouwenhoven, L. P. (1997). Electron transport in quantum dots. In B. L. Sohn et al. (Eds.), *Mesoscopic Electron Transfer* (pp. 105–215). Dordrecht: Kluwer, Dordrecht. doi:10.1007/978-94-015-8839-3_4

Krishnamurthy, K. (2012). A Method for Estimating the Lyapunov Exponents of Chaotic Time Series Corrupted by Random Noise Using Extended Kalman Filter. In *Mathematical Modelling and Scientific Computation* (pp. 237–244). Springer Berlin Heidelberg.

Ku, C., Hung, K., Wu, T., & Wang, H. (2010). Wavelet-based ECG data compression system with linear quality control scheme. *IEEE Transactions on Bio-Medical Engineering*, *57*(6), 1399–1409. doi:10.1109/TBME.2009.2037605 PMID:20142155

Kulkarni, P. K., Kumar, V., & Verma, H. K. (1997). ECG data compression using fast Walsh transform and its clinical acceptability. *International Journal of Systems Science*, *28*(8), 831–836. doi:10.1080/00207729708929443

Kumar, K. S., Bhowmik, D., & Duraivel, S. (2014). Hypertension Epidemic in India-A Comprehensive Review of Clinical Features, Management and Remedies. Academic Press.

Kumar, R., Kumar, A., & Kumar, R. (2012). Electrocardiogram Signal Compression Using Beta Wavelets. *Journal of Mathematical Modelling and Algorithms*, *11*(3), 235–248. doi:10.1007/s10852-012-9181-9

Kumar, V., Saxena, S. C., & Giri, V. K. (2006). Direct data compression of ECG signal for telemedicine. *International Journal of Systems Science*, *37*(1), 45–63. doi:10.1080/00319100500412337

Kumar, V., Saxena, S. C., Giri, V. K., & Singh, D. (2005). Improved modified AZTEC technique for ECG data compression: Effect of length of parabolic filter on reconstructed signal. *Computers & Electrical Engineering*, *31*(4-5), 334–344. doi:10.1016/j.compeleceng.2005.02.002

Kumbhar, A. D., & Kulkarni, A. V. (2011). Magnetic Resonant image segmentation using trained K-means clustering. *World Congress on Information and Communication Technologies (WICT)*. doi:10.1109/WICT.2011.6141301

Kuo, R. J., Lin, S. Y., & Shih, C. W. (2007). Mining association rules through integration of clustering analysis and ant colony system for health insurance database in Taiwan. *Expert Systems with Applications*, *33*(3), 794–808. doi:10.1016/j.eswa.2006.08.035

Kurylyak, Y., Lamonaca, F., & Grimaldi, D. (2013). A neural network-based method for continuous blood pressure estimation from a ppg signal. In *Instrumentation and Measurement Technology Conference (I2MTC), 2013 IEEE International*.

La Rovere, M. T., Pinna, G. D., & Raczak, G. (2008). Baroreflex sensitivity: Measurement and clinical implications. *Annals of Noninvasive Electrocardiology*, *13*(2), 191–207. PMID:18426445

La Scala, B. F., & Bitmead, R. R. (1996). Design of an extended Kalman filter frequency tracer. *IEEE Transactions on Signal Processing*, *44*(3), 739–742. doi:10.1109/78.489052

Lane, J. D., Greenstadt, L., Shapiro, D., & Rubinstein, E. (1983). Pulse transit time and blood pressure: An intensive analysis. *Psychophysiology*, *20*(1), 45–49. PMID:6828611

Lass, J., Meigas, K., Karai, D., Kattai, R., Kaik, J., & Rossmann, M. (2004). Continuous blood pressure monitoring during exercise using pulse wave transit time measurement. In *Engineering in Medicine and Biology Society, 2004. IEMBS '04. 26th Annual International Conference of the IEEE*.

Lázaro, J., Gil, E., Bailn, R., Minchol, A., & Laguna, P. (2013). Deriving respiration from photoplethysmographic pulse width. *Medical & Biological Engineering & Computing*, *51*(1-2), 233–242. PMID:22996834

Leandro dos Santos, C. (2010). Gaussian quantum-behaved particle swarm optimization approaches for constrained engineering design problems. *Expert Systems with Applications*, *37*(2), 1676–1683. doi:10.1016/j.eswa.2009.06.044

Lee, H., & Buckley, K. M. (1999). ECG data compression using cut and align beats approach and 2-D transforms. *IEEE Transactions on Bio-Medical Engineering*, *46*(5), 556–564. doi:10.1109/10.759056 PMID:10230134

Lee, J. O., Kang, S. G., Kim, S. H., Park, S. J., & Song, S. W. (2011). The Relationship between Menopausal Symptoms and Heart Rate Variability in Middle Aged Women. *Korean Journal of Family Medicine*, *32*(5), 299–305. doi:10.4082/kjfm.2011.32.5.299 PMID:22745867

Lee, K. C., Lee, N., & Lee, H. (2012). Multi-agent knowledge integration mechanism using particle swarm optimization. *Journal of Technological Forecasting and Social Change*, *79*(3), 469–484. doi:10.1016/j.techfore.2011.08.004

Lee, M. S., Ju, H., Song, J. W., & Park, C. G. (2015). Kinematic model-based pedestrian dead reckoning for heading correction and lower body motion tracking. *Sensors (Basel, Switzerland)*, *15*(11), 28129–28153. doi:10.3390/s151128129 PMID:26561814

Lee, Q. Y., Redmond, S. J., Chan, G. S., Middleton, P. M., Steel, E., Malouf, P., & …, Lovell, N. H. (2013). Estimation of cardiac output and systemic vascular resistance using a multivariate regression model with features selected from the finger photoplethysmogram and routine cardiovascular measurements. *Biomedical Engineering Online*, *12*(19), 16. PMID:23452705

Lee, S., Kim, J., & Lee, M. (2011). A real-time ECG data compression and transmission algorithm for an e-health device. *IEEE Transactions on Bio-Medical Engineering*, *58*(9), 2448–2455. doi:10.1109/TBME.2011.2156794 PMID:21606020

Leicht, A., Hirning, D., & Allen, G. (2003). Heart rate variability and endogenous sex hormones during the menstrual cycle in young women. *Experimental Physiology*, *88*(3), 441–446. doi:10.1113/eph8802535 PMID:12719769

Leier, C. V. (2001). Nuggets, pearls, and vignettes of master heart failure clinicians. *Congestive Heart Failure (Greenwich, Conn.)*, *7*(6), 297–308. PMID:11828174

Levy, J. A. (1994). Long-term survivors of HIV infection. *Hospital Practice (Office Ed.)*, *29*(10), 41–44. doi:10.1080/21548331.1994.11443088 PMID:7929674

Lewicki, P., & Hill, T. (2006). *Statistics: methods and applications.* Tulsa, OK. Statsoft.

Lewis, R. J. (2000). *An introduction to classification and regression tree (CART) analysis*. Academic Press.

Lewis, R. P., Rittogers, S. E., Froester, W. F., & Boudoulas, H. (1977). A critical review of the systolic time intervals. *Circulation*, *56*(2), 146–158. PMID:872305

Li, Y, Yanmei, L., Hailun, F. (2010). Study on the methods of image enhancement for liver CT images. *Optik - International Journal for Light and Electron Optics, 121*, 1752-1755.

Li. (2012, May). Genetic Particle Filtering for Denoising of ECG Corrupted by Muscle Artifacts. In *Natural Computation (ICNC)* (pp. 562-565).

Liang, H., Miao, H., & Wu, H. (2010). Estimation of constant and time-varying dynamic parameters of HIV infection in a nonlinear differential equation model. *The Annals of Applied Statistics*, *4*(1), 460–483. doi:10.1214/09-AOAS290 PMID:20556240

Li, J. K.-J., Cui, T., & Drzewiecki, G. (1990). A nonlinear model of the arterial system incorporating a pressure-dependent compliance. Biomedical Engineering. *IEEE Transactions on*, *37*(7), 673–678.

Li, J., & Li. (2008, May). Home healthcare platform based on Wireless Sensor Networks. In *5th International Conference on Informational Technology and Application in Biomedicine*, China (pp. 263-266). doi:10.1109/LATINCOM.2009.5305161

Lillacci, G., & Khammash, M. (2010). Parameter Identification of Biological Networks Using Extended Kalman Filtering and X2 Criteria.*49th IEEE Conference on Decision and Control*. doi:10.1109/CDC.2010.5717460

Lim, K. H., Shin, Y. D., Park, S. H., Bae, J. H., Lee, H. J., Kim, S. J., & Choi, Y. J. et al. (2013). Correlation of blood pressure and the ratio of s1 to s2 as measured by esophageal stethoscope and wireless bluetooth transmission. *Pakistan Journal of Medical Sciences*, *4*(29), 1023–1027. PMID:24353680

Lin, C. J. (2008). An efficient immune-based symbiotic particle swarm optimization learning algorithm for TSK-type neuro-fuzzy networks design. *Journal on Fuzzy Sets and Systems*, *159*(21), 2890–2909. doi:10.1016/j.fss.2008.01.020

Lindberg, B., Nilsson, C., Zotterman, D., Soderberg, S., & Skar, L. (2013). Using Information and Communication Technology in home care for communication between patients, family members, and healthcare professionals: A systematic review. *International Journal of Telemedicine and Applications*, *2013*, 1–31. doi:10.1155/2013/461829 PMID:23690763

Linyi, L., & Deren, L. (2008). Fuzzy entropy image segmentation based on particle swarm optimization. *Progress in Natural Science*, *18*(9), 1167–1171. doi:10.1016/j.pnsc.2008.03.020

Litvack, D. A., Oberlander, T. F., Carney, L. H., & Saul, J. P. (1995). Time and frequency domain methods for heart rate variability analysis: A methodological comparison. *Psychophysiology*, *32*(5), 492–504. doi:10.1111/j.1469-8986.1995.tb02101.x PMID:7568644

Liu, C., & He, B. (2011). Noninvasive estimation of global activation sequence using the extended Kalman filter. *Biomedical Engineering. IEEE Transactions on*, *58*(3), 541–549.

Liu, Q., Yan, B., Yu, C.-M., Zhang, Y.-T., & Poon, C. (2014). Attenuation of systolic blood pressure and pulse transit time hysteresis during exercise and recovery in cardiovascular patients. Biomedical Engineering. *IEEE Transactions on*, *61*(2), 346–352.

Liu, Y., Dong, X., & Chen, P. (2012). Biological and chemical sensors based on graphene materials. *Chemical Society Reviews*, *41*(6), 2283–2307. doi:10.1039/C1CS15270J PMID:22143223

Ljung, L. (1979). Asymptotic behavior of the extended Kalman filter as a parameter estimator for linear systems. *Automatic Control. IEEE Transactions on*, *24*(1), 36–50.

Lo, Thiemjarus, King, & Yang. (n.d.). *Body Sensor Network – A Wireless Sensor Platform For Pervasive Healthcare Monitoring*. Academic Press.

Logier, R., De Jonckheere, J., Delecroix, M., Keribedj, A., Jeanne, M., Jounwaz, R., & Tavernier, B. (2011). Heart rate variability analysis for arterial hypertension etiological diagnosis during surgical procedures under tourniquet. In *Engineering in Medicine and Biology Society,EMBC, 2011 Annual International Conference of the IEEE.*

Longhini, C., Baracca, E., Brunazzi, C., Vaccari, M., Longhini, L., & Barbaresi, F. (1991). A new noninvasive method for estimation of pulmonary arterial pressure in mitral stenosis. *The American Journal of Cardiology*, *68*(4), 398–401. PMID:1858684

Luk, J. M., Lam, B. Y., Lee, N. P. Y., Ho, D. W., Sham, P. C., Chen, L., & Fan, S.-T. et al. (2007). Artificial neural networks and decision tree model analysis of liver cancer proteomes. *Journal of Biochemical and Biophysical Research Communications*, *361*(1), 68–73. doi:10.1016/j.bbrc.2007.06.172 PMID:17644064

Lu, Z., Kim, D. Y., & Pearlman, W. A. P. (2000). Wavelet compression of ECG signals by set partitioning in hierarchical trees algorithm. *IEEE Transactions on Bio-Medical Engineering*, *47*(7), 849–856. doi:10.1109/10.846678 PMID:10916255

Lyon, A. (2014). Why are Normal Distributions Normal? *The British Journal for the Philosophy of Science*, *65*(3), 621–649. doi:10.1093/bjps/axs046

Ma, T., & Zhang, Y. (2005). A correlation study on the variabilities in pulse transit time, blood pressure, and heart rate recorded simultaneously from healthy subjects. In *Engineering in Medicine and Biology Society, 2005. IEEE-EMBS 2005. 27th Annual International Conference of the.*

Maestri, R., Pinna, G. D., Accardo, A., Allegrini, P., Balocchi, R., D'Addio, G., & Cerutti, S. et al. (2007). Nonlinear indices of heart rate variability in chronic heart failure patients: Redundancy and comparative clinical value. *Journal of Cardiovascular Electrophysiology*, *18*(4), 425–433. doi:10.1111/j.1540-8167.2007.00728.x PMID:17284264

Mahmoodabadi, S., Ahmadian, A., Abolhasani, M., Eslami, M., & Bidgoli, J. (2006). *ECG feature extraction based on multiresolution wavelet transform*. Academic Press.

Ma, J., Zhang, T., & Dong, M. (2015). A Novel ECG data compression method using adaptive fourier decomposition with security guarantee in e-Health applications. *IEEE Journal of Biomedical and Health Informatics*, *19*(3), 986–994. PMID:25222961

Mallat, S. (2009). A wavelet tour of signal processing (S. Mallat, Ed.). Academic Press.

Mallat, S. (1999). *A wavelet tour of signal processing*. Academic Press.

Mamaghanian, Khaled, Atienza, & Vandergheynst. (2011, September). Compressed Sensing for Real Time Energy Efficient ECG Compression on Wireless Body Sensor Nodes. *IEEE Transactions on Biomedical Engineering, 58*(9), 2457-2466.

Maneesha, V., Ramesh, R. G. R., & Abhishek, T. K. (2012). Low Power Intelligent Wearable Cardiac Sensor Using Discrete Wavelet Compression. In *International Conference on Advances in Mobile Network, Communication and its Application* (pp. 107-110). IEEE.

Manickavasagam, K., Sutha, S., & Kamalanand, K. (2014). Development of Systems for Classification of Different Plasmodium Species in Thin Blood Smear Microscopic Images. *Journal of Advanced Microscopy Research*, *9*(2), 86–92. doi:10.1166/jamr.2014.1194

Manikandan, M. S., & Dandapat, S. (2006). Wavelet threshold based ECG compression using USZZQ and Huffman coding of DSM. *Biomedical Signal Processing and Control*, *1*(4), 261–270. doi:10.1016/j.bspc.2006.11.003

Manimegalai, J., & Thanushkodi. (2012). Estimation of cardiovascular parameters from ECG and PPG signals. *Bioengineering Conference (NEBEC), 2012 38th Annual Northeast*. IEEE. doi:10.1109/eTELEMED.2009.35

Manimegalai, P., Jacob, D., & Thanushkodi, K. (2012, March). Estimation of cardiovascular parameters from ECG and PPG signals. In *Bioengineering Conference (NEBEC), 2012 38th Annual Northeast* (pp. 237-238). IEEE. doi:10.1109/NEBC.2012.6207051

Mannar Jawahar, P., & Kamalanand, K. (2013). Computational Techniques for Infectious Diseases and Clinical Research. *European Journal for Biomedical Informatics*, *9*(2), 1-2.

Mansier, P., Clairambault, J., Charlotte, N., Medigue, C., Vermeiren, C., LePape, G., & Swynghedauw, B. et al. (1996). Linear and non-linear analyses of heart rate variability: A minireview. *Cardiovascular Research*, *31*(3), 371–379. doi:10.1016/0008-6363(96)00009-0 PMID:8681324

Maolong, X., Jun, S., & Wenbo, X. (2008). An Improved quantum-behaved particle swarm optimization algorithm with weighted mean best position. *Applied Mathematics and Computation*, *205*(2), 751–759. doi:10.1016/j.amc.2008.05.135

Marčelja, S. (1980). Mathematical description of the responses of simple cortical cells*. *JOSA*, *70*(11), 1297–1300. doi:10.1364/JOSA.70.001297 PMID:7463179

Martis, R. J., Krishnan, M. M. R., Chakraborty, C., Pal, S., Sarkar, D., Mandana, K. M., & Ray, A. K. (2012). Automated Screening of Arrhythmia Using Wavelet Based Machine Learning Techniques. *Journal of Medical Systems*, *36*(2), 677–688. doi:10.1007/s10916-010-9535-7 PMID:20703662

Masek, O. (2009). *Heart Rate Variability Analysis*. (Diploma Thesis). Czech Technical University in Prague, Prague, Czech Republic.

Masè, M., Mattei, W., Cucino, R., Faes, L., & Nollo, G. (2011). Feasibility of cuff-free measurement of systolic and diastolic arterial blood pressure. *Journal of Electrocardiology*, *44*(2), 201–207. PMID:21353067

Mashhoori, A., & Jahromi, M. Z. (2013). Block-wise two-directional 2DPCA with ensemble learning for face recognition. *Neurocomputing*, *108*, 111–117. doi:10.1016/j.neucom.2012.12.005

Maurer, U., Rowe, A., Smailagic, A., & Siewiorek, D. (2006). Location and activity recognition using eWatch: a wearable sensor platform. Lecture Notes in Computer Science, 3864, 86–102.

McAdams, E., Gehin, C., Massot, B., & McLaughlin, J. (2012). The challenges Facing Wearable Sensor Systems.*International Conference on Wearable Micro and Nano Technologies for Personalized Health.*

McCarthy, B. M., O'Flynn, B., & Mathewson, A. (2011, August). An investigation of pulse transit time as a non-invasive blood pressure measurement method. Journal of Physics, 307(1). doi:10.1088/1742-6596/307/1/012060

McCarthy, J. (2012). *Down for the count: 9 high-profile cloud outages*. Available at: http://www.crn.com/slide-shows/cloud/240012554/down-for-the-count-9-high-profilecloud outages. htm?pgno=4

Mckinley, P., King, A., Shapiro, P., Slavov, I., Fang, Y., Chen, I., & Sloan, R. et al. (2009). The impact of menstrual cycle phase on cardiac autonomic regulation. *Psychophysiology*, *46*(4), 904–911. doi:10.1111/j.1469-8986.2009.00811.x PMID:19386049

McLachlan, G., & Krishnan, T. (1997). *The EM Algorithm and Extensions*. John Wiley & Sons.

McNab, P., Castro, P., Verdejo, H., & Martinez, G. (2010). Estimacionauscultatoria de la presionsistolica dearteria pulmonar: Esfactible? correlacioncondeterminacionecocardiografica. *Revista Medica de Chile*, *138*, 1351–1356. PMID:21279246

McNames, J., & Aboy, M. (2008). Statistical modeling of cardiovascular signals and parameter estimation based on the extended Kalman filter. *Biomedical Engineering. IEEE Transactions on*, *55*(1), 119–129.

Mease, D., Wyner, A. J., & Buja, A. (2007). Boosted classification trees and class probability/quantile estimation. *Journal of Machine Learning Research*, *8*, 409–439.

Meigas, K., Lass, J., Karai, D., Kattai, R., & Kaik, J. (2007). Pulse wave velocity in continuous blood pressure measurements. In *World Congress on Medical Physics and Biomedical Engineering 2006*. Springer Berlin Heidelberg.

Meirav, U., & Foxman, E. B. (1995). Single-electron phenomena in semiconductors. *Semiconductor Science and Technology*, *10*, 255–284.

Messidor Project. (2004). Retrieved from http://messidor.crihan.fr/download-en.php

MESSIDOR. (2013). *Methods to evaluate segmentation and indexing techniques in the field of retinal ophthalmology*. Retrieved from http://messidor.crihan.fr/

Meste, O., Rix, H., Jané, R., & Caminal, P. (1991). Détection battement par battement de potentiels tardifs dans les electrocardiogrammes à haute amplification. *Innovation et technologie en biologie et médecine, 12*(5), 517-531.

Meyer, C., Morren, G., Muehlsteff, J., Heiss, C., Lauer, T., Schauerte, P., & Kelm, M. et al. (2011). Predicting neurally mediated syncope based on pulse arrival time: Algorithm development and preliminary results. *Journal of Cardiovascular Electrophysiology*, *22*(9), 1042–1048. PMID:21410580

Meyer, Y. (1995). *Wavelets and operators* (Vol. 1). Cambridge university press.

MIAS. (2013). *Mammographic Image Analysis Society*. Retrieved from http://peipa.essex. ac.uk/info/mias.html

Mico, W., & Carmen, P. (2009). An evaluation of the cuffless blood pressure estimation based on pulse transit time technique: A half year study on normotensive subjects. *Cardiovascular Engineering: An International Journal*, *9*(1), 32–38. PMID:19381806

Mikkelsen, G., & Aasly, J. (2001). Concordance of information in parallel electronic and paper based patient records. *International Journal of Medical Informatics*, *63*(3), 123–131. doi:10.1016/S1386-5056(01)00152-6 PMID:11502428

Millasseau, S. C., Stewart, A. D., Patel, S. J., Redwood, S. R., & Chowienczyk, P. J. (2005). Evaluation of carotid-femoral pulse wave velocity influence of timing algorithm and heart rate. *Hypertension*, *45*(2), 222–226. PMID:15642772

Miller, J. D., Beazer, M. S., & Hahn, M. E. (2013). Myoelectric walking mode classification for transtibial amputees. *IEEE Transactions on Bio-Medical Engineering*, *60*(10), 2745–2750. doi:10.1109/TBME.2013.2264466 PMID:23708765

Ming, Z., Youfu, L., Qinghao, M., Ting, Y., & Jian, L. (2012). Improving histogram-based image contrast enhancement using gray-level information histogram with application to X-ray images. *Optik-International Journal for Light and Electron Optics*, *123*(6), 511–520. doi:10.1016/j.ijleo.2011.05.017

Misiti, M., Misiti, Y., Oppenheim, G., & Poggi, J.-M. (1997). Wavelet toolbox. Matlab User's Guide, 64.

Mitra, B. (2002). Gaussian based edge-detection methods: A survey. *IEEE Transactions on Systems, Man and Cybernetics. Part C, Applications and Reviews*, *32*(3), 252–260. doi:10.1109/TSMCC.2002.804448

Moavenian, M., & Khorrami, H. (2010). A qualitative comparison of Artificial Neural Networks and Support Vector Machines in ECG arrhythmias classification. *Expert Systems with Applications*, *37*(4), 3088–3093. doi:10.1016/j.eswa.2009.09.021

Monte-Moreno, E. (2011). Non-invasive estimate of blood glucose and blood pressure from a photoplethysmograph by means of machine learning techniques. *Artificial Intelligence in Medicine*, *53*(2), 127–138. PMID:21696930

Moodithaya, S., & Sandhya, T. (2009). Comparison of Cardiac Autonomic Activity between Pre and Post Menopausal Women using Heart Rate Variability. *Indian Journal of Physiology and Pharmacology*, *53*, 227–234. PMID:20329369

Moody, J., & Darken, C. J. (1989). Fast learning in networks of locally-tuned processing units. *Neural Computation*, *1*(2), 281–294. doi:10.1162/neco.1989.1.2.281

Moonchai, S., Lenbury, Y., & Triampo, W. (2010). Cellular automata simulation modeling of HIV infection in lymph node and peripheral blood compartments. *International Journal of Mathematics and Computers in Simulation*, *4*, 124.

Mousavirad, S. J., & Ebrahimpour-Komleh, H. (2014). A Comparative Study on Medical Diagnosis Using Predictive Data Mining: A Case Study. *Data Mining and Analysis in the Engineering Field*, 327.

Muehlsteff, J., Aubert, X., & Morren, G. (2008). Continuous cuff-less blood pressure monitoring based on the pulse arrival time approach: The impact of posture. In *Engineering in Medicine and Biology Society, 2008. EMBS 2008. 30th Annual International Conference of the IEEE.*

Muehlsteff, J., Aubert, X., & Schuett, M. (2006). Cuffless estimation of systolic blood pressure for short effort bicycle tests: The prominent role of the pre-ejection period. In *Engineering in Medicine and Biology Society, 2006. EMBS '06. 28th Annual International Conference of the IEEE.*

Mueller, W. C. (1977). Arrhythmia detection program for an ambulatory ECG monitor. *Biomedical Sciences Instrumentation, 14*(1), 81–85. PMID:687739

Mukhopadhyay, S. K., Mitra, S., & Mitra, M. (2011). A lossless ECG data compression technique using ASCII character encoding. *Computers & Electrical Engineering, 37*(4), 486–497. doi:10.1016/j.compeleceng.2011.05.004

Mukhopadhyay, S. K., Mitra, S., & Mitra, M. (2012). An ECG signal compression technique using ASCII character encoding. *Measurement, 45*(6), 1651–1660. doi:10.1016/j.measurement.2012.01.017

Mukhopadhyay, S. K., Mitra, S., & Mitra, M. (2013). ECG signal compression using ASCII character encoding and transmission via SMS. *Biomedical Signal Processing and Control, 8*(4), 354–363. doi:10.1016/j.bspc.2013.02.007

Murdoch, T. B., & Detsky, A. S. (2013). The inevitable application of big data to health care. *Journal of the American Medical Association, 309*(13), 1351–1352. doi:10.1001/jama.2013.393 PMID:23549579

Muthulakshmi, S., & Latha, K. (2012). Classification of ECG Waveform Using Feature Selection Algorithm. In *International Conference on Advanced Communication Control and Computing Technologies* (pp. 162-165). IEEE.

Nahar, J., Imam, T., Tickle, K. S., & Chen, Y. P. (2013). Association rule mining to detect factors which contribute to heart disease in males and females. *Expert Systems with Applications, 40*(4), 1086–1093. doi:10.1016/j.eswa.2012.08.028

Nakagawa, M., Ooie, T., Takahashi, N., Taniguchi, Y., Anan, F., Yonemochi, H., & Saikawa, T. (2006). Influence of menstrual cycle on QT interval dynamics. *Pacing and Clinical Electrophysiology, 29*(6), 607–613. doi:10.1111/j.1540-8159.2006.00407.x PMID:16784426

Nandagopalan, S., Adiga, B. S., & Dhanalakshmi, C., & Deepak. (2010). Automatic Segmentation and ventricular border detection of 2D echocardiography images combining K-Means clustering and active contour model. Second International Conference on Computer and Network Technology (ICCNT).

Nandagopalan, S., Dhanalakshmi, C., Adiga, B.S., & Deepak, N. (2010). A Fast K-Means algorithm for the segmentation of echocardiographic images using DBMS-SQL. *The 2ndInternational Conference Computer and Automation Engineering* (ICCAE).

Nanda, S. J., & Panda, G. (2012). Accurate partitional clustering algorithm based on Immunized PSO.*IEEE International Conference on Advances in Engineering, Science and Management.*

Naschitz, J., Bezobchuk, S., Mussafia-Priselac, R., Sundick, S., Dreyfuss, D., Khorshidi, I., & Gaitini, L. et al. (2004). Pulse transit time by r-wave-gated infrared photoplethysmography: Review of the literature and personal experience. *Journal of Clinical Monitoring and Computing, 18*(5-6), 333–342. PMID:15957624

Natteshan, N. V. S., & Angel Arul Jothi, J. (2014). Automatic classification of brain MRI Images using SVM and neural network classifiers. *Advances in Intelligent Systems and Computing, 311*, 157–166.

Nave, G., & Cohen, A. (1993). ECG compression using long-term prediction. *IEEE Transactions on Bio-Medical Engineering, 40*(9), 877–885. doi:10.1109/10.245608 PMID:8288278

Neeraj, S., & Lalit, M. (2010). Automated medical image segmentation techniques. *Journal of Medical Physics*, *35*(1), 3–14. doi:10.4103/0971-6203.58777 PMID:20177565

Neves, V. F., Silva de Sa, M. F., Gallo, L. J. Jr, Catai, A. M., Martins, L. E., Crescencio, J. C., & Silva, E. et al. (2007). Autonomic modulation of heart rate of young and postmenopausal women undergoing estrogen therapy. *Brazilian Journal of Medical and Biological Research*, *40*(4), 491–499. doi:10.1590/S0100-879X2007000400007 PMID:17401492

Newlin, D. B. (1981). Relationships of pulse transmission times to pre-ejection period and blood pressure. *Psychophysiology, 18*, 316-321.

Ng, H. P., Ong, S. H., Foong, K. W. C., Goh, P. S., & Nowinski, W. L. (2006). Image Segmentation Using K-Means Clustering and Improved Watershed Algorithm.*IEEE Southwest Symposium on Image Analysis and Interpretation*. doi:10.1109/SSIAI.2006.1633722

Nichols, M., Townsend, N., Scarborough, P., & Rayner, M. (2014). Cardiovascular disease in Europe: Epidemiological update. *European Heart Journal*, *35*(42), 3028–3034. doi:10.1093/eurheartj/ehu299 PMID:24014390

Niemeijer, M., Staal, J., van Ginneken, B., Loog, M., & Abramoff, M. D. (2004). *Comparative study of retinal vessel segmentation methods on a new publicly available database*. Paper presented at the Medical Imaging 2004. doi:10.1117/12.535349

Niskanen, J. P., Tarvainen, M. P., Ranta-Aho, P. O., & Karjalainen, P. A. (2004). Software for advanced HRV analysis. *Computer Methods and Programs in Biomedicine*, *76*(1), 73–81. doi:10.1016/j.cmpb.2004.03.004 PMID:15313543

Nualnim, N., Parkhurst, K., Dhindsa, M., Tarumi, T., Vavrek, J., & Tanaka, H. (2012). Effects of swimming training on blood pressure and vascular function in adults> 50 years of age. *The American Journal of Cardiology*, *109*(7), 1005–1010. doi:10.1016/j.amjcard.2011.11.029 PMID:22244035

O'Brien, E., Atkins, N., Stergiou, G., Karpettas, N., Parati, G., Asmar, R., & Shennan, A. et al. (2010). on behalf of the working group on blood pressure monitoring of the european society of hypertension, european society of hypertension international protocol revision 2010 for the validation of blood pressure measuring devices in adults. *Blood Pressure Monitoring*, *15*(1), 23–38. PMID:20110786

O'Brien, E., Pickering, T., Asmar, R., Myers, M., Parati, G., Staessen, J., & Palatini, P. et al. (2002). on behalf of the working group on blood pressure monitoring of the european society of hypertension, working group on blood pressure monitoring of the european society of hypertension international protocol for validation of blood pressure measuring devices in adults. *Blood Pressure Monitoring*, *7*(1), 3–17. PMID:12040236

Ojala, T., Pietikäinen, M., & Mäenpää, T. (2002). Multiresolution gray-scale and rotation invariant texture classification with local binary patterns. *Pattern Analysis and Machine Intelligence. IEEE Transactions on*, *24*(7), 971–987.

Okano, A. H., Fontes, E. B., Montenegro, R. A., Farinatti, P. d. T. V., Cyrino, E. S., Li, L. M., et al. (2013). Brain stimulation modulates the autonomic nervous system, rating of perceived exertion and performance during maximal exercise. *British Journal of Sports Medicine*.

Olesen, Cordero, & Zeng. (2009). Auto-Clustering using particle swarm optimization and bacterial foraging, in: Agents and Data Mining Interaction. Lecture Notes in Computer Science, 5680, 69–83.

Olivier, L., & Truchetet, F. (2010). A nonlinear derivative scheme applied to edge detection. *IEEE Transactions on Pattern Analysis and Machine Intelligence*, *32*(2), 242–257. doi:10.1109/TPAMI.2008.282 PMID:20075456

Ottesen, J., & Danielsen, M. (2003). Modeling ventricular contraction with heart rate changes. *Journal of Theoretical Biology*, *222*(3), 337–346. PMID:12732480

Ouadfel, S., Batouche, M., & Teleb-Ahmed, A. (2010). A modified particle swarm optimization algorithm for automatic image clustering.*Proceedings of the 1st International Symposium on Modeling and Implementing Complex Systems.*

Ouattara, D. A. (2005, September). Mathematical analysis of the HIV-1 infection: Parameter estimation, therapies effectiveness, and therapeutical failures. In *27th Annual International Conference of the IEEE Engineering in Medicine and Biology Society, Shanghai, China*. doi:10.1109/IEMBS.2005.1616541

Ozyilmaz, L., & Yildirim, T. (2003). *Artificial neural networks for diagnosis of hepatitis disease*. Academic Press.

Paggetti, C., Lusini, M., Varanini, M., Taddei, A., Marchesi, C., & Sistemi, D. (1994). *A Multichannel Template Based Data Compression Algorithm*. Academic Press.

Palladino, J., Mulier, J., & Noordergraaf, A. (1996). An alternative to time-varying elastance descriptions of the heart. In *Engineering in Medicine and Biology Society, 1996. Bridging Disciplines for Biomedicine.Proceedings of the 18th Annual International Conference of the IEEE.*

Paloheimo, M. P. J., Sahanne, S., & Uutela, K. H. (2010). Autonomic nervous system state: The effect of general anaesthesia and bilateral tonsillectomy after unilateral infiltration of lidocaine. *British Journal of Anaesthesia*, *104*(5), 587–895. PMID:20354006

Pan, J., & Tompkins, W. J. (1985). A real-time QRS detection algorithm. *Biomedical Engineering, IEEE Transactions on*, (3), 230-236.

Pandeya, S., Voorsluys, W., Niua, S., Khandokerb, A., & Buyyaa, R. (2012). An autonomic cloud environment for hosting ECG data analysis services. *Future Generation Computer Systems*, *28*(1), 147–154. doi:10.1016/j.future.2011.04.022

Pandian, P., Mohanavelu, K., Safeer, K., Kotresh, T., Shakunthala, D., Gopal, P., & Padaki, V. (2008). Smart vest: Wearable multi-parameter remote physiological monitoring system. *Medical Engineering & Physics*, *30*(4), 466–477. PMID:17869159

Pan, J., & Tompkins, W. J. (1985). A real-time QRS detection algorithm. *IEEE Transactions on Bio-Medical Engineering*, *32*(3), 230–236. doi:10.1109/TBME.1985.325532 PMID:3997178

Panos, M., Pardalos, H., Romeijn, & Tuy. (2000). Recent developments and trends in global optimization. *Journal of Computational and Applied Mathematics*, *124*(1-2), 209–228.

Panov, P., Dzeroski, S., & Soldatova, L. (2008). OntoDM: An ontology of data mining.*IEEE International Conference on Data Mining Workshops.*

Papoulis, A. (1965). Probability, random variables and stochastic processes. New York: McGraw-Hill.

Park, J. W., Harley, R., & Venayagamoorthy, G. (2002). *Comparison of MLP and RBF neural networks using deviation signals for on-line identification of a synchronous generator*. Academic Press.

Parkka, J., Ermes, M., Korpipaa, P., Mantyjarvi, J., Peltola, J., & Korhonen, I. (2006). Activity classification using realistic data from wearable sensors. *IEEE Transactions on Information Technology in Biomedicine*, *10*(1), 119–128. doi:10.1109/TITB.2005.856863 PMID:16445257

Patel, P., Pathak, A., Texeira, T., & Issarny, V. (2011). Towards application development for the Internet of Things. In *Proceedings of the 8th Middleware Doctoral Symposium (MDS '11)*. ACM. doi:10.1145/2093190.2093195

Patolsky, F., Timko, B. P., Yu, G., Fang, Y., & Greytak, A. B. et al.. (2006). Detection, stimulation, and inhibition of neuronal signals with high-density nanowire transistor arrays. *Science*, *313*(5790), 1100–1104. doi:10.1126/science.1128640 PMID:16931757

Paul, S. (2002). Addison, The illustrated wavelet transform handbook. *Institute of Physics, 1*, 117–154.

Payne, R. A., Symeonides, C. N., Webb, D. J., & Maxwell, S. R. J. (2005). Pulse transit time measured from the ecg: An unreliable marker of beat-to-beat blood pressure. *Journal of Applied Physiology, 100*(1), 136–141. PMID:16141378

Pellegrino, F., Vanzella, W., & Torre, V. (2004). Edge detection revisited. *IEEE Transactions on Systems, Man, and Cybernetics. Part B, Cybernetics, 34*(3), 1500–1518. doi:10.1109/TSMCB.2004.824147 PMID:15484920

Penaz, J., ... (1973). Photoelectric measurement of blood pressure, volume and flow in the finger. In *Digest of the 10th international conference on medical and biological engineering*. International Federation for Medical and Biological Engineering.

Peng, F., Yingjun, P., Biao, W., Wei, J., & Deling, M. (2007). Enhancing retinal image by the contourlet transform. *Pattern Recognition Letters, 28*(4), 516–522. doi:10.1016/j.patrec.2006.09.007

Perelson, A. S., Kirschner, D. E., & De Boer, R. (1993). Dynamics of HIV infection of CD4+ T cells. *Mathematical Biosciences, 114*(1), 81–125. doi:10.1016/0025-5564(93)90043-A PMID:8096155

Peretto, L., Poletti, G., Longhini, L., Vitolo, A., & Santini, C. (2011). A comparison study of two indirect methods for measuring the systolic pulmonary arterial pressure. In *Medical Measurements and Applications Proceedings (MeMeA), 2011 IEEE International Workshop on.*

Peter, L., Noury, N., & Cerny, M. (2014). A review of methods for non-invasive and continuous blood pressure monitoring: Pulse transit time method is promising?. *IRBM, 35*(5), 271–282.

Phan, T. H. (2009). Vessel enhancement filter using directional filter bank. *Computer Vision and Image Understanding, 113*(1), 101–112. doi:10.1016/j.cviu.2008.07.009

PHIL. (2012). *Public Health Image Library*. Retrieved from http://phil.cdc.gov/phil

Pickering, T. G., Hall, J. E., Appel, L. J., Falkner, B. E., Graves, J., Hill, M. N., & Roccella, E. J. et al. (2005). Recommendations for blood pressure measurement in humans and experimental animals: Part 1: Blood pressure measurement in humans: A statement for professionals from the subcommittee of professional and public education of the American heart association council on high blood pressure research. *Hypertension, 45*(1), 142–161. PMID:15611362

Pincus, S. M. (1991). Approximate entropy as a measure of system complexity. *Proc. Natl Acad., 88*(March), 2297–2301. doi:10.1073/pnas.88.6.2297 PMID:11607165

Pincus, S. M., Goldberger, A. L. R. Y. L., Steven, M., & Goldberger, A. L. R. Y. L. (1994). Physiological time-series analysis: What does regularity quantify? *The American Journal of Physiology, 266*(4 Pt 2), H1643–H1656. Retrieved from http://www.pubmedcentral.nih.gov/articlerender.fcgi?artid=1332574&tool=pmcentrez&rendertype=abstract PMID:8184944

Pinz, A., Bernögger, S., Datlinger, P., & Kruger, A. (1998). Mapping the human retina. *Medical Imaging. IEEE Transactions on, 17*(4), 606–619.

Pitson, D., & Stradling. (1998). Value of beat-to-beat blood pressure changes, detected by pulse transit time, in the management of the obstructive sleep apnoea/hypopnoea syndrome. *The European Respiratory Journal, 12*(3), 685–692. PMID:9762800

Pober, D. M., Staudenmayer, J., Raphael, C., & Freedson, P. S. (2006). Development of novel techniques to classify physical activity mode using accelerometers. *Medicine and Science in Sports and Exercise, 38*(9), 1626–1634. doi:10.1249/01.mss.0000227542.43669.45 PMID:16960524

Polat, K., & Güneş, S. (2006). Hepatitis disease diagnosis using a new hybrid system based on feature selection (FS) and artificial immune recognition system with fuzzy resource allocation. *Digital Signal Processing*, *16*(6), 889–901. doi:10.1016/j.dsp.2006.07.005

Polat, K., & Güneş, S. (2007). Breast cancer diagnosis using least square support vector machine. *Digital Signal Processing*, *17*(4), 694–701. doi:10.1016/j.dsp.2006.10.008

Polat, K., Güneş, S., & Tosun, S. (2006). Diagnosis of heart disease using artificial immune recognition system and fuzzy weighted pre-processing. *Pattern Recognition*, *39*(11), 2186–2193. doi:10.1016/j.patcog.2006.05.028

Pollak, M. H., & Obrist, P. A. (1983). Aortic-radial pulse transit time and ecg q-wave to radial pulse wave interval as indices of beat-by-beat blood pressure change. *Psychophysiology*, *20*, 21–28. PMID:6828608

Poon, C. C. Y., & Zhang, Y. (2005). Cuff-less and noninvasive measurements of arterial blood pressure by pulse transit time. In *Engineering in Medicine and Biology Society, 2005. IEEE-EMBS 2005. 27th Annual International Conference of the*.

Pratt, W. K. (2004). *Digital Image Processing*. New York: John Wiley and Sons.

Princi, T., Parco, S., Accardo, A., Radillo, O., Seta, F., & Guaschino, S. (2005). Parametric evaluation of heart rate variability during the menstrual cycle in young women. *Biomedical Sciences Instrumentation*, *41*, 340–345. PMID:15850129

Proença, J., Muehlsteff, J., Aubert, X., & Carvalho, P. (2010). Is pulse transit time a good indicator of blood pressure changes during short physical exercise in a young population? In *Engineering in Medicine and Biology Society (EMBC), 2010 Annual International Conference of the IEEE*.

Pui, T. S., Sudibya, H. G., Luan, X., Zhang, Q., Ye, F., Huang, Y., & Chen, P. (2010). Non-invasive detection of cellular bioelectricity based on carbon nanotube devices for high-throughput drug screening. *Advanced Materials*, *22*(29), 3199–3203. doi:10.1002/adma.201000548 PMID:20533507

Putter, H., Heisterkamp, S. H., Lange, J. M. A., & De Wolf, F. (2002). A Bayesian approach to parameter estimation in HIV dynamical models. *Statistics in Medicine*, *21*(15), 2199–2214. doi:10.1002/sim.1211 PMID:12210633

Pyle, D. (1999). *Data Preparation for Data Mining*. Morgan Kaufmann.

Qi, L. P., Wakeling, J. M., Green, A., Lambrecht, K., & Ferguson-Pell, M. (2011). Spectral properties of electromyographic and mechanomyographic signals during isometric ramp and step contractions in biceps brachii. *Journal of Electromyography and Kinesiology*, *21*(1), 128–135. doi:10.1016/j.jelekin.2010.09.006 PMID:21067944

Rahman, F., Pechnik, S., Gross, D., Sewell, L., & Goldstein, D. S. (2011). Low frequency power of heart rate variability reflects baroreflex function, not cardiac sympathetic innervation. *Clinical Autonomic Research*, *21*(3), 133–141. doi:10.1007/s10286-010-0098-y PMID:21279414

Rakesh, R. R., Probal, C., & Murthy, C. A. (2004). Thresholding in edge detection: A statistical approach. *IEEE Transactions on Image Processing*, *13*(7), 927–936. doi:10.1109/TIP.2004.828404 PMID:15648859

Rakshit, M., Panigrahy, D., & Sahu, P. K. (2015). EKF with PSO Technique for Delineation of P And T Wave In Electrocardiogram (ECG) Signal.*2nd International Conference Signal Processing and Integrated Networks (SPIN)*. doi:10.1109/SPIN.2015.7095293

Ramakrishnan, A. G., Prathosh, A. P., & Ananthapadmanabha, T. V. (2014). Threshold-independent QRS detection using the dynamic plosion index. *IEEE Signal Processing Letters*, *21*(5), 554–558. doi:10.1109/LSP.2014.2308591

Ramakrishnan, A. G., & Saha, S. (1997). ECG Coding by Wavelet-Based Linear Prediction. *IEEE Transactions on Bio-Medical Engineering*, *44*(12), 1253–1261. doi:10.1109/10.649997 PMID:9401225

Rashid, A., & Rahim, S. & Mahalin. (2008, December). Home healthcare via Wireless Biomedical Sensor Network. In *IEEE International Rf And Microwave Conference Proceedings* (pp. 511-514). IEEE.

Reddy, B. R. S., & Murthy, I. S. N. (1986). ECG data compression using Fourier descriptors. *IEEE Transactions on Bio-Medical Engineering*, *33*(4), 428–434. doi:10.1109/TBME.1986.325799 PMID:3957398

Reed, M. A. (1997). Conductance of a Molecular Junction. *Science*, *278*(5336), 252–254. doi:10.1126/science.278.5336.252

Regtien, P., Van Der Heijden, F., Korsten, M. J., & Otthius, W. (2004). *Measurement science for engineers*. Elsevier.

Reid, J. G. (1987). Normal functions of normal random variables. *Computers & Mathematics with Applications (Oxford, England)*, *14*(3), 157–160. doi:10.1016/0898-1221(87)90147-7

Ribeiro, T. F., Azevendo, G. D., Crescencio, J. C., Maraes, V. R., Papa, V., Catai, A. M., & Siliva, E. et al. (2001). Heart rate variability under resting conditions in post menopausal and young women. *Brazilian Journal of Medical and Biological Research*, *34*(7), 871–877. doi:10.1590/S0100-879X2001000700006 PMID:11449305

Richards, A., Nicholls, M., Yandle, T., Ikram, H., Espiner, E., Turner, J., & Smyth, D. W. et al. (1999). Neuroendocrine prediction of left ventricular function and heart failure after acute myocardial infarction. *Heart (British Cardiac Society)*, *81*(2), 114–120. doi:10.1136/hrt.81.2.114 PMID:9922344

Richman, J. S., & Moorman, J. R. (2000). Physiological time-series analysis using approximate entropy and sample entropy. *American Journal of Physiology. Heart and Circulatory Physiology*, *278*(6), 2039–2049. PMID:10843903

Rigatos, G. G., Rigatou, E. G., & Djida, J. D. (2015). Change detection in the dynamics of an intracellular protein synthesis model using nonlinear Kalman filtering. *Mathematical Biosciences and Engineering*, *12*(5), 1017–1035. doi:10.3934/mbe.2015.12.1017 PMID:26280184

Roche, A., Lahaye, P. J., & Poline, J. B. (2004, April). Incremental activation detection in fMRI series using kalman filtering. In *Biomedical Imaging: Nano to Macro, 2004. IEEE International Symposium on* (pp. 376-379). IEEE. doi:10.1109/ISBI.2004.1398553

Rodriguez, B., Jane, R., & Brooks, D. (2000). *Ventricular tachycardia risk detection using wavelet decomposition of the signal averaged ECG*. Academic Press.

Rodriguez-Galiano, V., Ghimire, B., Rogan, J., Chica-Olmo, M., & Rigol-Sanchez, J. (2012). An assessment of the effectiveness of a random forest classifier for land-cover classification. *ISPRS Journal of Photogrammetry and Remote Sensing*, *67*, 93–104. doi:10.1016/j.isprsjprs.2011.11.002

Rolim, C. O., Koch, F. L., Westphall, C. B., Werner, J., Fracalossi, A., & Salvador, G. S. (2010). A Cloud Computing Solution for Patient's Data Collection in Health Care Institutions. In *Proceedings of 2nd International Conference on eHealth, Telemedicine and social Medicine* (ETRLEMED' 10). IEEE Computer Society. doi:10.1109/eTELEMED.2010.19

Rosimini, C. (2003). Benefits of swim training for children and adolescents with asthma. *Journal of the American Academy of Nurse Practitioners*, *15*(6), 247–252. doi:10.1111/j.1745-7599.2003.tb00394.x PMID:12861890

Rotariu & Manta. (2012). Wireless System for Remote Monitoring of Oxygen Saturation and Heart Rate. In *Proceedings of Federated Conference on Computer Science and Information System* (pp. 193-196). IEEE.

Sabarimalai Sur, M., & Dandapat, S. (2014). Wavelet-based electrocardiogram signal compression methods and their performances: A prospective review. *Biomedical Signal Processing and Control*, *14*(1), 73–107. Retrieved from http://linkinghub.elsevier.com/retrieve/pii/S1746809414000998

Sabatini, A. M., Martelloni, C., Scapellato, S., & Cavallo, F. (2005). Assessment of walking features from foot inertial sensing. *IEEE Transactions on Bio-Medical Engineering*, *52*(3), 486–494. doi:10.1109/TBME.2004.840727 PMID:15759579

Saeki, Y., Atogami, F., Takahashi, K., & Yoshizawa, T. (1997). Reflex control of autonomic function induced by posture change during the menstrual cycle. *Journal of the Autonomic Nervous System*, *66*(1-2), 69–74. doi:10.1016/S0165-1838(97)00067-2 PMID:9334995

Salarian, A., Russmann, H., Vingerhoets, F. J. G., Burkhard, P. R., & Aminian, K. (2007). Ambulatory monitoring of physical activities in patients with Parkinson's disease. *IEEE Transactions on Bio-Medical Engineering*, *54*(12), 2296–2299. doi:10.1109/TBME.2007.896591 PMID:18075046

Salgado, P., & Igrejas, G. (2012). A PCA-fuzzy clustering algorithm for contours analysis. *Advances in Intelligent and Soft Computing*, *107*, 305–311. doi:10.1007/978-3-642-24001-0_28

Sameni, R., Shamsollahi, M. B., & Jutten, C. (2005). Filtering electrocardiogram signals using the extended Kalman filter. In *Engineering in Medicine and Biology Society, 2005. IEEE-EMBS 2005. 27th Annual International Conference of the* (pp. 5639-5642). IEEE. doi:10.1109/IEMBS.2005.1615765

Sandryhaila, A., Saba, S., & Kovacevic, J. (2012). Efficient Compression of QRS Complexes Using Hermite Expansion. *IEEE Transactions on Signal Processing*, *60*(2), 947–955. doi:10.1109/TSP.2011.2173336

Saravanakumar, S. (2006). A Luminance- and contrast-invariant edge-similarity measure. *IEEE Transactions on Pattern Analysis and Machine Intelligence*, *28*(12), 2042–2048. doi:10.1109/TPAMI.2006.236 PMID:17108378

Sato, N., & Miyake, S. (2004). Cardiovascular reactivity to mental stress: Relationship with menstrual cycle and gender. *Journal of Physiological Anthropology and Applied Human Science*, *23*(6), 215–223. doi:10.2114/jpa.23.215 PMID:15599065

Sato, N., Miyake, S., Akatsu, J., & Kumashiro, M. (1995). Power spectral analysis of heart rate variability in healthy young women during the normal menstrual cycle. *Psychosomatic Medicine*, *57*(4), 331–335. doi:10.1097/00006842-199507000-00004 PMID:7480562

Sawane, M. V., & Gupta, S. S. (2015). Resting heart rate variability after yogic training and swimming: A prospective randomized comparative trial. *International Journal of Yoga*, *8*(2), 96.

Sayood, K. (2010). Introduction to data compression. (K. Sayood, Ed.). Elsevier Inc.

Schmitt, L., Hellard, P., Millet, G., Roels, B., Richalet, J., & Fouillot, J. (2006). Heart rate variability and performance at two different altitudes in well-trained swimmers. *International Journal of Sports Medicine*, *27*(3), 226–231. doi:10.1055/s-2005-865647 PMID:16541379

Sehgal, A., Perelman, V., Kuryla, S., & Schonwalder, J. (2012). Management of Resource Constrained Devices in the Internet of Things. *IEEE Communications Magazine*, *50*(12), 144–149. doi:10.1109/MCOM.2012.6384464

Senthilnath, J., Omkar, S. N., & Mani, V. (2011). Clustering using firefly algorithm: Performance study. *Swarm and Evolutionary Computation*, *1*(3), 164–171. doi:10.1016/j.swevo.2011.06.003

Shaou-Gang, M., & Yen, H.-L. (2001). Multichannel ECG compression using multichannel adaptive vector quantization. *IEEE Transactions on Bio-Medical Engineering*, *48*(10), 1203–1207. doi:10.1109/10.951524 PMID:11585045

Sharwood-Smith, G., Bruce, J., & Drummond, G. (2006). Assessment of pulse transit time to indicate cardiovascular changes during obstetric spinal anaesthesia. *British Journal of Anaesthesia*, *96*(1), 100–105. PMID:16257996

Shasidha, M., & Sudheer Raja, V., & Kumar. (2011). MRI Brain image segmentation using modified fuzzy c-means clustering algorithm. *International Conference on Communication Systems and Network Technologies*.

Sheema, U. K., Sarwari, K. N., & Malipatil, B. S. (2014). Influence of different phases of the menstrual cycle on heart rate variability. *International Journal of Basic and Applied Medical Sciences*, *4*(3), 168-172.

Shepp, L. (1964). Normal functions of normal random variables. *SIAM Review*, *6*(4), 459–460. doi:10.1137/1006100

Sherry, J., & Salvador, T. (2001). Running and grimacing: the struggle for balance in mobile work. In B. Brown, N. Green, & R. Harper (Eds.), *Wireless World: Social and Interactional Aspects of the Mobile Age* (pp. 108–120). Berlin, Germany: Springer.

Sherwood, A., Allen, M. T., Fahrenberg, J., Kelsey, R. M., Lovallo, W. R., & van Doornen, L. J. (1990). Methodological guidelines for impedance cardiography. *Psychophysiology*, *27*(1), 1–23. PMID:2187214

Shillabeer, A., & Roddick, J. (2007). Establishing a lineage for medical knowledge discovery. In *Proceedings of the 6th Australasian Conference of Data Mining and Analytics (AusDM '07)*. Darlinghurst, Australia: Australian Computer Society.

Shimamoto, H., Adachi, Y., Takahashi, M., & Tanaka, K. (1998). Low impact aerobic dance as a useful exercise mode for reducing body mass in mildly obese middle-aged women. *Applied Human Science*, *17*(3), 109–114. doi:10.2114/jpa.17.109 PMID:9682520

Shin, K., Minamitani, H., Onishi, S., Yamazaki, H., & Lee, M. (1993). *The power spectral analysis of heart rate variability in athletes during exercise*. Academic Press.

Shiraz, M., Gani, A., Khokhar, R. H., & Buyya, R. K. (2013). A Review on Distributed Application Processing Frameworks in Smart Mobile Devices for Mobile Cloud Computing. *IEEE Communications Society*, *15*(3), 1294–1313. doi:10.1109/SURV.2012.111412.00045

Shriram, R., Wakankar, A., Daimiwal, N., & Ramdasi, D. (2010, April). Continuous cuffless blood pressure monitoring based on PTT. In *Bioinformatics and Biomedical Technology (ICBBT), 2010 International Conference on* (pp. 51-55). IEEE. doi:10.1109/ICBBT.2010.5479013

Silberman, N., Ahrlich, K., Fergus, R., & Subramanian, L. (2010). *Case for Automated Detection of Diabetic Retinopathy*. Paper presented at the AAAI Spring Symposium: Artificial Intelligence for Development.

Simon, D. (2006). *Optimal state estimation: Kalman, H infinity, and nonlinear approaches*. John Wiley & Sons. doi:10.1002/0470045345

Simon, M. K. (2007). *Probability distributions involving Gaussian random variables: A handbook for engineers and scientists*. Springer Science & Business Media.

Singh, B. N., & Tiwari, A. K. (2006). Optimal selection of wavelet basis function applied to ECG signal denoising. *Digital Signal Processing*, *16*(3), 275–287. doi:10.1016/j.dsp.2005.12.003

Singh, B., & Singh, D. (2012). Effect of threshold value r on multiscale entropy based heart rate variability. *Cardiovascular Engineering and Technology*, *3*(2), 211–216. doi:10.1007/s13239-012-0082-x

Singh, B., Singh, D., Jaryal, A. K., & Deepak, K. K. (2012). Ectopic beats in approximate entropy and sample entropy-based HRV assessment. *International Journal of Systems Science*, *43*(5), 884–893. doi:10.1080/00207721.2010.543478

Smith, E. M. (2007). Nano panelist sees molecular devices as next step toward smaller, cheaper, faster devices (James J. Marek, Jr.). *ASME NEWS.* Retrieved from http://www.asmenews.org/archives/backissues/aug01/features/nanopan.html

Smith, R. P., Argod, J., Ppin, J.-L., & Lvy, P. A. (1999). Pulse transit time: An appraisal of potential clinical applications. *Thorax, 54*(5), 452–457. PMID:10212114

Smith, R., & Ventura, D. (2013). A general model for continuous noninvasive pulmonary artery pressure estimation. *Computers in Biology and Medicine, 43*(7), 904–913. PMID:23746733

Sola, J., Chetelat, O., Sartori, C., Allemann, Y., & Rimoldi, S. (2011). Chest pulse-wave velocity: A novel approach to assess arterial stiffness. Biomedical Engineering. *IEEE Transactions on, 58*(1), 215–223.

Sola, J., Proenc¸a, M., Ferrario, D., Porchet, J.-A., Falhi, A., Grossenbacher, O., & Sartori, C. et al. (2013). Noninvasive and nonocclusive blood pressure estimation via a chest sensor. Biomedical Engineering. *IEEE Transactions on, 60*(12), 3505–3513.

Sola, J., Vetter, R., Renevey, P., Chatelat, O., Sartori, C., & Rimoldi, S. F. (2009). Parametric estimation of pulse arrival time: A robust approach to pulse wave velocity. *Physiological Measurement, 30*(7), 603. PMID:19491457

SoteraWireless (2015). *Visi mobile.* Author.

Spulak, D., Cmejla, R., & Fabian, V. (2011). Parameters for mean blood pressure estimation based on electrocardiography and photoplethysmography. In *Applied Electronics (AE), 2011 International Conference on.*

Staal, J. J., Abramoff, M. D., Niemeijer, M., Viergever, M. A., & Ginneken, B. (2004). Ridge based vessel segmentation in color images of the retina. *IEEE Transactions on Medical Imaging, 23*(4), 501–509. doi:10.1109/TMI.2004.825627 PMID:15084075

STARE. (2013). *STructured Analysis of the Retina project.* Retrieved from http://www.ces.clemson.edu/~ahoover/stare/

Stephen, P. (2009). Activity identification using body-mounted sensors-a review of classification techniques. *Journal of Physiological Measurement, 30*(4), R1–R33. doi:10.1088/0967-3334/30/4/R01 PMID:19342767

Suarjaya. (2012). A New Algorithm for Data Compression Optimization. *International Journal of Advanced Computer Science and Applications, 3*(8), 14-17. doi:10.1109/ICACCCT.2012.6320762

Sullivan, M. J., & Knight, J. D., & Cobb, F. R. (1989). Relation between central and peripheral hemodynamics during exercise in patients with chronic heart failure. muscle blood flow is reduced with maintenance of arterial perfusion pressure. *Circulation, 80*, 769–781. PMID:2791242

Sundaram, M., Ramar, K., Arumugam, N., & Prabin, G. (2011). Histogram Modified Local Contrast Enhancement for mammogram images. *Applied Soft Computing, 11*(8), 5809–5816. doi:10.1016/j.asoc.2011.05.003

Sup, F., Bohara, A., & Goldfrab, M. (2008). Design and control of a powered transfemoral prosthesis. *The International Journal of Robotics Research, 27*(2), 263–273. doi:10.1177/0278364907084588 PMID:19898683

Suzuki, S., & Oguri, K. (2008). Cuffless and non-invasive systolic blood pressure estimation for aged class by using a photoplethysmograph. In *Engineering in Medicine and Biology Society, 2008. EMBS 2008. 30th Annual International Conference of the IEEE.*

Suzuki, S., & Oguri, K. (2009). Cuffless blood pressure estimation by error-correcting output coding method based on an aggregation of adaboost with a photoplethysmograph sensor. In *Engineering in Medicine and Biology Society, 2009. EMBC 2009. Annual International Conference of the IEEE.*

Sztajzel, J. (2004). Heart rate variability: A noninvasive electrocardiographic method to measure the autonomic nervous system. *Swiss Medical Weekly*, *134*, 514–522. PMID:15517504

Talbi, E. (2002). A Taxonomy of hybrid metaheuristics. *Journal of Heuristics*, *8*(5), 541–564. doi:10.1023/A:1016540724870

Tang, X. (1998). Texture information in run-length matrices. *Image Processing. IEEE Transactions on*, *7*(11), 1602–1609.

Tan, H. H. Y. (2012). A two-stage genetic algorithm for automatic clustering. *Neurocomputing*, *81*(1), 49–59.

Taubman, D. S., Marcellin, M. W., & Rabbani, M. (2002). JPEG2000: Image compression fundamentals, standards and practice. *Journal of Electronic Imaging*, *11*(2), 286. doi:10.1117/1.1469618

Tavel, M. E. (2006). Cardiac auscultation: A glorious pastand it does have a future! *Circulation*, *113*(9), 1255–1259. PMID:16520426

Tay, P. C., Garson, C. D., Acton, S. T., & Hossack, J. A. (2010). Ultrasound despeckling for contrast enhancement. *IEEE Transactions on Image Processing*, *19*(7), 1847–1860. doi:10.1109/TIP.2010.2044962 PMID:20227984

Teng, X. F., & Zhang, Y. T. (2003). Continuous and noninvasive estimation of arterial blood pressure using a photoplethysmographic approach. In *Engineering in Medicine and Biology Society, 2003.Proceedings of the 25th Annual International Conference of the IEEE.*

Testani, J. M., Sutton, M. G. S. J., Wiegers, S. E., Khera, A. V., Shannon, R. P., & Kirkpatrick, J. N. (2010). Accuracy of noninvasively determined pulmonary artery systolic pressure. *The American Journal of Cardiology*, *105*(8), 1192–1197. PMID:20381676

Thakor, N., Gramatikov, B., & Mita, M. (1993). *Multiresolution wavelet analysis of ECG during ischemia and reperfusion.* Academic Press.

Tian, B., Cohen-karni, T., Qing, Q., Duan, X., Xie, P., & Lieber, C. M. (2010). Three-dimensional, flexible nanoscale field-effect transistors as localized bioprobes. *Science*, *329*(5993), 830–834. doi:10.1126/science.1192033 PMID:20705858

Tian, J., & Zeng, J. (2009). 2D Fuzzy Maximum Entropy Image Threshold Segmentation Method Based on QPSO. *Computer Engineering.*, *35*(3), 230–232.

Time. (1974). Mini-mini Components: Turning Individual Molecules into Electronic Components. *Time Magazine*, *103*, 97.

Toh, Do, Chung, & Lee. (2009). Health Decision Support for Biomedical Signals Monitoring System over a WSN. In *2nd International Symposium on Electronic Commerce and Security* (pp. 605-608). IEEE.

Tompkins, W. J. (1993). *Biomedical digital signal processing.* Editorial Prentice Hall.

Tranulis, C., Durand, L., Senhadji, L., & Pibarot, P. (2002). Estimation of pulmonary arterial pressure by a neural network analysis using features based on time-frequency representations of the second heart sound. *Medical & Biological Engineering & Computing*, *40*(2), 205–212. PMID:12043802

Trigo, F. C., Gonzalez-Lima, R., & Amato, M. B. P. (2004). Electrical impedance tomography using the extended Kalman filter. *Biomedical Engineering. IEEE Transactions on*, *51*(1), 72–81.

Tseng, Tsai, Lai, & Fang. (2009). *A Wireless Biomedical Sensor Network using IEEE802.15.4.* IEEE.

Tucker, M. R., Olivier, J., Pagel, A., Bleuler, H., Bouri, M., Lambercy, O., & Gassert, R. et al. (2015). Control strategies for active lower extremity prosthetics and orthotics: A review. *Journal of Neuroengineering and Rehabilitation*, *12*(1), 1–29. doi:10.1186/1743-0003-12-1 PMID:25557982

Tuomi, I. (2002). The Lives and Death of Moore's Law. *First Monday*, *7*(11). doi:10.5210/fm.v7i11.1000

Tuomikoski, P., Ylikorkala, O., & Mikkola, T. S. (2011). Menopausal hot flushes and vascular health. *Annals of Medicine, 43*(4), 283–291. doi:10.3109/07853890.2010.546364 PMID:21254907

Uguz, H. (2012). A hybrid system based on information gain and principal component analysis for the classification of transcranial Doppler signals. *Computer Methods and Programs in Biomedicine, 107*(3), 598–609. doi:10.1016/j.cmpb.2011.03.013 PMID:21524813

Vahid, F., & Gholam Ali, M. (2013). An Improvement in RBF learning algorithm based on PSO for real time applications. *Neurocomputing, 111*, 169–176. doi:10.1016/j.neucom.2012.12.024

Valens, C.A., & Valens C. (1999). *Really friendly guide to wavelets*. Academic Press.

Valentine, E., & Evans, C. (2001). The effects of solo singing, choral singing and swimming on mood and physiological indices. *The British Journal of Medical Psychology, 74*(1), 115–120. doi:10.1348/000711201160849

Van Der Heijden, F., Duin, R., De Ridder, D., & Tax, D. M. (2005). *Classification, parameter estimation and state estimation: an engineering approach using MATLAB*. John Wiley & Sons.

Vatanparast, M., & Harati, A. (2012). *A feasibility study on detection of Neovascularization in retinal color images using texture*. Paper presented at the Computer and Knowledge Engineering (ICCKE), 2012 2nd International eConference on. doi:10.1109/ICCKE.2012.6395382

Vaz de Almeida, M. D., Graça, P., Afonso, C., D'Amicis, A., Lappalainen, R., & Damkjaer, S. (1999). Physical activity levels and body weight in a nationally representative sample in the European Union. *Public Health Nutrition, 2*(1a), 105–114. doi:10.1017/S1368980099000154 PMID:10933630

Venkatesh, T., Premkumar, N., & Sivaguru, G. (2013). Efficient cloud platform providing an omnipresent healthcare services. *International Journal of Innovative Research in Computer and communication Engineering, 1*(2), 193-199. Retrieved from http://www.rroij.com/open-access/efficient-cloud-platform-providing-anomnipresent-healthcare-services.pdf

Vetterli, M., & Herley, C. (1992). Wavelets and filter banks: Theory and design. *Signal Processing. IEEE Transactions on, 40*(9), 2207–2232. doi:10.1109/78.157221

Vinet, A., Beck, L., Nottin, S., & Obert, P. (2005). Effect of intensive training on heart rate variability in prepubertal swimmers. *European Journal of Clinical Investigation, 35*(10), 610–614. doi:10.1111/j.1365-2362.2005.01557.x PMID:16178879

Vishrutha, K., Harini, N., Ganaraja, B., Pavanchand, A., & Susheela, V. (2012). A study of cardiac autonomic control and pulmonary functions in different phases of menstrual cycle. *International Journal of Applied Biology and Pharmaceutical Technology, 3*(3), 306–311.

Visvanathan, A., Sinha, A., & Pal, A. (2013). Estimation of blood pressure levels from reflective photoplethysmograph using smart phones. In *Bioinformatics and Bioengineering (BIBE), 2013 IEEE 13th International Conference on.*

Von Tscharner, V., & Goepfert, B. (2006). Estimation of the interplay between groups of fast and slow muscle fibers of the tibialis anterior and gastrocnemius muscle while running. *Journal of Electromyography and Kinesiology, 16*(2), 188–197. doi:10.1016/j.jelekin.2005.07.004 PMID:16139523

Vu, T. H. N., & Park, N. (2010). *Heart rate variability pattern recognition in ambulatory environments*. Academic Press.

Wacker, M., & Witte, H. (2013). Time-frequency Techniques in Biomedical Signal Analysis A Tutorial Review of Similarities and Differences. *Methods of Information in Medicine, 52*(4), 279–296. doi:10.3414/ME12-01-0083 PMID:23703538

Wagner, D., Roesch, N., Harpes, P., Krtke, H., Plumer, P., Saberin, A., & Bhm, M. et al. (2010). Relationship between pulse transit time and blood pressure is impaired in patients with chronic heart failure. *Clinical Research in Cardiology; Official Journal of the German Cardiac Society*, *99*(10), 657–664. PMID:20473677

Wakeling, J. M., Uehli, K., & Rozitis, A. I. (2006). Muscle fibre recruitment can respond to the mechanics of the muscle contraction. *Journal of the Royal Society, Interface*, *3*(9), 533–544. doi:10.1098/rsif.2006.0113 PMID:16849250

Wakeling, J., Delaney, R., & Dudkiewicz, I. (2007). A method for quantifying dynamic muscle dysfunction in children and young adults with cerebral palsy. *Gait & Posture*, *25*(4), 580–589. doi:10.1016/j.gaitpost.2006.06.009 PMID:16876416

Walter, T., Klein, J.-C., Massin, P., & Erginay, A. (2002). A contribution of image processing to the diagnosis of diabetic retinopathy-detection of exudates in color fundus images of the human retina. *Medical Imaging. IEEE Transactions on*, *21*(10), 1236–1243.

Wan, E., & Van Der Merwe, R. (2000). The unscented Kalman filter for nonlinear estimation. In *Adaptive Systems for Signal Processing, Communications, and Control Symposium 2000. AS-SPCC. The IEEE 2000* (pp. 153-158). IEEE. doi:10.1109/ASSPCC.2000.882463

Wang, Shiqin, & Xu. (2007). Scalability of hybrid fuzzy C-Means algorithm based on quantum-behaved PSO. *Fourth International Conference on Fuzzy Systems and Knowledge Discovery.*

Wang, G., Krueger, G. R., & Buja, L. M. (2004). A simple model to simulate cellular changes in the T cell system following HIV-1 infection. *Anticancer Research*, *24*(3A), 1689–1698. PMID:15274342

Wang, X., & Meng, J. (2008). A 2-D ECG compression algorithm based on wavelet transform and vector quantization. *Digital Signal Processing*, *18*(2), 179–188. doi:10.1016/j.dsp.2007.03.003

Wang, Z., Bovik, A. C., Sheikh, H. R., & Simoncelli, E. P. (2004). Image quality assessment: From error measurement to structural similarity. *IEEE Transactions on Image Processing*, *13*(4), 600–612. doi:10.1109/TIP.2003.819861 PMID:15376593

Wanpeng, C., Rensheng, C., & Dong, Y. (2008). An illumination-independent edge detection and fuzzy enhancement algorithm based on wavelet transform for non-uniform weak illumination images. *Pattern Recognition Letters*, *29*(3), 192–199. doi:10.1016/j.patrec.2007.09.012

Ward, J. H. Jr. (1963). Hierarchical grouping to optimize an objective function. *Journal of the American Statistical Association*, *58*(301), 236–244. doi:10.1080/01621459.1963.10500845

Ward, M., & Langton, J. A. (2007). Blood pressure measurement. *Continuing Education in Anaesthesia Critical Care & Pain*, *7*(4), 122–126. doi:10.1093/bjaceaccp/mkm022

Webster, J. G. (Ed.). (2006). *Encyclopedia of Medical Devices and Instrumentation* (2nd ed.). Wiley-Interscience.

Weiderpass, H. A., Pachi, C. G. F., Yamamoto, J. F., Hamamoto, A., Onodera, A. N., & Sacco, I. C. N. (2013). Time-frequency analysis methods for detecting effects of diabetic neuropathy. *International Journal for Numerical Methods in Biomedical Engineering*, *29*(9), 1000–1010. doi:10.1002/cnm.2545 PMID:23620093

Wei, J. J., Chang, C. J., Chou, N. K., & Jan, G. J. (2001). ECG data compression using truncated singular value decomposition. *IEEE Transactions on Information Technology in Biomedicine*, *5*(4), 290–299. doi:10.1109/4233.966104 PMID:11759835

Welch, G., & Bishop, G. (2006). *An introduction to the kalman filter. 2006*. Chapel Hill, NC: University of North Carolina.

WHO. (2004). *eHealth for Health-care Delivery: Strategy 2004-2007*. Geneva, Switzerland: WHO. Retrieved from http://www.who.int/eht/en/eHealth_HCD.pdf

WHO. (2008). *Report on the global tobacco epidemic*. Retrieved from http://www.who.int/tobacco/mpower/mpower_report_full_2008.pdf

Wibmer, T., Doering, K., Kropf-Sanchen, C., Rdiger, S., Blanta, I., Stoiber, K., & Schumann, C. et al. (2014). Pulse transit time and blood pressure during cardiopulmonary exercise tests. *Physiological Research*, *63*(3), 287–296. PMID:24564606

Wilkie, R. M., Kountouriotis, G. K., Merat, N., & Wann, J. P. (2010). Using vision to control locomotion: Looking where you want to go. *Experimental Brain Research*, *204*(4), 539–547. doi:10.1007/s00221-010-2321-4 PMID:20556368

Wilkie, R. M., Wann, J. P., & Robert, S. (2008). Active Gaze, Visual Look-Ahead and locomotor control. *Journal of Experimental Psychology. Human Perception and Performance*, *34*(5), 1150–1164. doi:10.1037/0096-1523.34.5.1150 PMID:18823202

Winchell, R. J., & Hoyt, D. B. (1996). Spectral analysis of heart rate variability in the ICU: A measure of autonomic function. *The Journal of Surgical Research*, *63*(1), 11–16. doi:10.1006/jsre.1996.0214 PMID:8661164

Wong, M., Zhang, X., & Zhang, Y. (2006). The cuffless arterial blood pressure estimation based on the timing- characteristics of second heart sound. In *Engineering in Medicine and Biology Society, 2006. EMBS '06. 28th Annual International Conference of the IEEE*.

Wong, Y., & Zhang, Y. (2005). The effects of exercises on the relationship between pulse transit time and arterial blood pressure. In *Engineering in Medicine and Biology Society, 2005. IEEE-EMBS 2005. 27th Annual International Conference of the*.

Wooldridge, L., Lissina, A., Vernazza, J., Gostick, E., Laugel, B., Hutchinson, S. L., & Sewell, A. K. et al. (2007). Enhanced immunogenicity of CTL antigens through mutation of the CD8 binding MHC class I invariant region. *European Journal of Immunology*, *37*(5), 1323–1333. doi:10.1002/eji.200636765 PMID:17429845

Wu, D., Zhang, M., Liu, J.-C., & Bauman, W. (2006). On the adaptive detection of blood vessels in retinal images. *Biomedical Engineering. IEEE Transactions on*, *53*(2), 341–343.

Wu, H., Ding, A. A., & De Gruttola, V. (1998). Estimation of HIV dynamic parameters. *Statistics in Medicine*, *17*(21), 2463–2485. doi:10.1002/(SICI)1097-0258(19981115)17:21<2463::AID-SIM939>3.0.CO;2-A PMID:9819839

Wu, H., Zhu, H., Miao, H., & Perelson, A. S. (2008). Parameter identifiability and estimation of HIV/AIDS dynamic models. *Bulletin of Mathematical Biology*, *70*(3), 785–799. doi:10.1007/s11538-007-9279-9 PMID:18247096

Wu, W. H., Bui, A. A., Batalin, M. A., Liu, D., & Kaiser, W. J. (2007). Incremental diagnosis method for intelligent wearablesensor systems. *IEEE Transactions on Information Technology in Biomedicine*, *11*(5), 553–562. doi:10.1109/TITB.2007.897579 PMID:17912972

Xia, X. (2003). Estimation of HIV/AIDS parameters. *Automatica*, *39*(11), 1983–1988. doi:10.1016/S0005-1098(03)00220-6

Xie, H. B., Guo, T. R., Sivakumar, B., Liew, A. W. C., & Dokos, S. (2014). Symplectic geometry spectrum analysis of nonlinear time series. *Proceedings of the Royal Society a-Mathematical Physical and Engineering Sciences, 470*(2170). doi:10.1098/rspa.2014.0409

Xie, Y., Schreier, G., Chang, D.C., Neubauer, S., Liu, Y., Redmond, S.J., & Lovell, N.H. (2015). Predicting Days in Hospital Using Health Insurance Claims. *IEEE Journal of Biomedical and Health Informatics*, *19*(4), 1224-1233. doi:10.d109/JBHI.2015.2402692

Xie, H. B., & Dokos, S. (2013a). A hybrid symplectic principal component analysis and central tendency measure method for detection of determinism in noisy time series with application to mechanomyography. *Chaos, 23*(2). doi. *Artn, 023131*. doi:10.1063/1.4812287

Xie, H. B., & Dokos, S. (2013b). A symplectic geometry-based method for nonlinear time series decomposition and prediction. *Applied Physics Letters, 103*(5). doi:10.1063/1.4817181

Xie, H. B., & Wang, Z. Z. (2006). Mean frequency derived via Hilbert-Huang transform with application to fatigue EMG signal analysis. *Computer Methods and Programs in Biomedicine, 82*(2), 114–120. doi:10.1016/j.cmpb.2006.02.009 PMID:16616796

Xie, H. B., Zheng, Y. P., & Guo, J. Y. (2009). Classification of the mechanomyogram signal using a wavelet packet transform and singular value decomposition for multifunction prosthesis control. *Physiological Measurement, 30*(5), 441–457. doi:10.1088/0967-3334/30/5/002 PMID:19349648

Xie, H. B., Zheng, Y. P., Guo, J. Y., Chen, X., & Shi, J. (2009). Estimation of wrist angle from sonomyography using support vector machine and artificial neural network models. *Medical Engineering & Physics, 31*(3), 384–391. doi:10.1016/j.medengphy.2008.05.005 PMID:18586548

Xu, L., Guo, X., Yang, F., Yin, S., Zhang, X., & Meng, M. Q. H. (2012, June). Implementation of cuff-less continuous blood pressure measurement system based on Android. In *Information and Automation (ICIA), 2012 International Conference on* (pp. 552-556). IEEE. doi:10.1109/ICInfA.2012.6246866

Xu, J., Durand, L.-G., & Pibarot, P. (2001). Extraction of the aortic and pulmonary components of the second heart sound using a nonlinear transient chirp signal model. Biomedical Engineering. *IEEE Transactions on, 48*(3), 277–283.

Xu, J., Durand, L.-G., & Pibarot, P. (2002). A new, simple, and accurate method for non-invasive estimation of pulmonary arterial pressure. *Heart (British Cardiac Society), 88*, 76–80. PMID:12067952

Xu, S., & McCusker, J. (1968-70). Yale Image Finder (YIF): A new search engine for retrieving biomedical images. *Journal of Bioinformatics, 24*(17). doi:10.1093/bioinformatics/btn340

Yang, F., Sun, T., & Zhang, C. (2009). An efficient hybrid data clustering method based on K-harmonic means and Particle Swarm Optimization. *Expert Systems with Applications, 36*(6), 9847–9852. doi:10.1016/j.eswa.2009.02.003

Yang, J., Zhang, D., Frangi, A. F., & Yang, J. Y. (2004). Two-dimensional PCA: A new approach to appearance-based face representation and recognition. *IEEE Transactions on Pattern Analysis and Machine Intelligence, 26*(1), 131–137. doi:10.1109/TPAMI.2004.1261097 PMID:15382693

Yang, Y., Su, Z., & Sun, L. (2010). Medical image enhancement algorithm based on wavelet transform. *IET Electronics Letters, 46*(2), 120–121. doi:10.1049/el.2010.2063

Yang, Z. R. (2004). Biological applications of support vector machines. *Briefings in Bioinformatics, 5*(4), 328–338. doi:10.1093/bib/5.4.328 PMID:15606969

Yildirir, A., Kabakci, G., Akgul, E., Tokgozoglu, L., & Oto, A. (2002). Effects of menstrual cycle on cardiac autonomic innervation as assessed by heart rate variability. *Annals of Noninvasive Electrocardiology, 7*(1), 60–63. doi:10.1111/j.1542-474X.2001.tb00140.x PMID:11844293

Yinggan, T., Qiuyan, D., Xinping, G., & Fucai, L. (2008). Threshold Selection Based on Fuzzy Tsallis Entropy and Particle Swarm Optimization. *NeuroQuantology, 6*(4), 412–419. doi:10.14704/nq.2008.6.4.197

Yoon, Hwang, Noh, Cheol, & Royoon. (2010, July). Comparison Of Cwt With Dwt For Detecting QRS Complex On Wearable Ecg Recorder. In *IEEE, International Conference on Wavelet Analysis and Pattern Recognition, Qingdao* (pp. 300-303). IEEE.

Yoon, Y., Cho, J., & Yoon, G. (2009). Non-constrained blood pressure monitoring using ecg and ppg for personal healthcare. *Journal of Medical Systems*, *33*(4), 261–266. PMID:19697692

Younessi, H. M., Khalilzadeh, M. A., & Joharinia, S. (2014). Continuous and Cuffless Blood Pressure Monitoring Based on ECG and SpO2 Signals ByUsing Microsoft Visual C Sharp. *Journal of Biomedical Physics & Engineering*, *4*(1), 27–32. PMID:25505765

Yu, Yang, & Chong. (2010). ECG Monitoring over Bluetooth: Data Compression and Transmission. In *Communication Society WCNC Proceedings*. IEEE.

Yu, R. L., Kuo, L. C., Guei, Y. L., & Chyou, H. C. (2012). Gaussian mixture modelling of histograms for contrast enhancement. *Expert Systems with Applications*, *39*(8), 6720–6728. doi:10.1016/j.eswa.2011.12.018

Zahhad, Ahmed, & Zakaria. (2012). Electrocardiogram Signals Compression Technique Based on QRS.Complex Estimation and 2.D DWT. In ICCIT (pp. 554-559).

Zahl, H. A. (1968). *Electrons Away, or Tales of a Government Scientist*. New York: Vintage.

Zatout, Y. (2012). Using Wireless Technologies for Healthcare Monitoring at Home: a Survey. In 14th International Conference on e.Health Networking, Applications and Services (pp. 383-386). IEEE.

Zhang, X.-Y., & Zhang, Y.-T. (2006). A model-based study of relationship between timing of second heart sound and systolic blood pressure. In *Engineering in Medicine and Biology Society, 2006. EMBS '06. 28th Annual International Conference of the IEEE.*

Zhang, Y., de Peuter, O. R., Kamphuisen, P. W., & Karemaker, J. M. (2013). Search for HRV-parameters that detect a sympathetic shift in heart failure patients on β-blocker treatment. *Frontiers in Physiology, 4.*

Zhang, D. Q., & Zhou, Z. H. (2005). (2D)(2)PCA: Two-directional two-dimensional PCA for efficient face representation and recognition. *Neurocomputing*, *69*(1-3), 224–231. doi:10.1016/j.neucom.2005.06.004

Zhang, G., Gao, M., Xu, D., Olivier, N. B., & Mukkamala, R. (2011). Pulse arrival time is not an adequate surrogate for pulse transit time as a marker of blood pressure. *Journal of Applied Physiology*, *111*(6), 1681–1686. PMID:21960657

Zhang, X., Liu, Y., Zhang, F., Ren, J., Sun, Y. L., & Yang, Q. (2012). On design and implementation of neural-machine interface for artificial legs. *IEEE Trans IndInf*, *8*(2), 418–429.

Zhang, X.-Y., MacPherson, E., & Zhang, Y.-T. (2008). Relations between the timing of the second heart sound and aortic blood pressure. Biomedical Engineering. *IEEE Transactions on*, *55*(4), 1291–1297.

Zhang, X., & Zhou, P. (2012). High-Density Myoelectric Pattern Recognition Toward Improved Stroke Rehabilitation. *IEEE Transactions on Bio-Medical Engineering*, *59*(6), 1649–1657. doi:10.1109/TBME.2012.2191551 PMID:22453603

Zhang, Y., Yu, R., Xie, S., Yao, W., Xiao, Y., & Guizani, M. (2011). Home M2M networks: Architectures, standards, and QoS improvement. *IEEE Communications Magazine*, *49*(4), 44–52. doi:10.1109/MCOM.2011.5741145

Zheng, Y.-L., Ding, X.-R., Poon, C., Lo, B., Zhang, H., Zhou, X.-L., & Zhang, Y.-T. et al. (2014). Unobtrusive sensing and wearable devices for health informatics. Biomedical Engineering. *IEEE Transactions on*, *61*(5), 1538–1554.

Zheng, Y.-L., Yan, B., Zhang, Y.-T., & Poon, C. (2014b). An armband wearable device for overnight and cuffless blood pressure measurement. Biomedical Engineering. *IEEE Transactions on*, *61*(7), 2179–2186.

Zhide, L., Jiabin, C., & Chunlei. (2009). A New RBF Neural Network with GA-based Fuzzy C-Means Clustering Algorithm for SINS Fault Diagnosis. C*hinese Control and Decision Conference*. doi:10.1109/CCDC.2009.5195114

Zhiguo, G., & Yi, L. (2011). An image sharpening algorithm based on fuzzy logic. *International Journal for Light and Electron Optics*, *122*(8), 697–702. doi:10.1016/j.ijleo.2010.05.010

Zhu, W., Nah, F. F. H., & Zhao, F. (2003). Factors influencing user adoption of mobile computing. In J. Mariga (Ed.), Managing e-commerce and mobile computing technologies (pp. 260-271). Hershey, PA: Iron Mountain Incorporated (IRM) Press. doi:10.4018/978-1-93177-746-9.ch018

Zissis, D., & Lekkas, D. (2012). Addressing cloud computing security issues. *Journal of Future Generation Computer Systems*, *28*(3), 583–592. doi:10.1016/j.future.2010.12.006

Zuiderveld, K. (1994). Contrast Limited Adaptive Histogram Equalization. Cambridge, MA: Academic Press. doi:10.1016/B978-0-12-336156-1.50061-6

About the Contributors

Butta Singh received his Bachelor's degree in Electronics and Communication Engineering from Guru Nanak Dev Engineering College, Ludhiana, Punjab, India in 2002, Master's degree in Instrumentation and Control Engineering from Sant Longowal Institute of Engineering and Technology, Longowal, Sangrur, Punjab, India in 2005 and PhD degree from National Institute of Technology, Jalandhar, Punjab, India. He is serving as a Asst professor in the Department of Electronics and Communication Engineering, Guru Nanak Dev University, Regional Campus, Jalandhar, Punjab, India. His professional research interests are in signal processing, in particular, applied to biomedical applications. He has published over 40 research articles in internationally reputed journals and conference proceedings.

* * *

Azam Asilian Bidgoli was born in Kashan, Iran, in 1983. She graduated from Azad University of Kashan in 2005. She received MA degree from Kashan University, Iran in 2011 & started his Ph.D. at Computer engineering Department in the University of Kashan, Iran, in 2014. His main research interests are Pattern Recognition, Data mining and Image processing. She has published several research papers in National and International journals and conferences. Presently, She is working in the area of Image processing and data mining.

Paulo de Carvalho received his PhD in Informatics Engineering in 2002 from the University of Coimbra, where is an Associate Professor. His main research interests are adaptive computational techniques with application to bio-signals, pattern recognition, modelling and Clinical Informatics. His publications include several book chapters and over 150 papers in refereed international journals and conferences. He served the organization committees of several international conferences. He was the co-founder of the Clinical Informatics research track at CISUC. He is a member of the IFMBE Working Group on Clinical Informatics.

Ana Castro received the Ph.D. degree on Biomedical Engineering from the Faculty of Engineering, University of Porto, Portugal, in 2012. After finishing her degree on Applied Mathematics (Faculty of Science, University of Porto, 2006), she pursued her work on the analysis and control of nociception during anesthesia, receiving the 2012 Pain Award, by the Grünenthal Portuguese Foundation. She is now a researcher at the Faculdade de Ciências da Universidade do Porto, and her research interests are focused on the signal processing of biomedical signals, and patient monitoring in hospital and home-based scenarios. Main lines of work include acute and chronic pain assessment, monitoring in anesthesia (electroencephalogram, evoked potentials, electrocardiogram, photoplethysmography, e.g.), heart sound analysis for cardiac disease detection, and blood pressure estimation through non-invasive methods.

Biswajeet Champaty received the B.Tech degree in Biomedical Engineering from Trident Academy of Technology, Bhubaneswar, Odisha, India in 2010, M.Tech degree in Biomedical Engineering from SRM University, Chennai, India in 2012. Currently, he is pursuing his PhD degree in Biomedical Engineering from the National Institute of Technology, Rourkela, India. His area of research includes biomedical instrumentation and signal processing for designing human-computer interface devices mainly for rehabilitation and assistive purposes.

Miguel Coimbra is one of the founders and the current director of IT Porto, in which he founded and coordinates the Interactive Multimedia group, personally leading a team of 1 post-doc researcher, 5 PhD students and various MSc and BSc researchers. Leads and participates in various projects involving engineering and medicine, namely cardiology and gastroenterology, with current and past cooperations with hospitals in Portugal, Brazil (Pernambuco, Paraíba, Minas Gerais, São Paulo), Germany and Sweden. The nearly 10 years of experience in biomedical signal processing and interactive systems for healthcare have led to the development and deployment of systems for the collection and analysis of auscultation signals, echocardiography image processing for rheumatic fever screening, monitoring of stress and fatigue of firefighters in action, endoscopy signal analysis for cancer detection, computer assisted decision systems for capsule endoscopy, and quantification of 3d motion patterns for epilepsy, among others. Prof. Coimbra has 76 total scientific publications, 10 of which in high-impact scientific journals, and has attracted and managed a total of 1M€ in research funding, over a total of 11 research projects acting as the PI or co-PI of the Instituto de Telecomunicações team. He is the current Director of the Master in Medical Informatics of the University of Porto, a Technical Advisor of the Portugal Chapter of the IEEE Engineering and Medicine Society, and a EURASIP Local Liason Officer. Finally, Prof. Coimbra is a co-founder of IS4H - Interactive Systems for Healthcare, a spin-off company of the University of Porto, which has licensed and is selling products based on all the interactive auscultation technologies developed by his team.

Tianruo Guo received Ph.D degree in biomedical engineering from University of New South Wales (UNSW), Sydney, Australia, in 2015. He is currently a Postdoctoral Research Fellow with the Graduate School of Biomedical Engineering, UNSW. His research interests include large-scale optimization for developing accurate ionic models of cardiac myocytes and neural cells, and biomedical signal processing.

Michael E. Hahn received the B.S. degree from Colorado Mesa University, the M.S. degree from Iowa State University, and the Ph.D. from the University of Oregon. He is currently an Assistant Professor in the Department of Human Physiology at the University of Oregon, Eugene, OR.

Deepak Joshi received PhD from IIT Delhi. He was a research engineer in National University of Singapore before joining Institute of Neuroscience, Newcastle University (United Kingdom) as a visiting scholar. He was a postdoctoral from University of Oregon in United States of America. He has published in journals of repute like IEEE, Elsevier, and Taylor and Francis. He is a visiting research scientist at All India Institute of Medical Sciences(AIIMS) New Delhi. He was awarded from Intellectual Ventures Asia for his innovations in prosthetics design. He is a member of American Association for the advancement of Science (AAAS). Currently, he is working as an Assistant Professor at centre for biomedical engineering, Indian Institute of Technology (IIT) Delhi in India.

Pankaj Deep Kaur is working as an Assistant Professor in the Department of Computer Science and Engineering, Guru Nanak Dev University, RC, Jalandhar, India. She received her Bachelor's Degree in Computer Applications (2000) and Master's Degree in Information Technology (2003) from Guru Nanak Dev University, Amritsar, India. She completed her Ph.D. in Resource Scheduling in Cloud Computing from Thapar University, Patiala (2014) and has over ten years of teaching and research experience. She has been a university position holder in her graduation studies and received Gold Medal for her excellent performance in her Post Graduation studies. She is a recipient of Junior Research Fellowship from Ministry of Human Resource and Development, Govt. of India. Her research interests include Cloud Computing and Big data.

Kamalanand Krishnamurthy is an Assistant Professor at the Department of Instrumentation Engineering, Madras Institute of Technology Campus, Anna University, Chennai, India. His research focuses on mathematical analysis of biological and psychological systems. Recently, along with Prof. Dr. P Mannar Jawahar, he served as a guest editor for a special issue of the European Journal for Biomedical Informatics, entitled 'Applications of computational techniques in infectious diseases and clinical research'.

Dilip Kumar received the B.E. degree in electronics and telecommunication engineering from the Army Institute of Technology, University of Pune, India, in 2000, the M. E. degree in electronics product design and technology from the Panjab University, Chandigarh, India, in 2013 and the Ph.D. degree in faculty of engineering and technology from the M.M. University, Mullana, India, in 2010. In 2005, he joined the Centre for Department of Advanced Computing (CDAC) Mohali, India as a Design Engineer, and in 2009 became a Senior Design Engineer. He joined SLIET Longowal, Deemed University, India, in February 2014. Since 2014, he has been with the Department of Electronics and Communication Engineering, SLIET Longowal, Deemed University, where he is currently an Associate Professor. His current research interests include embedded systems, electronic system design, wireless sensor networks, and vehicular ad hoc networks. He has published more than 60 research papers in reputed international journals and conferences. Currently, he was the recipient of the 2015 Premium Award for Best Paper in IET Wireless Sensor Systems.

Rajeev Kumar received M.tech from Guru Nanak Dev University. He is currently pursuing PHD in Computer Science and Engineering from Punjab Technical Universities.He has 17 national and international research papers.

Sandra S. Mattos is a Pediatric Cardiologist and the Director of the Maternal-Fetal Cardiac Unit of the Royal Portuguese Hospital, Recife, Brazil. She is also the President of the The Heart CirCle of Pernambuco and a Researcher of the Keiso Asami Immunopathology Lab of the Federal University of Pernambuco, Recife, Brazil.

Seyed Jalaleddin Mousavirad was born in Neishabour, Iran, in 1986. He graduated from Azad University of Mashhad in 2007. He received MA degree from Kurdistan University, Iran in 2011 & started his Ph.D. at Computer Engineering Department in the University of Kashan, Iran, in 2012. His main research interests are Metaheuristic algorithms, Pattern Recognition, and Image processing. He has published about 15 research papers in National and International journals and conferences. Presently, He is working in the area of Metaheuristic algorithms and Image processing.

Jens Muehlsteff is Principal Scientist Philips Research.

Suraj Kumar Nayak received his B. Tech in Electrical Engineering from Government College of Engineering Keonjhar, Odisha, India (formerly known as OSME Keonjhar) and M. Tech in Biomedical Engineering from National Institute of Technology Rourkela, Odisha, India. Currently, he is pursuing his PhD degree in Biomedical Engineering from National Institute of Technology Rourkela, Odisha, India. His research interests include Biomedical Instrumentation, Biomedical Signal & Image Processing, Artificial Neural Network and Trans-dermal Drug Delivery.

Kunal Pal is an Asst. Professor in the department of Biotechnology and Medical Engg., NIT Rourkela.

Anukul Pandey was born in Jamui, Bihar, India in 1990. He received his B.Tech Degree in Electronics and Communication Engineering from Biju Patnaik University of Technology (BPUT), Rourkela, Orissa in 2011 and M.Tech degree in Electronics and Communication Engineering from Dr. B. R. Ambedkar National Institute of Technology Jalandhar, India in 2013.Currently, he is pursuing Ph.D. Degree in Electronics and Communication Engineering department from Dr B R Ambedkar National Institute of Technology Jalandhar. His research interests include the areas Biomedical Signal Processing, Wireless Communications.

Deep Kamal Kaur Randhawa is an engineering educationist. She is B.Eng. (PU Chandigarh), M.Tech (PTU Jalandhar) and PhD in Engg (GNDU Amritsar). She has been associated with teaching and research since 1993. Presently she is teaching in the ECE department of Guru Nanak Dev University, Regional Campus, Jalandhar. Her research interests include study and analysis of nanomaterials for use in nanoelectronics.

Kirti Rawal was born in Panipat, India. She received her B.Tech degree in Electronics & Communication Engineering from IITT college of Engineering, Pojewal, India in 2005 and then obtained her M.Tech degree in Electronics & Communication Engineering from BBSBEC Fatehgarh Sahib, Punjab. Presently, she is pursuing her Ph.D. in the area of Biomedical Signal Processing from Dr B R Ambedkar National Institute of Technology Jalandhar, since 2011.

Anupama Ray is a full-time Ph.D student with the Dept. of Electrical Engineering, Indian Institute of Technology Delhi, India. Her current research interests include pattern recognition, machine learning, document analysis and computer vision. This was a part of her Masters thesis from the Department of Biotechnology & Medical Engineering, National Institute of Technology Rourkela, India.

Anand S. completed B.E. (Electronics and Communication Engineering) in 1991 from University of Madras, M.E. (Communication System) from Madurai Kamaraj University and PhD from Anna University, Chennai with 22 years of teaching experience. Area of Research includes Digital Image

Processing, Medical Image Enhancement and Fractal Antenna Design. 45 Research Papers are published in International Journals and Conferences.

B. S. Saini was born in Jalandhar, India, in 1970. He received his B.Tech degree in Electronics & Communication Engineering from Gulbarga University, India in 1994, M.Tech. degree in Electronics & Communication Engineering from Kurukshetra University, India in 1996 and Ph.D. degree in the area of Signal Processing of heart rate variability from NIT Jalandhar, India, in 2009. He is serving as Associate Professor in Electronics & Communication Engineering Department, NIT Jalandhar, India from last 15 years. His research interests include Biomedical Signal Processing, Image Processing, Microprocessors & Microcontrollers, and Soft Computing. He is a member of IEEE, IEEE EMBS, and Fellow IETE. He has guided more that 30 MTech students and guiding 07 PhD research scholars. He has published more that 20 research papers in International Journals of repute.

Indu Saini was born in Ferozepur, India, in 1971. She received her B.Tech degree in Electronics & Communication Engineering from Guru Nanak Dev University, India in 1994 and then obtained her M.Tech(by Research) degree and Ph. D. degree in Electronics & Communication Engineering from National Institute of Technology Jalandhar, where she is also serving as Assistant Professor in Electronics & Communication Engineering Department since 2002.

Pallavi Sharma is currently pursuing her Master's Degree in Computer Science and Engineering from Guru Nanak Dev University, RC, Jalandhar, India. She received her Bachelor's Degree in the discipline of Computer Science and Engineering (2014) in First Division with Distinction from Rayat Bahra College of Engineering & Nano Technology, Hoshiarpur, India. Her research work includes Data Mining in Healthcare.

Harinderjit Singh was born in Chandigarh, India. He received the B.Tech. degree in electronics and communication engineering from Punjab Technical University, Jalandhar, India in 2012, the M.Tech. degree in electronics product design and technology from C-DAC, Mohali, India in 2014. He has held Embedded Design Engineer at TCILIT, Mohali, India. He is currently a Project Fellow at UIET, Panjab University, Chandigarh. His research interests cover the noninvasive cuffless blood pressure monitoring system and signal processing.

Tony Singla received B.Tech degree from Punjabi University Patiala. He is currently pursuing M.tech in Computer Science and Engineering from Punjab Technical University. He has published one research paper in International journal.

Neetu Sood works as assistant professor at NIT Jalandhar since 2007. Her research area includes wireless system design, channel modelling, OFDM based systems.

D. N. Tibarewala is presently a Professor of Biomedical Engineering since August 1996 and has earlier served as Director in the School of Bioscience & Engineering at Jadavpur University, Kolkata, India during the period May 2004-November 2011. He did his BSc (Honours) in 1971 and B. Tech (Applied Physics) in 1974 from the Calcutta University, India. He was admitted to the Ph.D. (Tech) degree of the same University in 1980. Having professional, academic and research experience of more than 35 years, Dr. Tibarewala has contributed about 250 research papers in the areas of Rehabilitation Technology, Biomedical Instrumentation and, related branches of Biomedical Engineering.

Anusuya S. Venkatesan is currently employed as Associate Professor at Saveetha School of Engineering, Saveetha University, Chennai. She was awarded Doctor of Philosophy in the year 2015. Her area of interests includes Data Mining, Image Processing, Neural Networks and Fuzzy Logic.

Hongbo Xie received his PhD in biomedical engineering from Shanghai Jiao Tong University, Shanghai, China, in 2006. He is currently a Vice Chancellor's Research Fellow in the ARC Centre of Excellence for Mathematical and Statistical Frontiers, Queensland University of Technology. His research interests include neuromuscular bioelectronics, human- computer interfaces, biomedical signal and image processing, and nonlinear time series analysis.

Index

O

P

Q

R

S

T

V

W

X

Y

Z

www.ingramcontent.com/pod-product-compliance
Lightning Source LLC
LaVergne TN
LVHW060401300926
849162LV00006B/1319
9781522506607